Medical Management of Thyroid Disease

Medical Management of Thyroid Disease

Third Edition

Edited by

David S. Cooper and Jennifer A. Sipos

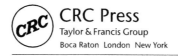

CRC Press
Taylor & Francis Group
Boca Raton London New York

CRC Press is an imprint of the
Taylor & Francis Group, an **informa** business

CRC Press
Taylor & Francis Group
6000 Broken Sound Parkway NW, Suite 300
Boca Raton, FL 33487-2742

First issued in paperback 2020

ISBN 13: 978-0-367-57063-7 (pbk)
ISBN 13: 978-1-138-57723-7 (hbk)

Library of Congress Cataloging-in-Publication Data

Names: Cooper, David S. (Physician), editor. | Sipos, Jennifer, editor.
Title: Medical management of thyroid disease / [edited by] David S.Cooper and
Jennifer Sipos.
Description: Third edition. | Boca Raton : Taylor & Francis, 2019. | Includes
bibliographical references and index.
Identifiers: LCCN 2018030183| ISBN 9781138577237 (hardback : alk. paper) |
ISBN 9781351267489 (ebook)
Subjects: | MESH: Thyroid Diseases--therapy | Thyroid Diseases--diagnosis
Classification: LCC RC655 | NLM WK 267 | DDC 616.4/4--dc23
LC record available at https://lccn.loc.gov/2018030183

Visit the Taylor & Francis Web site at
http://www.taylorandfrancis.com

and the CRC Press Web site at
http://www.crcpress.com

Contents

Preface   vii

Editors   ix

Contributors   xi

1   The laboratory and imaging approaches to thyroid disorders   1
    Jacqueline Jonklaas and David S. Cooper
2   The diagnostic evaluation and management of hyperthyroidism due to Graves' disease,
    toxic nodules, and toxic multinodular goiter   37
    David S. Cooper
3   Thyroiditis   81
    Robert C. Smallridge and Victor Bernet
4   Rare forms of hyperthyroidism   97
    Nicole O. Vietor and Henry B. Burch
5   Drug-induced thyroid dysfunction   107
    Victor Bernet and Robert C. Smallridge
6   Hypothyroidism   129
    Michael T. McDermott
7   Thyroid nodules and multinodular goiter   159
    Poorani N. Goundan and Stephanie L. Lee
8   Differentiated thyroid carcinoma   181
    Carolyn Maxwell and Jennifer A. Sipos
9   Medullary thyroid carcinoma in medical management of thyroid disease   225
    Mimi I. Hu, Elizabeth G. Grubbs, and Julie Ann Sosa
10 Anaplastic thyroid carcinoma and thyroid lymphoma   243
    Ashish V. Chintakuntlawar and Keith C. Bible
11 Surgical approach to thyroid disorders   261
    Vaninder K. Dhillon and Ralph P. Tufano
12 Thyroid disease and pregnancy   275
    Alisha N. Wade and Susan J. Mandel

Index   297

Preface

It has been more than 10 years since the second edition of *Medical Management of Thyroid Disease* was published. When I was asked by the publisher to edit this third edition of the text, I invited Dr. Jennifer Sipos from The Ohio State University to be my coeditor. Together, we have continued the tradition of this book, which was initially developed to be a practical guide on the management of both common and uncommon thyroid problems. We have tried, as much as possible, to limit the discussion to the clinical manifestations, diagnostic procedures, and treatment of the gamut of thyroid disorders in adults. As before, to the greatest degree possible, all of the recommendations in the text are "evidence-based" or recapitulate evidence-based clinical practice guidelines. We have invited a number of new authors to provide a fresh approach to some of the topics.

Since the last edition of this text was published in 2008, there have been remarkable strides in our ability to care for thyroid patients. In the realm of benign thyroid disease, we now recognize that drug-induced thyroid dysfunction includes a large array of new drugs that inhibit tyrosine kinases, have effects on the immune system as "checkpoint inhibitors," or have other more ill-defined effects. An entire chapter is devoted to this topic, in recognition of its importance. In the treatment of hypothyroidism, clinicians are now feeling more justified in using T4/T3 combination therapy in some patients, reflecting a better understanding that T4 monotherapy may not recapitulate the serum hormonal profile of the thyroid gland itself. There has been a revolution in the management of thyroid nodules, including a new classification for cytopathology (the Bethesda system), as well as the development of molecular testing for improved diagnosis of indeterminate thyroid nodules. There has also been a sea change in the way low-risk thyroid cancer is managed, based on the 2015 American Thyroid Association clinical practice guidelines. Instead of a "one-size-fits-all" approach, we now have a more personalized set of management strategies, based on the recognition that more aggressive treatment (i.e., total thyroidectomy, radioiodine ablation, and full suppression of serum TSH) is not necessary for the vast majority of thyroid cancer patients. Furthermore, there are now a number of randomized clinical trials which have helped to define the best management for advanced thyroid cancers.

Dr. Sipos and I want to thank the contributors to this text for their time and expertise. We also want to express our gratitude to two of our mentors, Dr. E. Chester Ridgway and Dr. Ernest Mazzaferri. Both were giants in the field of thyroidology, both contributed to the first and second editions of this text, and both have sadly passed away in the last several years. We wish to recognize them for their guidance, and for being inspiring role models and colleagues. Finally, we hope that practitioners will benefit from reading this textbook, but we understand that the ultimate beneficiaries of the knowledge gained will be the millions of patients suffering from thyroid disease around the world.

David S. Cooper, MD
The Johns Hopkins University School of Medicine

Jennifer A. Sipos, MD
The Ohio State University Wexner Medical Center

Editors

David S. Cooper, MD, MACP, received his medical degree from Tufts University School of Medicine and completed his endocrinology fellowship training at the Massachusetts General Hospital/Harvard Medical School. He is Professor of Medicine and Radiology at The Johns Hopkins University School of Medicine and Director of The Johns Hopkins Thyroid Clinic. He serves as editor-in-chief for endocrinology at *Up-to-Date*. He is a former contributing editor at *JAMA* and former deputy editor of the *Journal of Clinical Endocrinology and Metabolism*. He is the past chair of the Subspecialty Board for Endocrinology, Diabetes, and Metabolism of the American Board of Internal Medicine. Dr. Cooper is the past president of the American Thyroid Association and the recipient of the American Thyroid Association's Distinguished Service Award and its Paul Starr Award. He is also the recipient of the Distinction in Clinical Endocrinology Award from the American College of Endocrinology and the Endocrine Society's 2016 Outstanding Scholarly Physician Award.

Jennifer A. Sipos, MD, is a Professor of Medicine and Director of the Benign Thyroid Disorders Program at The Ohio State University. She obtained her medical degree and received her internal medicine residency training at Wake Forest University. She completed her endocrinology and metabolism fellowship at the University of North Carolina in Chapel Hill. Dr. Sipos has developed an interest in the use of ultrasonography for the diagnosis and management of thyroid cancer and has taught and served as a course director for numerous ultrasound courses nationally and internationally, including meetings for the Endocrine Society, American Thyroid Association, European Thyroid Association, American Association for Clinical Endocrinologists, Asia and Oceania Thyroid Association, Indian Endocrine Society, and International Congress for Endocrinology. Additionally, she is actively involved in several clinical research projects with a particular interest in factors implicated in the development of salivary damage after radioiodine therapy. She also participates in clinical trials for the evaluation of multikinase inhibitor therapies in refractory thyroid cancer and the diagnostic use of molecular markers in thyroid nodules.

Contributors

Victor Bernet
Mayo Clinic
Jacksonville, Florida

Keith C. Bible
Mayo Clinic
Rochester, Minnesota

Henry B. Burch
National Institutes of Health
Bethesda, Maryland

Ashish V. Chintakuntlawar
Mayo Clinic
Rochester, Minnesota

David S. Cooper
The Johns Hopkins University School of Medicine
Baltimore, Maryland

Vaninder K. Dhillon
The Johns Hopkins University
Baltimore, Maryland

Poorani N. Goundan
Boston Medical Center
Boston, Massachusetts

Elizabeth G. Grubbs
The University of Texas MD Anderson Cancer
    Center
Houston, Texas

Mimi I. Hu
The University of Texas MD Anderson Cancer
    Center
Houston, Texas

Jacqueline Jonklaas
Georgetown University School of Medicine
Washington, DC

Stephanie L. Lee
Boston Medical Center
Boston, Massachusetts

Susan J. Mandel
University of Pennsylvania
Philadelphia, Pennsylvania

Carolyn Maxwell
Stony Brook University Hospital
Stony Brook, New York

Michael T. McDermott
University of Colorado Denver School of
    Medicine
Denver, Colorado

Jennifer A. Sipos
The Ohio State University
Columbus, Ohio

Robert C. Smallridge
Mayo Clinic
Jacksonville, Florida

Julie Ann Sosa
University of California at San Francisco
San Francisco, California

Ralph P. Tufano
The Johns Hopkins University
Baltimore, Maryland

Nicole O. Vietor
Walter Reed National Military Medical Center
Bethesda, Maryland

Alisha N. Wade
University of the Witwatersrand
Johannesburg, South Africa

The laboratory and imaging approaches to thyroid disorders

JACQUELINE JONKLAAS AND DAVID S. COOPER

Introduction	1	Screening and case findings	16
Physiology of the hypothalamic-pituitary-		Imaging approach to thyroid disease	17
thyroid axis	2	Ultrasonography and nuclear medicine studies	17
Laboratory evaluation of thyroid function	3	Ultrasonography	17
Assays of thyroid hormones	3	Technique	17
Total serum iodothyronine concentrations	3	Indications	17
Determination of free T4 and T3		Normal thyroid appearance	17
concentrations	4	Diffuse thyroid disease	17
Causes of increased T4 and/or T3		Thyroid nodules	21
concentrations	6	Risk stratification systems for thyroid nodules	21
Causes of decreased T4 and/or T3		Lymph nodes	23
concentrations	9	Nuclear medicine studies	23
Assays of thyroid-stimulating hormones	10	Technique	23
Causes of hypothyrotropinemia	12	Indications	24
Causes of hyperthyrotropinemia	12	Normal thyroid appearance	25
Specialized studies of thyroid function	13	Diffuse thyroid disease	26
Thyroglobulin	13	Thyroid nodules	27
Thyroid autoantibodies	14	Ectopic thyroid tissue	27
Tissue responses to thyroid hormone action	15	Thyroid cancer	27
Laboratory evaluation for thyroid disease	15	References	28

INTRODUCTION

The central role of the thyroid gland in controlling metabolism was recognized in the 19th century, but evaluation of the function of the thyroid remains an evolving science. Initial approaches to the assessment of thyroid function centered on measuring end-organ responses as biological markers of thyroid hormone actions. Development of in vitro competitive binding assay methods allowed the direct quantification of hormone levels in serum, and sensitive immunoassays have demonstrated the subtleties of pituitary and hypothalamic control of the thyroid. Abnormalities of hormone binding by serum proteins necessitated sensitive estimation of free hormone levels. With the detection of serum markers of autoimmune and malignant diseases of the thyroid gland, earlier diagnosis and improved monitoring of these conditions have been achieved, often with greater sensitivity than may be clinically relevant. Limitations to the measurement methods utilized exist, however, particularly when underlying assumptions about the comparability of patient and control specimens are invalid. Nonetheless, the clinician can now effectively confirm suspected diagnoses of thyroid dysfunction, cost-effectively screen asymptomatic populations for common diseases, and appropriately monitor the treatment of patients with disorders of the thyroid.

PHYSIOLOGY OF THE HYPOTHALAMIC-PITUITARY-THYROID AXIS

Excellent reviews and books provide detailed explorations of the physiology of the hypothalamic-pituitary-thyroid axis, and the reader is invited to delve into those worthwhile sources (1). For the purposes of this chapter, a brief review of the biosynthesis and transport of thyroid hormones and the regulation of thyroid function by the hypothalamic-pituitary complex will suffice (Figure 1.1).

The synthesis of thyroxine (T4) and triiodothyronine (T3) begins with the active transport of iodide into the cell via a sodium-iodine symporter located in the basal membrane. Following oxidation by thyroid peroxidase, the iodide moiety is covalently attached to tyrosyl residues of thyroglobulin, and the resulting iodotyrosines are coupled and cleaved from thyroglobulin to form T4 and T3, normally in a 10:1 ratio. Thyroid hormone secretion requires endocytosis and degradation of iodinated thyroglobulin, followed by the release of T4 and T3 into the circulation. This process results in the total daily output of 80 to 100 µg of T4. In contrast, only 20% of the circulating T3 is produced by the thyroid, the remaining 80% is derived from the enzymatic outer-ring or 5'-monodeiodination of T4 in extrathyroidal tissues such as the liver, kidney, brain, muscle, and skin. Removal of the inner-ring or 5-iodine of T4 forms the inactive metabolite reverse T3 (rT3). Other inactivating pathways for T4 and T3 include glucuronidation, sulfation, deamination, and cleavage. The normal daily fractional turnover rates for T4 and T3 are 10% and 75%, respectively.

In serum, at least 99.95% of T4 and 99.5% of T3 molecules are bound by the transport proteins thyroxine-binding globulin (TBG), transthyretin (thyroxine-binding prealbumin [TBPA]), and

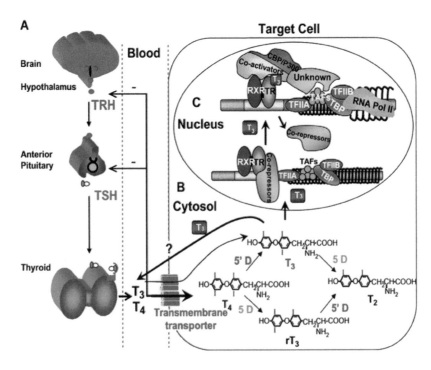

Figure 1.1 The hypothalamic pituitary thyroid axis. (From Refetoff S, Dumitrescu A. *Best Pract Res Clin Endocrinol Metab.* 2007;21:277–305. Used with permission.)

albumin. Although TBG is present in lower concentrations than either transthyretin or albumin, its greater affinity for thyroid hormones makes it the predominant serum carrier of T4 and T3. Variations in binding characteristics among normal and abnormal thyroid hormone-binding proteins are responsible for much of the methodologic limitations in assays that attempt to measure concentrations of free T4 and T3. This large pool of protein-bound hormone provides a stable reservoir that maintains the supply of free, unbound hormone available for transport into the cells. Once within target cells, T4 is further deiodinated to T3, which in the nucleus binds to the thyroid hormone receptor, modulating the transcription of thyroid hormone-responsive genes and producing most of the clinical effects recognized as the metabolic effects of thyroid hormones.

The primary regulatory influence on thyroid gland function is the circulating level of thyrotropin (thyroid stimulating hormone, or TSH). Produced by thyrotroph cells of the anterior pituitary, TSH is a two-subunit glycoprotein, the specificity of which is conferred by its β-subunit; the α-subunit is structurally similar to that of follicle-stimulating hormone, luteinizing hormone, and human chorionic gonadotropin. Negative feedback by T4 and T3 influences TSH synthesis and release, as evidenced by a complex inverse relationship between the concentrations of TSH and free iodothyronine (2, 3). It is likely that each individual has a genetically determined set-point for this TSH/free T4 relationship, based on twin studies (4, 5). TSH levels peak just before nocturnal sleep, and the nadir occurs in the late afternoon; this nocturnal surge is lost early in the course of nonthyroidal illness. TSH levels in various populations conform best to a log-Gaussian rather than Gaussian distribution (6). The hypothalamic tripeptide thyrotropin-releasing hormone (TRH) stimulates TSH secretion and modulates thyrotroph response to altered thyroid hormone levels. In conjunction with the suppressive effects of dopamine, corticosteroids, somatostatin, androgens, and endogenous opioids, TRH may be responsible for modulating the setpoint for the negative feedback loop that controls thyroid hormone levels. Hypothalamic production of TRH itself is regulated by circulating thyroid hormones, as well as by multiple central nervous system factors.

LABORATORY EVALUATION OF THYROID FUNCTION

Assays of thyroid hormones

TOTAL SERUM IODOTHYRONINE CONCENTRATIONS

When concentrations and binding affinities of thyroid hormone-binding proteins are normal, there exists at physiologic equilibrium a direct relationship between levels of total hormone and free hormone (7). Thus, measurement of total iodothyronine concentration can provide a reasonable surrogate for estimating the amount of free iodothyronine present. Either serum or plasma can be used to assay hormone concentrations, although serum is generally preferred. The most commonly employed technique for the determination of total T4 (TT4) and T3 (TT3) concentrations is competitive immunoassay, using either polyclonal or monoclonal "capture" antibodies directed against the specific iodothyronine. To ensure measurement of bound as well as free hormones, inhibitors of iodothyronine binding are added—e.g., 8-anilino-1-naphthalene sulfonic or salicylic acids for TBG and barbital for TBPA. These agents successfully dissociate the hormone from binding proteins without interfering with hormone binding to immunoglobulin.

Radioimmunoassay (RIA) depends upon measurement of the distribution of a tracer quantity of radiolabeled hormone that competes with the endogenous hormone in the patient's specimen for binding to a capture antibody. The higher the serum hormone concentration, the lower the amount of radiolabel that binds to the antibody. Following the addition of a limited amount of capture antibody and the radiolabeled iodothyronine to be measured, the antibody-antigen complexes are separated from the serum. Separation techniques vary, including ammonium sulfate or second antibody precipitation. Newer methods that facilitate automated separation include attachment of the anti-T4 antibody to a solid phase, such as the wall of the assay tube or magnetizable particles. The concentration of either TT4 or TT3 is then determined by comparison of the amount of antibody-bound radiolabel with a simultaneously derived standard curve. A fundamental assumption, therefore, is that there is no difference in the assay conditions (including protein binding and other constituents found in the serum) between the patient's sample and the control standards, an assumption that is often invalid.

Nonisotopic methods avoid reliance upon radioactive reagents and are now the most commonly used assays. The heterogeneous enzyme-linked immunosorbent assay (ELISA) incorporates enzymes, fluorescent, or chemiluminescent molecules that create a quantitative signal when interacting with a specific enzyme bound to the tracer hormone—e.g., alkaline phosphatase, horseradish peroxidase, or glucose-6-phosphate dehydrogenase. As in RIA, numerous physical and chemical approaches exist for separating signal bound to the anti-iodothyronine antibody from unbound signal. In contrast, homogeneous enzyme immunoassays do not require a separation step. Instead, the binding of the antibody to a tracer hormone directly affects the activity of the signal-generating enzyme bound to the tracer. Other technologies, such as liquid chromatograph-tandem mass spectroscopy (LC-MS/MS) have also been applied to provide greater specificity and less analytical interference (8).

Due to common alterations in serum TBG levels, TT4 and TT3 are generally not used as stand-alone tests in clinical practice, but are combined with direct measurements of TBG or TBG-binding capacity, which can then be used to calculate a Free Thyroxine Index (see below).

Reference ranges vary to some degree, but commonly cited ranges are 4.5–12.6 mcg/dL (58–160 nmol/L) for TT4 and 80–180 ng/dL (1.2–2.7 nmol/L) for TT3 (9). As developed by their manufacturers, these assay techniques have similar performance characteristics, although each may be affected by different sources of interference. TT4 assays tend to be more reliable than TT3 assays. For example, in a recent study, in which 11 TT4 and 12 TT3 assays were compared, with LC-MS/MS values as the reference serum concentrations, only 4/10 TT4 assays and 4/11 TT3 assays failed to agree to within 10% of the reference concentrations, with greater deviation seen with the TT3 assay (10). Contributing factors to measurement error include qualitative differences between the protein constituents of sample diluents used for calibration and those found in patient sera, leading to differential dissociation of hormone from binding proteins.

DETERMINATION OF FREE T4 AND T3 CONCENTRATIONS

Because T4 and T3 are highly bound to serum proteins, alterations in either the levels of these proteins or their binding characteristics can significantly alter the concentration of total hormone. As it is the free hormone that is biologically active, however, techniques are required to permit either direct measurement or estimation of the serum free hormone levels. All methods that have been developed face the identical problem: distinguishing between the 3–4 orders of magnitude difference in the concentrations of the free and the protein-bound hormones. In all free hormone assays, the central assumption is that the effectiveness of separating the free from the bound hormone is identical in both the patient samples and the standards used to calibrate the assay, an assumption that is difficult to validate in all potential clinical situations. As a result, in a study comparing the results of 15 FT4 and 13 FT3 immunoassays to values obtained by the reference method equilibrium dialysis-LC-MS/MS, all the FT4 immunoassays and 9 of the FT3 immunoassays produced results that were outside the 10% agreement with the reference method (11).

Direct methods for measuring FT4 and FT3 include equilibrium dialysis, ultrafiltration, and gel filtration to separate the free hormone from its binding proteins. In the case of equilibrium dialysis, undiluted patient serum is dialyzed overnight across a membrane with pores that allow free but not protein-bound hormone to partition, allowing equilibration of the free hormone concentration across the membrane. A highly sensitive RIA, capable of detecting nanogram (or picomole) quantities of hormones, is then used to measure the hormone content of the protein-free dialysate, comparing to a standard curve generated with gravimetrically determined amounts of hormone (12). Faster turnaround can be achieved by using ultrafiltration rather than equilibrium dialysis, but greater variability can result from minimal amounts of serum proteins that leak through the filtration device as well as a hormone that is adsorbed to either the membrane or container surface. Such direct measurements are generally expensive, time consuming, and not widely used commercially. Expected adult values for these direct methods are about 0.8 to 2.3 ng/dL for free T4 and 210 to 440 pg/dL for free T3. As mentioned above, the LC-MS/MS assay used above as the reference method for assessing FT4 and FT3 assays employed separation by equilibrium dialysis (11). Separation by ultrafiltration has also been combined with LC-MS/MS (13). The LC-MS/MS technique to measure free T4 levels provides high specificity; hence its use as a reference assay (11). LC-MS/MS can also offer simultaneous measurement of other thyroid analytes (13).

Immunoassay methods for estimation of free hormone concentration are now widely used. In the "analogue" or "one-step" free T4 method, a labeled T4 analogue that does not bind to serum-binding proteins is added to serum and the mixture is either incubated with an anti-T4 antibody or allowed to bind to antibody attached to a solid phase. At equilibrium, the amount of analogue complexed to the antibody is inversely proportional to the amount of free T4 that is available. One-step methods require structurally modified analogues that do not displace hormone from protein-binding sites, but a complete lack of displacement is rarely achieved. Therefore, these methods depend on the assumption that there is no difference in hormone-binding affinity for proteins between the sample to be measured and the assay controls or calibrators, both for the actual analyte as well as the analogue. This assumption is particularly at risk when there are circulating inhibitors of hormone binding in serum, such as occurs in renal failure or other nonthyroidal illnesses, or major alterations in hormone-binding protein concentrations (14). Because the analogues used generally bind to albumin, although not with the same kinetics as T4 or T3, this method may not correct for abnormalities in albumin binding.

In "two-step" assays, serum is exposed to a solid phase containing an anti-T4 antibody, binding a certain amount of free hormone to the solid phase. By diluting the specimen and limiting the duration of incubation, there should be minimal disruption of endogenous hormone binding to serum proteins (12). After removal of the serum and its proteins, a tracer quantity of radiolabeled T4 is incubated with the solid phase, equilibrating with the remaining unoccupied antibody molecules. The amount of radiolabeled T4 complexed to the solid phase is thus inversely proportional to the free T4 concentration of the serum. Because the label is unable to interact with serum-binding proteins or endogenous inhibitors of hormone binding to protein (due to the physical separation step), the

"two-step" method has a good correlation with the free T4 determined by direct equilibrium dialysis. Nonradioactive assays have also been developed, and automated two-step procedures are in common use.

For free T3 measurements, methods that rely upon physical separation of bound from free hormones, such as dialysis or ultrafiltration, are not generally commercially available. The same technology for "one-step" assays of free T4 is used to measure free T3. Interference from serum proteins and difficulty avoiding stripping T3 from its binding proteins is a greater problem than in free T4 assays (15). New methods that utilize tandem mass spectrometry following equilibrium dialysis or ultrafiltration may allow faster and more reliable assays (16).

The thyroid hormone-binding ratio (THBR), another calculated value proportional to the fraction of hormone that is free in circulation, derives from measurement of the availability of protein-binding sites in the patient's serum. In the traditional uptake method, a tracer quantity of radiolabeled iodothyronine is added to the serum and allowed to partition between unoccupied specific protein-binding sites and a nonsaturable adsorbent—e.g., talc, charcoal, resin, or anti-iodothyronine antibodies. T3 is generally preferred as the labeled ligand, as it has a lower affinity for TBG and therefore does not displace T4 from its binding sites. There is an inverse relationship between the amounts of radiolabel adsorbed by the inert solid phase and unoccupied serum protein-binding sites. The percent uptake derives from the ratio of tracer bound by the adsorbent to the tracer bound by serum proteins; an alternative but less reliable formula expresses the ratio as the amount of tracer attached to adsorbent to the amount initially added. The THBR is then calculated as the percent uptake in the patient's serum and normalized to that of a control or reference serum; the expected normal range is centered around unity. The THBR is increased when there are few endogenous binding sites, which can occur with an increased amount of T4 available to bind (thyrotoxicosis), the presence of competing ligands (certain drugs and nonthyroidal illness), or a decreased amount of binding protein (TBG deficiency). Conversely, hypothyroidism and TBG excess will produce an increased number of available binding sites, producing a decreased THBR. As a general rule, true thyroid function abnormalities produce concordant increases or decreases in the total serum T4 and THBR, whereas discordant changes in the two tests typically result from protein-binding abnormalities. Alternate methods use nonisotopic labels, such as enzyme-linked tracers and light emitters. These all rely on the similar principle of estimating the partitioning of the labeled hormone between serum-binding proteins and a solid phase. A free hormone index is estimated by multiplying the total serum hormone concentration by the THBR. In most conditions of endogenous thyroid function abnormalities or protein-binding alterations, the index corrects for effects of protein binding on total T4 levels, and correlates well with free T4 levels measured by reference methods.

Potential pitfalls in the interpretation of THBR tests occur when there is a ligand that can interfere with binding to both the solid phase and serum proteins, for example, nonthyroidal illness. Falsely elevated free thyroxine index values can also be present when the protein-binding abnormality is specific for T4 and masked by the use of T3 in the THBR—for example, familial dysalbuminemic hyperthyroxinemia, in which an abnormal albumin binds only thyroxine with high affinity. Similarly derived from the total T3, the "free T3 index" can be useful in evaluating cases of abnormal serum binding.

CAUSES OF INCREASED T4 AND/OR T3 CONCENTRATIONS

The majority of patients with hyperthyroidism, regardless of the etiology, have increased total serum concentrations of both T4 and T3, as well as high levels of the free hormones (Table 1.1). In a minority of cases, there may be an isolated elevation of either iodothyronine. T3-toxicosis is especially prominent in patients with mild and recurrent Graves' disease or hyperfunctioning adenomas and those patients overtreated with triiodothyronine-containing thyroid hormone preparations. The relative magnitude of T3 elevation is often greater than T4 in forms of hyperthyroidism caused by increased glandular synthesis of hormone; in Graves' disease, the proportion of circulating T3 that derives from thyroidal production nearly doubles (17). The opposite—that is, a lower T3:T4 ratio—is true in thyrotoxicosis due to an inflammatory thyroiditis, in which there is a release of the previously formed hormone, iodide-induced

Table 1.1 Causes of increased T4 and/or T3 concentrations

Thyrotoxicosis
Euthyroid hyperthyroxinemia
Increased binding to plasma proteins
Thyroxine-binding globulin excess
Congenital
Hyperestrogenemia: Exogenous, endogenous
Acute and chronic active hepatitis
Acute intermittent porphyria
HIV-1 infection
Familial dysalbuminemic hyperthyroxinemia
Transthyretin excess
Congenital
Paraneoplastic
Antithyroxine immunoglobulins
Impaired T4 to T3 conversion
Iodinated contrast agents
Amiodarone
Glucocorticoids
Propranolol
Congenital
Generalized resistance to thyroid hormones
Nonthyroidal illness
Acute psychosis
Acute medical/surgical illness
Hyperemesis gravidarum
Lead intoxication
Drugs
Clofibrate
5-fluorouracil
Perphenazine
Methadone
Heroin
L-thyroxine therapy

hyperthyroidism, and iatrogenic thyrotoxicosis due to exogenous levothyroxine administration. Mild hyperthyroxinemia can even be seen in patients being treated with exogenous levothyoxine for hypothyroidism but whose TSH levels are normal on therapy (18, 19) (Tables 1.2 and 1.3).

Increased total T4 concentrations without thyrotoxicosis, termed euthyroid hyperthyroxinemia, result from both acquired and congenital etiologies. One commonly encountered situation is acquired TBG excess due to hyperestrogenemia.

Table 1.2 Causes of decreased T4 and/or T3 concentrations

| Hypothyroidism |
| Euthyroid hypothyroxinemia |
| Decreased binding to serum proteins |
| Thyroxine-binding globulin deficiency |
| Chronic liver disease |
| Congenital |
| Cushing's syndrome |
| Drugs |
| L-Asparaginase |
| Androgens |
| Nicotinic acid |
| Growth hormone excess |
| Nephrosis |
| Protein-losing enteropathy |
| Thyroxine-binding globulin and transthyretin variants with reduced affinity |
| Inhibition of T4 binding by drugs |
| Carbamazepine |
| Diphenylhydantoin |
| Fenclofenac |
| Furosemide |
| Heparin |
| Meclofenamic acid |
| Mefenamic acid |
| Salicylates |
| Sertraline |
| Nonthyroidal illnesses |

Table 1.3 How various serum constituents are altered in hyperthyroidism and hypothyroidism

Increased	Decreased
Hyperthyroidism	
Alkaline phosphatase	Cholesterol (total, LDL)
Angiotensin-converting enzyme	Apolipoprotein b, apo (a)
Calcium	Corticosteroid-binding globulin
Factor VIII	
Ferritin	
Osteocalcin	
Sex hormone-binding globulin	
Urine nitrogen excretion	
Urine pyridinoline cross links	
Hypothyroidism	
Carcinoembryonic antigen	Aldosterone
Cholesterol (LDL and HDL fractions)	Angiotensin-converting enzyme
Creatine phosphokinase	Factor VIII
Creatinine	Osmolarity
Lactic dehydrogenase	Sex hormone-binding globulin
Myoglobin	Corticosteroid-binding globulin
Norepinephrine	
Prolactin	

Elevated hepatic exposure to estrogen leads to increased sialylation of carbohydrate side chains of TBG, thereby decreasing the clearance of the glycoprotein and increasing serum TBG levels. This effect is seen within several weeks of the onset of hyperestrogenemia and can occur with exogenous administration of estrogens, increased endogenous production—for example, pregnancy—and even administration of selective estrogen receptor modulators, such as tamoxifen and raloxifene (20, 21). Exogenous estrogen administered transdermally, by avoiding first pass metabolism in the liver, does not cause elevated TBG levels and hyperthyroxinemia (22). Acquired TBG excess may also be responsible for the slight increase in T4 levels reported in male cigarette smokers (23). X-linked inherited TBG excess occurs with a frequency of 1 in 25,000 newborns, and can cause up to 2.5-fold elevations

in the total serum concentration of T4. Other abnormal serum-binding proteins can contribute to euthyroid hyperthyroxinemia. In the autosomal dominant condition familial dysalbuminemic hyperthyroxinemia (FDH), one or more abnormal species of albumin contain a high-affinity binding site for thyroxine. Because the defect is specific for T4 and does not affect T3 binding, these patients have an elevated total T4; a normal THBR using T3, but a decreased THBR using T4 as the ligand; a normal total T3; and either a normal or increased free T4, depending on the type of direct assay used. Equilibrium dialysis typically yields normal levels of free T4 in this syndrome. The diagnosis is established by paper or gel electrophoresis of serum enriched with radiolabeled T4, which permits identification of the abnormal binding proteins.

Elevations of free T4 concentrations can occur as a result of interference in binding to serum proteins. In vivo, hormones can be displaced from protein by medications such as furosemide, causing a true, albeit rapidly reversible, minimal hyperthyroxinemia after rapid intravenous administration of the diuretic. Activation of lipases by both low- and high-molecular-weight heparins leads to increased levels of free fatty acids that displace thyroid hormones ex vivo, causing an artefactual elevation of measured free hormone (24).

In autoimmune thyroid diseases and monoclonal gammopathies, endogenous serum anti-T4 or anti-T3 antibodies bind thyroid hormones, increasing the serum concentrations of protein-bound hormones. More commonly, however, anti-iodothyronine autoantibodies have negligible in vivo effects on hormone binding, but interfere with immunoassay measurements (25). In a classic RIA for total hormone concentration, the autoantibody will compete with the capture antibody for the radiolabeled ligand, reducing the amount of signal available to be measured and leading to a false high value. A similar spuriously increased result can occur in the one-step free T4 assay, in which the autoantibody binds the labeled T4 analogue, preventing it from being measured and yielding a falsely increased free T4 level; this is avoided in a two-step assay in which the labeled ligand is unable to interact with the serum autoantibodies. Another autoantibody that interferes with immunoassays is the rheumatoid factor, an

IgM directed against the Fc fragment of human IgG. Because rheumatoid factor is weakly heterophilic, it appears to bind to the nonhuman capture antibody, preventing interaction with the radiolabeled ligand and leading to a falsely increased hormone concentration (26). Preincubation of the serum specimen with a nonspecific animal immunoglobulin, ethanol, or polyethylene glycol reduces this antibody-mediated interference.

Assay interference by biotin supplements is a recently recognized cause of artefact in a number of thyroid-related assays that employ biotinylated components, potentially falsely decreasing results in sandwich immunoassays or falsely increasing results in competitive immunoassays (27). Thus, depending on the assay system, biotin ingestion can cause falsely elevated or falsely low serum FT4, FT3, and TSH, and even falsely increased levels of thyroid-stimulating antibodies mimicking Graves' disease (28) (Table 1.4).

Decreased function of the 5'-monodeiodinase causes impaired conversion of T4 to T3, decreasing T4 clearance and increasing T4 levels. Iodinated radiocontrast dyes—for example, sodium ipodate—are potent inhibitors of T4 to T3 conversion and have been used therapeutically in severely hyperthyroid patients, but are no longer commercially available in the United States. Amiodarone, a highly iodinated antiarrhythmic agent, also interferes with T4 deiodination. Since amiodarone-induced

Table 1.4. Biotin-related assay interference

Type of assay	Relationship between signal and analyte concentration	Impact on signal	Type of potential error	Example of analyte
Competitive	Signal intensity of washed solid phase is inversely proportional to analyte concentration	Biotin interferes with binding of antigen antibody complexes to solid phase	Overestimation of concentration of analyte	FT4 FT3 TRAb
Non-competitive, Sandwich	Signal intensity of washed solid phase is proportional to analyte concentration	Biotin interferes with binding of sandwich to solid phase	Underestimation of concentration of analyte	TSH hCG Thyroglobulin

hyperthyroidism can also occur, great care must be taken in interpreting hyperthyroxinemia in patients receiving iodinated medications (29). An inherited defect in 5'-monodeiodinase function, due to a mutation in a selenocysteine insertion sequence binding protein, has recently been described, and is probably responsible for hyperthyroxinemia observed in these patients (30).

Patients with resistance to thyroid hormones have an inherited partial defect in tissue responsiveness to thyroid hormones. Serum concentrations of total and free thyroid hormones are both increased as compensation for partial resistance. Most kindreds that have been evaluated have been found to have a dominant negative mutation in a single allele of the thyroid hormone receptor beta gene. Although affected individuals are generally described as being clinically euthyroid, considerable variation exists in the measurable degrees of hormone resistance among specific target organs for thyroid hormone (31).

Transient elevations of total serum T4 and, less frequently, free T4 levels occur in patients with acute medical and psychiatric illnesses. Although some patients develop increased levels of both T4 and T3 when the nonthyroidal illness resolves, consistent with coexistent hyperthyroidism, in most of these patients normal thyroid hormone levels are restored with recovery (32). Transient increases in total and free T4 and T3 can be seen in 8 to 33% of patients admitted for acute psychiatric disorders (33, 34). TSH concentrations have been reported as increased in up to 10% of acutely psychotic patients (35), but they are frequently suppressed in severely depressed outpatients as well as those suffering from post-traumatic stress disorders (36, 37).

CAUSES OF DECREASED T4 AND/OR T3 CONCENTRATIONS

Reduced serum levels of total and free T4 and T3 are typically seen in patients with overt hypothyroidism, reflecting impairment of hormone synthesis and release by the gland (Table 1.2). Due to TSH stimulation of residual gland function and elevation in the fractional conversion of T4 to T3 by 5'-monodeiodinase in both thyroid and peripheral tissues, 30% of patients with primary hypothyroidism maintain normal T3 levels despite decreases in T4. Thyroxine synthesis is also suppressed in patients receiving T3 exogenously or with autonomous T3 overproduction.

Euthyroid hypothyroxinemia can be due to a variety of mechanisms. Analogous to the abnormalities that can cause hyperthyroxinemia, defects in hormone binding to serum proteins can lead to decreases in T4 levels. Partial deficiency of TBG, caused by impaired production or accelerated degradation of unstable variants, occurs in 1 in 4,000 births. X-linked complete TBG deficiency is less common, found in 1 in 15,000 male births; female heterozygotes have TBG levels that are partially reduced. Numerous variants of TBG with reduced affinity for thyroid hormones have been described, with varying frequencies in different populations (38). Acquired impairment of hormone binding develops secondary to decreases in binding protein levels, due to either reduced production (as occurs in hyperthyroidism) or increased clearance (as from nephrotic syndrome). In most patients with quantitative or qualitative defects in TBG, direct and indirect estimates of free T4 levels are normal. In the extreme case of complete deficiency, lack of a linear relationship between free T4 fraction and THBR leads to falsely low free T4 index results, and values of free T4 can be either normal or underestimated by two-step and direct measurements.

Hypothyroxinemia and hypotriiodothyroninemia are common findings in patients with nonthyroidal illness, with more severe reductions in total hormone levels associated with more severe or critical illness (39, 40). Milder degrees of illness are typically accompanied by reductions in T4 to T3 conversion, resulting in a low T3 state but the preservation of T4 levels. In addition to deficiency of albumin and transthyretin, another proposed mechanism includes the inhibition of hormone binding to TBG, perhaps due to certain free fatty acids released from damaged tissues or cytokines, such as tumor necrosis factor (41). Numerous medications interfere with thyroid hormone binding to serum proteins, including diphenylhydantoin, furosemide, heparin, sertraline, and certain non-steroidal anti-inflammatory agents (42, 43). Inhibition of 5'-monodeiodinase activity in nonthyroidal tissues accelerates clearance of T4 through nondeiodinative mechanisms, particularly in nonthyroidal illness and starvation, and may be secondary to increased levels of interleukin-6; the production rate of T3 declines as a result of this monodeiodinase inhibition, but no change is seen in T3 metabolic clearance (44). Medications such as glucocorticoids, amiodarone, oral radiocontrast agents, gold, and high-dose pro-pranolol and propylthiouracil (PTU) also inhibit T4 deiodination to T3; however, clinical signs of hypothyroidism are unlikely to develop, except with unmonitored PTU use. Hypothyroxinemia has been described in patients treated with novel anti-cancer agents that inhibit vascular endothelial growth factor receptors, with evidence of multiple potential mechanisms that include primary thyroid dysfunction, but also effects on either thyroid hormone absorption or metabolic clearance (45, 46). Pituitary TSH production is suppressed by endogenous and/or exogenous glucocorticoids, dopamine, somatostatin, and endorphins and may also be mediated by reduced hypothalamic TRH secretion (47). Alteration of TSH sialylation and bioactivity may occur in critical illness as well (48). However, in general, the serum TSH is the most reliable measure of thyroid function in this patient population. With increasing severity of nonthyroidal illness, all of the proposed mechanisms presumably result in a low T4, low T3 state. Often, the decrease in protein binding is reflected by a decreased T4 and increased THBR, yielding a normal free thyroxine index. However, in many instances, the presence of a binding inhibitor (such as heparin or free fatty acids released in inflammation) interferes with hormone attachment to the solid phase, leading to a slightly lower value for the THBR and a falsely low estimate of the free thyroxine index. Most analogue and some two-step procedures for measuring free T4 are also adversely affected by binding inhibition in nonthyroidal illness (7, 14). These laboratory abnormalities reverse with recovery from the nonthyroidal illness or discontinuation of the interfering medication. Although most of the effects of nonthyroidal illness may represent energy-conserving adaptive mechanisms, the traditional view of these patients as being euthyroid is not universally held (49). However, no benefit from thyroid hormone supplementation has yet been demonstrated.

Low serum FT4 levels are often encountered in the second and third trimester of pregnancy, a finding which is thought to be a methodological artefact related to expanded plasma volume, high serum TBG serum levels, and other unknown factors (50). Since a low FT4 and a normal serum TSH suggest central hypothyroidism, it is important to be aware of this pitfall. Many experts recommend using the total T4 with or without serum TBG assessment, as a more reliable assessment of thyroid hormone levels in the second and third trimesters, taking into account the normal elevation of T4 because of higher serum TBG concentrations (50).

Assays of thyroid-stimulating hormones

Early TSH assays utilized a single polyclonal antibody in a radioimmunoassay and were capable of detecting elevated levels of TSH in patients who have primary hypothyroidism. With a sensitivity of about 1 mU/L, these tests were unable to distinguish the low-normal TSH levels in serum of 25% of euthyroid individuals from subnormal concentrations. With the introduction of immunometric (IMA) methods that use two or more antibodies directed at different antigenic determinants on the TSH molecule, assay sensitivities have been improved by 10- to 200-fold. The first antibody, usually a mouse monoclonal construct, is linked to a solid phase, permitting the target molecule to be separated from the serum with high affinity; the second antibody, which may be polyclonal, is labeled, providing a signal proportional to the amount of ligand bound. With these more sensitive assays, hyperthyroid patients can be identified on the basis of low or undetectable levels of TSH in IMAs, analogous to detection of primary hypothyroidism with elevated TSH levels. Even more sensitive determinations of low TSH values have been obtained in an assay utilizing a chemiluminescent acridinium ester to generate the antibody-linked signal. High intraassay and interassay precision with chemiluminometric methods may permit routine detection of TSH levels as low as 0.01 mU/L or lower.

The ability of TSH assays to accurately measure low concentrations of the hormone is termed the "functional sensitivity" of the assay, defined as the concentration at which the interassay coefficient of variation is 20%. This contrasts with the "analytical sensitivity," which is based on intraassay measurements of the blank calibrator, and does not reflect a clinically meaningful result (9). Whereas the original RIA methods have been termed "first generation" assays, the newer, more sensitive TSH assays, which provide a sufficient separation in serum TSH values between hyperthyroid and euthyroid patients, are defined as "second generation" when the functional sensitivity is 0.1 mU/L, and "third generation" when the functional sensitivity is 0.01 mU/L (51).

Multiple sources contribute to the total variation observed in TSH assay results (52). Endogenous, biologic variation exists due to the heterogeneity of TSH isoforms, based on posttranslational modifications that can alter the immunoreactivity as well as the bioactivity of the molecule; this potentially may be overcome with the use of variants of recombinant TSH that mimic these individual modifications (53, 54). Circadian and seasonal effects contribute to within-person variation as well. But, within-person variation during serial measurements is relatively minimal compared with between-person variation, raising concern that population reference standards may be inadequate to distinguish a healthy from diseased state (52, 55, 56).

Debate now exists about the optimal reference range for TSH assays. Typically, the lower and upper limits of a population reference range of the analyte's concentrations are the 2.5th and 97.5th percentiles (the 95% confidence interval), measured in a rigorously defined normal cohort without any evidence of relevant disease. Applying this criterion to TSH levels, as determined in the U.S. National Health and Nutrition Examination Survey (NHANES III), the population reference range would be 0.45–4.12 mU/L (57). Similar ranges have been reported in other populations, differing to some degree due to variations in iodine intake, race, age, gender, and even the time of day that blood is sampled (58). As most functional thyroid disorders are due to autoimmune thyroid disease, the relationship between levels of thyroid autoantibodies and TSH has also been evaluated, demonstrating a U-shaped curve with the lowest prevalence of autoantibodies at TSH levels between 0.1 and 1.5 mU/L in women and 0.1 and 2.0 mU/L in men (59). Additionally, the likelihood of eventual development of overt primary hypothyroidism has been reported to be markedly higher in the setting of a TSH level of at least 2.0 mU/L and elevated levels of antithyroid peroxidase antibodies (60). Therefore, it has been proposed that the upper limit of the population reference range should in fact be as low as 2.5 or 3.0 mU/L (61, 62). Other studies have suggested that age-specific reference ranges would be appropriate, with the 97.5th percentile being well above 4.5 mU/L with successively increasing deciles of age (63). However, in the absence of definitive evidence that defining hypothyroidism as a TSH greater than 2.5 mU/L leads to unequivocal clinical benefit from treatment with thyroid hormone, and given the overall concern that the population reference range may not be optimal for defining a disease state when inter-individual variation is relatively large, changes in the TSH reference range have not been made, and is generally in the 0.4–4.5 mU/L range in most laboratories (64).

During pregnancy, the placenta is responsible for the production of high levels of hCG, a glycoprotein hormone sharing a common alpha subunit with TSH. While there is no cross-reactivity of hCG in TSH immunometric assays, hCG in high serum concentrations can stimulate the thyroid to produce thyroid hormone, thereby lowering serum TSH concentrations. Most laboratories have now established trimester specific TSH serum concentrations that, in general, are decreased by 0.1–0.2 mU/L and 1 mU/L at the low- and high-end, respectively, of the usual TSH reference range of 0.4–4 mU/L in nonpregnant women (65). Indeed, levels less than 0.1 mU/L in the first trimester can be seen in about 10% of normal women (66). Since serum hCG levels peak at the end of the first trimester, the effect on serum TSH wanes, so that the TSH reference range becomes closer to the normal nonpregnant range by the third trimester.

Interference with TSH immunoassays is uncommon. Patients with endogenous heterophilic antibodies directed against mouse immunoglobulin can have falsely elevated TSH levels, as the heterophilic antibody can substitute for TSH and bridge between the two antibodies in the assay (67). This problem has been eliminated from most commercially available kits by addition of an excess of mouse immunoglobulin. If interference with the assay is suspected, measurement of serial dilutions of the sample may show a non-linear relationship; alternatively, the sample can be tested using another manufacturer's assay (9, 67). MacroTSH, in which TSH is complexed to immunoglobulins to form a high molecular weight species with no biological activity, is another cause of artefactually elevated serum TSH, analogous to the case of macroprolactin (68). In this case, serial dilution of the sample is linear for TSH, and the presence of macroTSH in the serum needs to be detected by measuring TSH in the supernatant after polyethylene glycol precipitation (68).

CAUSES OF HYPOTHYROTROPINEMIA

In severe hyperthyroidism, serum TSH levels remain below the functional sensitivity of even third or fourth generation assays, but such degrees of suppression are not seen in other causes of low TSH levels. Subnormal but detectable TSH levels can be seen in patients who have mild or asymptomatic hyperthyroidism of any etiology, or they may be due to TSH suppression from nonthyroidal illness. More sensitive TSH immunoassays provide adequate separation between hospitalized hyperthyroid patients with medical illness, in whom basal TSH levels generally remain undetectably low, and euthyroid patients with nonthyroidal illness, in whom basal TSH levels are usually but not always >0.01 mU/L.

In hypothyroidism due to hypothalamic or pituitary disease, low levels of basal TSH may occur. Hypothyroidism due to pituitary or hypothalamic disease can also present with inappropriately normal or even slightly elevated levels of immunologically intact but biologically inactive TSH secondary to alternative glycosylation of the protein (69, 70). Among the drugs that can affect TSH production, the rexinoid bexarotene appears to suppress TSH gene transcription directly and causes a dose-dependent central hypothyroidism (71, 72). The hypoglycemic drug metformin has been reported to lower TSH levels by an as yet unknown mechanism (73).

CAUSES OF HYPERTHYROTROPINEMIA

Elevated serum TSH values are the cornerstone of the diagnosis of primary hypothyroidism. Due to the extreme sensitivity of the hypothalamic-pituitary-thyroid negative feedback loop, small decrements in circulating thyroid hormone levels produce logarithmic increases in serum TSH levels (51). At one end of the spectrum are patients with frankly symptomatic thyroid hormone deficiency, whose free T4 levels are subnormal and whose TSH levels are typically >20 mU/L. But, even patients with the earliest stages of thyroid gland impairment can have elevated TSH concentrations. These patients with so-called subclinical hypothyroidism have T4 and T3 levels within the normal range associated with increased serum TSH concentrations. Although the clinical management of such patients remains controversial, those individuals with a predisposition to developing clinical hypothyroidism—for example, those with autoimmune thyroiditis or a history of thyroid irradiation or surgery, should be treated or followed longitudinally for development of overt hypothyroidism (74). Medications that have been associated with hyperthyrotropinemia include cytokines that can cause autoimmune thyroiditis (such as interferon-α), and antineoplastic agents such as tyrosine kinase inhibitors, and immune checkpoint inhibitors (45). In neonates, various maternal causes of fetal distress, including preeclampsia and gestational diabetes mellitus, are associated with elevated TSH levels in cord blood, but whether this reflects transient primary hypothyroidism or a central stimulation of TSH production is unknown (75).

The differential diagnosis of hyperthyrotropinemia also includes conditions associated with inappropriate TSH secretion, as in patients whose TSH levels are higher than would be predicted from their circulating free thyroid hormone levels. Patients with TSH-secreting pituitary adenomas may have normal or increased TSH levels in the setting of increased T4 concentrations. These patients usually present with a goiter and clinical evidence of thyrotoxicosis, with or without clinical evidence of a sellar mass lesion. In half of the cases, there is co-secretion of other anterior pituitary hormones (e.g., growth hormone or prolactin) and the α-subunit of TSH is commonly overproduced. A molar ratio of α-subunit to intact TSH that is greater than unity is strongly suggestive of a pituitary adenoma (76). Resistance to thyroid hormone (RTH) is a rare inherited disorder characterized by reduced responsiveness of target tissues to thyroid hormone due to mutations in the thyroid hormone receptor gene (77). The diagnosis of RTH should be considered when thyroid function tests reveal elevated T4 and T3 levels and a non-suppressed TSH. Due to very similar thyroid function test abnormalities, RTH must be distinguished from a TSH-producing adenoma. RTH patients exhibit normal α-subunit and a normal molar ratio of α-subunit to intact TSH of ≤ 1.

The resistance of the thyroid to TSH, presenting with nongoitrous congenital hypothyroidism and elevated TSH levels, has been described both in isolated form as well as in pseudohypoparathyroidism type Ia (78). In this latter congenital condition, deficiency of the stimulatory subunit of the guanine nucleotide-binding proteins that mediate activation of adenylate cyclase can cause resistance to multiple hormones, including TSH and parathyroid hormone.

In infants, exposure to cold temperatures immediately following birth or during hypothermic surgery causes TSH concentrations to rise as high as 50 to 100 mU/L, which is thought to reflect the immaturity of the hypothalamic-pituitary-thyroid axis (79). Adults, on the other hand, do not demonstrate altered TSH levels after brief periods of cold exposure, despite increases in the concentrations and fractional clearance rates of circulating free T4 and T3. However, seasonal changes in serum TSH (i.e., during colder vs warmer temperatures) have been recently observed (80).

Specialized studies of thyroid function

THYROGLOBULIN

In most forms of thyroid disease, thyroglobulin (Tg) is released from thyroid follicular cells proportional to the synthesis and release of T4 and T3, increasing size of the gland, and the degree of cytotoxic inflammation. The reference range in subjects with intact thyroid glands and normal TSH levels is about 3 to 40 ng/mL. Markedly elevated levels are seen in most patients with hyperthyroidism and thyroiditis, but mild increases are also observed in cigarette smokers despite slightly lower TSH levels (81). In determining the cause of hyperthyroidism, an undetectable serum Tg suggests factitious or iatrogenic thyrotoxicosis. Undetectable levels are also seen in hypothyroid patients with congenital or acquired absence of the thyroid gland. Presently, the primary indication for measurement of serum Tg concentrations is as a tumor marker for the longitudinal follow-up of patients with differentiated thyroid carcinoma, which necessitates greater functional sensitivity at lower concentrations than the euthyroid reference range (82). Although introduced more than 15 years ago, these assays are now being increasingly used to detect Tg in fine needle aspirations of neck masses or cystic lesions as an adjunct to cytologic interpretation to diagnose recurrent or metastatic cancer (83).

Serum Tg is generally measured by either two-antibody immunometric assay or single-antibody immunoassay. The newer immunometric assays require shorter incubation times and have greater sensitivity ($\leq$1 ng/mL) than the immunoassays, but several problems persist. The greatest limitation is the potential for interference by anti-Tg autoantibodies, which can be found in up to 25% of patients with differentiated thyroid carcinoma. In the immunometric assays, the serum Tg concentration can be falsely lowered by autoantibodies that bind Tg and effectively remove it from the serum, thus making it incapable of binding to the assay's reporter antibodies. Detecting the presence and degree of autoantibody interference in an immunoassay may also be difficult (84). Conversely, in radioimmunoassays, anti-Tg autoantibodies can cause falsely high values because they bind radiolabeled Tg; as a result, less is available to bind to the assay antibody. Thus, in the presence of anti-Tg antibodies, discordant findings of an undetectable Tg in an immunometric assay and a concentration of at least 2 ng/dL in a radioimmunoassay may suggest the presence of antibody interference, but cannot be used to quantify the problem. A measure of serum Tg should therefore always be preceded by a test for anti-Tg antibodies, and it is recommended that laboratories withhold reporting low results of Tg immunometric assays when autoantibodies are identified (9). Of note, recent reports demonstrate that the presence of anti-Tg antibodies may not preclude identification of the high concentration of Tg seen in fine needle aspiration specimens (85).

Despite a trend toward assay standardization, the variability of results using differing Tg assays remains at at least 25% due to variations in the anti-thyroglobulin antibodies used and the molecular heterogeneity of Tg. Occasionally, immunometric assays may fail to detect very high serum Tg concentrations due to the so-called hook effect, in which the high concentrations of Tg bind to one antibody, preventing the formation of the two-antibody sandwich upon which the assay depends. If this effect is suspected, the sample should be reanalyzed after dilution. Another cause of a false-negative Tg in patients with differentiated thyroid cancer can be tumor production of variants of Tg that fail to be recognized by the antibodies used in an assay (86). Recently, thyroglobulin LC-MS/MS assays have been introduced that purport to circumvent the problem of anti-Tg antibody interference (87). However, recent data suggest that these assays are still capable of generating falsely low serum Tg levels in patients with known residual disease (88).

Measurement of serum Tg has become a cornerstone of differentiated thyroid cancer follow-up (89). There is a very high negative predictive value of an undetectable TSH-stimulated serum Tg level to identify those patients with differentiated thyroid cancer who have no evidence of disease. Recent data suggest that similar high negative predictive values of an non-TSH-stimulated serum Tg <0.1 are seen using a second-generation Tg immuno-chemiluminometric assay (ICMA) with a functional sensitivity of 0.05 ng/mL (90).

Alternatively, the positive predictive value is limited in the presence of remnant normal thyroid cells left after thyroidectomy, and thus one indication for postsurgical adjuvant radioiodine therapy is to eliminate such normal sources of Tg (89). However, in most patients who have not undergone remnant ablation after total thyroidectomy, serum Tg levels are generally <1–2 ng/ml, and a rising serum Tg is still useful in the detection of recurrent disease (91). The thyroglobulin doubling time, analogous to the calcitonin doubling time in medullary thyroid cancer, is a useful prognostic parameter to monitor in patients with known residual disease (92). False positive Tg results can also be caused by heterophilic antibodies, a problem in many immunometric assays that has only been partially resolved by the addition of blocking antibodies, but rare false-negative results have also been reported (93, 94).

THYROID AUTOANTIBODIES

Antibodies directed against the cell surface (TSH receptor), intracellular components (microsomal membranes, thyroglobulin), and extracellular antigens (T4, T3) are often found in sera of patients with autoimmune thyroid diseases. Although autoantibodies tend to target fewer antigenic epitopes than heterologous antibodies, these autoantibodies can still be quite a heterogeneous mixture of proteins, leading to problems with both specificity and sensitivity in assays.

In Hashimoto's disease, cytotoxic antibodies may bind to a thyroid microsomal antigen that is expressed on the apical cell surface, and these antibodies subsequently fix complement. These antithyroid microsomal antibodies can be detected by sensitive hemagglutination techniques in the sera of 95% of patients with histologically proven Hashimoto's disease, as compared with only 55% for non-complement-fixing antithyroglobulin antibodies. Among commercially available assays, immunometric procedures, including RIA, immunoradiometric assay, and enzyme-linked and fluorescent methods are superior to routine hemagglutination techniques. Improvements in

sensitivity and specificity have been obtained using monoclonal antibodies directed against thyroid peroxidase (TPO), and purified or recombinant TPO in the assay systems (95, 96). International standardization now exists against a specific reference preparation, MRC 66/387, permitting reporting of results in "international units," but concordance among multiple assays remains suboptimal (97). Reference ranges vary widely among different assays, with manufacturers often citing levels greater than 10 kIU/L as being clinically relevant predictors of autoimmune thyroid disease. However, long-term follow-up studies that identified anti-microsomal antibodies as being predictive of eventual hypothyroidism were likely based on far less sensitive assays, and similar studies will be required to determine whether such minimally detectable levels are also predictive (60, 98).

Antithyroglobulin antibodies are less specific for autoimmune thyroiditis but have achieved greater significance for their potential to interfere with thyroglobulin assays in patients with thyroid cancer. Contemporary immunoassays are considerably more sensitive and specific than older, agglutination methods, and can detect antithyroglobulin antibodies in up to 10% of the clinically disease-free population and 3.4% of those who lack anti-TPO antibodies (57). Nevertheless, reference preparations for standardization of these assays still vary considerably, and even use of the accepted international standard reference MRC 65/93 has not resulted in the interchangeability of assays (99). As with anti-TPO antibody measurements, differences exist in the definitions used for reference ranges. Assays that report detectable levels of antithyroglobulin antibodies below 10 kIU/L as abnormal may have low specificity both for actual pathology and for antibodies that can interfere with thyroglobulin assays (99).

No correlation exists between the severity of hypothyroidism and titers of antithyroid antibodies, and low levels can be seen in patients with no demonstrable thyroid dysfunction. Anti-TPO and antithyroglobulin antibodies are also present in Graves' disease, albeit less frequently (85% and 25%, respectively), and may predict the subsequent development of hypothyroidism in some patients with this condition. With appropriate treatment of the thyroid hormone excess or deficiency, antithyroid antibody titers often decrease but are not clinically useful measures of disease activity.

Multiple procedures have been developed to measure the TSH-receptor stimulatory immunoglobulins that are pathogenetic for Graves' disease, detecting either stimulation of biochemical functions in thyroid cells (thyroid-stimulating immunoglobulins) or blockade of receptor binding by TSH (TSH-binding inhibitors). The original long-acting thyroid stimulator (LATS) assay of Adams and Purves had been largely replaced by quantitation of cyclic AMP production, typically by Chinese hamster ovary cells transfected with human TSH receptors or chimeric human/rat TSH receptors (100). TSH-binding inhibitors can be detected by quantitation of radiolabeled TSH binding to recombinant human TSH receptors in the presence of serum, followed by polyethylene glycol precipitation to separate bound from unbound radiolabel (101). Alternatively, recombinant TSH receptors can be affinity-immobilized on an antibody-coated tube, which is then incubated with TSH with an attached radioactive or chemiluminescent label (102). In general, the most sensitive of these assays can detect thyroid-stimulating immunoglobulins in up to 95% of hyperthyroid Graves' sera, and TSH-binding inhibitors in 60 to 85%. In general, there is an excellent correlation between the bioassay methods and the TSH receptor–based assays (103). However, thyroid-stimulating immunoglobulins levels may be more useful for identifying Graves' disease as the cause of exophthalmos (104). Blocking antibodies that bind to but do not stimulate the TSH receptor have also been identified in hypothyroid and euthyroid patients with autoimmune thyroiditis or Graves' disease.

The measurement of thyroid autoantibodies is of value in selected clinical situations. The presence of thyroid-stimulating immunoglobulins in patients in whom the etiology of hyperthyroidism is uncertain can lead to a diagnosis of Graves' disease. Current third generation TRAb assays have a 95% sensitivity and specificity for diagnosing Graves' disease (105). Assessment of anti-TSH receptor antibody levels before treatment can be predictors of the likelihood of remission after a course of antithyroid drug therapy or the development of Graves' ophthalmopathy (106). Persistence of high levels of thyroid-stimulating immunoglobulins in Graves' disease following therapy is associated with increased rates of recurrence (107, 108). When detected during the third trimester of pregnancy in a woman with Graves' disease, significant increases in either TSH-binding inhibitors or thyroid-stimulating immunoglobulins titers correlate with the development of intrauterine and neonatal hyperthyroidism due to transplacental passage of immunoglobulins (109).

TISSUE RESPONSES TO THYROID HORMONE ACTION

Before the availability of hormone immunoassays, measurement of the end-organ responses—for example, the basal metabolic rate—was the primary means of evaluating thyroid hormone function. Today, regulation of serum TSH levels by T4 and T3 is the most precisely measurable and useful response by tissues to the action of thyroid hormones. Measurements of thyroid hormone effects in extrapituitary tissues are occasionally used to evaluate patients in whom there is a discordance among the clinical evaluation, thyroid hormone levels, and the concentration of TSH (110).

Numerous serum constituents have altered levels in hyperthyroidism and hypothyroidism, mostly reflecting changes in synthesis and/or clearance of these substances (Table 1.3). There is considerable overlap between the normal ranges and values seen in thyroid gland dysfunction. However, they remain useful markers of thyroid hormone effects, especially with serial determination during therapy of underlying thyroid disorders and in the evaluation of patients with discordant thyroid function tests. Combinations of biophysical and serum parameters of thyroid hormone action are particularly useful in the evaluation of patients with possible thyroid hormone resistance states. To characterize the presence and extent of resistance, parameters of pituitary and peripheral tissue response are measured before and during the administration of increasing doses of T3 (50, 100, and 200 µg per day). Among the various tests performed, changes in sex hormone-binding globulin, basal metabolic rate, and body weight provide the strongest distinction between normal responsiveness and generalized resistance to thyroid hormones (111).

LABORATORY EVALUATION FOR THYROID DISEASE

Distinct strategies for use of thyroid function tests should be designed to satisfy four distinct purposes: screening for the presence of clinically unsuspected disease in an asymptomatic general population, case finding to detect thyroid disease in patients whose symptoms and signs are sufficiently subtle that the examining clinician may not suspect thyroid dysfunction as the etiology, diagnosis to prove the presence of clinically suspected disease, and optimization of management of proven thyroid disease.

Screening and case findings

Population screening is generally warranted if the prevalence of such disease is not small, the health consequences of undiagnosed disease are substantial, and the treatment is effective. With these criteria in mind, there is considerable controversy about the appropriateness of screening asymptomatic adults for thyroid dysfunction (112–114). The Whickham study demonstrated an annual incidence of thyroid hormone excess and deficiency of 0.5% in women and 0.06% in men in the United Kingdom (60). The hazard rate for developing thyroid dysfunction was higher in women with advancing age, but not men. Using a logit model to evaluate contributors to risk, only the presence of antithyroid antibodies and a baseline TSH of at least 2.0 mU/L were predictive of eventual overt hypothyroidism. More at issue than prevalence, however, is the question of whether undiagnosed mild hypothyroidism or hyperthyroidism has significant enough consequences to justify the costs of screening. Using a decision analysis model, adding a serum TSH determination to the quintennial cholesterol screening recommended starting at age 35 was found to be reasonably cost-effective (115). Deferring periodic TSH screening until older ages and decreasing cost for TSH assays are key factors in improving cost-effectiveness even further. As a result, three endocrine professional organizations (the American Thyroid Association, American Association of Clinical Endocrinologists, and The Endocrine Society) all support routine screening of asymptomatic adults (116). Conversely, other organizations with a broader focus than these endocrine groups do not recommend screening for thyroid dysfunction, including the U.S. Preventive Services Task Force, American College of Physicians, Royal College of Physicians, and Institute of Medicine (113, 117, 118).

There is uniform agreement, however, that screening for neonatal hypothyroidism is necessary (119). Neonatal hypothyroidism occurs with a frequency of 1 in 4,000 live births and is associated with significant neurological and developmental morbidity, much of which can be prevented by early treatment with thyroid hormone replacement. Mandatory neonatal screening is based either upon the measurement of total (not free) T4 or TSH in whole blood collected on filter paper. In strategies that measure T4 first, determination of the TSH concentration is performed if the T4 level is below the 10th percentile, and serum assays are then used to confirm a diagnosis of hypothyroidism. The advantage of a T4-first strategy is the ability to detect central hypothyroidism and minimized impact of the neonatal TSH surge (120). An alternative strategy employs primary TSH screening, followed by confirmatory T4 testing; this approach is more commonly used in Europe and in areas of iodine deficiency (121).

Case findings are best reserved for patients whose clinical assessment may be sufficiently complex as to obscure suspicion for thyroid dysfunction. Often, these patients are elderly, and their symptoms may be primarily constitutional, neuropsychiatric, or cardiovascular. Although dementia is an uncommon presentation of hypothyroidism, the relative ease of diagnosis and treatment of this condition warrants inclusion of a thyroid function test in the evaluation of such patients. As an initial test for case finding, a sensitive TSH assay has excellent sensitivity and specificity for both hyperthyroidism and hypothyroidism. In contrast, hospitalized patients with acute illnesses have a high frequency of transient thyroid function abnormalities and are unlikely to have primary thyroid disease diagnosed on the basis of routine tests. In the absence of strong clinical evidence of thyroid dysfunction, patients hospitalized with acute illnesses should probably not undergo thyroid testing for case finding (39).

Postpartum women have a high frequency of transient thyroid dysfunction, especially those with pre-existing euthyroid autoimmune thyroiditis. Within the first 3 months after delivery, at least 5% of women develop postpartum thyroiditis, a painless inflammatory condition that can cause thyrotoxicosis and/or hypothyroidism. More than one-half of these patients require therapeutic intervention. Furthermore, 25% of women with postpartum thyroiditis eventually develop chronic hypothyroidism requiring lifelong therapy. Case finding with serum TSH measurements 3 and 6 months after delivery is recommended for women with type 1 diabetes mellitus, personal history of postpartum thyroiditis, or those known to have elevated levels of anti-TPO antibodies (122).

IMAGING APPROACH TO THYROID DISEASE

Ultrasonography and nuclear medicine studies

Two imaging modalities have proven to be of considerable utility for the evaluation of thyroid disease. These modalities are ultrasonography, which has become the gold standard for the initial evaluation of diffuse and nodular thyroid disease, and radioiodine scanning and uptake, which are of crucial importance for the diagnosis and management of hyperthyroidism and thyroid cancer.

Ultrasonography

TECHNIQUE

Ultrasound (US) examination of the thyroid gland is performed using high-frequency sound waves (10–15 MHz) generated by a linear transducer. The reflections of the sound waves are used to generate an image which can then be displayed. The magnitude of the echo from each point in the field of view is mapped to the gray level or brightness of the corresponding pixel in the image (B-mode, grayscale image). In order to perform a US assessment, the patient is placed in a supine position with the neck extended. Axial (or horizontal or transverse) scans of the whole thyroid gland are obtained at the upper, middle, and lower poles, with a comparison of the size and echogenicity of each lobe and documentation of their width and anterior-posterior diameters (123). Longitudinal (or sagittal) scans provide the length of the lobes. Focal lesions are then documented and described using standardized reporting criteria (123, 124). The following characteristics of nodules are reported: size, location, shape, composition, description of any calcifications, echogenicity, and vascular pattern. The vascularity of the lobes and the associated nodules is also depicted using color Doppler imaging, in which blood flow information is color-coded and superimposed on the B-mode grayscale image.

INDICATIONS

In addition to documenting the presence of thyroid nodules, US can also provide information about their risk of malignancy. The nodule characteristics described above are used to assign a risk of malignancy. For those nodules with a significant risk of malignancy, US can also be used to guide fine needle aspiration biopsy. Nodules that are determined not to be malignant can be monitored by US for changes in their size and other characteristics. Other roles for US examination are to document cervical lymphadenopathy, evaluate other thyroid lesions, and evaluate changes in the thyroid parenchyma. US is also invaluable for monitoring the post-thyroidectomy neck for tumor recurrence or suspicious lymph nodes in a patient being followed after initial treatment of thyroid cancer.

NORMAL THYROID APPEARANCE

The normal thyroid gland consists of right and left lobes and a connecting isthmus. A normal thyroid gland weighs approximately 30 gm, but the size, shape, and volume of the gland vary with age and sex. Measurement of the width, depth, and length of each thyroid lobe can be used to calculate thyroid volume. Normal volumes are 10–15 ml and 12–18 ml for females and males, respectively. The echogenicity of a normal thyroid gland is greater than the echogenicity of the surrounding muscles. The normal gland appears homogeneous with a "ground glass" appearance (123) (see Figure 1.2).

DIFFUSE THYROID DISEASE

US can be used to document a diffusely enlarged thyroid gland and can document extension into the superior mediastinum. It can also document the parenchymal changes associated with various diffuse thyroid diseases based on the echogenicity compared with the normal thyroid gland (123). A gland affected by Hashimoto's thyroiditis can appear heterogeneous with multiple hypoechoic micronodular areas (see Figure 1.3a), as compared with the more homogeneous appearance of normal thyroid parenchyma (Figures 1.2d and 1.2e). As the disease progresses, the parenchymal fibrosis is manifest as linear bands of echogenicity. Vascularity, as indicated by color Doppler imaging, is usually normal or increased early in the disease course (see Figure 1.3b) and reduced in the later

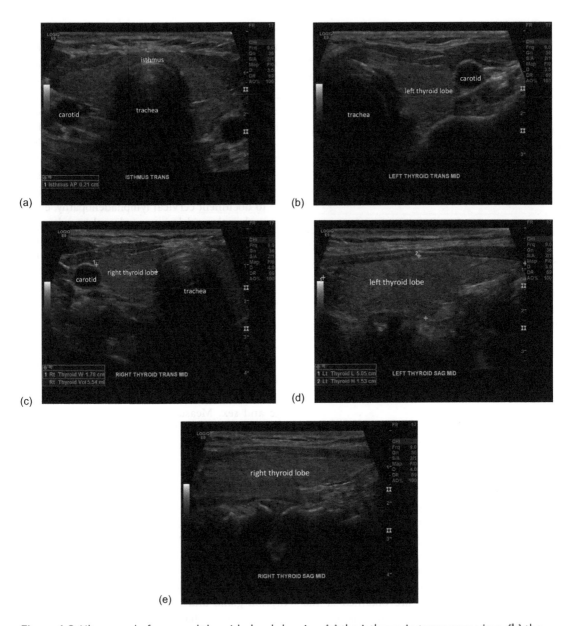

Figure 1.2 Ultrasound of a normal thyroid gland showing **(a)** the isthmus in transverse view, **(b)** the left thyroid in transverse view, **(c)** the right thyroid lobe in transverse view, **(d)** the left thyroid lobe in sagittal view, **(e)** the right thyroid lobe in sagittal view.

atrophic stage. In the case of Graves' disease, the gland is enlarged and lobulated with reduced echogenicity secondary to increased blood flow and decreased colloid (see Figure 1.4a), as compared with normal thyroid gland parenchyma (Figures 1.2d and 1.2e). In comparison to Hashimoto's thyroiditis, the gland is less heterogeneous, and when color Doppler imaging is employed, has increased vascularity and increased blood flow (see

Figure 1.4b). Subacute granulomatous thyroiditis is characterized by ill-defined patchy hypoechoic areas in the thyroid gland. The thyroid gland in both silent and postpartum thyroiditis appears either diffusely hypoechoic or has multiple areas of low echogenicity throughout both lobes. Riedel's thyroiditis appears as an enlarged hypoechoic gland that has a coarse echotexture with linear echogenic streaks corresponding with fibrotic

(a)

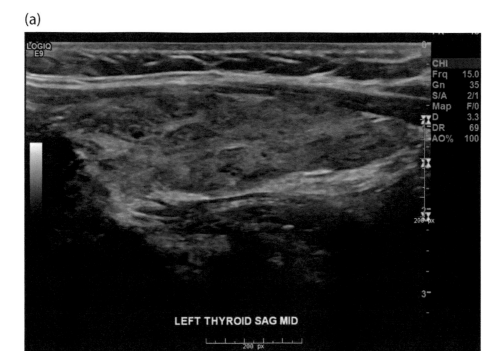

(b)

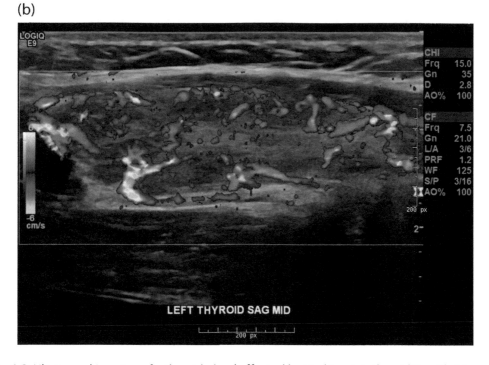

Figure 1.3 Ultrasound imaging of a thyroid gland affected by Hashimoto's thyroiditis with (a) gray scale imaging showing hypoechoic micronodular areas and (b) color Doppler showing increased vascularity.

(a)

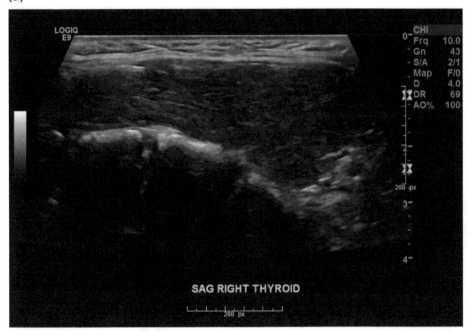

(b)

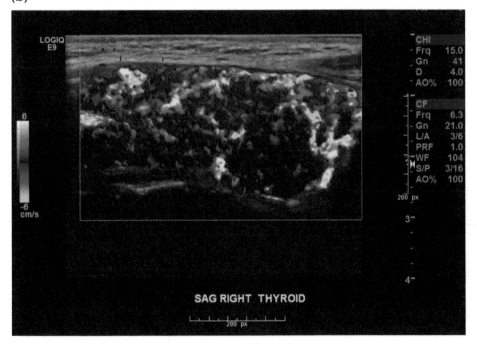

Figure 1.4 Ultrasound imaging of a thyroid gland affected by Graves' disease with (a) grayscale imaging showing reduced echogenicity and less heterogeneity than Hashimoto's thyroiditis and (b) color Doppler showing increased vascularity and blood flow.

bands. Color Doppler imaging has been used to distinguish the causes of amiodarone-induced thyrotoxicosis, as type 1 disease is characterized by increased blood flow and type 2 disease is associated with normal or decreased flow.

THYROID NODULES

US has become a key tool for determining whether a thyroid nodule, which has been found by palpation or incidentally by imaging, requires biopsy to exclude malignancy (124). Benign thyroid nodules are generally isoechoic or hyperechoic. Pure cysts are anechoic and are always benign and do not require biopsy. Spongiform nodules containing scattered microcystic structures also have a very low (<3%) risk of malignancy. The most common thyroid malignancy, papillary thyroid cancer, is generally hypoechoic, with other features such as irregular margins, microcalcifications, a "taller than wide" configuration in the transverse view, and internal vascularity. Follicular thyroid cancers are often hypoechoic with a rounded shape. Anaplastic thyroid cancer is typically hypoechoic, with irregular margins and areas of necrosis. Medullary thyroid cancer is also hypoechoic in appearance and may have echogenic foci due to amyloid deposition. US can also provide information about the number and characteristics of additional nodules, in addition to the index nodule. The presence of multiple nodules within the thyroid gland is associated with a very slightly reduced overall risk of thyroid cancer for the individual patient (125).

RISK STRATIFICATION SYSTEMS FOR THYROID NODULES

Systems used to stratify the risk of malignancy within a thyroid nodule have been based on a description of the individual ultrasound features, or various scoring systems that accommodate the US patterns or number of suspicious ultrasound features (126). A 2005 guideline recommended biopsy with different size cut-off criteria based on individual US features (127). A recent meta-analysis examining the predictive value of individual US features using combined data from 31 studies suggested that the highest diagnostic odds ratio for malignancy of 11.14 (CI 6.6–18.9) was provided by the taller than wide characteristic (128). Other individual predictive features were infiltrative margins, internal calcifications, hypoechogenicity,

and a solid nodule. However, each of these individual features had relatively modest likelihood ratios, and when the prevalence of thyroid cancer was taken into account, they resulted in a relatively modest post-test probability of thyroid cancer being present. Other meta-analyses have produced similar conclusions (129). Thus, the use of a single US feature does not take into account the alteration in risk that can occur with a combination of features, nor does it incorporate individual patient risk factors.

Combinations or patterns of US features have higher predictive value for thyroid cancer (126) compared with individual features. The American Thyroid Association (ATA) has developed criteria for assessment of the risk of malignancy within a nodule using the pattern of sonographic features (89) (see Figure 1.5). Using this system, a solid hypoechoic nodule that also has either irregular margins, microcalcifications, a taller-than-wide shape, an extrusive soft-tissue component, or extra thyroidal extension is considered to be high suspicion and to have at least a 70–90% risk of malignancy. Figure 1.6 shows a nodule with high-risk ATA sonographic features that was found to be papillary thyroid cancer when subject to biopsy. Solid hypoechoic nodules without these additional features are considered to be intermediate risk with a 10–20% risk of malignancy. Isoechoic or hyperechoic nodules without these features have a low risk (5–10%) of malignancy. A hyperechoic nodule with low-risk features is shown in Figure 1.7. Spongiform nodules have very low (<3%) risk of malignancy, whereas purely cystic lesions are considered benign with <1% risk of malignancy. Based on these differing assessments of the risk of thyroid cancer, different size criteria are suggested by the ATA for making a decision to pursue fine needle aspiration biopsy. For example, nodules with high and intermediate risk sonographic patterns are recommended for biopsy if they are greater than 1 cm in size, whereas low risk nodules are recommended for biopsy if they are greater than 1.5 cm in dimension.

Several other systems for assessing the risk of a thyroid nodule harboring malignancy have been developed. Some of these are quantitative and are based on calculating the number of suspicious US features and generating a risk score. The Thyroid Imaging Reporting and Data Systems (TIRADS), originally formulated in 2009 (130), has since been

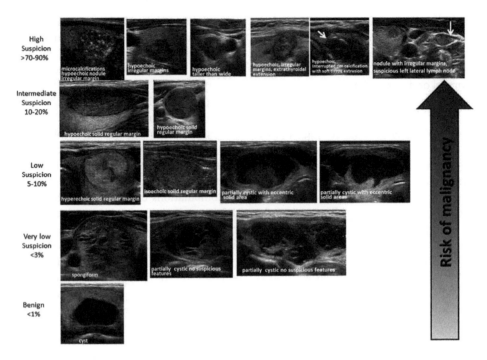

Figure 1.5 Risk stratification of thyroid nodules as proposed by the American Thyroid Association (ATA) 2016 Guidelines.

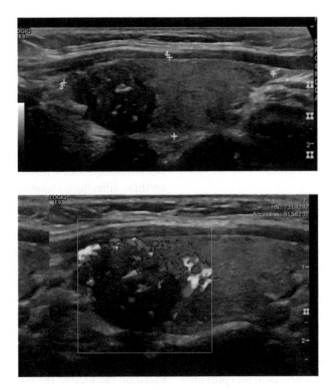

Figure 1.6 Nodule with ATA high suspicion sonographic pattern. (Right upper pole nodule is solid and hypoechoic with irregular margins and multiple microcalcifications. Color flow is present. Nodule is taller than it is wide. No extrathyroidal extension.)

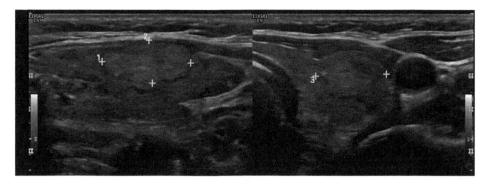

Figure 1.7 Nodule with ATA low suspicion sonographic pattern. (Left mid-lower pole solid hyperechoic elongated nodule has no microcalcifications or extrathyroidal extension.)

proposed in many different iterations (131–135). The significance of sonographic features and combinations of features are similar to the ATA schema (89), but size cutoffs for fine needle aspiration and need for a follow-up sonography are slightly different.

Thyroid nodules can also be assessed using strain elastography that employs an US transducer, which is used to compress and decompress the thyroid nodule(s) being examined (136). The change in signal measures the tissue stiffness, which is usually displayed as a continuum of colors. The greater the stiffness of thyroid tissue, the greater the likelihood of malignancy. However, at this time, this technique has not been sufficiently standardized to be in general use. Computer-aided diagnostic systems have also been studied for the assessment of thyroid nodules. Although this type of artificial intelligence does not currently perform any better than an experienced radiologist, producing similar sensitivity, but lesser specificity and accuracy (137), such algorithms may be refined in the future.

Sonographic patterns can also be used to guide the follow-up of thyroid nodules that are found to have benign cytology after biopsy (89). If a nodule has a high suspicion US pattern, follow-up US and biopsy within 12 months is indicated. Nodules with intermediate or low-risk patterns merit a follow-up US examination at 12–24 months and a repeat biopsy if there are new suspicious sonographic features or growth. Benign nodules with very low suspicion features may not require sonographic surveillance, or can be reimaged after 24 months.

LYMPH NODES

US is also of considerable value in identifying abnormal cervical lymph nodes in individuals being evaluated for a possible thyroid cancer diagnosis, for those undergoing evaluation prior to thyroid surgery for known thyroid cancer, and for surveillance of the thyroid bed and neck in patients after surgery for thyroid cancer. Benign lymph nodes are usually oval with a preserved hilum (see Figures 1.8a and 1.8b), whereas lymph nodes containing metastatic thyroid cancer are more likely to have a rounded shape, loss of their fatty hilum, cystic change, microcalcifications, or irregular internal hypervascularity (see Figure 1.8c)

Nuclear medicine studies

TECHNIQUE

The thyroid has the ability to concentrate iodine and incorporate it into thyroid hormone. In fact, adequate supplies of iodine are essential for normal thyroid function and a euthyroid status. Iodine is transported into the thyroid gland via the sodium-iodide symporter (NIS), a transporter whose activity is stimulated by thyroid stimulating hormone or thyrotropin (TSH) and iodine depletion. Radioactive iodine is taken up and incorporated into the thyroid gland in an identical manner to "cold" iodine. Radioiodine isotopes used in evaluating thyroid disease include iodine-123 (I-123) and iodine-131 (I-131). Technetium-99m (Tc-99m), a manmade element, is another radiopharmaceutical used in thyroid imaging. Tc-99m can be considered to

Figure 1.8 **(a)** Benign 0.5 cm lymph node with normal fatty hilum, **(b)** morphologically normal 0.9 cm lymph node, **(c)** 1.6 cm lymph node with eccentric cystic component, abnormal vascularity and abnormal echogenicity.

be an iodine analogue which is trapped within thyroid follicular cells by NIS, but, unlike iodine, is not incorporated into thyroid hormone (138). Radioiodine imaging utilizes a gamma camera which detects the gamma rays (photons) emitted by both I-123 and I-131. Gamma rays from I-123 have a low energy (159 KeV) and are detected by a low energy collimator, whereas gamma rays from I-131 include primary photons of higher energy (364 KeV) that are detected by a high energy collimator (139). Radioactive iodine is usually administered orally and is typically visualized 4 and 24 hours after administration. Photons emanating from the thyroid interact with the crystal within the gamma camera to produce scintillations that are converted into light and displayed as an image that can be digitally enhanced. Two pieces of information are useful: these are the pattern and the amount of radioiodine accumulated by the thyroid gland. The uptake at 24 hours is most useful for assessing thyrotoxicosis, whereas uptake may be studied at various times when imaging the whole body in a patient with thyroid cancer. The half-life of I-123 is 13 hours, compared with 8 days for I-131, and 6 hours for Tc-99m

(139). I-131 emits beta particles, as well as gamma photons. These particles have an average energy of 192 KeV and will destroy cells they are trapped within, which is the reason that I-131 is currently used almost exclusively for therapy rather than imaging. Tc-99m is also a gamma emitter, and is readily available and much less expensive than I-123. Tc-99m is administered intravenously and imaging typically occurs 20 minutes later, with an uptake in the 0.4–1% range.

INDICATIONS

I-131 was one of the first isotopes used in medicine beginning in the 1940s and is useful for evaluating and treating hyperthyroidism and thyroid cancer. Once a patient has been diagnosed with hyperthyroidism, a thyroid scan and uptake may be helpful in determining etiology, depending on the accompanying clinical presentation. In a patient in whom the clinical and laboratory constellation of findings is indicative of Graves' disease, a thyroid scan and uptake may not be necessary, although the radioiodine uptake is usually needed if therapy with I-131 is selected. However, in a patient with thyrotoxicosis in whom the underlying etiology is not immediately obvious, a thyroid scan and uptake is useful in distinguishing between Graves' disease, thyroiditis, and iatrogenic thyrotoxicosis. In the case of a patient with a multinodular gland or a solitary thyroid nodule, the pattern of a scan with I-123 or Tc-99m can identify autonomous nodules that are responsible for the hyperthyroidism. Sometimes hypofunctioning nodules that require further evaluation by US, due to their potential for malignancy, are also identified. Potential findings from a thyroid scan and uptake are shown in Table 1.5. I-123 and I-131 also have key roles in the imaging and treatment of thyroid cancer, as cancerous tissue retains the ability to concentrate iodine, although to lesser and varying degrees. Following thyroidectomy, I-123 can be used to detect both remnant normal thyroid tissues and thyroid cancer metastases. I-131 can be administered to achieve ablation of these normal and malignant tissues and to image them thereafter.

NORMAL THYROID APPEARANCE

A normal thyroid gland has a smooth appearance and homogeneous tracer distribution. There may be relatively less activity at the periphery of the lobes (see Figure 1.9a). The two thyroid lobes may not be symmetrical as asymmetry of lobe size is a normal variant. Normal radioactive iodine uptake values vary according to the population's iodine intake and the individual nuclear medicine

Table 1.5. Diagnosis of hyperthyroidism based on thyroid scan and uptake

Diagnosis	Uptake	Pattern	Depiction of scan
Graves' disease	Elevated	Diffuse	
Toxic multinodular goiter	Usually elevated	Heterogeneous	
Toxic nodule	May be elevated	Focal, potential suppression of the rest of the gland	
Thyroiditis	Low	May be patchy	
Exogenous thyroid hormone	Low	Uniform	
Ectopic thyroid tissue	May be elevated	Outside of the thyroid gland	

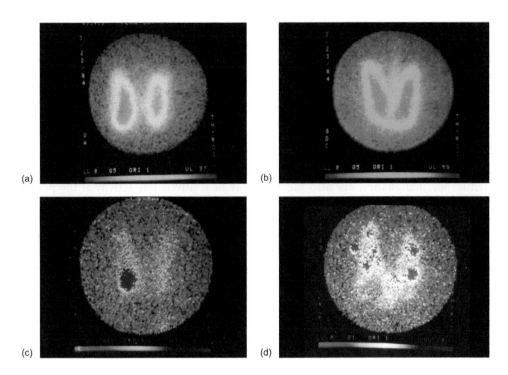

Figure 1.9 Thyroid radioisotope scans may be helpful in assessing certain patients with hyperthyroidism. (a) Demonstrates symmetrical isotope distribution (123I) in a normal individual. (b) Demonstrates an enlarged gland with diffuse uptake consistent with Graves' disease. (c) Demonstrates a solitary functioning thyroid nodule. There is intense activity in the right-lobe nodule with diminished activity in the rest of the gland because of suppression of TSH by thyroid hormone secretion of the nodule. (d) Shows a toxic multinodular goiter. Radioactive isotope activity is heterogeneous, with areas of intense activity interspersed with areas of reduced activity.

facility's established reference range. The values also vary over time after the administration of the dose of radioisotope. Normal radioiodine uptake values are approximately 5–15% at 4 hours and 15–30% at 24 hours (140). The Tc-99m uptake is much lower (138) and is assessed approximately 20 minutes after injection of the radiotracer.

DIFFUSE THYROID DISEASE

Thyroid scanning and measurement of uptake using I-123 are useful for the differential diagnosis of Graves' disease (140). Thyroid gland uptake is increased over the normal range in Graves' disease (see Table 1.5 and Figure 1.9b), which is the most common cause of thyrotoxicosis. The pattern of uptake is homogeneous, and a pyramidal lobe may be visible (139). If treatment with I-131 is the selected therapy for Graves' disease, the therapy may be given using one of a variety of calculations to determine the appropriate administered activity (see Chapter 2, "The Diagnostic Evaluation and

Management of Hyperthyroidism due to Graves' Disease").

In subacute or silent thyroiditis, despite the laboratory evidence of thyrotoxicosis, there is low uptake of radioiodine (or Tc-99m) by the gland (Table 1.5) (139). This decreased uptake may give way to a patchy pattern of uptake as the gland recovers from the thyroiditis. Low radioiodine uptake over the thyroid gland may also be seen in a patient with thyrotoxicosis when the cause of the problem is thyroid hormone ingestion or iodine excess. Low uptake is typically seen in a hypothyroid patient with Hashimoto's thyroiditis. Rarely, this low uptake may be preceded by a period of diffusely increased uptake and hyperthyroidism in the early stage of Hashimoto's disease (so called "Hashitoxicosis") (140). Other rare situations in which there may be low or absent radioiodine uptake in the neck in a hyperthyroid patient include struma ovarii, where there is increased uptake of the tracer in the pelvis, and functioning metastatic thyroid cancer.

THYROID NODULES

Thyroid nodules may be present in a euthyroid, hypothyroid, or hyperthyroid patient. In the first two instances, the primary means of nodule evaluation is with US. In the case of a patient with both nodular disease and hyperthyroidism, a thyroid scan and uptake will help determine whether autonomously functioning nodular thyroid tissue is the cause of the hyperthyroidism (see Table 1.5) (139). The greater the size of a solitary nodule, the greater the likelihood that it will cause hyperthyroidism. As the adenoma grows over time, its hyperfunction may lead to suppression of endogenous TSH secretion with concomitant suppression of radioiodine uptake by the rest of the gland (140) (see Figure 1.9c). Almost all hyperfunctioning nodules are benign. However, rarely, a malignant nodule may appear to be functioning with Tc-99m when the scan is performed at 20 minutes, but the nodule will be nonfunctioning with I-123 at 24 hours. Such cancers can "trap" Tc 99m and I-123, but cannot further process ("organify") the iodine into thyroid hormone, and will therefore appear nonfunctioning or "cold" on the scan done at 24 hours. Therefore, patients with nodules that are functioning on pertechnetate imaging should undergo I-123 imaging to verify that they are functioning (141). A multinodular gland may contain both hyperfunctioning and hypofunctioning nodules (see Figure 1.9d). Before considering I-131 treatment of a toxic multinodular goiter, the non-functioning nodules should undergo examination by US, and sonographically suspicious nodules should be subject to fine needle aspiration biopsy to exclude malignancy.

ECTOPIC THYROID TISSUE

Radiotracer scanning may identify thyroid tissue that is not present in the usual location (138, 140). Examples include a thyroglossal duct cyst and a lingual thyroid, which are present in the midline along the normal course of the embryologic descent of the thyroid gland. Other potential findings include a substernal goiter and ectopic thyroid tissue within the chest.

THYROID CANCER

A diagnosis of differentiated thyroid cancer typically leads to thyroidectomy or lobectomy. If a thyroidectomy is pursued, depending on the size of the tumor and other features such as cervical node involvement, lymphatic or vascular invasion, or extrathyroidal extension, whole body scanning with I-123, and adjuvant or therapeutic I-131 administration might also be employed (89, 139). Malignant thyroid tissue does not take up iodine as effectively as normal thyroid tissue. Therefore, manipulations, including iodine depletion employing a low iodine diet, and elevation of serum TSH, either through injection of recombinant human TSH (rhTSH, Thyrogen®) or withdrawal from thyroid hormone therapy, are required (89). Poorly differentiated thyroid cancers do not accumulate iodine effectively and have minimal response to I-131 therapy. Anaplastic thyroid cancer also does not effectively accumulate iodine. Medullary thyroid cancer cells do not have an iodine transporter and are not treated with I-131 at all. PET scanning using 18-F-fluorodeoxyglucose is another imaging modality that may be useful for assessing thyroid cancers which do not concentrate iodine efficiently.

A diagnostic whole-body iodine scan is usually performed following I-123 administration, and the pattern and amount of uptake can be used to tailor the patient's I-131 therapy. The administered activity of I-123 is usually approximately 3 mCi, and scanning is performed approximately 24 hours after oral administration of the tracer dose. In addition to uptake within any remnant thyroid tissue within the neck, there will also be a demonstration of physiologic iodine uptake or distribution within salivary glands, liver, gastrointestinal tract, and bladder. Metastatic disease within cervical or mediastinal lymph nodes, lungs, or the skeleton may also be demonstrated. Depending upon the histopathologic features of the patient's tumor, combined with the pattern and degree of uptake documented on the diagnostic scan, a therapeutic activity of I-131, varying from 30 to 200 mCi, is selected. The beta particles from the I-131 will destroy any benign or malignant tissue which accumulates the isotope. A post-therapy scan is recommended 3–7 days after administration of I-131 therapy. Such scans may demonstrate additional sites of disease that were not identified by the diagnostic (or pre-therapy) scan (see Figure 1.10, which shows uptake within cervical and pulmonary metastases only appreciated after therapy). "False positive" areas of iodine uptake may also be seen associated with physiologic or non-thyroid cancer pathologic processes. These include uptake in the thymus, breast, endometrium, and pleural effusions (142).

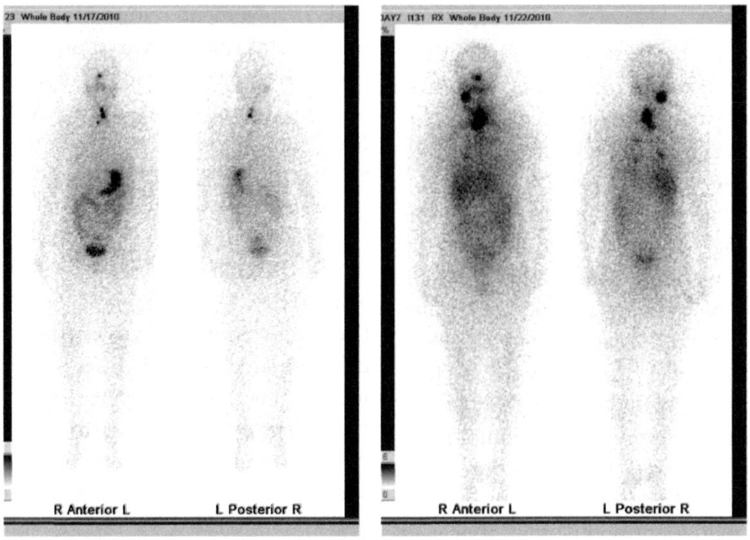

(a) (b)

Figure 1.10 (a) Diagnostic whole-body scan after 3 mCi I-123 showing 3 foci within the thyroid bed and right lower lung field uptake, (b) post-therapy scan showing thyroid bed foci, right lower lung uptake, and additionally right cervical uptake and left lung uptake.

REFERENCES

1. Ortiga-Carvalho TM, Chiamolera MI, Pazos-Moura CC, Wondisford FE. Hypothalamus-pituitary-thyroid axis. *Compr. Physiol.* 2016;6(3):1387–428.

2. Burmeister LA, Goumaz MO, Mariash CN, Oppenheimer JH. Levothyroxine dose requirements for thyrotropin suppression in the treatment of differentiated thyroid cancer. *J. Clin. Endocrinol. Metab.* 1992;75(2):344–50.

3. Hoermann R, Eckl W, Hoermann C, Larisch R. Complex relationship between free thyroxine and TSH in the regulation of thyroid function. *Eur. J. Endocrinol.* 2010;162(6):1123–9.

4. Meikle AW, Stringham JD, Woodward MG, Nelson JC. Hereditary and environmental influences on the variation of thyroid hormones in normal male twins. *J. Clin. Endocrinol. Metab.* 1988;66(3):588–92.

5. Hansen PS, Brix TH, Iachine I, Sorensen TI, Kyvik KO, Hegedus L. Genetic and environmental interrelations between measurements of thyroid function in a healthy Danish twin population. *Am. J. Physiol. Endocrinol. Metab.* 2007;292(3):E765–70.

6. Jensen E, Hyltoft Petersen P, Blaabjerg O, Hansen PS, Brix TH, Kyvik KO, et al. Establishment of a serum thyroid stimulating hormone (TSH) reference interval in healthy adults. The importance of environmental factors, including thyroid antibodies. *Clin. Chem. Lab. Med.* 2004;42(7):824–32.

7. Midgley JE. Direct and indirect free thyroxine assay methods: Theory and practice. *Clin. Chem.* 2001;47(8):1353–63.

8. van Deventer HE, Soldin SJ. The expanding role of tandem mass spectrometry in optimizing diagnosis and treatment of thyroid disease. *Adv. Clin. Chem.* 2013;61:127–52.

9. Baloch Z, Carayon P, Conte-Devolx B, Demers LM, Feldt-Rasmussen U, Henry JF, et al. Laboratory medicine practice guidelines. Laboratory support for the diagnosis and monitoring of thyroid disease. *Thyroid* 2003;13(1):3–126.

10. Thienpont LM, Van Uytfanghe K, Beastall G, Faix JD, Ieiri T, Miller WG, et al. Report of the IFCC Working Group for

Standardization of Thyroid Function Tests; part 3: Total thyroxine and total triiodothyronine. *Clin. Chem.* 2010;56(6):921–9.

11. Thienpont LM, Van Uytfanghe K, Beastall G, Faix JD, Ieiri T, Miller WG, et al. Report of the IFCC Working Group for Standardization of Thyroid Function Tests; part 2: Free thyroxine and free triiodothyronine. *Clin. Chem.* 2010;56(6):912–20.

12. Holm SS, Hansen SH, Faber J, Staun-Olsen P. Reference methods for the measurement of free thyroid hormones in blood: Evaluation of potential reference methods for free thyroxine. *Clin. Biochem.* 2004;37(2):85–93.

13. Soldin OP, Soldin SJ. Thyroid hormone testing by tandem mass spectrometry. *Clin. Biochem.* 2011;44(1):89–94.

14. Wang R, Nelson JC, Weiss RM, Wilcox RB. Accuracy of free thyroxine measurements across natural ranges of thyroxine binding to serum proteins. *Thyroid* 2000;10(1):31–9.

15. Toldy E, Locsei Z, Szabolcs I, Bezzegh A, Kovacs GL. Protein interference in thyroid assays: An in vitro study with in vivo consequences. *Clin. Chim. Acta* 2005; 352 (1–2): 93–104.

16. Wu AH, French D. Implementation of liquid chromatography/mass spectrometry into the clinical laboratory. *Clin. Chim. Acta* 2013;420:4–10.

17. Woeber KA. Triiodothyronine production in Graves' hyperthyroidism. *Thyroid* 2006;16(7):687–90.

18. Ito M, Miyauchi A, Morita S, Kudo T, Nishihara E, Kihara M, et al. TSH-suppressive doses of levothyroxine are required to achieve preoperative native serum triiodothyronine levels in patients who have undergone total thyroidectomy. *Eur. J. Endocrinol.* 2012;167(3):373–8.

19. Jonklaas J, Davidson B, Bhagat S, Soldin SJ. Triiodothyronine levels in athyreotic individuals during levothyroxine therapy. *JAMA* 2008;299(7):769–77.

20. Ceresini G, Morganti S, Rebecchi I, Bertone L, Ceda GP, Bacchi-Modena A, et al. A one-year follow-up on the effects of raloxifene on thyroid function in postmenopausal women. *Menopause* 2004;11(2):176–9.

21. Brent GA. Maternal thyroid function: Interpretation of thyroid function tests in pregnancy. *Clin. Obstet. Gynecol.* 1997;40(1):3–15.

22. Shifren JL, Desindes S, McIlwain M, Doros G, Mazer NA. A randomized, open-label, crossover study comparing the effects of oral versus transdermal estrogen therapy on serum androgens, thyroid hormones, and adrenal hormones in naturally menopausal women. *Menopause* 2007;14(6):985–94.

23. Fisher CL, Mannino DM, Herman WH, Frumkin H. Cigarette smoking and thyroid hormone levels in males. *Int. J. Epidemiol.* 1997;26(5):972–7.

24. Stevenson HP, Archbold GP, Johnston P, Young IS, Sheridan B. Misleading serum free thyroxine results during low molecular weight heparin treatment. *Clin. Chem.* 1998;44(5):1002–7.

25. Klee GG. Interferences in hormone immunoassays. *Clin. Lab. Med.* 2004;24(1):1–18.

26. Norden AG, Jackson RA, Norden LE, Griffin AJ, Barnes MA, Little JA. Misleading results from immunoassays of serum free thyroxine in the presence of rheumatoid factor. *Clin. Chem.* 1997;43(6 Pt 1):957–62.

27. Li D, Radulescu A, Shrestha RT, Root M, Karger AB, Killeen AA, et al. Association of biotin ingestion with performance of hormone and nonhormone assays in healthy adults. *JAMA* 2017;318(12):1150–60.

28. Barbesino G. Misdiagnosis of Graves' disease with apparent severe hyperthyroidism in a patient taking biotin megadoses. *Thyroid* 2016;26(6):860–3.

29. Martino E, Bartalena L, Bogazzi F, Braverman LE. The effects of amiodarone on the thyroid. *Endocr. Rev.* 2001;22(2):240–54.

30. Dumitrescu AM, Liao XH, Abdullah MS, Lado-Abeal J, Majed FA, Moeller LC, et al. Mutations in SECISBP2 result in abnormal thyroid hormone metabolism. *Nat. Genet.* 2005;37(11):1247–52.

31. Refetoff S, Dumitrescu AM. Syndromes of reduced sensitivity to thyroid hormone: Genetic defects in hormone receptors, cell transporters and deiodination. *Best Pract. Res. Clin. Endocrinol. Metab.* 2007;21(2):277–305.

32. Attia J, Margetts P, Guyatt G. Diagnosis of thyroid disease in hospitalized patients: A systematic review. *Arch. Intern. Med.* 1999;159(7):658–65.

33. Chopra IJ, Solomon DH, Huang TS. Serum thyrotropin in hospitalized psychiatric patients: Evidence for hyperthyrotropinemia as measured by an ultrasensitive thyrotropin assay. *Metabolism* 1990;39(5):538–43.

34. Nader S, Warner MD, Doyle S, Peabody CA. Euthyroid sick syndrome in psychiatric inpatients. *Biol. Psychiatry* 1996;40(12):1288–93.

35. Woolf PD, Nichols D, Porsteinsson A, Boulay R. Thyroid evaluation of hospitalized psychiatric patients: The role of TSH screening for thyroid dysfunction. *Thyroid* 1996;6(5):451–6.

36. Brouwer JP, Appelhof BC, Hoogendijk WJ, Huyser J, Endert E, Zuketto C, et al. Thyroid and adrenal axis in major depression: A controlled study in outpatients. *Eur. J. Endocrinol.* 2005;152(2):185–91.

37. Olff M, Guzelcan Y, de Vries GJ, Assies J, Gersons BP. HPA- and HPT-axis alterations in chronic posttraumatic stress disorder. *Psychoneuroendocrinology* 2006;31(10):1220–30.

38. Schussler GC. The thyroxine-binding proteins. *Thyroid* 2000;10(2):141–9.

39. Langton JE, Brent GA. Nonthyroidal illness syndrome: Evaluation of thyroid function in sick patients. *Endocrinol. Metab. Clin. North Am.* 2002;31(1):159–72.

40. Adler SM, Wartofsky L. The nonthyroidal illness syndrome. *Endocrinol. Metab. Clin. North Am.* 2007;36(3):657–72, vi.

41. Feelders RA, Swaak AJ, Romijn JA, Eggermont AM, Tielens ET, Vreugdenhil G, et al. Characteristics of recovery from the euthyroid sick syndrome induced by tumor necrosis factor alpha in cancer patients. *Metabolism* 1999;48(3):324–9.

42. Harel Z, Biro FM, Tedford WL. Effects of long term treatment with sertraline (Zoloft) simulating hypothyroidism in an adolescent. *J. Adolesc. Health* 1995;16(3):232–4.

43. Samuels MH, Pillote K, Asher D, Nelson JC. Variable effects of nonsteroidal antiinflammatory agents on thyroid test results. *J. Clin. Endocrinol. Metab.* 2003;88(12):5710–6.

44. Torpy DJ, Tsigos C, Lotsikas AJ, Defensor R, Chrousos GP, Papanicolaou DA. Acute and delayed effects of a single-dose injection of interleukin-6 on thyroid function in healthy humans. *Metabolism* 1998;47(10):1289–93.

45. Torino F, Barnabei A, Paragliola R, Baldelli R, Appetecchia M, Corsello SM. Thyroid dysfunction as an unintended side effect of anticancer drugs. *Thyroid* 2013;23(11):1345–66.

46. Tamaskar I, Bukowski R, Elson P, Ioachimescu AG, Wood L, Dreicer R, et al. Thyroid function test abnormalities in patients with metastatic renal cell carcinoma treated with sorafenib. *Ann. Oncol.* 2008;19(2):265–8.

47. Fliers E, Alkemade A, Wiersinga WM. The hypothalamic-pituitary-thyroid axis in critical illness. *Best Pract. Res. Clin. Endocrinol. Metab.* 2001;15(4):453–64.

48. Magner J, Roy P, Fainter L, Barnard V, Fletcher P, Jr. Transiently decreased sialylation of thyrotropin (TSH) in a patient with the euthyroid sick syndrome. *Thyroid* 1997;7(1):55–61.

49. DeGroot LJ. "Non-thyroidal illness syndrome" is functional central hypothyroidism, and if severe, hormone replacement is appropriate in light of present knowledge. *J. Endocrinol. Invest.* 2003;26(12):1163–70.

50. Lee RH, Spencer CA, Mestman JH, Miller EA, Petrovic I, Braverman LE, et al. Free T4 immunoassays are flawed during pregnancy. *Am. J. Obstet. Gynecol.* 2009;200(3):260 e1–6.

51. Spencer CA, Schwarzbein D, Guttler RB, LoPresti JS, Nicoloff JT. Thyrotropin (TSH)-releasing hormone stimulation test responses employing third and fourth generation TSH assays. *J. Clin. Endocrinol. Metab.* 1993;76(2):494–8.

52. Andersen S, Bruun NH, Pedersen KM, Laurberg P. Biologic variation is important for interpretation of thyroid function tests. *Thyroid* 2003;13(11):1069–78.

53. Persani L, Borgato S, Romoli R, Asteria C, Pizzocaro A, Beck-Peccoz P. Changes in the degree of sialylation of carbohydrate chains modify the biological properties of circulating thyrotropin isoforms

in various physiological and pathological states. *J. Clin. Endocrinol. Metab.* 1998;83(7):2486–92.

54. Donadio S, Pascual A, Thijssen JH, Ronin C. Feasibility study of new calibrators for thyroid-stimulating hormone (TSH) immunoprocedures based on remodeling of recombinant TSH to mimic glycoforms circulating in patients with thyroid disorders. *Clin. Chem.* 2006;52(2):286–97.

55. Harris EK. Effects of intra- and inter-individual variation on the appropriate use of normal ranges. *Clin. Chem.* 1974;20(12):1535–42.

56. Brabant G, Beck-Peccoz P, Jarzab B, Laurberg P, Orgiazzi J, Szabolcs I, et al. Is there a need to redefine the upper normal limit of TSH? *Eur. J. Endocrinol.* 2006;154(5):633–7.

57. Hollowell JG, Staehling NW, Flanders WD, Hannon WH, Gunter EW, Spencer CA, et al. Serum TSH, T(4), and thyroid antibodies in the United States population (1988 to 1994): National Health and Nutrition Examination Survey (NHANES III). *J. Clin. Endocrinol. Metab.* 2002;87(2):489–99.

58. Jensen E, Blaabjerg O, Petersen PH, Hegedus L. Sampling time is important but may be overlooked in establishment and use of thyroid-stimulating hormone reference intervals. *Clin. Chem.* 2007;53(2):355–6.

59. Spencer CA, Hollowell JG, Kazarosyan M, Braverman LE. National Health and Nutrition Examination Survey III thyroid-stimulating hormone (TSH)-thyroperoxidase antibody relationships demonstrate that TSH upper reference limits may be skewed by occult thyroid dysfunction. *J. Clin. Endocrinol. Metab.* 2007;92(11):4236–40.

60. Vanderpump MP, Tunbridge WM, French JM, Appleton D, Bates D, Clark F, et al. The incidence of thyroid disorders in the community: A twenty-year follow-up of the Whickham Survey. *Clin. Endocrinol. (Oxf).* 1995;43(1):55–68.

61. Baskin HJ, Cobin RH, Duick DS, Gharib H, Guttler RB, Kaplan MM, et al. American association of clinical endocrinologists medical guidelines for clinical practice for the evaluation and treatment of hyperthyroidism and hypothyroidism. *Endocr. Pract.* 2002;8(6):457–69.

62. Wartofsky L, Dickey RA. The evidence for a narrower thyrotropin reference range is compelling. *J. Clin. Endocrinol. Metab.* 2005;90(9):5483–8.

63. Surks MI, Hollowell JG. Age-specific distribution of serum thyrotropin and anti-thyroid antibodies in the US population: Implications for the prevalence of sub-clinical hypothyroidism. *J. Clin. Endocrinol. Metab.* 2007;92(12):4575–82.

64. Biondi B, Cooper DS. The clinical significance of subclinical thyroid dysfunction. *Endocr. Rev.* 2008;29(1):76–131.

65. Stricker R, Echenard M, Eberhart R, Chevailler MC, Perez V, Quinn FA, et al. Evaluation of maternal thyroid function during pregnancy: The importance of using gestational age-specific reference intervals. *Eur. J. Endocrinol.* 2007;157(4):509–14.

66. Casey BM, Dashe JS, Wells CE, McIntire DD, Leveno KJ, Cunningham FG. Subclinical hyperthyroidism and pregnancy outcomes. *Obstet. Gynecol.* 2006;107(2 Pt 1):337–41.

67. Despres N, Grant AM. Antibody interference in thyroid assays: A potential for clinical misinformation. *Clin. Chem.* 1998;44(3):440–54.

68. Hattori N, Ishihara T, Shimatsu A. Variability in the detection of macro TSH in different immunoassay systems. *Eur. J. Endocrinol.* 2016;174(1):9–15.

69. Persani L, Ferretti E, Borgato S, Faglia G, Beck-Peccoz P. Circulating thyrotropin bioactivity in sporadic central hypothyroidism. *J. Clin. Endocrinol. Metab.* 2000;85(10):3631–5.

70. Oliveira JH, Persani L, Beck-Peccoz P, Abucham J. Investigating the paradox of hypothyroidism and increased serum thyrotropin (TSH) levels in Sheehan's syndrome: Characterization of TSH carbohydrate content and bioactivity. *J. Clin. Endocrinol. Metab.* 2001;86(4):1694–9.

71. Sherman SI, Gopal J, Haugen BR, Chiu AC, Whaley K, Nowlakha P, et al. Central hypothyroidism associated with retinoid X receptor-selective ligands. *N. Engl. J. Med.* 1999;340 (14):1075–9.

72. Golden WM, Weber KB, Hernandez TL, Sherman SI, Woodmansee WW, Haugen BR. Single-dose rexinoid rapidly and specifically suppresses serum thyrotropin in normal subjects. *J. Clin. Endocrinol. Metab.* 2007;92(1):124–30.

73. Vigersky RA, Filmore-Nassar A, Glass AR. Thyrotropin suppression by metformin. *J. Clin. Endocrinol. Metab.* 2006;91(1):225–7.

74. Peeters RP. Subclinical hypothyroidism. *N. Engl. J. Med.* 2017;376 (26):2556–65.

75. Chan LY, Chiu PY, Lau TK. Cord blood thyroid-stimulating hormone level in high-risk pregnancies. *Eur. J. Obstet. Gynecol. Reprod. Biol.* 2003;108(2):142–5.

76. Amlashi FG, Tritos NA. Thyrotropin-secreting pituitary adenomas: Epidemiology, diagnosis, and management. *Endocrine* 2016;52(3):427–40.

77. Refetoff S, Bassett JH, Beck-Peccoz P, Bernal J, Brent G, Chatterjee K, et al. Classification and proposed nomenclature for inherited defects of thyroid hormone action, cell transport, and metabolism. *Thyroid* 2014;24(3):407–9.

78. Beck-Peccoz P, Persani L, Calebiro D, Bonomi M, Mannavola D, Campi I. Syndromes of hormone resistance in the hypothalamic-pituitary-thyroid axis. *Best Pract. Res. Clin. Endocrinol. Metab.* 2006;20(4):529–46.

79. Fisher DA, Nelson JC, Carlton EI, Wilcox RB. Maturation of human hypothalamic-pituitary-thyroid function and control. *Thyroid* 2000;10(3):229–34.

80. Kim TH, Kim KW, Ahn HY, Choi HS, Won H, Choi Y, et al. Effect of seasonal changes on the transition between subclinical hypothyroid and euthyroid status. *J. Clin. Endocrinol. Metab.* 2013;98(8):3420–9.

81. Bertelsen JB, Hegedus L. Cigarette smoking and the thyroid. *Thyroid* 1994;4(3):327–31.

82. Netzel BC, Grebe SK, Carranza Leon BG, Castro MR, Clark PM, Hoofnagle AN, et al. Thyroglobulin (Tg) testing revisited: Tg assays, TgAb assays, and correlation of results with clinical outcomes. *J. Clin. Endocrinol. Metab.* 2015;100(8):E1074–83.

83. Grani G, Fumarola A. Thyroglobulin in lymph node fine-needle aspiration wash-out: A systematic review and meta-analysis of diagnostic accuracy. *J. Clin. Endocrinol. Metab.* 2014;99(6):1970–82.

84. Spencer CA, Lopresti JS. Measuring thyroglobulin and thyroglobulin autoantibody in patients with differentiated thyroid cancer. *Nat. Clin. Pract. Endocrinol. Metab.* 2008;4(4):223–33.

85. Boi F, Baghino G, Atzeni F, Lai ML, Faa G, Mariotti S. The diagnostic value for differentiated thyroid carcinoma metastases of thyroglobulin (Tg) measurement in washout fluid from fine-needle aspiration biopsy of neck lymph nodes is maintained in the presence of circulating anti-Tg antibodies. *J. Clin. Endocrinol. Metab.* 2006;91(4):1364–9.

86. Prentice L, Kiso Y, Fukuma N, Horimoto M, Petersen V, Grennan F, et al. Monoclonal thyroglobulin autoantibodies: Variable region analysis and epitope recognition. *J. Clin. Endocrinol. Metab.* 1995;80(3):977–86.

87. Clarke NJ, Zhang Y, Reitz RE. A novel mass spectrometry-based assay for the accurate measurement of thyroglobulin from patient samples containing antithyroglobulin autoantibodies. *J. Investig. Med.* 2012;60 (8):1157–63.

88. Azmat U, Porter K, Senter L, Ringel MD, Nabhan F. Thyroglobulin liquid chromatography-tandem mass spectrometry has a low sensitivity for detecting structural disease in patients with antithyroglobulin antibodies. *Thyroid* 2017;27(1):74–80.

89. Haugen BR, Alexander EK, Bible KC, Doherty GM, Mandel SJ, Nikiforov YE, et al. 2015 American thyroid association management guidelines for adult patients with thyroid nodules and differentiated thyroid cancer: The American thyroid association guidelines task force on thyroid nodules and differentiated thyroid cancer. *Thyroid* 2016;26(1):1–133.

90. Spencer C, Fatemi S, Singer P, Nicoloff J, Lopresti J. Serum Basal thyroglobulin measured by a second-generation assay correlates with the recombinant

human thyrotropin-stimulated thyroglobulin response in patients treated for differentiated thyroid cancer. *Thyroid* 2010;20(6):587–95.

91. Durante C, Montesano T, Attard M, Torlontano M, Monzani F, Costante G, et al. Long-term surveillance of papillary thyroid cancer patients who do not undergo postoperative radioiodine remnant ablation: Is there a role for serum thyroglobulin measurement? *J. Clin. Endocrinol. Metab.* 2012;97(8):2748–53.

92. Miyauchi A, Kudo T, Miya A, Kobayashi K, Ito Y, Takamura Y, et al. Prognostic impact of serum thyroglobulin doubling-time under thyrotropin suppression in patients with papillary thyroid carcinoma who underwent total thyroidectomy. *Thyroid* 2011;21(7):707–16.

93. Giovanella L, Ghelfo A. Undetectable serum thyroglobulin due to negative interference of heterophile antibodies in relapsing thyroid carcinoma. *Clin. Chem.* 2007;53(10):1871–2.

94. Preissner CM, O'Kane DJ, Singh RJ, Morris JC, Grebe SK. Phantoms in the assay tube: Heterophile antibody interferences in serum thyroglobulin assays. *J. Clin. Endocrinol. Metab.* 2003;88(7):3069–74.

95. La'ulu SL, Slev PR, Roberts WL. Performance characteristics of 5 automated thyroglobulin autoantibody and thyroid peroxidase autoantibody assays. *Clin. Chim. Acta* 2007;376(1–2):88–95.

96. Sinclair D. Analytical aspects of thyroid antibodies estimation. *Autoimmunity* 2008;41(1):46–54.

97. Tozzoli R, D'Aurizio F, Ferrari A, Castello R, Metus P, Caruso B, et al. The upper reference limit for thyroid peroxidase autoantibodies is method-dependent: A collaborative study with biomedical industries. *Clin. Chim. Acta* 2016;452:61–5.

98. Huber G, Staub JJ, Meier C, Mitrache C, Guglielmetti M, Huber P, et al. Prospective study of the spontaneous course of subclinical hypothyroidism: Prognostic value of thyrotropin, thyroid reserve, and thyroid antibodies. *J. Clin. Endocrinol. Metab.* 2002;87(7):3221–6.

99. Spencer CA, Takeuchi M, Kazarosyan M, Wang CC, Guttler RB, Singer PA, et al. Serum thyroglobulin autoantibodies: Prevalence, influence on serum thyroglobulin measurement, and prognostic significance in patients with differentiated thyroid carcinoma. *J. Clin. Endocrinol. Metab.* 1998;83(4):1121–7.

100. Kamijo K, Murayama H, Uzu T, Togashi K, Olivo PD, Kahaly GJ. Similar clinical performance of a novel chimeric thyroid-stimulating hormone receptor bioassay and an automated thyroid-stimulating hormone receptor binding assay in Graves' disease. *Thyroid* 2011;21(12):1295–9.

101. Schott M, Feldkamp J, Bathan C, Fritzen R, Scherbaum WA, Seissler J. Detecting TSH-receptor antibodies with the recombinant TBII assay: Technical and clinical evaluation. *Horm. Metab. Res.* 2000;32(10):429–35.

102. Costagliola S, Morgenthaler NG, Hoermann R, Badenhoop K, Struck J, Freitag D, et al. Second generation assay for thyrotropin receptor antibodies has superior diagnostic sensitivity for Graves' disease. *J. Clin. Endocrinol. Metab.* 1999;84(1):90–7.

103. Gupta MK. Thyrotropin-receptor antibodies in thyroid diseases: Advances in detection techniques and clinical applications. *Clin. Chim. Acta* 2000; 293(1–2):1–29.

104. Yamano Y, Takamatsu J, Sakane S, Hirai K, Kuma K, Ohsawa N. Differences between changes in serum thyrotropin-binding inhibitory antibodies and thyroid-stimulating antibodies in the course of antithyroid drug therapy for Graves' disease. *Thyroid* 1999;9(8):769–73.

105. Barbesino G, Tomer Y. Clinical review: Clinical utility of TSH receptor antibodies. *J. Clin. Endocrinol. Metab.* 2013;98(6):2247–55.

106. Carella C, Mazziotti G, Sorvillo F, Piscopo M, Cioffi M, Pilla P, et al. Serum thyrotropin receptor antibodies concentrations in patients with Graves' disease before, at the end of methimazole treatment, and after drug withdrawal: Evidence that the activity of thyrotropin receptor antibody and/or thyroid response modify during the observation period. *Thyroid* 2006;16(3):295–302.

107. Schott M, Morgenthaler NG, Fritzen R, Feldkamp J, Willenberg HS, Scherbaum WA, et al. Levels of autoantibodies against human TSH receptor predict relapse of hyperthyroidism in Graves' disease. *Horm. Metab. Res.* 2004;36(2):92–6.

108. Laurberg P, Wallin G, Tallstedt L, Abraham-Nordling M, Lundell G, Torring O. TSH-receptor autoimmunity in Graves' disease after therapy with anti-thyroid drugs, surgery, or radioiodine: A 5-year prospective randomized study. *Eur. J. Endocrinol.* 2008;158(1):69–75.

109. Chan GW, Mandel SJ. Therapy insight: Management of Graves' disease during pregnancy. *Nat. Clin. Pract. Endocrinol. Metab.* 2007;3(6):470–8.

110. Klein I. Clinical, metabolic, and organ-specific indices of thyroid function. *Endocrinol. Metab. Clin. North Am.* 2001;30(2):415–27, ix.

111. Refetoff S. Resistance to thyroid hormone. *Clin. Lab. Med.* 1993;13(3):563–81.

112. Surks MI, Ortiz E, Daniels GH, Sawin CT, Col NF, Cobin RH, et al. Subclinical thyroid disease: Scientific review and guidelines for diagnosis and management. *JAMA* 2004;291(2):228–38.

113. LeFevre ML, Force USPST. Screening for vitamin D deficiency in adults: U.S. Preventive Services Task Force recommendation statement. *Ann. Intern. Med.* 2015;162(2):133–40.

114. Cappola AR, Cooper DS. Screening and treating subclinical thyroid disease: Getting past the impasse. *Ann. Intern. Med.* 2015;162(9):664–5.

115. Danese MD, Powe NR, Sawin CT, Ladenson PW. Screening for mild thyroid failure at the periodic health examination: A decision and cost-effectiveness analysis. *JAMA* 1996;276(4):285–92.

116. Gharib H, Tuttle RM, Baskin HJ, Fish LH, Singer PA, McDermott MT. Subclinical thyroid dysfunction: A joint statement on management from the American Association of Clinical Endocrinologists, the American Thyroid Association, and the Endocrine Society. *J. Clin. Endocrinol. Metab.* 2005;90(1):581–5; discussion 6–7.

117. Stone M, Wallace R. *Committee on the Medicare Coverage of Routine Thyroid Screening BoHCS.* Institute of Medicine. Medicare Coverage of Routine Screening for Thyroid Dysfunction. Washington, DC: National Academies Press; 2003.

118. Vanderpump MP, Ahlquist JA, Franklyn JA, Clayton RN. Consensus statement for good practice and audit measures in the management of hypothyroidism and hyperthyroidism. The Research Unit of the Royal College of Physicians of London, the Endocrinology and Diabetes Committee of the Royal College of Physicians of London, and the Society for Endocrinology. *BMJ* 1996;313(7056):539–44.

119. La Franchi S, Dussault J, Fisher D, Foley Jr T, Mitchell M. American Academy of Pediatrics AAP Section on Endocrinology and Committee on Genetics, and American Thyroid Association Committee on Public Health: Newborn screening for congenital hypothyroidism: Recommended guidelines. *Pediatrics* 1993;91(6):1203–9.

120. Hanna CE, Krainz PL, Skeels MR, Miyahira RS, Sesser DE, LaFranchi SH. Detection of congenital hypopituitary hypothyroidism: Ten-year experience in the Northwest Regional Screening Program. *J. Pediatr.* 1986;109(6):959–64.

121. Delange F. Screening for congenital hypothyroidism used as an indicator of the degree of iodine deficiency and of its control. *Thyroid* 1998;8(12):1185–92.

122. Alexander EK, Pearce EN, Brent GA, Brown RS, Chen H, Dosiou C, et al. 2017 Guidelines of the American Thyroid Association for the diagnosis and management of thyroid disease during pregnancy and the postpartum. *Thyroid* 2017;27(3):315–89.

123. Dighe M, Barr R, Bojunga J, Cantisani V, Chammas MC, Cosgrove D, et al. Thyroid ultrasound: State of the art part 1 – Thyroid ultrasound reporting and diffuse thyroid diseases. *Med. Ultrason.* 2017;19(1):79–93.

124. Dighe M, Barr R, Bojunga J, Cantisani V, Chammas MC, Cosgrove D, et al. Thyroid ultrasound: State of the Art. Part 2 – Focal thyroid lesions. *Med. Ultrason.* 2017;19(2):195–210.

125. Brito JP, Yarur AJ, Prokop LJ, McIver B, Murad MH, Montori VM. Prevalence of thyroid cancer in multinodular goiter versus single nodule: A systematic review and meta-analysis. *Thyroid* 2013;23(4):449–55.

126. Ha EJ, Baek JH, Na DG. Risk stratification of thyroid nodules on ultrasonography: Current status and perspectives. *Thyroid* 2017;27(12):1463–8.

127. Frates MC, Benson CB, Charboneau JW, Cibas ES, Clark OH, Coleman BG, et al. Management of thyroid nodules detected at US: Society of Radiologists in Ultrasound consensus conference statement. *Radiology* 2005;237(3):794–800.

128. Brito JP, Gionfriddo MR, Al Nofal A, Boehmer KR, Leppin AL, Reading C, et al. The accuracy of thyroid nodule ultrasound to predict thyroid cancer: Systematic review and meta-analysis. *J. Clin. Endocrinol. Metab.* 2014;99(4):1253–63.

129. Remonti LR, Kramer CK, Leitao CB, Pinto LC, Gross JL. Thyroid ultrasound features and risk of carcinoma: A systematic review and meta-analysis of observational studies. *Thyroid* 2015;25(5):538–50.

130. Horvath E, Majlis S, Rossi R, Franco C, Niedmann JP, Castro A, et al. An ultrasonogram reporting system for thyroid nodules stratifying cancer risk for clinical management. *J. Clin. Endocrinol. Metab.* 2009;94(5):1748–51.

131. Kwak JY, Han KH, Yoon JH, Moon HJ, Son EJ, Park SH, et al. Thyroid imaging reporting and data system for US features of nodules: A step in establishing better stratification of cancer risk. *Radiology* 2011;260(3):892–9.

132. Russ G, Royer B, Bigorgne C, Rouxel A, Bienvenu-Perrard M, Leenhardt L. Prospective evaluation of thyroid imaging reporting and data system on 4550 nodules with and without elastography. *Eur. J. Endocrinol.* 2013;168(5):649–55.

133. Kwak JY, Jung I, Baek JH, Baek SM, Choi N, Choi YJ, et al. Image reporting and characterization system for ultrasound features of thyroid nodules: Multicentric Korean retrospective study. *Korean J. Radiol.* 2013;14(1):110–7.

134. Shin JH, Baek JH, Chung J, Ha EJ, Kim JH, Lee YH, et al. Ultrasonography diagnosis and imaging-based management of thyroid nodules: Revised Korean Society of Thyroid Radiology Consensus Statement and Recommendations. *Korean J. Radiol.* 2016;17(3):370–95.

135. Tessler FN, Middleton WD, Grant EG, Hoang JK, Berland LL, Teefey SA, et al. ACR Thyroid Imaging, Reporting and Data System (TI-RADS): White Paper of the ACR TI-RADS Committee. *J. Am. Coll. Radiol.* 2017;14(5):587–95.

136. Cosgrove D, Barr R, Bojunga J, Cantisani V, Chammas MC, Dighe M, et al. WFUMB guidelines and recommendations on the clinical use of ultrasound elastography: Part 4. Thyroid. *Ultrasound Med. Biol.* 2017;43(1):4–26.

137. Choi YJ, Baek JH, Park HS, Shim WH, Kim TY, Shong YK, et al. A computer-aided diagnosis system using artificial intelligence for the diagnosis and characterization of thyroid nodules on ultrasound: Initial clinical assessment. *Thyroid* 2017;27(4):546–52.

138. Intenzo CM, Dam HQ, Manzone TA, Kim SM. Imaging of the thyroid in benign and malignant disease. *Semin. Nucl. Med.* 2012;42(1):49–61.

139. Griggs WS, Divgi C. Radioiodine imaging and treatment in thyroid disorders. *Neuroimaging Clin. North Am.* 2008;18(3):505–15, viii.

140. Smith JR, Oates E. Radionuclide imaging of the thyroid gland: Patterns, pearls, and pitfalls. *Clin. Nucl. Med.* 2004;29(3):181–93.

141. Shambaugh GE, 3rd, Quinn JL, Oyasu R, Freinkel N. Disparate thyroid imaging. Combined studies with sodium pertechnetate Tc 99m and radioactive iodine. *JAMA* 1974;228(7):866–9.

142. Chudgar AV, Shah JC. Pictorial review of false-positive results on radioiodine scintigrams of patients with differentiated thyroid cancer. *Radiographics* 2017;37(1):298–315.

The diagnostic evaluation and management of hyperthyroidism due to Graves' disease, toxic nodules, and toxic multinodular goiter

DAVID S. COOPER

Graves' disease	38	Subclinical hyperthyroidism	58
Introduction	38	Diagnosis	58
Epidemiology	38	Treatment	59
Pathophysiology	38	Thyroid storm	59
Diagnosis	38	Treatment	60
Signs and symptoms	38	Solitary toxic nodules	61
Laboratory diagnosis	42	Introduction	61
Thyroid hormone and TSH levels	42	Pathology	61
24-hour radioiodine uptake	43	Pathogenesis	62
TSH receptor antibody measurements	44	Clinical considerations	62
Pitfalls	44	Diagnosis	62
Treatment	45	Treatment	63
Antithyroid drug therapy	45	Other treatment modalities: Percutaneous	
Beta-adrenergic antagonist drugs	51	ethanol injection (PEI), radiofrequency	
Potassium iodide therapy	51	ablation (RFA), and laser therapy	64
Radioiodine (^{131}I) therapy for Graves' disease	51	Toxic multinodular goiter	64
Thyroidectomy for Graves' disease	55	Introduction	64
Choice of therapy for Graves' disease:		Pathogenesis	64
Summary	55	Diagnosis	65
Treatment of Graves' ophthalmopathy and		Treatment	65
pretibial myxedema	56	References	66

GRAVES' DISEASE

Introduction

Graves' disease is an autoimmune thyroid disorder characterized by clinical hyperthyroidism and the presence of autoantibodies directed against the thyrotropin (TSH) receptor (1). The presentation of this disease varies with age. Younger patients manifest nervousness, weight loss, anxiety, heat intolerance, hyperdefecation, inability to concentrate, and tremulousness, while older patients may manifest few if any of these typical symptoms (2). Circulating TSH receptor–stimulating antibodies are present in at least 90% of patients and are responsible, in large part, for the thyroidal hyperactivity (3). An interesting aspect of Graves' disease is its association with ophthalmopathy, which can cause tearing, burning, itching, proptosis, double vision, and/or (rarely) visual impairment (4). The etiology of Graves' hyperthyroidism and ophthalmopathy remains unclear. There are abnormalities in T-cell function that allow the TSH receptor antibodies to develop; these antibodies not only stimulate TSH receptor action in thyrocytes but may cross-react with orbital antigens (e.g., fibroblasts and adipocytes) as well (5).

Epidemiology

Although it may present in patients of any age, Graves' disease occurs more commonly in women than men, especially in women between the ages of about 20 and 50 years (6). Graves' disease is rare in young children; when it occurs in neonates, it is almost always related to transplacental passage of TSH receptor–stimulating immunoglobulins, a condition that typically persists for several weeks until the IgG antibodies are cleared from the neonate's circulation (7). In adults, the annual incidence of new cases of Graves' disease is 1 to 10 per 100,000, although, of course, these numbers vary depending upon the method of detection and the iodine content in the geographic area (8). People living in all areas of the world are affected by Graves' disease. It is believed that the incidence correlates directly with the amount of iodine in the diet. Increased iodine intake has been shown to be associated with an increased frequency of hyperthyroidism (9). Cigarette smoking and stressful life events have also been linked to the etiology of Graves' disease (9).

The use of certain drugs, especially interferon-alpha, has been associated with the development of Graves' disease during therapy (10).

Pathophysiology

Although much has been learned about the immune dysregulation that characterizes Graves' disease, the precise cause is unknown. There are defects in antigen-specific T cells that result in B-cell production of many antibodies, most notably stimulatory TSH receptor antibodies. The thyroid glands of patients with Graves' disease are infiltrated with these antigen-specific T cells. Whether the disease is caused by abnormal clones of autoreactive T cells or the initial trigger is abnormal antigen presentation by thyrocytes is not known (11). It is thought that the same anti-TSH receptor antibodies are responsible for Graves' ophthalmopathy (GO, also called thyroid eye disease [TED]) (Figures 2.1a, 2.1b, and 2.2).

Diagnosis

SIGNS AND SYMPTOMS

The typical signs and symptoms of Graves' hyperthyroidism do not differ significantly from those of any other type of hyperthyroidism (Table 2.1) (3). The main features of hyperthyroidism relate to the action of excess thyroid hormone at the cellular level and enhanced beta-adrenergic activity. Typical manifestations include weakness, fatigue, anxiety, tremulousness, heat intolerance, and weight loss. Any organ system may be involved. The skin may be warm, smooth, and moist. Tachycardia is common, but atrial arrhythmias, heart block, or high or low cardiac output may occur, especially in older individuals (12). Mitral valve prolapse, a systolic flow murmur, an S3 gallop, or a Means–Lerman "scratch" murmur may be present. The latter systolic sound is best heard along the left intercostal space during expiration. It is thought to result from either turbulent pulmonic artery blood flow or to friction between the pericardial and pleural surface in a hyperdynamic heart. Recent studies have also shown that older patients with thyrotoxicosis may develop congestive heart failure with evidence of a reversible cardiomyopathy and normal or low ejection fraction (13). In addition, some patients may develop reversible, usually asymptomatic, pulmonary hypertension

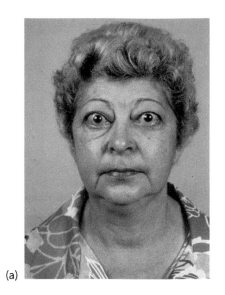

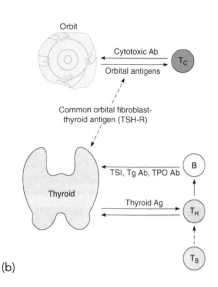

(a) (b)

Figure 2.1 **(a)** Patient with Graves' disease and ophthalmopathy demonstrating proptosis and periorbital edema. **(b)** One theory of the pathogenesis of Graves' disease. There is a defect in suppressor T lymphocytes (Ts) that allows helper T lymphocytes (TH) to stimulate B lymphocytes (B) to synthesize thyroid auto-antibodies. The thyroid-stimulating immunoglobulin (TSI) is the driving force for thyrotoxicosis. The inflammatory process in the orbital muscles may be due to sensitization of cytotoxic T lymphocytes (Tc), or killer cells, to orbital antigens in association with cytotoxic antibodies. The thyroid and the eye are linked by a common antigen, the TSH-R, found in thyroid follicular cells and orbital fibroblasts. It is not yet clear what triggers this immunologic cascade. (Tg Ab, thyroglobulin antibody; TPO Ab, thyroperoxidase or microsomal antibody; Ag, antigen; Ab, antibody.) (From *Greenspan's Basic and Clinical Endocrinology*, Gardner D and Shoback D, eds. McGraw-Hill 2016.)

related to increased cardiac output or to left atrial diastolic dysfunction (14).

Patients may complain that they are eating voraciously but are still losing weight; hyperdefecation is more frequent than frank diarrhea. Some patients may actually gain weight due to an enhanced appetite. Anorexia may be encountered in elderly patients where hyperthyroidism can masquerade as an occult malignancy (15). Liver function tests may be elevated secondary to the hyperthyroid process or—less frequently—to related autoimmune disorders, such as primary biliary cirrhosis, systemic lupus erythematosus, or scleroderma (16). Additional manifestations of hyperthyroidism actually relate to the underlying immunological abnormalities. Vitiligo and/or prematurely gray hair may be present, indicating the presence of antimelanocyte autoantibodies. Patients with Graves' ophthalmopathy may present with or have burning, itching, proptosis, photophobia, or diplopia. Uncommonly, there may be proptosis or optic nerve compression, resulting in decreased visual acuity (Figure 2.3).

Elevated serum calcium, probably related to a direct effect of thyroid hormones on osteoclasts, may occur in about 10% of patients. Even mildly elevated thyroid hormone levels or subclinical hyperthyroidism may be associated with decreased bone mineral density, most notably in postmenopausal women, as shown in population-based studies and a meta-analysis (17–20). Hand tremor and generalized proximal muscle weakness are common. Rarely, hypokalemic periodic paralysis may occur, most frequently in Asian males (21). Attacks are precipitated by high carbohydrate intake and heavy exercise. The precise pathophysiology of these events is unknown, but patients may have a genetic predisposition to activation of Na/K-ATPase activity, which is enhanced in hyperthyroidism (22). One suggested treatment regimen is to administer 10 mEq KCL IV or 2 gm KCL every 2 hours with close monitoring of serum potassium and cardiac status, as rebound hyperkalemia occurs commonly (23). Propranolol, 3–4 mg/kg orally, can reverse or

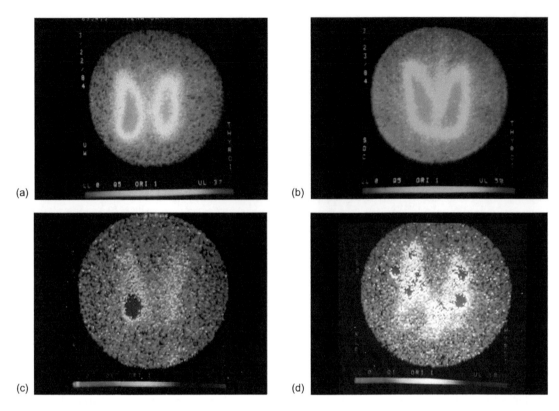

Figure 2.2 **(a–d)** Thyroid radioisotope scans may be helpful in assessing certain patients with hyperthyroidism. **(a)** Demonstrates symmetrical isotope distribution (^{123}I) in a normal individual. **(b)** Demonstrates an enlarged gland with diffuse uptake consistent with Graves' disease. **(c)** Demonstrates a solitary functioning thyroid nodule. There is intense activity in the right-lobe nodule with diminished activity in the rest of the gland because of suppression of TSH by thyroid hormone secretion of the nodule. **(d)** Shows a toxic multinodular goiter. Radioactive isotope activity is heterogeneous, with areas of intense activity interspersed with areas of reduced activity.

prevent attacks (21). Restoration of the euthyroid state prevents future attacks.

The central nervous system (CNS) manifestations of Graves' hyperthyroidism are varied but include restlessness, irritability, nervousness, and impatience. Some patients may realize that they have a decreased ability to concentrate and remember facts; occasionally, they may have demonstrable personality changes (24). These features may be difficult to quantify, but relatives may help to identify them. Cognitive function may be impaired, especially in hospitalized elderly patients, and seizures and coma can be the presenting features of "thyroid storm" (see section on Thyroid Storm). Depression and irrational or even criminal behavior are very unusual. It is difficult to prove that serious personality disorders or criminal behavior are directly associated with hyperthyroidism per se,

although hyperthyroidism has been implicated in these circumstances (25). Suicide does not seem to be more common in hyperthyroidism (26). Rarely, hyperthyroid patients may present with other neurological findings, such as chorea (27).

Women may have irregular menses and decreased fertility, but amenorrhea is rare (28). Men may have decreased libido and gynecomastia, thought to be related to increased estrogen production (Figure 2.4) (29). Total serum estrogen levels are usually increased, in part related to increased sex hormone–binding globulin levels. Serum LH concentrations are increased and there may be Leydig cell failure associated with impaired spermatogenesis (27). One study suggested that up to 50% of hyperthyroid men have some aspect of sexual dysfunction that is recovered with therapy (30). Generalized lymphadenopathy,

Table 2.1 Clinical effects of hyperthyroidism*

System	Effects
General	Nervousness, insomnia, fatigue, tremulousness, heat intolerance, weight loss
Skin	Warmth, moistness, hyperidrosis, alopecia, increased pigmentation, onycholysis, acropachy*, pretibial myxedema*, urticaria, pruritus, vitiligo*
Eyes	Exophthalmos*, conjunctivitis*, chemosis*, diplopia*, decreased vision*
Cardiovascular	Tachycardia, dyspnea, palpitations, atrial fibrillation, heart block, congestive failure, angina pectoris
Gastrointestinal	Hyperphagia, diarrhea or hyperdefecation, elevated liver function tests, hepatosplenomegaly
Metabolic	Elevated serum calcium, decreased serum magnesium, increased bone alkaline phosphatase, hypercalciuria
Neuromuscular	Fine hand tremor, proximal muscle weakness, myopathy, muscle atrophy, creatinuria, periodic paralysis
Osseous	Osteoporosis, osteopenia
Neurological	Fever, delirium, stupor, coma, syncope, choreoathetosis, hemiballismus
Reproductive/sexual	Irregular menses, amenorrhea, gynecomastia, decreased fertility
Hematopoietic	Normochromic normocytic anemia, lymphocytosis, lymphadenopathy, enlarged thymus*, splenomegaly*
Mental	Restlessness, irritability anxiety, inability to concentrate, emotional lability, depression, psychosis

This table is not intended to be all-inclusive but rather representative.
*Indicates findings seen only in Graves' disease.

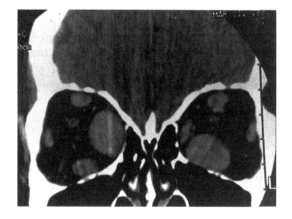

Figure 2.3 An orbital CT scan (coronal view) showing diffuse orbital muscle involvement with enlargement, most notably of the right medial and left inferior recti muscles in a patient with Graves' ophthalmopathy.

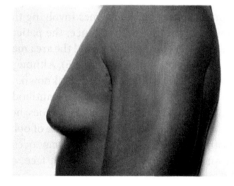

Figure 2.4 A patient with Graves' disease showing gynecomastia. The cause of gynecomastia in this circumstance is thought to be related to increased conversion of testosterone to estradiol. Other causes of gynecomastia, such as hCG-secreting tumors, should also be considered.

splenomegaly, and thymic enlargement may occur, although other causes should be excluded (31). A normochromic normocytic anemia has been described, probably related to decreased ability to incorporate iron into red blood cell precursors. A macrocytic anemia should prompt an evaluation for gastric achlorhydria and possible vitamin B12 deficiency (32).

Pretibial myxedema results from excessive lymphocyte infiltration in the pretibial area, with resultant mucopolysaccharide deposition by fibroblasts (33, 34). The clinical result may simply be a small area of raised discoloration in the pretibial

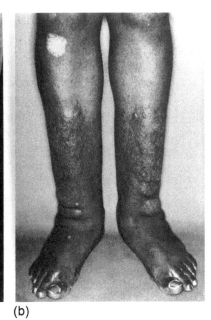

(a)   (b)

Figure 2.5 Two different patients with pretibial myxedema demonstrating varying degrees of involvement. (a) Illustrates more minimal involvement with skin thickening, while (b) shows severe thickening, which would make daily activities, such as walking with shoes, difficult. The patient on the right also has a patch of vitiligo.

area. Rarely, a large area of induration and nonpitting edema may develop, sometimes involving the entire lower leg. In this circumstance, the patient may have difficulty wearing shoes and the area may be pruritic and even painful (Figure 2.5). Although the cause of pretibial myxedema is unknown, it seems to be related to anti-TSH receptor antibody levels (63). Pretibial myxedema usually does not occur unless a patient has clinical evidence of ophthalmopathy, and pretibial myxedema may occur in other anatomic sites, such as the feet, face, or preradial area. Topical steroids, usually recommended to be used under an occlusive dressing, is the most effective therapy, but the response is poor in patients with more severe disease. Thyroid acropachy, which is clubbing of the fingers and toes, occurs rarely in Graves' disease and develops almost exclusively in patients with concomitant ophthalmopathy and dermopathy (Figure 2.6). The etiology is unknown (32).

The manifestations of Graves' hyperthyroidism that occur in younger individuals may be different from those in older subjects (35). Younger patients tend to have more classic findings, such as nervousness, weight loss, anxiousness, tachycardia, and heat intolerance. Older patients may have none of these manifestations but may only present with weight loss or a cardiac abnormality, especially atrial fibrillation. The explanation for these differences is unknown, and, of course, these comments should be taken as generalizations with many exceptions.

Laboratory diagnosis

THYROID HORMONE AND TSH LEVELS

In the past, common thyroid hormone measures included total T4, total T3, resin T3 uptake, and TSH. However, recent advances in techniques now allow the direct measurement of free T4 (FT4). This analysis is preferred to the total T4, as >99% of T4 is bound to circulating proteins (thyroxine-binding globulin, albumin, and prealbumin) and <1% is unbound and available to enter cells and, after conversion to T3, bind specific nuclear receptors and mediate biological activity. Total T4 measurements are affected by factors that influence thyroid hormone–binding proteins, including drugs (estrogens, birth control pills, androgens, opiates) and medical conditions such as hepatitis, cirrhosis, and nephrotic syndrome. FT4 levels remain normal in these situations. Total T3 is

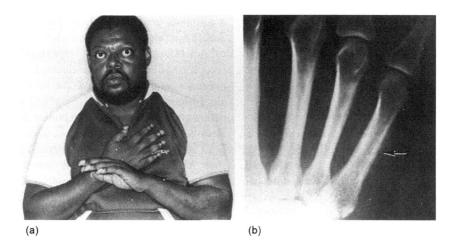

Figure 2.6 A patient with Graves' disease demonstrating bilateral exophthalmos and acropachy (clubbing) (a). (b) Shows a radiograph of the same patient demonstrating phalangeal periosteal reaction (arrow).

preferred by many experts because FT3 still may not be measured in most laboratories in a reliable, precise, cost-effective manner. Approximately 5% of patients will have a normal serum free T4 level and elevated serum T3 level ("T3 toxicosis") (36), and some patients, especially the elderly can have "T4 toxicosis" with normal serum T3 levels (37). Like total T4, total T3 levels are altered by situations that change thyroid hormone–binding proteins. Sensitive TSH assays can measure <0.01 mU/L in serum, with the normal range being about 0.5 to 4.5 mU/L. These improvements in sensitivity result from utilizing chemiluminescence and other techniques. All patients with conventional forms of hyperthyroidism should have an undetectable TSH level in third-generation assays, although many commercial laboratories only report that a value is <0.01 mU/L.

24-HOUR RADIOIODINE UPTAKE

Serum measurements of thyroid hormone and TSH are the cornerstone in the diagnosis of hyperthyroidism, but they do not assess biological activity or the tissue effects of the circulating thyroid hormone levels. The capacity of the thyroid gland to concentrate radioactive iodine is a physiological test representing in vivo events. A normal subject will concentrate about 8% to 30% of radioactive iodine administered when determined at 24 hours. Patients with hyperthyroidism will usually concentrate higher amounts of radioactive iodine than normal, reflecting the heightened ability of the

gland to concentrate iodine. On the other hand, patients with thyrotoxicosis and a low radioiodine uptake (RAIU) generally have a problem associated with increased release into the circulation of preformed thyroid hormone, for example, the various form of thyroiditis (see Chapter 3, "Thyroiditis"). Radiocontrast dyes and other sources of exogenous iodine such as amiodarone will interfere with this test because the enormous amounts of unlabeled iodine in these compounds dilute out the radioactive label, resulting in less radioactive iodine being concentrated by the thyroid gland and a very low 24-hour uptake. Since dietary iodine intake in the United States has decreased over time, the normal range for the 24-hour uptake may have increased compared to values obtained 20 or 30 years ago. Variations in geographic and individual dietary iodine intake of bread, pastry, seafood, salt, and dairy products may also contribute to changes in the 24-hour uptake. Most institutions have not reassessed their normal range for this test in many years, mainly because it is difficult to justify the administration of radioactive materials to normal subjects. Therefore, the normal range should be considered as a guide and not an absolute limit. Some clinicians feel that a scan should be performed whenever a radioiodine uptake is ordered to assess whether an undetected cold nodule also may be present. In addition to the radioiodine uptake, a scan of the thyroid can also be obtained, generally performed at 24 hours with [123]I. This can provide additional information about the size of the thyroid gland, whether the uptake is diffuse or focal, with one or more discrete areas of increased uptake, as well as the presence of areas of decreased activity which may require further evaluation with ultrasound (Figures 2.2 a–d).

TSH RECEPTOR ANTIBODY MEASUREMENTS

If the cause of hyperthyroidism is uncertain, measurement of anti-TSH receptor antibodies (TRAb; also called TSI and TBII) can be performed. Anti-TSH receptor antibody measurements can be performed with one of two possible assays (3). Stimulatory TSH receptor immunoglobulins (TSI) are measured in vitro by testing the ability of serum or IgG from a possible Graves' patient to stimulate cells transfected with the TSH receptor to generate cyclic adenosine monophosphate (cAMP) (3). These responses are compared to those of normal control serum or IgG. A >50% increase above control serum is considered to be a positive cAMP response. Usually, sera from Graves' disease patients will stimulate cAMP by more than two- or threefold. The advantage of the TSI assay is that it measures TSH receptor–stimulating antibodies, which are relevant to hyperthyroidism. Another test, called a thyrotropin-binding inhibitory immunoglobulin assay (TBII assay), measures the total conglomerate amount of TSH receptor antibodies in serum. The ability of serum or IgG from hyperthyroid patients to inhibit radiolabeled TSH binding to recombinant TSH receptors is compared to control normal serum (3). The potential disadvantage of TBII measurements is that they do not distinguish stimulatory from inhibitory or "blocking" antibodies. To date, there are no commercial assays that can measure inhibitory antibodies. Both assay methods have comparable sensitivity and specificity for the diagnosis of Graves' disease (3).

The measurement of TSH receptor antibodies is useful in several clinical settings (3). Their presence will differentiate Graves' disease from other causes of hyperthyroidism when this differentiation cannot be made clinically. Anti-TSH receptor antibody measurements may also be useful to help confirm the presence of Graves' ophthalmopathy from other nonendocrine causes of proptosis in euthyroid patients (so-called "euthyroid Graves' disease"). Anti-TSH receptor antibody measurements may also help predict if a patient with Graves' disease is in remission at the end of

a course of antithyroid drug therapy (ATD) (38), and this strategy is recommended in recent clinical practice guidelines (39). Importantly, anti-TSH receptor antibodies may be elevated in the sera of pregnant women who have (or have had) active autoimmune thyroid disease, such as Graves' disease. If the TSH receptor antibodies are markedly elevated (e.g., two- to threefold above the upper limit of normal), there is an increased likelihood that these IgG antibodies will cross the placenta and cause neonatal hyperthyroidism (40).

Anti-TSH receptor antibodies can be found in the sera of pregnant women with Graves' disease, but they may also be present in the sera of patients who have had Graves' disease and are hypothyroid after radioiodine therapy (41). Many experts suggest measuring these antibodies in the third trimester in women with active Graves' disease or Graves' ophthalmopathy and in women treated for Graves' disease in the recent past, or remotely if they were treated with radioiodine (39).

PITFALLS

There are several pitfalls that should be avoided in the laboratory assessment of Graves' disease patients. The assays for iodothyronines and TSH are specific and accurate; as a result, there are few reasons for artifactual results except for mislabeling and rare laboratory errors. Specific antibodies against T3 or T4 may alter their respective measurements. Although unusual, such antibodies can occur in patients with autoimmune thyroid disease, in those who work with animals, and, occasionally, for no apparent reason. In a study of 115 patients with antithyroid hormone autoantibodies, about 42% of patients had antibodies against triiodothyronine, 33% against thyroxine, and 25% of patients had both anti-T3 and anti-T4 antibodies (42). Although 44% of these patients were considered to be euthyroid, 16% were hyperthyroid and almost 40% were hypothyroid. While the effect of antibodies on T4 and T3 measurements depends upon the method of measurement, in general, they cause a laboratory result that is incongruent with the clinical state (40).

It is important to ensure that patients with Graves' hyperthyroidism have an undetectable serum TSH level so that rare individuals with peripheral hormone resistance or TSH-secreting pituitary tumors are not misdiagnosed as having Graves' disease. Also, certain patients may harbor heterophilic antibodies that can result in falsely elevated serum TSH levels, causing diagnostic confusion in patients with hyperthyroidism (43). Biotin ingestion can also cause a falsely low serum TSH and elevated levels of FT4 and FT3 in assays that use streptavidin–biotin detection systems, mimicking the biochemical profile of hyperthyroidism (44).

It is also important to exclude other coexistent autoimmune disorders that may be confusing the clinical picture. For example, a patient with Graves' hyperthyroidism who complains of inordinate weakness and tiredness may, in fact, have coexistent hypoadrenalism due to Addison's disease; a patient with persistent gastrointestinal symptoms may have occult celiac disease (45).

The patient's clinical assessment and history must be integrated with the thyroid function tests. Thyroid function tests should ideally be determined twice prior to treatment and, when possible, measurement of FT4 and T3 is preferred. In patients with mild hyperthyroidism and no clinical features of Graves' disease, it is important to obtain a radioactive iodine uptake test or TRAb prior to treatment to confirm high-uptake thyroid disease (i.e., Graves' disease). Even if the diagnosis of Graves' disease seems obvious, at least one TSH measurement should be obtained to rule out the unlikely TSH-secreting pituitary tumor.

Treatment

Ideally, the treatment of any medical condition is directed at its cause, but the proximate cause of the immune dysregulation in Graves' disease remains obscure (11). Therefore, the available treatments are directed at the thyroid gland rather than the underlying autoimmunity. The therapies that are available to the clinician in the twenty-first century are the same as those that were available almost 80 years ago: antithyroid drugs, radioiodine, and surgery (39). Although some patients, especially those who are relatively asymptomatic, may wonder whether specific treatment is necessary, overtly hyperthyroid individuals usually require restoration of a euthyroid state because of potentially deleterious skeletal, cardiovascular, and psychological effects.

ANTITHYROID DRUG THERAPY

Antithyroid drugs remain the first choice for initial therapy of children, adolescents, and young adults in the United States (46). They are the usual treatment for almost all patients in the rest of the world (44, 47) and perhaps for most patients in the United States as well (48). Antithyroid drugs are generally safe and effective in controlling the hyperthyroid state. However, they have limitations and toxicities that are important to recognize, and their proper use requires knowledge of their pharmacology as well as clinical experience.

Clinical pharmacology of antithyroid drugs

Antithyroid drugs do not directly affect iodine uptake or hormone release by the thyroid; hence, contrary to popular belief, the 24-hour radioiodine uptake is not affected very much by antithyroid drug therapy (49).

Within the thyroid, both propylthiouracil (PTU) and methimazole (Tapazole) inhibit thyroid hormone synthesis by interfering with intrathyroidal iodine utilization and the iodotyrosine coupling reaction, both of which are catalyzed by thyroid peroxidase. Extrathyroidally, PTU, but not methimazole, inhibits the conversion of T4 to T3 in peripheral tissues. Although some feel that this difference confers an advantage to PTU over methimazole in severe hyperthyroidism or thyroid storm, there are no comparative data to support this supposition. In controlled trials in outpatients, methimazole generally normalizes serum T4 and T3 levels faster than PTU (50). There are also in vitro and in vivo data pointing to possible beneficial effects of both drugs on the immune system, although it is far from clear whether this is important clinically in terms of remission rates with antithyroid drug therapy (47, 51).

Antithyroid agents are well absorbed from the gastrointestinal tract. In the circulation, PTU is heavily protein-bound, mainly to albumin, while methimazole binding to proteins is negligible. However, both drugs appear to cross the placenta equally well (52, 53). The serum half-lives of PTU and methimazole are 1 and 4 to 6 hours, respectively. However, the intrathyroidal duration of action of both drugs is longer than that, making the determination of drug blood levels not particularly helpful clinically. Although both drugs are metabolized in the liver and metabolites are excreted by the kidney, in the absence of data to the contrary, the doses used to treat hyperthyroidism do not generally need to be altered in patients with liver or kidney disease.

Antithyroid drugs in clinical practice

Antithyroid drugs are used in two ways in the therapy of hyperthyroidism (47). They can be employed as primary therapy and are usually given for 1 to 2 years in the hope that the patient will achieve remission (remission is usually defined arbitrarily as biochemical euthyroidism for 1 year following cessation of the antithyroid drug), or they are used for a few months to "cool the patient down" prior to ablative therapy with radioiodine or surgery. Unfortunately, patients are often started on antithyroid drugs without a clear goal in mind and then remain on them either continuously or intermittently for protracted periods of time. Antithyroid drugs are also mistakenly used in the long-term treatment of toxic nodules or toxic multinodular goiter, situations in which remission is highly unlikely.

Antithyroid drugs for primary therapy of Graves' disease

Prior to initiating antithyroid drug therapy, the physician should carefully discuss the options with patients and their family (54). Unlike radioiodine and surgery, antithyroid drug treatment will not cause permanent hypothyroidism, but the chances of remission are <50% for the average patient. Even if remission occurs, the chances of permanent remission are <50%, and late hypothyroidism may develop in up to 20% (39, 55). Also, the potential for allergic reactions is often underestimated or not discussed (56). Patient preferences are important to take into consideration, even if the decision for or against a particular therapy seems to be based more on emotion than fact. No therapy has been shown to be superior to any other in terms of efficacy or patient satisfaction (57). However, the physician can help the patient make an informed choice. In a recent meta-analysis (58), orbitopathy, smoking, goiter size, thyroid hormone levels, and levels of anti-TSH receptor antibodies were all significantly associated with relapse. A prior history of multiple relapses is another factor that would argue against antithyroid drug use as first-line therapy. On the other hand, a small gland and mild biochemical changes would favor remission, and in some studies the rates may be as high as 70 to 90%. A negative thyroid-stimulating immunoglobulin (TSI) titer at the beginning of therapy has been shown to predict a high rate of remission (59), but negative titers occur in only about 10% of patients, so it is probably not cost-effective to order TSI titers routinely. Age, sex, family history of Graves' disease, the presence of ophthalmopathy, and smoking behavior are not reliably or consistently predictors of remission.

Family planning is another factor that should be considered in women. First, many clinicians feel that if pregnancy is desired in the following 1 to 2 years, antithyroid drugs are less appropriate, since the patient may be pregnant while taking a drug that could harm the fetus. Also, in patients who are in remission after a course of antithyroid drugs, relapse is very common in the postpartum period (60). Therefore, some clinicians feel that women desirous of pregnancy in the near future are not optimal candidates for long-term antithyroid drug treatment (see Chapter 12, "Thyroid Disease and Pregnancy") (61).

Once antithyroid drugs are selected as initial treatment, methimazole (or carbimazole in the United Kingdom and certain other countries) has emerged as the preferred therapy because of potentially life-threatening hepatotoxicity with PTU (62). Methimazole has a number of other advantages over PTU. First, it is a once-a-day drug, which improves compliance, and the number of methimazole tablets that a typical patient takes daily is fewer, which is important to some patients. Also, the toxicity of methimazole is more predictable, in that the frequency of side effects is dose-related; many patients can be treated with doses as low as 5 to 15 mg/day, a dose range in which side effects are few (63). PTU may be preferable in "thyroid storm" or severe hyperthyroidism because of its ability to block T4-to-T3 conversion (47). PTU could be considered in patients with a mild drug reaction to methimazole (e.g., a drug eruption) that does not respond to antihistamines and who reject definitive therapy with either radioiodine or surgery (39).

In mild to moderate thyrotoxicosis, methimazole is usually started at a dose of 10 to 30 mg/day as a single daily dose. The rapidity of response depends on the severity of the underlying thyroid problem, the size of the gland and its hormonal stores, the dose and frequency of the drugs, and, of course, compliance. Most patients become euthyroid within 6 to 12 weeks; it is important to monitor both T3 and FT4 levels, as serum T3 may take longer to normalize than the FT4 (48). In general,

Table 2.2 Methimazole dosing in hyperthyroidism

Free T4 levels (fold above the upper limit of the reference range, typically 1.8 ng/dl)	Methimazole starting dose (mg/day)
FT4 = 2–3 ng/dl (1–1.5 fold)	5–10
FT4 = 3–4 ng/dl (1.5–2 fold)	10–20
FT4 = >4 ng/dl (>2 fold)	20–40

Data based on recommendations in (39).

the methimazole dose is related to the severity of the underlying thyrotoxicosis (Table 2.2) (39).

Although it may take longer to achieve control than with higher doses (48), initial doses as low as 10 mg/day can control hyperthyroidism in many patients (61). Once antithyroid drugs have been started, thyroid function should be monitored every 4 to 6 weeks at least for the first 6 months and less frequently thereafter. During treatment, some patients can have startling degrees of "T3 predominance," with serum T3 levels two to three times above the upper limit of normal and serum T4 values that are subnormal (64). Also, the serum TSH level can remain suppressed long after the patient has become euthyroid or even hypothyroid, which limits its value early in the course of treatment. In many patients, the drug can be tapered to a lower dose after a few months, once the patient has become biochemically euthyroid. If this tapering is not done, hypothyroidism will often ensue (65). In patients who are hyperthyroid on a low drug dose but hypothyroid on a larger dose, some physicians use a "block-replacement" regimen. In this method, a dose of antithyroid drug that would cause hypothyroidism is employed in conjunction with thyroxine supplementation to maintain a euthyroid state. This method of treating patients may also be useful in the pediatric population but has not gained wider acceptance (66).

Once a patient has been placed on long-term therapy with an antithyroid drug, what is the optimal duration of therapy before a remission has been achieved and the drug can be discontinued? Older retrospective data suggested that the longer a person remained on therapy, the more likely a remission would be achieved once the drug was stopped. More recently, prospective trials have not shown longer treatment periods (e.g., >12–18 months) to be more effective (e.g., [67]). Therefore, treatment for 12–18 months is reasonable, but data supporting longer periods of time are lacking.

After 1 to 2 years of therapy, a large goiter, continued requirement for a large dose of methimazole (e.g., greater than 10 mg a day), and a persistently high T3/T4 ratio or low TSH are all poor prognostic signs for remission. Anti-TSH receptor antibody testing (TRAb) should be performed, and if persistently positive, the chances of remission are very low (<10%), but even in patients with normal levels, there is a 20% to 30% chance of eventual relapse (68, 38). In patients whose TRAb levels are normal and the drug discontinued, thyroid function should be monitored every 2–3 months, as relapses in this situation occur over months to years, rather than weeks to months (3). During this time, patients are not necessarily seen for an office visit unless they become hyperthyroid, or at 6–12 months if they remain normal. T3 thyrotoxicosis frequently occurs during a relapse, so that serum T3 should be monitored along with the serum T4 levels. In contrast, relapses are most likely to occur within the first 6 months after drug discontinuation if the drug is stopped in the face of positive TSAb (69).

Some patients have persistent subclinical hyperthyroidism after antithyroid drug cessation, with normal serum T4 and T3 values but suppressed serum TSH concentrations. While the chances that such patients will have a full-fledged relapse are greater (70), relapse is not inevitable. Some experts treat patients with subclinical hyperthyroidism (i.e., suppressed TSH, normal FT4 and T3) as if they had relapsed and recommend another trial of antithyroid drug therapy or radioiodine. Others simply observe them expectantly and only recommend treatment if and when overt hyperthyroidism develops. A persistently fully suppressed serum TSH (i.e., <0.1 mU/l) is of more concern in the elderly (see section on Subclinical Hyperthyroidism) (71).

Remissions are not necessarily lifelong, but long-term follow-up studies have shown that some patients have durable remissions that apparently last for many years (72). A strategy for treatment of relapse should be discussed with the patient in advance. Some patients will opt for another course of antithyroid drug, even though more than one prior relapse is associated with continued relapse. Other patients will wish to move on to definitive radioiodine therapy, or, more uncommonly, to surgery. Some patients prefer chronic antithyroid drug treatment, often for decades (73, 74). As noted previously, some patients eventually develop spontaneous hypothyroidism, so that lifelong follow-up is necessary.

Antithyroid drug side effects

The side effects of antithyroid drugs are usually classified as "minor" or "major," depending on the level of potential harm to the patient (Table 2.3) (47, 75). Many side effects appear to be "allergic" or "immune," and one preliminary report suggested that patients with Graves' disease were more likely to have adverse reactions than hyperthyroid patients with nodular thyroid disease (76). Overall, side effects develop in 5% to 25% of patients and are among the most frequent reasons for abandoning drug therapy. As noted previously, methimazole-related drug reactions are dose-related, but this does not appear to be the case for PTU. The commonest minor reactions are fever, rash, pruritus, arthralgias, gastrointestinal distress, and nausea. Rashes can be urticarial, macular, or morbilliform. In one prospective trial, rash developed in about 20% of patients treated with 30 mg of methimazole versus 6.6% with 15 mg of methimazole daily (48). If a rash develops, it will sometimes resolve spontaneously (even with continued use) with or without the use of antihistamines to treat associated itching. Although switching to the alternative drug is another possibility, the cross-reaction rate may be as high as 50% (77). Some patients may simply elect to stop the offending drug and accept a definitive form of therapy. Loss of sense of taste, sometimes

Table 2.3 Side effects of antithyroid drugs (49, 76)

	Overall frequency[a]	Comments
Minor side effects		
Skin reactions (pruritic rash)	4–6%	Dose-related for MMI; possibly more common with MMI
Arthralgias	1–5%	Gastrointestinal 1–5%
Hair loss	4%	Possibly related to change in thyroid function (hypothyroidism)
Abnormal taste/smell 0.3%		Only reported with MMI/CBZ
Sialadenitis	Very rare	
Major side effects		
Severe polyarthritis	1–2%	
Agranulocytosis	0.1–0.5%	
Aplastic anemia	Rare	
Vasculitis	Rare	May be ANCA + drug-induced SLE and other immune syndromes also reported
Severe hepatitis	0.1–0.01	Almost exclusively PTU; transient increases in transaminases seen in 30%
Cholestasis	Rare	Almost exclusively seen with MMI or CBZ. No deaths reported
Hypoprothrombinemia	Rare	No case reports since 1982
Insulin-autoimmune syndrome	Rare	Seen almost exclusively in Asians

Key: MMI, methimazole; CBZ, carbimazole; PTU, propylthiouracil; ANCA, antineutrophil cytoplasmic antibody.
[a] Rate of side effects (minor and major) is greater at high doses of MMI and may approach 30% at high doses.

associated with anosmia, is a rare minor side effect reported only with methimazole (73). It develops suddenly after 1 to 2 months of therapy and resolves after the drug is stopped (Table 2.3).

Fever and arthralgias, while technically minor side effects, warrant drug discontinuation since they may be the harbinger of more serious problems, such as vasculitis. Similarly, leukopenia, defined as a white blood cell (WBC) count $<4 \times 10^9/L$, occurs in up to 10% of patients. Leukopenia requires follow-up and prompt cessation of the antithyroid drug if the WBC count falls below $3 \times 10^9/L$, since leukopenia may precede the development of full-blown agranulocytosis. Antithyroid drug–related leukopenia should be distinguished from the leukopenia that can be seen in Graves' disease and in healthy African Americans by obtaining a baseline WBC count (39). A white blood cell count and differential should be obtained prior to initiating therapy, and the use of methimazole should be reconsidered if the granulocyte count is $<1.5 \times 10^9/L$ (39).

The major side effects are quite rare, but the most frequent are agranulocytosis, vasculitis and drug-induced lupus, and hepatic damage (hepatitis and cholestasis). Agranulocytosis develops in approximately 0.2% to 0.5% of patients. In one case series, agranulocytosis developed in 12 of 2190 (0.55%) patients taking PTU and 43 of 13,208 (0.31%) patients taking methimazole (78). Agranulocytosis is usually defined as an absolute granulocyte count $<0.5 \times 10^9/L$, but most patients have granulocyte counts that are far lower, often close to zero. It should be distinguished from the exceedingly rare cases of antithyroid drug–induced aplastic anemia by a hematocrit $>30\%$ and a platelet count $100 \times 10^9/L$. Agranulocytosis is thought to be autoimmune in origin, developing because of antigranulocyte antibodies that are found in the serum of affected patients (79). Since the development of agranulocytosis may be HLA-linked (80), it might be reasonable to avoid giving antithyroid drugs to close relatives of a patient who has had this side effect.

Agranulocytosis typically develops in the first 3 months of therapy, but there are notable exceptions (81, 82). Older patients may be more susceptible, and it can develop after one or more prior innocuous exposures to the drugs (83). Routine monitoring of the WBC count has not been recommended because it is not cost-effective, but some patients do have a slow decline in leukocyte counts that is the harbinger of agranulocytosis (75, 79). Although current guidelines do not recommend monitoring of the white blood cell count (39), some clinicians monitor the complete blood count and liver function tests in patients taking antithyroid agents, both prior to and periodically during this treatment (44).

Patients with agranulocytosis may be afebrile until they develop an infection. The typical patient has severe malaise, oropharyngitis and odynophagia, and high fever. Immediate cessation of the antithyroid drug, hospitalization, and administration of broad-spectrum antibiotics is mandatory, with coverage for *Pseudomonas aeruginosa* which is frequently isolated from the blood in affected patients (84). Although most patients recover, it should be recalled that agranulocytosis is associated with a mortality rate as high as 5–10% in recent series (85, 86). A bone marrow examination may provide helpful prognostic information; an extreme loss of myeloid precursors suggests a longer time to recovery (87), as well as the potential for a poorer response to granulocyte colony-stimulating factor (G-CSF) therapy (88). The use of G-CSF has become standard in the management of drug-induced agranulocytosis (82). A randomized controlled trial of G-CSF in antithyroid drug-induced agranulocytosis found no statistically significant difference in the mean time to recovery from G-CSF compared to conservative therapy (89). However, this trial has been criticized because the dose of G-CSF was thought to be too low (100–200 mcg/day) versus the now standard dose of 300 mcg/day (86). If thyrotoxicosis requires treatment during the acute episode of agranulocytosis, beta-adrenergic blocking drugs, lithium, or iodinated contrast agents can be used. Attempting to switch to the other antithyroid drug is not recommended, as cross-sensitivity has been reported. In this situation, plasmapheresis should be considered (90), although PTU could be used for a few days with close monitoring of the granulocyte count.

An antithyroid drug–related syndrome that includes renal failure, vasculitic skin changes, pulmonary and respiratory tract involvement, arthritis, and positive circulating anticytoplasmic neutrophil antibodies (ANCAs) has been described, mainly in Asian patients (91). Anticytoplasmic neutrophil antibodies have typically been associated with Wegener's granulomatosis and polyarteritis nodosa, but they may also be present in drug allergy. In the antithyroid drug–related cases, the antibodies are of the pericytoplasmic variety (so-called pANCAs, with myeloperoxidase being the putative antigen), and the vast majority, but not all, have been patients exposed to PTU. Although the syndrome usually resolves after a few weeks, some patients with severe renal dysfunction or pulmonary involvement have required high-dose glucocorticoid therapy or cyclophosphamide, and several patients have needed short-term hemodialysis. In some antithyroid drug-treated patients, ANCAs are present, but patients remain asymptomatic (92).

Some patients develop a condition that has been termed the "antithyroid arthritis syndrome" (93, 94). The frequency of this side effect is in the range of 1% to 2%, and it usually develops within 60 days of initiating therapy. The syndrome is characterized by hot, swollen, tender joints involving multiple sites. Patients with this syndrome do not have positive ANCAs. Symptoms usually resolve after 1 to 2 weeks of therapy with nonsteroidal anti-inflammatory drugs; glucocorticoid therapy may be necessary in severe cases.

Liver toxicity is a rare but serious side effect of antithyroid drug therapy (95, 96). Hepatic involvement with PTU typically presents as clinical hepatitis with malaise, anorexia, jaundice, and tender hepatomegaly. Laboratory data and liver biopsy histology are consistent with hepatocellular injury. The following criteria for the diagnosis of PTU-induced hepatitis have been proposed: clinical and laboratory evidence of hepatocellular damage; temporal relationship to PTU therapy; exclusion of known infectious agents, drugs, or toxins; and absence of shock or sepsis (97). Over 50 cases of PTU-related hepatitis have been reported in the literature, with fatalities and some patients requiring liver transplant (98). The mean duration of PTU therapy in reported cases is 3 months, with a range of 2 days to 1 year; the average age of affected individuals in one review was 28 years (99). Young African American females may be at higher risk (100). Once the syndrome is recognized, immediate cessation of the drug is mandatory. Expert management of potential complications and hepatic failure is essential. Although glucocorticoid therapy has been used, there is no evidence that it decreases the time to recovery or survival, and glucocorticoids are not recommended. There

have been patients whose ongoing hyperthyroidism has been managed successfully with methimazole (e.g., [101]); other options would include beta-adrenergic blocking drugs, saturated solution of potassium iodide (SSKI) and definitive therapy with radioiodine or surgery.

Approximately one-third of PTU-treated patients develop asymptomatic two- to sixfold elevations of serum transaminases within 2 months of starting the drug, which then resolve despite continued therapy (103). Also, up to 35% of patients with Graves' disease have elevations of liver function tests at baseline (104). In one report, PTU therapy led to normalization of liver function tests in two-thirds of patients, while the remaining one-third had a further elevation before levels returned to baseline (100). These data suggest that abnormal liver function tests are not an absolute contraindication to PTU therapy, although a serious discussion of these issues must be held with the patient. All patients about to embark on a course of PTU should be warned about the possibility of hepatitis and told to discontinue the drug if malaise, jaundice, dark urine, or light-colored stools develop. Routine monitoring of liver function is controversial but is suggested by some thyroidologists (44).

Similar to the case with PTU, methimazole therapy results in the normalization of abnormal liver function tests in most patients (105). Methimazole therapy has not been associated with potentially lethal hepatic involvement. Rather, a cholestatic picture is characteristic, with severe hyperbilirubinemia, bile duct stasis, and preserved hepatocellular architecture on biopsy (92, 93). One review collected 30 cases in the literature (106), but there are probably many cases that go unreported, as with PTU-induced hepatitis. The syndrome usually resolves slowly over a period of several months after the drug is stopped. In one case report of methimazole-related hepatotoxicity, PTU was substituted for methimazole without sequelae (107). Extreme caution should be used when employing one antithyroid agent in a situation in which the alternative agent has caused hepatic abnormalities. Recent studies from Asia suggest that methimazole can also be associated with laboratory abnormalities that are more consistent with hepatocellular damage than cholestasis (108, 109). Further studies in other populations are necessary to document whether this is true in other ethnic groups. As noted previously, some patients with hyperthyroidism have abnormal liver function tests, and pre-existing liver disease per se is not a contraindication to antithyroid drug therapy; however, transaminases more than fivefold above the upper limit of the reference range should prompt consideration of other therapies (39).

BETA-ADRENERGIC ANTAGONIST DRUGS

Beta-adrenergic antagonist drugs play an important role in the management of thyrotoxicosis (110). Blockade of adrenergic receptors provides patients with considerable relief from adrenergic symptoms such as tremor, palpitation, anxiety, and heat intolerance. Small decreases in serum T3 concentrations occur in patients treated with large doses of selected beta-adrenergic antagonist drugs (propranolol) because of inhibition of extrathyroidal conversion of T4 to T3 (111), but these are probably clinically insignificant.

Although beta blockers improve the negative nitrogen balance and decrease heart rate, cardiac output, and oxygen consumption in thyrotoxic patients, these measurements seldom become normal except in the mildest cases. Therefore, these drugs are used as primary therapy only in patients with self-limited forms of thyrotoxicosis (e.g., the various forms of subacute thyroiditis). They are most often used in Graves' disease as an adjunct to alleviate symptoms during the diagnostic evaluation, while awaiting the effects of antithyroid drugs, the results of ablative therapy with radioiodine, or to prepare patients for surgery.

Although propranolol was the drug originally used by most clinicians for therapy of thyrotoxicosis, other beta blockers have a longer duration of action (e.g., long-acting propranolol, atenolol, metoprolol, and nadolol) or are more cardioselective (atenolol and metoprolol). The usual starting dose of propranolol is in the range of 80 to 160 mg/day; similar effects are produced by 50 to 200 mg/day of atenolol or metoprolol or 40 to 80 mg/day of nadolol. Large doses (e.g., 360 to 480 mg/day of propranolol) are sometimes necessary for optimum clinical effects, possibly because of accelerated drug clearance (112). Propranolol and esmolol can be given intravenously to patients who are acutely ill (see discussion of thyroid storm).

Beta-adrenergic antagonist drugs are well tolerated. Common side effects include nausea, headache, fatigue, insomnia, and depression. Rash, fever, agranulocytosis, and thrombocytopenia

are rare. Undesirable effects related to the beta-adrenergic antagonist effects are far more common. Patients with a clear history of asthma should not receive these drugs; a cardioselective drug could be used cautiously in patients with mild asthma. Patients with a history of congestive heart failure should not receive a beta-adrenergic blocking drug except when the heart failure is clearly rate-related or caused by atrial fibrillation. Even then, the drug should be given cautiously, preferably with digoxin. Beta blockers are also relatively contraindicated in insulin-treated diabetic patients, in whom hypoglycemic symptoms may be masked. They should not be given to patients with bradyarrhythmias or Raynaud's phenomenon or patients being treated with a monoamine oxidase inhibitor; they should also probably not be given routinely to pregnant patients.

The potential usefulness of diltiazem in thyrotoxicosis has been studied (113). This calcium channel blocking agent reduced resting heart rate by 17%, comparable to what can be achieved with a beta-adrenergic antagonist drug. Calcium channel blockers should be considered in patients with severe tachycardia in whom beta blockers are contraindicated—for example, in patients with both asthma and thyrotoxicosis.

POTASSIUM IODIDE THERAPY

Potassium iodide (KI) has been used in the past to treat mild hyperthyroidism due to Graves' disease (114), but it has fallen out of favor because of concern that continued use might lead to an exacerbation of thyrotoxicosis due to an "escape" from the inhibitory effects on thyroid hormone synthesis. However, two recent Japanese reports found that KI can be useful in patients with mild thyrotoxicosis, especially in those who are allergic to antithyroid drugs (100, 115). In one report, patients treated with a dose of 50–100 mg KI daily had control of their hyperthyroidism that was comparable to a control group treated with low-dose methimazole (116), and some patients (38% of a group of 29 patients treated for a mean of 7.4 years) achieved remission (100).

RADIOIODINE (^{131}I) THERAPY FOR GRAVES' DISEASE

[131]I therapy has been utilized for approximately 70 years for patients with Graves' disease; it is

considered safe and effective (116, 117). The goal of therapy is to render the patient permanently hypothyroid, a process that typically takes about 3 months. In the past, radioiodine therapy was considered to be first-line therapy in most adults with thyrotoxic Graves' disease in the United States, but this may longer be the case (46). Patients and their families must be counseled about the advantages and disadvantages of radioiodine therapy and must participate in the decision process. Elderly or severely thyrotoxic patients considered too ill to undergo the therapeutic manipulations inherent in the process of giving ^{131}I are usually initially treated with antithyroid agents to render them euthyroid, at which time a decision can be made with regard to definitive radioiodine therapy.

If the diagnosis of Graves' disease is clear, a 24-hour radioactive iodine uptake test is not absolutely required before administering ^{131}I therapy, but many experts believe that it is important to document that the uptake is sufficiently elevated to administer ^{131}I. On rare occasions, a patient will have had exposure to radiocontrast dye or compounds containing sufficient iodine to suppress the radioactive iodine uptake. In this circumstance, giving a therapeutic dose of ^{131}I would fail to treat the patient and exposure him or her unnecessarily to radiation. ^{131}I therapy should not be given to a breastfeeding woman or a patient who may be pregnant. Therefore, a careful medical history and a serum beta-hCG should be obtained within 5 to 7 days prior to giving the therapy. A woman of childbearing age should be counseled not to become pregnant for 6 months after ^{131}I therapy (39). This time period is chosen based on the biological half-life of the radioiodine, as well as the desire for the patient to be euthyroid prior to becoming pregnant. Careful radiation safety procedures must be followed by the patient and his or her family for about a week following ^{131}I therapy (118). For example, if a patient has young children in the house, they should not share eating utensils or be kissed or held closely. The individual instructions vary from institution to institution and with the family situation.

There are two general approaches to deciding on the appropriate therapeutic dose of ^{131}I for a patient with Graves' disease (116, 117). The first method attempts to determine the most appropriate dose for an individual by estimating the size of the thyroid gland and delivering approximately 80–200 µC of ^{131}I per gram of thyroid tissue. The estimated thyroid gland size is multiplied by the desired delivered dose per gram of tissue (100 to 120 µC of ^{131}I), and this number is divided by the 24-hour uptake expressed as a decimal (e.g., 80% uptake is converted to 0.80). This method appears to be more quantitative than it actually is because clinicians tend to underestimate the size of large thyroid glands and overestimate the size of smaller ones, and it is impossible to predict radiation sensitivity of a specific thyroid gland (119). Alternatively, a second method of treatment is to use "fixed doses" of ^{131}I. With this approach, the physician arbitrarily picks a given ^{131}I dose that is used in all patients with hyperthyroid Graves' disease. A typical fixed dose would be 10 to 15 mCi ^{131}I. This practice has the advantage of simplicity—but, of course, it does not take into account the size or activity of the thyroid gland. Retrospective and prospective studies have not shown major differences in outcomes for the two methods of dose determination (120, 121). In randomized trials, both methods have similar outcomes at 6–12 months, in terms of rates of hypothyroidism and persistent hyperthyroidism, with approximately 80% of patients being either hypothyroid or euthyroid, and about 20% having persistent hyperthyroidism (120, 121). There is a clear increase in the risk of worsening of thyroid eye disease (see below). Most studies have not found an increase in malignancy after radioiodine therapy for Graves' disease (see the section below on radioiodine and cancer).

The follow-up evaluation of a patient after ^{131}I therapy varies between institutions and physicians, and, of course, depends upon the clinical circumstances and goals of treatment. In the typical patient with Graves' disease, ^{131}I is given in order to induce permanent hypothyroidism. In this circumstance, following a therapeutic dose of ^{131}I, serum FT4 and total T3 levels are determined periodically, perhaps every 3 to 6 weeks, depending upon the clinical context. After several months, when the thyroid function tests are decreased to the normal range and the patient is being evaluated for possible hypothyroidism, serum TSH is also determined. Some patients develop transient central hypothyroidism following radioiodine therapy, with subnormal serum TSH that usually, but not always, evolves into permanent primary hypothyroidism (122). Approximately 10–20% of patients will require a second dose of ^{131}I, and about 1% of patients require a third dose. It is prudent to wait 6 to 12 months for the full effects of the initial dose to be manifest before another dose is considered. Overall, about 50% of patients become permanently hypothyroid after one year, with the rate being dependent on the radioiodine dose, with another 2–3% developing hypothyroidism in the ensuing years (121). Thus, patients who do not become hypothyroid early require lifelong follow-up to monitor for the development of hypothyroidism.

Prior to definitive therapy, most patients will be given a beta blocker when the diagnosis of thyrotoxicosis is made, the goal being amelioration of symptoms and a pulse rate <100 beats per minute. Young patients who are mildly to moderately thyrotoxic (e.g., minimal symptoms, otherwise healthy, minimal elevations of T4 and T3) do not require methimazole pretreatment before ^{131}I treatment, although they usually will continue their beta blocker or be prescribed one. There is a possibility of worsening of thyroid function in the weeks following radioiodine therapy (123), likely due to a transient increase in TRAb (124). Therefore, older patients with moderate hyperthyroidism or patients with more severe disease (e.g., presence of coexisting medical conditions, elevated FT4 and total T3 perhaps 3–4 times above normal), are commonly given antithyroid agents before and continued after radioiodine therapy to maintain normal thyroid hormone levels (125, 126). The drug is tapered as the thyroid function tests normalize and then stopped when the tests show the development of hypothyroidism. Continued methimazole therapy interferes with the efficacy of radioiodine therapy and needs to be stopped at the time of therapy (127). Most endocrinologists provide a window of about 2 to 5 days prior to and after ^{131}I therapy when the patient does not receive antithyroid drugs; 3 days is sufficient (128).

In a meta-analysis of studies that examined outcomes of patients either pretreated or not pretreated with antithyroid drugs prior to radioiodine (129), new-onset atrial fibrillation was reported in 1/660 (0.2%) patients pretreated with ATDs vs. 3/646 patients without ATDs (0.5%). Death after radioiodine was reported in 1/660 (0.2%) pretreated with antithyroid agent and in 6/646 (0.9%) without adjunctive drug therapy. Clearly, the routine use of antithyroid drugs in this context is unnecessary and potentially exposes patients to drug toxicity.

Antithyroid drug pretreatment may interfere with the efficacy of radioiodine, perhaps by acting as free radical scavengers within the irradiated gland. An older meta-analysis ascertained that both antithyroid drugs lower the success rate whether they are used before or after radioiodine treatment (126), but randomized trials have not shown a significant effect on efficacy from methimazole or carbimazole (130, 131).

Radioiodine and Graves' ophthalmopathy

[131]I therapy is believed to exacerbate existing ophthalmopathy (132, 133), at least when it is more than minimally active on clinical grounds (134); thus, it is important to take a relevant history and perform a thorough ophthalmological examination. If there is moderately severe ophthalmopathy or if it seems to be progressive, it is important to obtain an ophthalmology consultation, and an orbital computed tomography (CT) scan (without contrast) or magnetic resonance imaging (MRI) should be considered to evaluate the presence and extent of disease. These radiological studies may be required only in selected patients, but they do provide quantitative, reliable information regarding proptosis, muscle size, and possible optic nerve compression that can be used for comparative purposes later.

Tallstedt et al. (132) studied 168 patients with Graves' hyperthyroidism divided into age group 1 (20 to 34 years; $n = 54$ patients) and age group 2 (35 to 55 years; $n = 114$ patients). The patients in group 1 were randomly assigned to receive either methimazole treatment for 18 months or subtotal thyroidectomy, while those in group 2 were to receive either of these two treatments or, alternatively, ^{131}I therapy. All patients were studied for at least 24 months. During the period of evaluation, ophthalmopathy developed for the first time in 22 patients (13%) and worsened in 8 patients (5%). The likelihood of the development or worsening of ophthalmopathy was comparable among the patients in group 1 (medical therapy, 15%, and surgery, 11%). In group 2, ophthalmopathy developed or worsened in 10% of patients treated medically, in 16% treated surgically, and in 33% of patients treated with [131]I ($p = 0.02$).

Bartalena (133) studied 443 patients with Graves' hyperthyroidism that had either no ophthalmopathy or minimal disease. Patients were randomly assigned to receive radioiodine, radioiodine followed by a 3-month course of prednisone, or methimazole for 18 months. The initial dose of prednisone was 0.4 to 0.5 mg/kg/day starting 2 to 3 days after ^{131}I therapy and continuing for 1 month. The dose was tapered and discontinued after 2 months. Patients were followed closely biochemically and clinically for 12 months. In patients treated with radioiodine alone ($n = 150$), ophthalmopathy developed or worsened in 15% within 6 months after treatment. No patient in this group had an improvement in ophthalmopathy. In marked contrast, in the group treated with radioiodine and prednisone, 50 of the 75 (67%) with ophthalmopathy at baseline had improvement, and no patient had progression. Of the 148 patients treated with methimazole, 3 (2%) who had ophthalmopathy at baseline improved, 4 (3%) had worsening of eye disease, and the remaining 141 had no change. These data clearly show that prednisone therapy can help prevent radioiodine-associated deterioration in ophthalmopathy. Ideally, glucocorticoid therapy should be considered as a team decision among the patient, endocrinologist, and ophthalmologist.

Taking into account various regimens in the literature, one reasonable approach in patients with mild–moderate ophthalmopathy is to administer prednisone in doses of 40 to 60 mg prednisone daily starting several days prior to or on the day of ^{131}I therapy and continuing for several weeks, trying to taper the drug completely by 6 to 8 weeks (39). Corticosteroid therapy is reserved for patients with mild or moderate ophthalmopathy, and lower doses (e.g., 0.2–0.3 mg/kg of prednisone) may be effective in patients with mild disease (39, 135). Recent American Thyroid Association guidelines recommend against using radioiodine therapy in patients with active moderate to severe ophthalmopathy (39). Tallstedt et al. noted that the initial serum T3 level was an independent risk factor for the development of ophthalmopathy and that post-ablative hypothyroidism should be avoided (136). Bartelena et al. (137) also showed that cigarette smoking was a potent independent risk factor for the worsening of ophthalmopathy after radioiodine therapy, and patients with Graves' disease who smoke should be advised to discontinue. Whether cigarette smokers without eye disease should be treated with glucocorticoids after radioiodine has not been studied, and ATA guidelines make no recommendation in this situation (39). To complicate matters, a randomized trial showed that radioiodine therapy was capable of inducing eye disease in patients presenting without clinical findings (138). In this report, 18% (23 of 131) of patients treated with methimazole had development of ophthalmopathy compared to 38% (53 0f 141) of radioiodine-treated patients. Although for the most part, the eye disease was mild, this study indicates that even patients without clinical eye involvement need to be informed about the increased risk of eye disease developing following radioiodine therapy, especially if they are cigarette smokers.

Radioiodine and cancer

A number of older studies have failed to show a definitive causal relationship between radioiodine therapy for hyperthyroidism and the subsequent development of thyroid cancer, leukemia, or other malignancies. For example, Ron et al. (139) retrospectively analyzed 35,593 hyperthyroid patients (91% had Graves' disease) who had been treated with radioiodine, antithyroid drugs, or surgery between 1946 and 1954. Some 65% of these patients were treated with radioactive iodine, thus allowing long-term comparison of results between various therapeutic modalities. When studied in December 1990, about half of the patients had died. The total number of cancer deaths in all hyperthyroid patients was comparable in patients treated with radioactive iodine and those treated with surgery or antithyroid agents, although there was a slight excess of cancer-related mortality from lung, breast, kidney, and thyroid. Starting at least 1 year after treatment, an enhanced risk of cancer mortality was also seen in hyperthyroid patients treated with antithyroid drugs. After more than 5 years following therapy, radioactive iodine therapy was associated with an increased risk of thyroid cancer mortality, but only in patients with toxic multinodular goiter. Overall, the risk of thyroid cancer in patients treated with radioactive iodine resulted from a small absolute excess in actual patient deaths.

Franklyn et al. (140) suggested that ^{131}I therapy was associated with a higher incidence of thyroid cancer. They retrospectively studied 7417 patients treated in Birmingham, England, with radioiodine for Graves' disease. On analyzing 72,073 person-years of follow-up, 634 cancer diagnoses were found as compared with an expected number of 761. The relative risk of cancer mortality was also decreased, and incidence of cancers of the pancreas, bronchus, trachea, bladder, and lymphatic and hematopoietic systems was decreased. However, there were significant increases in incidence and mortality for cancers of the small bowel and thyroid, although the absolute risk of these cancers was small. In this English study, the goal of radioiodine therapy had been euthyroidism rather than hypothyroidism. The destruction of all residual thyroid tissue would be expected to lessen the possibility of thyroid cancer. In another population-based study of 3888 patients treated for hyperthyroidism, there was no increase in cancer mortality over 8 years of follow up, but the method of treatment was not specified (141). In a similar study of 2973 patients treated with radioiodine with a 9-year follow-up, there was an increase in overall and cancer mortality (adjusted RR 1.36; 95% CI 1.12–1.65), mainly due to cancer of the stomach, kidney, and breast, chiefly in elderly patients with nodular thyroid disease rather than Graves' disease (142). However, in another larger case control study from the same group, comparing cancer incidence among patients with hyperthyroidism treated with either surgery or radioiodine versus matched controls, there was no difference (143).

THYROIDECTOMY FOR GRAVES' DISEASE

A total or near total thyroidectomy is also a reasonable therapeutic option for selected patients with Graves' disease (39, 144, 145). This therapy is generally reserved for patients who are not well controlled on or allergic to antithyroid agents and do not want radioiodine therapy; who have a particular reason for surgery—for example, a very large goiter, co-existing hyperparathyroidism, a thyroid nodule with suspicious aspirate; and those who prefer this therapy after a careful consideration of each option. Thyroidectomy must be performed by an experienced thyroid surgeon, although there is still a risk of temporary or permanent hypocalcemia secondary to injury of the parathyroid glands. Hoarseness also may occur as a result of injury to the recurrent laryngeal nerve (146). These two serious complications occur in approximately 1% of patients treated surgically (147). Vitamin D status should be checked preoperatively and replenished in the case of deficiency, since this is a risk factor for postoperative hypocalcemia (39). In most

circumstances, a euthyroid state should be established prior to surgery with antithyroid agents, although more rapid preparation with beta-adrenergic blocking drugs and SSKI has been used as well (148). SSKI (10 drops three times a day) given daily for 10 days prior to surgery has been shown to decrease intraoperative blood loss in two randomized trials (149, 150) and may decrease complication rates (151). If there is no immediate need for surgery, antithyroid drug therapy is probably safer, as postoperative fever and tachycardia more commonly develop after preparation with beta blockers alone or with SSKI (152).

Rapid preparation of patients for surgery is occasionally necessary. In one series of ten patients with significant hyperthyroidism and antithyroid drug–induced agranulocytosis, beta blocking drugs, SSKI, and glucocorticoids have been successfully used to prepare patients for surgery (153). Cholestyramine has also been used to rapidly lower thyroid hormone levels in this setting (154). Despite optimal care, perioperative thyroid storm may still occur, and patients should be treated aggressively if signs or symptoms are present (155). Obviously, patients become hypothyroid immediately following surgery and require lifelong thyroxine therapy. Levothyroxine at a dose of 1.6 mcg/kg should be started on discharge from the hospital; slightly lower doses are appropriate for the elderly.

CHOICE OF THERAPY FOR GRAVES' DISEASE: SUMMARY

Antithyroid drugs are a reasonable choice for first-line therapy in patients with small goiters and mild disease or in those whose TSI levels are normal. Also, children and adolescents are traditionally treated initially with antithyroid drugs. Because of concern that radioiodine can worsen underlying ophthalmopathy, some clinicians recommend antithyroid drugs or surgery in patients with significant eye disease, even when the biochemical abnormalities are more severe. In the future, costs may become more important in the management of hyperthyroidism. In studies that examined costs of care, radioiodine therapy was the least expensive alternative compared to antithyroid drugs and surgery (156, 157). Computer-simulated cost-effectiveness analyses reached the same conclusion, with antithyroid drug therapy also being cost-effective (158, 159). Patient satisfaction is also an important outcome that has only recently been studied. In the one report in which it was measured, antithyroid drugs, radioiodine, and surgery were equal in terms of patient satisfaction, whether a particular therapy would be recommended to friends or relatives, and in patients' concern about possible side effects (160). Patient involvement in the decision-making process is critical to improved satisfaction with therapy (52, 161).

Treatment of Graves' ophthalmopathy and pretibial myxedema

Although almost all patients with Graves' disease have radiologic evidence of eye muscle involvement, only approximately 30 percent of patients have obvious clinical disease (162). Several different methods for assessing disease severity have been described, but none of the classifications are perfect. The "NOSPECS" classification is still in wide use today (Table 2.4a), as is the Clinical Activity Score, which is more quantitative (Table 2.4b) (163). In general, the most common symptoms are related to soft tissue swelling due to orbital congestion, with irritation, tearing, burning, and a gritty sensation in the eyes. Diplopia is a more unusual and debilitating problem, and only rarely is vision threatened because of corneal exposure or optic nerve involvement. Symptoms and cosmetic concerns also significantly impact negatively on the quality of life of affected patients (164).

The symptoms and signs of Graves' ophthalmopathy are due to orbital inflammation, with the extraocular muscles and/or retro-orbital fibroblasts being the target of the autoimmune reaction (165–166). Glycosaminoglycans produced by fibroblasts responding to T-cell infiltration cause edema of the extraocular muscles, and further expansion of the retro-orbital tissues is due to increased orbital fat (168). Ultimately, fibrosis of the extraocular muscles can lead to diplopia, and severe enlargement of the muscles can cause an ischemic optic neuropathy due to compression of the optic nerve as it exits the apex of the orbit.

The primary autoimmune target in Graves' ophthalmopathy is unknown but probably is a cross-reacting antigen or antigens that are present in both in the orbit and the thyroid gland. The TSH receptor has been hypothesized to be the putative common antigen. TSH receptor

Table 2.4a "NO SPECS" classification of eye changes of Graves' disease

Class	Definition
O	No physical signs or symptoms
I	Only signs, no symptoms (e.g., upper lid retraction, stare, and eyelid lag)
II	Soft tissue involvement (symptoms and signs)
III	Proptosis
IV	Extraocular muscle involvement
V	Corneal involvement
VI	Sight loss (optic nerve involvement)

Adapted from Werner SC. Modification of the classification of the eye changes of Graves' disease: Recommendations of the Ad Hoc Committee of the American Thyroid Association. *J. Clin. Endocrinol. Metab.* 1977; 44: 203–4.

Table 2.4b Clinical activity score to assess thyroid eye disease

Clinical activity score	
Pain	Painful feeling behind the globe
	Pain on attempted up-, side-, or downward gaze
Redness	Redness of the eyelids
	Diffuse redness of the conjunctivae
Swelling	Chemosis
	Swelling of the caruncle
	Edema of the eyelids
	Increase in proptosis of ≥2 mm in 3 months
Impaired Function	Decrease in visual acuity or decrease in eye movements over 1–3 months

Each sign gets 1 point. The Clinical Activity Score is the sum of all the points.
Adapted from Mourits MP, Koornneef L, Wiersinga WM, Prummel MF, Berghout A, van der Gaag R. Clinical criteria for the assessment of disease activity in Graves' ophthalmopathy: A novel approach. *Br. J. Ophthalmol.* 1989; 73: 639–44.

transcripts have been isolated from extraocular muscle using polymerase chain reaction (PCR) (169) and TSH receptor protein has been identified in orbital tissues (170). Further, autoantibodies directed against TSH receptor or the insulin-like growth factor-1 (IGF-1) receptor may play a role in the development or progression of Graves' ophthalmopathy (171).

Since the cause of Graves' ophthalmopathy is unknown, treatment is directed at treating symptoms. In most patients, the problem is self-limited, often resolving as the hyperthyroidism is treated. Although most experts feel that it is best for the patient to be euthyroid, there is no consistent relationship between a patient's thyroid function and progression or regression of eye disease. There is good evidence that smoking exacerbates Graves' ophthalmopathy (172), and it is suggested that smoking cessation has a beneficial effect (173). The mechanism by which smoking affects Graves' ophthalmopathy is unknown. There is solid evidence that radioactive iodine therapy can exacerbate Graves' eye disease when it is moderately severe at baseline (130, 131), likely due to the increase in TRAb levels after treatment (39). When the condition is mild, symptoms such as irritation, tearing, and photophobia are easily treated with artificial tears and lubricating eye ointments. In more severe cases, high doses of glucocorticoids usually will result in prompt improvement in local symptoms and ocular motility. Data from randomized clinical trials have shown that intravenous pulse therapy with methylprednisolone is more effective and safer than high-dose oral therapy (174, 175). One commonly used regimen is methylprednisolone 500 mg IV weekly for 6 weeks followed by 250 mg IV for 6 weeks, which resulted in a 77% response rate and minimal toxicity (176). Unfortunately, as the glucocorticoid is tapered, the ophthalmopathy often flares up, so that other measures are sometimes needed.

In patients with persistent moderate to severe eye disease, orbital radiotherapy is usually the next step after glucocorticoid therapy (177). Treatment typically entails administering 200 cGy over 14 days for a total of 2000 Gy. Although somewhat controversial, orbital radiotherapy has been shown to be effective in several studies, including a randomized prospective trial in which half of the patients received sham irradiation (178). In this study, 60% of irradiated patients improved versus 31% of sham-irradiated patients. However, Gorman et al. (179) also performed a prospective, randomized, double-masked, internally controlled, clinical trial of external beam radiotherapy for patients with mild to moderate Graves' ophthalmopathy. When analyzed 6–12 months after

orbital radiation, there was no apparent clinical benefit identified. Subsequent systematic reviews of the literature have concluded that orbital radiotherapy may provide benefit, especially for diplopia, and that it is more effective when combined with glucocorticoid therapy, rather than as a standalone treatment (181–183). In general, orbital radiation is considered to be safe, although there may be an increased risk of retinopathy in patients with diabetes (183). Some experts recommend radiotherapy plus steroids earlier in the course of thyroid eye disease, in that it may permit earlier withdrawal of glucocorticoid therapy.

Patients who fail radiation therapy may require surgical decompression of the orbit if there is rapidly progressive visual loss due to optic neuropathy, steroid dependence, or continuing ocular motility problems. Surgery is also indicated to correct self-perceived cosmetic problems, particularly in patients with severe proptosis or lid retraction. Unfortunately, orbital decompression often results in more significant ocular motility problems that then require additional strabismus surgery for correction (184). There are a variety of surgical procedures, including transorbital and transantral (transmaxillary) approaches, but there is no consensus about the relative merits of one approach over the other.

More specific pharmacologic therapies for Graves' ophthalmopathy have been studied. There has been great interest in selenium supplementation since the publication of a report from Italy of a masked randomized controlled trial of selenium 100 mcg twice a day versus placebo for 6 months in mild thyroid eye disease (185). In this study, selenium therapy significantly improved ophthalmopathy scores and quality of life compared to placebo. The proposed underlying rationale is selenium's role as an antioxidant and free radical scavenger, decreasing oxidative stress to orbital fibroblasts (186). However, it is unclear whether selenium supplementation will benefit persons who do not live in relative selenium-deficient geographical areas, such as the United States (187). Rituximab, a mouse-human monoclonal antibody directed against the CD 20 antigen on B lymphocytes, has been shown to be effective versus glucocorticoids in one randomized trial (188) but not effective versus a placebo in another similarly designed trial (189). It has been hypothesized by Salvi et al. (190) that the difference in outcomes between the two trials might be explained by the younger age, lower levels of TRAb, and shorter duration of disease in the trial. Recently, favorable results were reported from a randomized placebo-controlled trial of the IGF-1 receptor blocking drug teprotumumab (191). Other potential targets in the treatment of thyroid eye disease include anti-interleukin-6 antibodies and somatostatin analogs (192).

The cause of pretibial myxedema remains obscure (193), but it probably shares common features with Graves' ophthalmopathy, including lymphocytic infiltration and a response by fibroblasts to the subsequent inflammation. The usual treatment is topical steroid cream with or without occlusion (194). Intralesional steroids have also been used, but in general glucocorticoid therapy has been ineffective (195). There are case reports of plasmapheresis being effective, combined with immunosuppressive therapy (196), as well as case reports of rituximab having efficacy in severe "elephantine" pretibial myxedema (197, 198).

SUBCLINICAL HYPERTHYROIDISM

Subclinical hyperthyroidism is a term generally utilized to describe patients with normal serum total and FT4 and T3 levels and a decreased serum TSH level (199). A recent consensus panel has published useful guidelines for approaching and treating patients with subclinical hyperthyroidism (200). This group classified subclinical hyperthyroidism into Grade 1, with serum TSH levels between 0.1 mU/l and 0.4 mU/l, and Grade 2, with serum TSH level 0.1 mU/l. This may have relevance, since lower serum TSH levels reflect higher levels of serum FT4 and T3, albeit within their respective reference ranges (201). The serum TSH level should be measured in a third-generation assay that is capable of discriminating degrees of low values, and the patient must not be taking or receiving any medications known to alter the hypothalamic–pituitary axis (such as corticosteroids and dopamine). High-dose biotin ingestion (5–10 mg a day) can result in falsely low serum TSH levels in some assays (202). TSH can be suppressed in the first trimester of some pregnant patients and the patient must have a normal pituitary–thyroid axis. In addition, serum TSH levels may be below the traditional reference range in some healthy persons of African descent (203). Further, the patient must be relatively healthy, without

serious systemic diseases, since the "euthyroid sick syndrome" may lower the serum TSH level. The patient with subclinical hyperthyroidism typically does not have significant signs or symptoms of hyperthyroidism, such as weight loss, nervousness, or palpitations (204). Some of the signs and symptoms of overt hyperthyroidism are vague and nonspecific and it may be difficult to determine if a patient is really asymptomatic (205). In a young patient with subclinical hyperthyroidism due to Graves' disease, the thyroid is either not palpable or mildly enlarged, but a multinodular goiter is often palpable in older patients with multinodular goiters. When patients with known thyroid disease are excluded, the incidence of subclinical hyperthyroidism is estimated to be about 2% (196) and is higher in iodine-deficient populations (206).

Sawin et al. (207) first determined that low serum thyrotropin concentrations are a risk factor for subsequent atrial fibrillation. Subsequent larger population-based studies have confirmed the strong relationship between subclinical hyperthyroidism and atrial fibrillation, as well as other adverse cardiovascular outcomes such as congestive heart failure and cardiac mortality (208–210). Some studies have shown that postmenopausal women with subclinical hyperthyroidism have lower bone mineral density as compared with age-matched control women, and recent meta-analyses have shown that there is a higher risk of fractures in older persons with subclinical hyperthyroidism (211, 212). Subclinical hyperthyroidism may progress to overt hyperthyroidism, in which the serum FT4 and/or T3 levels are above normal. The rate of recurrence depends on the baseline serum TSH: it is relatively low when the serum TSH is between 0.1 and 0.4 (about 0.7% over 7 years) (213), but it is higher (about 20% over 3 years) when the serum TSH is fully suppressed (214). The etiology of the subclinical hyperthyroidism also influences the risk of progression, with the risk being higher in patients with Graves' disease compared to those with a toxic multinodular goiter (215).

Diagnosis

The evaluation of a patient with subclinical hyperthyroidism may vary among physicians, but a reasonable approach in a typical asymptomatic patient is to perform a complete history and physical examination, ensure the thyroid function tests are measured in appropriately sensitive assays, and repeat the thyroid function tests monthly or every other month for 3–6 months. Thyroid function tests should include FT4 and FT3, since occasionally the free hormone levels may be increased disproportionately compared to the total hormone levels (216). If atrial fibrillation, cardiovascular disease, or other significant medical illnesses are present, earlier diagnosis and treatment are appropriate, so it is recommended to repeat thyroid function tests over a shorter period of time, such as 2 weeks. The suppressed TSH level may represent the initial manifestations of hyperthyroidism that will evolve into a more overt form over the ensuing months. Alternatively, the suppressed TSH may be transient and return to the normal range, as a suppressed TSH could represent an episode of transient thyroiditis (217). If this were correct, the TSH would be expected to return to normal within three months. Therefore, to ensure the stability of the laboratory tests and help exclude the possibility of a laboratory error, thyroid function tests are determined periodically prior to further evaluation. However, after stability in TSH levels is demonstrated, studies to determine the etiology of the mild thyroid dysfunction should be performed, including thyroid ultrasound, a radioactive iodine uptake and scan, and to consider measuring TSH receptor antibody levels (218). A thyroid sonogram may be useful to quantitate thyroid gland size and to determine the presence and characteristics of thyroid nodules. Frequently, the radioactive iodine uptake is at the upper range of normal or slightly higher, and TSAbs are also minimally elevated or normal, reflecting the minimal degree of hyperthyroidism. The radioactive iodine uptake is measured not only to assess the level of thyroidal activity but also to exclude painless thyroiditis.

Treatment

Unfortunately, there are no large randomized trials that examine the potential benefits of treating subclinical hyperthyroidism. Mudde et al. (219) and Faber et al. (220) showed a benefit of antithyroid drug therapy or radioiodine therapy on bone density values in patients with subclinical hyperthyroidism. Buscemi et al. showed that restoration of euthyroidism with antithyroid agents had a favorable effect on cardiac and bone parameters

(221). Once the tests are shown to be consistent with persistent subclinical hyperthyroidism, treatment options must be discussed. The first option is simply to continue to monitor the patient and thyroid levels indefinitely. This is a reasonable option in some patients, especially young premenopausal women and young men with Grade 1 subclinical hyperthyroidism. However, treatment is recommended by most experts, despite the absence of high-quality evidence of benefit, for older patients, especially those with serum TSH levels <0.1 mU/l (Grade 2 subclinical hyperthyroidism) because of the risk of progression to overt hyperthyroidism, osteoporosis and fractures, and atrial fibrillation (39, 193, 211) Since there are data supporting the idea that atrial fibrillation is more likely in patients aged >65 with Grade 1 subclinical hyperthyroidism (201), treatment should be considered in this age group if the TSH is persistently only mildly suppressed (193). The treatment should be directed toward the underlying etiology of the thyroid dysfunction: antithyroid drugs or radioiodine in patients with Graves' disease and radioiodine for patients with thyroid nodular disease. Surgery would also be an option in patients with very large goiters or who have suspicious thyroid nodules (193). Detailed randomized prospective studies are required regarding all aspects of subclinical hyperthyroidism to allow a more evidence-based approach to these patients.

THYROID STORM

The term *thyroid storm* refers to severe and exaggerated symptoms and signs of hyperthyroidism, usually in association with tachycardia, fever, diarrhea, vomiting, dehydration, disorientation, or mental confusion (206, 267). Patients usually experience severe restlessness and anxiety and may be unable to reason. There is a continuum between "routine" hyperthyroidism and thyroid storm, and different observers may vary in their definition of thyroid storm. There are generally accepted criteria for the diagnosis of thyroid storm (Table 2.5) (222, 223). Thyroid function tests—for example, FT4 and FT3—overlap between routine hyperthyroidism and thyroid storm, and mean values are similar in most studies (224). Lower socioeconomic status and lack of access to medical care may be another important predisposing factor (225).

Thyroid storm is typically precipitated by a specific event, such as surgery (especially patients

Table 2.5 Point scale for the diagnosis of thyroid storm (223)

Criteria points	Points	Criteria	Points
Thermoregulatory dysfunction		**Gastrointestinal–hepatic dysfunction**	
Temperature (°F)[a]		**Manifestation**	
99.0–99.9	5	Absent	0
100.0–100.9	10	Moderate (diarrhea, abdominal pain, nausea/vomiting)	10
101.0–101.9	15	Severe (jaundice)	20
102.0–102.9	20		
103.0–103.9	25		
≥104.0	30		
		Central nervous system disturbance	
Cardiovascular		**Manifestation**	
Tachycardia (beats per minute)		Absent	0
100–109	5	Mild (agitation)	10
110–119	10	Moderate (delirium, psychosis, extreme lethargy)	20
120–129	15	Severe (seizure, coma)	30
130–139	20		
≥140	25		
		Precipitant history	
Atrial fibrillation		**Status**	
Absent	0	Positive	10
Present	10	Negative	0
Congestive heart failure			
Absent	0		
Mild	5		
Moderate	10		
Severe	20		

Scores totaled: >45 Thyroid storm, 25–45 Impending storm, <25 storm unlikely.

[a] Celsius 37.2–37.7 (5), 37.8–38.3 (10), 38.3–38.8 (15), 38.9–39.4 (20), 39.4–39.9 (25), ≥40 (30 points).

having thyroid surgery without adequate preparation), severe systemic illness (e.g., pneumonia, pharyngitis), or parturition. It is important to prevent thyroid storm whenever possible by trying to predict circumstances in which it may occur. It is preferable, in general, to treat patients as if they had thyroid storm when it is suspected, rather than to delay therapy in the hope that thyroid storm will not develop or become fully manifest.

Treatment (Table 2.6)

Patients should be treated with antithyroid agents to restore euthyroidism prior to anticipated stressful events, such as surgery. As noted earlier, hyperthyroid patients should be prepared with antithyroid medications for several weeks prior to thyroidectomy. Treatment for a patient with severe thyrotoxicosis or thyroid storm should be more aggressive than that for a patient with less severe thyroid dysfunction (226). The doses of medications are higher in patients considered to have thyroid storm. Propylthiouracil, 100 to 200 mg q4h, or methimazole, 10 to 20 mg q4h, is recommended in conjunction with propranolol, 60 to 80 mg q8h. In unusual circumstances when patients cannot be administered oral medication effectively, propylthiouracil or methimazole can be given rectally or intravenously (227, 228). Due to the rarity of the condition, there are no randomized trials comparing PTU and methimazole in thyroid storm, but PTU has a theoretical

Table 2.6 Drugs used to treat thyroid storm

Drug class	Recommended drug	Dose	Mechanism of action
Beta-adrenergic blockers	Propranolol	40–80 mg po tid–qid	• Beta-adrenergic blockade • Decreased T4 to T3 conversion with high-dose propranolol
	Esmolol	50–100 mcg/kg/min	
Thionamides	Propylthiouracil	200 mg po q 4 h	• Inhibition of hormone synthesis • Decreased T4 to T3 conversion
	Methimazole	20 mg po q 4 h	Inhibition of hormone synthesis
Iodine	SSKI	2 drops po q 8 h	• Inhibition of hormone synthesis • Decreased release of thyroid hormone
	Lugol's solution	3–5 drops po q 8 h	
Glucocorticoids	Dexamethasone	2 mg po or IV q 6 h	• Improved vasomotor stability • Decreased T4 to T3 conversion
	Hydrocortisone	100 mg po or IV q 8 h	
Bile acid-binding resin	Cholestyramine	4 gm po q 6 h	Interference with enterohepatic circulation and reabsorption of thyroid hormones

advantage since it blocks T4 to T3 conversion (47). Propranolol can also be given intravenously (2–5 mg every 4 hours), and if there is a history of pulmonary disease, esmolol, at a dose of 50–100 μg/kg/min can be used. Hydrocortisone at 100 mg q8h is added to ensure adequate adrenal function, and an iodine-containing agent may also be employed. An intravenous preparation of sodium iodide is not available. Oral saturated solution of potassium iodide, 5 drops three times a day (tid), or Lugol's solution, 5 drops tid, contain sufficient iodine to reduce thyroid production and secretion of T4 and T3, and their effects can be seen within several days. Cholestyramine (or colestipol) administration can be effective as adjunctive therapy to lower serum thyroid hormone levels, as it decreases the enterohepatic circulation of T4 and T3 (229). Care must be exercised to separate the interval between the administration of cholestyramine (and colestipol) and other oral medications. Plasma exchange has also proven useful in refractory cases (230).

SOLITARY TOXIC NODULES

Introduction

A solitary autonomous thyroid nodule produces sufficient thyroid hormone to suppress TSH and cause overt or subclinical hyperthyroidism (231). Often, a thyroid nodule may be autonomous and not yet be sufficiently functional to suppress serum TSH. The capacity to secrete thyroid hormones varies with the size of the thyroid nodule, and those that are >3 cm in size are much more likely to produce hyperthyroidism (232). The percentage of autonomous nodules that secrete sufficient thyroid hormones to produce overt hyperthyroidism is relatively low, in the range of 30% (232).

Pathology

Histologically, autonomous nodules are cellular follicular lesions with frequent hemorrhage, fibrosis, calcification, and cysts. There is a dense fibrous capsule. The vast majority of solitary autonomous thyroid nodules are benign. In adults, as many as several percent of these nodules contain foci of papillary thyroid cancer, whereas in children and adolescents, the percentage of autonomous nodules that contain thyroid cancer is likely higher (e.g., 233). A fine needle aspiration biopsy of the nodule should be performed if there is any suspicion of cancer based on clinical, historical, sonographic, or laboratory studies. For example, the presence of associated cervical lymphadenopathy, recent growth (which could simply represent hemorrhage), or a history of neck radiation may increase the suspicion for associated cancer. The type of thyroid cancer found in this circumstance is usually papillary thyroid cancer, although other types, such as follicular or Hürthle cell cancer (234) may be identified. Earlier studies suggested that cytologists would read aspirates from autonomous nodules as suspicious for follicular thyroid cancer, given the cellular nature of these nodules. However, subsequent analyses show that the fine needle aspirations are rarely confusing and that the majority of autonomous nodules yield benign cells in the presence of colloid.

Pathogenesis

Autonomous function of the nodule is attributed to either a loss in suppression of normal cell function or a genetic defect in the TSH receptor or a downstream pathway (e.g., G protein), causing excess stimulation of the thyroid cell and unregulated thyroid hormone production. The majority of solitary autonomous thyroid nodule tissue contains mutations in the TSH receptor protein or, less often, in the stimulatory G protein (235). Several different mutations in the TSH receptor gene and the resultant mutated protein are associated with cAMP-dependent transcription independent of the presence of TSH. Mutated receptors retain a significant response to TSH stimulation, although it is decreased when compared to normal thyrocytes. The G_s protein regulates cell growth; when it becomes mutated, this protein acts as an oncogene, leading to abnormal cellular regulation. G_s mutations have been found in approximately 5% to 30% of toxic thyroid nodules (226).

Clinical considerations

It has traditionally been thought that autonomous thyroid nodules were a relatively unusual form of hyperthyroidism (223). However, in a recent epidemiological study from Sweden, patients with solitary toxic thyroid nodules accounted for 15% of all hyperthyroid patients (6). Patients with autonomous functioning thyroid nodules present most frequently with a neck mass but may also have subclinical hyperthyroidism. Overt symptoms of hyperthyroidism are uncommon. The frequency of toxic adenomas increases with age, and only about half of patients with autonomous nodules over the age of 60 years manifest clinical signs or symptoms of hyperthyroidism. Autonomous nodules are much more common in women. Patients with an autonomous nodule larger than 3 cm have approximately a 20% chance of progressing to overt hyperthyroidism over several years, with smaller lesions having a much lower progression rate (232). Toxic nodules may undergo cystic or necrotic degeneration with return to euthyroidism, and as many as 20% to 30% patients with solitary autonomous nodules may have a restoration of normal function secondary to hemorrhage (223). Iodine deficiency increases the risk of iodine-induced hyperthyroidism in patients with autonomous thyroid nodules. Even a small addition of iodine, perhaps 100 µg/day, to a low-iodine diet can initiate hyperthyroidism (236). Although iodine deficiency is not a problem in the United States, hyperthyroidism has been reported in patients with autonomous thyroid nodules within 1 to 2 months after exposure to radiocontrast dyes (237), as well as after exposure to iodine-containing drugs such as amiodarone (238).

Diagnosis

Autonomous thyroid nodules are usually diagnosed by integration of the history and physical exam with laboratory and nuclear medicine testing. The serum TSH level is usually suppressed and is often unmeasurable. Free/total T4 and T3 are usually normal or slightly elevated but may vary depending upon nodule size and iodine exposure. Preferential T3 secretion—that is, T3 toxicosis—may be more common in patients with autonomous nodules than in Graves' disease (239). The identification of an autonomous nodule on technetium-99m or radioiodine scintigraphic scanning is the sine qua non of the diagnosis. When a radionuclide scan is performed, the solitary autonomous thyroid nodule represents the only tissue that appears to be trapping the radioactive tracer with the remainder of the thyroid tissue being suppressed. However, an abnormal thyroid scan alone does not prove autonomous function, since there are technical factors that could make a dominant nodule appear to be the sole area that traps radioactive material. When an autonomous thyroid nodule is suspected, it may be appropriate to use radioiodine rather than technetium as the diagnostic agent. Occasionally, a nodule may appear to be "hot" with technetium, when it is actually a "cold" nodule with radioiodine. This discordance is thought to relate to the ability of iodine to be trapped and organified by thyroid tissue, whereas technetium can only be trapped.

Treatment

Therapeutic decisions regarding autonomous nodules depend upon a variety of factors, including patient age, the severity of hyperthyroidism, and associated medical conditions such as coronary artery disease and/or a history of cardiac arrhythmias. Patients with overt hyperthyroidism in the presence of an undetectable TSH and elevated FT4 and T3 should be treated. Older patients with undetectable TSH and normal FT4 and T3 should be strongly considered for treatment because of possible deleterious effects on bone metabolism and the heart (see section on Subclinical Hyperthyroidism). More controversial is whether young patients with subclinical hyperthyroidism or people with nodules >3 cm in diameter should be treated prophylactically. Some patients desire treatment for cosmetic reasons.

The most important therapeutic option is radioactive iodine ablation of the toxic adenoma. Radioactive iodine concentrates in the autonomous nodule and may accumulate in extranodular tissue, albeit to a much lesser extent. Although results are variable—based upon the size of the nodule, nodule uptake, dose administered, and tissue radiation sensitivity—a typical toxic nodule will shrink approximately 40% within 1 year following an ablative dose. Radioactive iodine ablation of an autonomous thyroid nodule may decrease the ability of that nodule to secrete excess thyroid hormones; but the nodule itself, although functionally inactive, may remain and must be monitored clinically over time by physical examination or ultrasound (223). The beneficial effects of radioiodine may not be maximal until 4 to 12 months after therapy. Thyroid function may normalize or decrease to below the normal range in this time period, but the nodule may still be palpable in perhaps half the patients. Occasionally, a second or even a third dose of radioiodine is required to render a patient euthyroid. It is recommended to wait at least 6 months after the initial dose before considering retreatment with radioiodine.

Following radioiodine therapy, hypothyroidism occurs at an average rate of approximately 10% within the first year, with an annual rate thereafter

of about 3% (240). This occurrence rate may relate to the fact that the contralateral normal tissue is exposed to significant amounts of radiation (241). Underlying autoimmune thyroid disease may also predispose to the development of hypothyroidism. Larger doses of ^{131}I appear to be a causative factor in studies finding a substantial rate of hypothyroidism. The dose per gram of thyroid tissue, percent of radioactive iodine uptake, and pre- and/or posttreatment with antithyroid medications (which might normalize the serum TSH, resulting in increased uptake by the contralateral lobe), all may affect the outcome. In general, higher activities are associated with more prompt achievement of euthyroidism or hypothyroidism. In a prospective randomized trial of differing regimens of radioiodine therapy, 97 patients were divided into 4 groups: high (22.5mCi) or low (13mCi) fixed activity versus a calculated activity that was either high (180–200 µCi/g) or low (90–100 µCi/g) and corrected for 24-hour RAIU and thyroid weight, yielding administered activities of 18.7 mCi and 10.5 mCi, respectively (242). All of the regimens resulted in cure of the hyperthyroidism; control of thyroid function was more rapid with the two high-activity regimens but at the cost of a higher rate of hypothyroidism which approached 60% versus 10% in patients receiving lower activities

Most studies had shown that ^{131}I is tolerated well by the majority of patients, but exacerbation of the underlying thyrotoxicosis can occur, so antithyroid drug pretreatment of elderly patients or those with comorbidities is recommended. However, normalization of the serum TSH should be avoided, as noted previously (39).

Surgery can also be performed to remove the affected lobe and isthmus, leaving the remaining uninvolved lobe intact (243). Thyroid function should be normalized prior to surgery with antithyroid drugs. Preoperative treatment with SSKI is not recommended because of the risk of exacerbating the underlying hyperthyroidism (244). Ultrasonography should be performed prior to surgery to assess the contralateral lobe for possible nodules that may require biopsy and autoimmune thyroid disease, which make postsurgical hypothyroidism more likely. In experienced hands, surgery has a low anesthetic risk and a low surgical complication rate of vocal cord paralysis and hypoparathyroidism, especially if only a lobectomy rather than a thyroidectomy is performed (234). Following surgery, thyroid function should be assessed at 6 weeks.

OTHER TREATMENT MODALITIES: PERCUTANEOUS ETHANOL INJECTION (PEI), RADIOFREQUENCY ABLATION (RFA), AND LASER THERAPY

Percutaneous ethanol injection (PEI) is an alternative therapeutic option in patients with an autonomous thyroid nodule. Ethanol (95 to 98%) is injected into the autonomous nodule using a 22-gauge needle under sonographic guidance (245, 246). Special attention is given to avoiding leakage of ethanol into the extranodular tissue, which, should it occur, may cause serious complications. Other potential complications of PEI include pain at the local injection site, dysphonia (usually transient), exacerbation of thyrotoxicosis, fever, and hematoma. Nodules >30 mL in volume are more resistant to this therapy, having almost half the cure rate of smaller nodules. Centers experienced in this modality note that approximately four to eight treatments may be required to achieve success. The total volume of ethanol delivered is usually 1½ times the nodule volume, and 1 to 8 mL is administered in weekly sessions over a 2- to 12-week time frame. A multicenter study (247) reported a success rate (defined as normalization of thyroid function) at 12 months of 83.4% and 66.5% for toxic and pretoxic adenomas, respectively. In a single center study of 125 patients treated with PEI followed for an average of 5 years, cure of hyperthyroidism and disappearance of the nodule were noted in >90% of patients. Complications occurred in 4% of patients, including transient recurrent nerve dysfunction (two patients), and abscess and hematoma (one patient each). There were four recurrences with subclinical hyperthyroidism (248). PEI is operator-dependent, requires multiple sessions, and requires more treatments with larger nodules. Also, there appears to be relatively little experience with this therapy in the United States. Therefore, its use should be limited to experienced clinicians and medical centers in selected circumstances.

Radiofrequency ablation (RFA) (249) and laser therapy (250) have also been used to treat toxic thyroid nodules. A recent systematic review and meta-analysis concluded that RFA was superior to laser therapy in terms of reduction in nodule volume (251). A retrospective study comparing outcomes in 200 patients who had undergone RFA and 200 patients who had undergone thyroid lobectomy and total thyroidectomy (for toxic multinodular goiter) found similar efficacy but more complications among patients who had undergone thyroid surgery (6% versus 1%) (252). Similar to PEI, experience with RFA and laser therapy is extremely limited in the United States. Other local procedures that are under investigation include the use of microwaves and high-intensity focused ultrasound (253).

TOXIC MULTINODULAR GOITER

Introduction

A toxic multinodular goiter is a thyroid gland that contains at least two autonomous functioning thyroid nodules that secrete excessive amounts of thyroid hormone, suppressing serum TSH and often causing typical symptoms and signs of hypermetabolism (235). These nodules may be more or less distinct on clinical examination and scan. Autonomous nodules require many years to develop and transition through a phase when the TSH is normal and then subnormal with minimal clinical evidence of hyperthyroidism (subclinical hyperthyroidism). Because of the time required for this process to develop, most patients with toxic multinodular goiter are over the age of 50 (Figure 2.7). Many clinical aspects of patients with toxic multinodular goiters are similar to those found in those with solitary autonomous nodules. For example, exogenous iodine exposure can precipitate or aggravate thyrotoxicosis (235, 254).

Pathogenesis

The pathogenesis of toxic multinodular goiter is not known, although it is believed that individual thyroid follicles preferentially proliferate. Follicular size, colloid content, and cellular characteristics vary widely in different parts of the multinodular goiter. Indeed, marked cellular variation is the hallmark of multinodular goiters. It is believed that most of these nodules are clonal in origin. It is unknown how particular nodules grow and become autonomous. The more widely held view is that several individual clones develop,

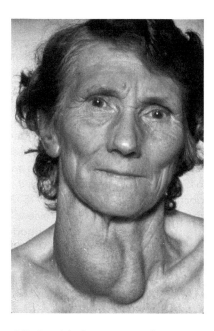

Figure 2.7 An elderly patient with a toxic multinodular goiter. It is frequently difficult to discern by clinical examination the extent of substernal extension of the thyroid gland.

perhaps related to a mutation in the TSH receptor gene, and that these cells gradually grow, become autonomous, and finally result in excess hormonal secretion (255, 256).

Diagnosis

Patients present with typical clinical and biochemical hyperthyroidism and small, medium-sized, or large multinodular goiters. There is nothing particularly unusual about their presentation, signs, or symptoms compared to patients with other causes of hyperthyroidism, except the nodules and goiter may be sufficiently large to cause local compressive symptoms. The radionuclide scan shows heterogeneous uptake with areas of hyper- and hypointensity. There is a spectrum of disease, ranging from minimal thyroid enlargement with small thyroid nodules only detected on scan or sonogram to markedly enlarged thyroid glands and large nodules. Color-flow Doppler sonography may also be useful, especially in helping to differentiate nodular variants of Graves' disease from toxic multinodular goiters that are non-autoimmune mediated (257). Some multinodular goiters have a significant substernal component.

Treatment

Radioiodine and surgery are the two major treatment modalities in patients with toxic multinodular goiters (39, 258). Because multinodular goiters are probably not responding to serum anti-TSH receptor immunoglobulins, it is not considered possible to induce a long-term remission with the chronic use of antithyroid agents. It may be appropriate to render a patient euthyroid with the use of antithyroid agents prior to radioiodine therapy, especially patients over age 60 or those with underlying heart disease. Selected patients can be maintained on these agents for an indefinite period of time—for example, elderly patients with accompanying serious medical disorders. However, this approach is applicable to a minority of patients with toxic multinodular goiters.

Radioiodine therapy is most often used to restore euthyroidism or induce hypothyroidism (114). ^{131}I therapy is generally thought to be less reliable in controlling the hyperthyroidism, compared with Graves' disease, and higher doses are usually required (approximately 20 to 30 mCi ^{131}I). The explanation for the difference in responses between Graves' disease and toxic multinodular goiter is unknown, but it probably relates to the fact that there are different degrees of autonomy and radiosensitivity among cells comprising the multinodular goiter. The dose of ^{131}I varies, but it is reasonable to attempt to deliver approximately 160 to 200 μC ^{131}I/g to the thyroid tissue. In one study, following ^{131}I treatment for a toxic multinodular goiter, 62% of patients were euthyroid, 19% hypothyroid, and 19% remained hyperthyroid. The mean size reduction overall was 32% (259). It is often difficult to estimate the size of multinodular goiters, especially because they may have a substernal component. A thyroid sonogram is helpful if the gland is cervical in location, and CT scanning (without intravenous contrast) is useful for estimating the size of a large multinodular goiter with substernal extension. Antithyroid drug pretreatment is recommended in the elderly and in patients with comorbidities (39), and such treatment has been shown to increase the 24-hour radioiodine uptake, thereby reducing the administered activity (260). A similar reduction in activity can be achieved using recombinant human TSH (rhTSH) (261). Unfortunately, rhTSH use in this clinical setting has been associated with a high frequency of post-therapy hyperthyroidism (262); therefore, its use in this clinical setting is not generally recommended, and it is not approved by the U.S. Food and Drug Administration for this indication.

It is difficult to predict the response to a given dose of ^{131}I; in one study, the cure rate was relatively similar to that seen in Graves' disease (263), but others have not found similar degrees of success (264). Release of preformed and stored thyroid hormones can occur after a dose of ^{131}I, so that these patients, who are typically older, should be carefully monitored. Not unexpectedly, smaller thyroid glands seem to respond more consistently than larger glands, although there is wide variation. Elderly patients or those with associated medical disorders or heart disease should be treated with antithyroid agents and beta blocking drugs prior to administering ^{131}I, as this is thought, but not proven, to reduce the chance of radioiodine-induced worsening of the hyperthyroidism (39). Similar to the situation with solitary toxic nodules, pretreatment with SSKI is contraindicated because of the potential for worsening of nodular hyperthyroidism (235).

A near total thyroidectomy represents an alternative therapeutic option. This procedure should be performed by an experienced thyroid surgeon (265), but even in this circumstance, there is a risk of hypocalcemia and recurrent laryngeal nerve paralysis as well as, in unusual circumstances, acute release of stored thyroid hormone, with an exacerbation of hyperthyroidism. A near total thyroidectomy is preferred to a subtotal thyroidectomy to reduce the recurrence rate (266).

Although therapy should be individualized and discussed with patients and their families as appropriate, most patients with hyperthyroidism due to a multinodular goiter should be treated with ^{131}I therapy. Antithyroid agent therapy may be useful for patients with smaller glands with less severe hyperthyroidism; long-term antithyroid agent therapy should be reserved for selected patients. Surgery addresses the problem expeditiously and can be used quite effectively; it should be considered for patients with very large thyroid glands since the likelihood of such patients responding to ^{131}I therapy is lower. Compressive symptoms such as hoarseness, superior vena cava syndrome, dysphagia, and/or dyspnea are additional indications for surgery. However, in patients who are not surgical candidates, radioiodine should be used.

REFERENCES

1. Morshed SA, Davies TF. Graves' disease mechanisms: The role of stimulating, blocking, and cleavage region TSH receptor antibodies. *Horm. Metab. Res.* 2015; 47(10): 727–34.
2. Boelaert K, Torlinska B, Holder RL, Franklyn JA. Older subjects with hyperthyroidism present with a paucity of symptoms and signs: A large cross-sectional study. *J. Clin. Endocrinol. Metab.* 2010; 95(6): 2715–26.
3. Barbesino G, Tomer Y. Clinical review: Clinical utility of TSH receptor antibodies. *J. Clin. Endocrinol. Metab.* 2013; 98(6): 2247–55.
4. Bahn RS. Graves' ophthalmopathy. *N. Engl. J. Med.* 2010; 362(8): 726–38.
5. Wiersinga WM. Advances in treatment of active, moderate-to-severe Graves' ophthalmopathy. *Lancet Diabetes Endocrinol.* 2017; 5(2): 134–42.
6. Abraham-Nordling M, Byström K, Törring O, Lantz M, Berg G, Calissendorff J, Nyström HF, et al. Incidence of hyperthyroidism in Sweden. *Eur. J. Endocrinol.* 2011; 165(6): 899–905.
7. Léger J. Management of fetal and neonatal Graves' disease. *Horm. Res. Paediatr.* 2017; 87(1): 1–6.
8. Carlé A, Krejbjerg A, Laurberg P. Epidemiology of nodular goiter. Influence of iodine intake. *Best Pract. Res. Clin. Endocrinol. Metab.* 2014; 28(4): 465–79.
9. Ferrari SM, Fallahi P, Antonelli A, Benvenga S. Environmental issues in thyroid diseases. *Front. Endocrinol. (Lausanne).* 2017; 8: 50.
10. Pastore F, Martocchia A, Stefanelli M, Prunas P, Giordano S, Toussan L, Devito A, Falaschi P. Hepatitis C virus infection and thyroid autoimmune disorders: A model of interactions between the host and the environment. *World J. Hepatol.* 2016; 8(2): 83–91.
11. Smith TJ, Hegedüs L. Graves' disease. *N. Engl. J. Med.* 2016;375(16):1552–65.
12. Jabbar A, Pingitore A, Pearce SH, Zaman A, Iervasi G, Razvi S. Thyroid hormones and cardiovascular disease. *Nat. Rev. Cardiol.* 2017; 14(1): 39–55.

13. Siu CW, Yeung CY, Lau CP, Kung AW, Tse HF. Incidence, clinical characteristics and outcome of congestive heart failure as the initial presentation in patients with primary hyperthyroidism. *Heart* 2007; 93(4): 483–7.

14. Siu CW, Zhang XH, Yung C, Kung AW, Lau CP, Tse HF. Hemodynamic changes in hyperthyroidism-related pulmonary hypertension: A prospective echocardiographic study. *J. Clin. Endocrinol. Metab.* 2007; 92(5): 1736–42.

15. Trivalle C, Doucet J, Chassagne P, Landrin I, Kadri N, Menard JF, Bercoff E. Differences in the signs and symptoms of hyperthyroidism in older and younger patients. *J. Am. Geriatr. Soc.* 1996; 44(1): 50–3.

16. Lin TY, Shekar AO, Li N, Yeh MW, Saab S, Wilson M, Leung AM. Incidence of abnormal liver biochemical tests in hyperthyroidism. *Clin. Endocrinol. (Oxf.)* 2017; 86(5): 755–9.

17. Vestergaard P, Mosekilde L. Hyperthyroidism, bone mineral, and fracture risk—A meta-analysis. *Thyroid* 2003; 13(6): 585–93.

18. Vestergaard P, Rejnmark L, Mosekilde L. Influence of hyper- and hypothyroidism, and the effects of treatment with antithyroid drugs and levothyroxine on fracture risk. *Calcif. Tissue Int.* 2005; 77(3): 139–44.

19. Ahmed LA, Schirmer H, Berntsen GK, Fonnebo V, Joakimsen RM. Self-reported diseases and the risk of non-vertebral fractures: The Tromsø study. *Osteoporos. Int.* 2006; 17(1): 46–53.

20. Abrahamsen B, Jørgensen HL, Laulund AS, Nybo M, Brix TH, Hegedüs L. Low serum thyrotropin level and duration of suppression as a predictor of major osteoporotic fractures—The OPENTHYRO register cohort. *J. Bone Miner. Res.* 2014; 29(9): 2040–50.

21. Chaudhry MA, Wayangankar S. Thyrotoxic periodic paralysis: A concise review of the literature. *Curr. Rheumatol. Rev.* 2016; 12(3): 190–4.

22. Maciel RM, Lindsey SC, Dias da Silva MR. Novel etiopathophysiological aspects of thyrotoxic periodic paralysis. *Nat. Rev. Endocrinol.* 2011; 7(11): 657–67.

23. Kung AW. Clinical review: Thyrotoxic periodic paralysis: A diagnostic challenge. *J. Clin. Endocrinol. Metab.* 2006; 91(7): 2490–5.

24. Feldman AZ, Shrestha RT, Hennessey JV. Neuropsychiatric manifestations of thyroid disease. *Endocrinol. Metab. Clin. North Am.* 2013; 42(3): 453–76.

25. Davis PJ, Rappeport JR, Lutz JH, Gregerman RI. Three thyrotoxic criminals. *Ann. Intern. Med.* 1971; 74(5): 743–5.

26. Abraham-Nordling M, Lönn S, Wallin G, Yin L, Nyren O, Tullgren O, Hall P, Törring O. Hyperthyroidism and suicide: A retrospective cohort study in Sweden. *Eur. J. Endocrinol.* 2009; 160(3): 437–41.

27. Baba M, Terada A, Hishida R, Matsunaga M, Kawabe Y, Takebe K. Persistent hemichorea associated with thyrotoxicosis. *Intern. Med.* 1992; 31(9): 1144–6.

28. Krassas GE, Poppe K, Glinoer D. Thyroid function and human reproductive health. *Endocr. Rev.* 2010; 31(5): 702–55.

29. Patel N, Kashanian JA. Thyroid dysfunction and male reproductive physiology. *Semin. Reprod. Med.* 2016; 34(6): 356–60.

30. Carani C, Isidori AM, Granata A, Carosa E, Maggi M, Lenzi A, Jannini EA. Multicenter study on the prevalence of sexual symptoms in male hypo- and hyperthyroid patients. *J. Clin. Endocrinol. Metab.* 2005; 90(12): 6472–9.

31. Dalla Costa M, Mangano FA, Betterle C. Thymic hyperplasia in patients with Graves' disease. *J. Endocrinol. Invest.* 2014; 37(12): 1175–9.

32. Hughes JW, Muegge BD, Tobin GS, Litvin M, Sun L, Saenz JB, Gyawali CP, McGill JB. High-risk gastric pathology and prevalent autoimmune diseases in patients with pernicious anemia. *Endocr. Pract.* 2017; 23(11): 1297–303.

33. Fatourechi V. Pretibial myxedema: Pathophysiology and treatment options. *Am. J. Clin. Dermatol.* 2005; 6(5): 295–309.

34. Bartalena L, Fatourechi V. Extrathyroidal manifestations of Graves' disease: A 2014 update. *J. Endocrinol. Invest.* 2014; 37(8): 691–700.

35. Trivalle C, Doucet J, Chassagne P, Landrin I, Kadri N, Menard JF, Bercoff E. Differences in the signs and symptoms of hyperthyroidism in older and younger patients. *J. Am. Geriatr. Soc.* 1996; 44(1): 50–3.

36. Figge J, Leinung M, Goodman AD, Izquierdo R, Mydosh T, Gates S, Line B, Lee DW. The clinical evaluation of patients with subclinical hyperthyroidism and free triiodothyronine (free T3) toxicosis. *Am. J. Med.* 1994; 96(3): 229–34.

37. Caplan RH, Pagliara AS, Wickus G. Thyroxine toxicosis. A common variant of hyperthyroidism. *JAMA* 1980; 244(17): 1934–8.

38. Carella C, Mazziotti G, Sorvillo F, Piscopo M, Cioffi M, Pilla P, Nersita R, et al. Serum thyrotropin receptor antibodies concentrations in patients with Graves' disease before, at the end of methimazole treatment, and after drug withdrawal: Evidence that the activity of thyrotropin receptor antibody and/or thyroid response modify during the observation period. *Thyroid* 2006;16 (3): 295–302.

39. Ross DS, Burch HB, Cooper DS, Greenlee MC, Laurberg P, Maia AL, Rivkees SA, et al. 2016 American Thyroid Association guidelines for diagnosis and management of hyperthyroidism and other causes of thyrotoxicosis. *Thyroid* 2016; 26(10): 1343–421.

40. Abeillon-du Payrat J, Chikh K, Bossard N, Bretones P, Gaucherand P, Claris O, Charrié A, et al. Predictive value of maternal second-generation thyroid-binding inhibitory immunoglobulin assay for neonatal autoimmune hyperthyroidism. *Eur. J. Endocrinol.* 2014; 171(4): 451–60.

41. Laurberg P, Wallin G, Tallstedt L, Abraham-Nordling M, Lundell G, Tørring O. TSH-receptor autoimmunity in Graves' disease after therapy with anti-thyroid drugs, surgery, or radioiodine: A 5-year prospective randomized study. *Eur. J. Endocrinol.* 2008; 158(1): 69–75.

42. Sakata S, Nakamura S, Miura K. Autoantibodies against thyroid hormones for iodothyronine: Implications in diagnosis, thyroid function, and pathogenesis. *Ann. Int. Med.* 1985; 103: 579–89.

43. Koulouri O, Moran C, Halsall D, Chatterjee K, Gurnell M. Pitfalls in the measurement and interpretation of thyroid function tests. *Best Pract. Res. Clin. Endocrinol. Metab.* 2013; 27(6): 745–62.

44. Barbesino G. Misdiagnosis of Graves' disease with apparent severe hyperthyroidism in a patient taking biotin megadoses. *Thyroid* 2016; 26(6): 860–3.

45. Ch'ng CL, Biswas M, Benton A, Jones MK, Kingham JG. Prospective screening for coeliac disease in patients with Graves' hyperthyroidism using anti-gliadin and tissue transglutaminase antibodies. *Clin. Endocrinol. (Oxf.)* 2005; 62(3): 303–6.

46. Burch HB, Burman KD, Cooper DS. A 2011 survey of clinical practice patterns in the management of Graves' disease. *J. Clin. Endocrinol. Metab.* 2012; 97(12): 4549–58.

47. Bartalena L, Burch HB, Burman KD, Kahaly GJ. A 2013 European survey of clinical practice patterns in the management of Graves' disease. *Clin. Endocrinol. (Oxf.)* 2016; 84(1): 115–20.

48. Brito JP, Schilz S, Singh Ospina N, Rodriguez-Gutierrez R, Maraka S, Sangaralingham LR, Montori VM. Antithyroid drugs-the most common treatment for Graves' disease in the United States: A nationwide population-based study. *Thyroid* 2016; 26(8): 1144–5.

49. Cooper DS. Antithyroid drugs. *N. Engl. J. Med.* 2005; 352(9): 905–17.

50. Nakamura H, Noh JY, Itoh K, Fukata S, Miyauchi A, Hamada N. Comparison of methimazole and propylthiouracil in patients with hyperthyroidism caused by Graves' disease. *J. Clin. Endocrinol. Metab.* 2007; 92(6): 2157–62.

51. Laurberg P. Remission of Graves' disease during anti-thyroid drug therapy. Time to reconsider the mechanism? *Eur. J. Endocrinol.* 2006; 155(6): 783–6.

52. Mortimer RH, Cannell GR, Addison RS, Johnson LP, Roberts MS, Bernus I. Methimazole and propylthiouracil equally cross the perfused human term placental lobule. *J. Clin. Endocrinol. Metab.* 1997; 82(9): 3099–102.

53. Momotani N, Noh JY, Ishikawa N, Ito K. Effects of propylthiouracil and methimazole on fetal thyroid status in mothers with Graves' hyperthyroidism. *J. Clin. Endocrinol. Metab.* 1997;82(11):3633–6.

54. Brito JP, Castaneda-Guarderas A, Gionfriddo MR, Ospina NS, Maraka S, Dean DS, Castro MR, et al. Development and pilot testing of an encounter tool for shared decision making about the treatment of Graves' disease. *Thyroid* 2015; 25(11): 1191–8.

55. Burch HB, Cooper DS. Management of Graves' disease: A review. *JAMA* 2015; 314(23): 2544–54.

56. Robinson J, Richardson M, Hickey J, James A, Pearce SH, Ball SG, Quinton R, et al. Patient knowledge of antithyroid drug-induced agranulocytosis. *Eur. Thyroid J.* 2014; 3(4): 245–51.

57. Abraham-Nordling M, Törring O, Hamberger B, Lundell G, Tallstedt L, Calissendorff J, Wallin G. Graves' disease: A long-term quality-of-life follow-up of patients randomized to treatment with antithyroid drugs, radioiodine, or surgery. *Thyroid* 2005;15(11): 1279–86.

58. Struja T, Fehlberg H, Kutz A, Guebelin L, Degen C, Mueller B, Schuetz P. Can we predict relapse in Graves' disease? Results from a systematic review and meta-analysis. *Eur. J. Endocrinol.* 2017; 176(1): 87–97.

59. Kawai K, Tamai H, Matsubayashi S, Mukata T, Morita T, Kubo C, Kuma K. A study of untreated Graves' patients with undetectable TSH binding inhibitor immunoglobulins and the effect of antithyroid drugs. *Clin. Endocrinol.* 1995: 551–6.

60. Pearce EN. Thyroid disorders during pregnancy and postpartum. *Best Pract. Res. Clin. Obstet. Gynaecol.* 2015; 29(5): 700–6.

61. Alexander EK, Pearce EN, Brent GA, Brown RS, Chen H, Dosiou C, Grobman WA, et al. 2017 Guidelines of the American Thyroid Association for the diagnosis and management of thyroid disease During pregnancy and the postpartum. *Thyroid* 2017; 27(3): 315–89.

62. Bahn RS, Burch HS, Cooper DS, Garber JR, Greenlee CM, Klein IL, Laurberg P, et al. The role of propylthiouracil in the management of Graves' disease in adults: Report of a meeting jointly sponsored by the American Thyroid Association and the Food and Drug Administration. *Thyroid* 2009; 19(7): 673–4.

63. Reinwein D, Benker G, Lazarus JH, Alexander WD. A prospective randomized trial of antithyroid drug dose in Graves' disease therapy. *J. Clin. Endocrinol. Metab.* 1993; 76(6): 1516–21.

64. Chen JJ, Ladenson PW. Discordant hypothyroxinemia and hypertriiodothyroninemia in treated patients with hyperthyroid Graves' disease. *J. Clin. Endocrinol. Metab.* 1986; 63(1):102–6.

65. Page SR, Sheard CE, Herbert M, Hopton M, Jeffcoate WJ. A comparison of 20 or 40 mg per day of carbimazole in the initial treatment of hyperthyroidism. *Clin. Endocrinol. (Oxf.)* 1996; 45(5): 511–6.

66. Abraham P, Avenell A, McGeoch SC, Clark LF, Bevan JS. Antithyroid drug regimen for treating Graves' hyperthyroidism. *Cochrane Database Syst. Rev.* 2010; 20(1): CD003420.

67. Maugendre D, Gatel A, Campion L, Massart C, Guilhem I, Lorcy Y, Lescouarch J, Herry JY, Allannic H. Antithyroid drugs and Graves' disease—Prospective randomized assessment of long-term treatment. *Clin. Endocrinol. (Oxf.)* 1999; 50(1):127–32.

68. Young ET, Steel NR, Taylor JJ, Stephenson AM, Stratton A, Holcombe M, Kendall-Taylor P. Prediction of remission after antithyroid drug treatment in Graves' disease. *Q. J. Med.* 1988; 66(250): 175–89.

69. Vitti P, Rago T, Chiovato L, Pallini S, Santini F, Fiore E, Rocchi R, Martino E, Pinchera A. Clinical features of patients with Graves' disease undergoing remission after antithyroid drug treatment. *Thyroid* 1997; 7(3): 369–75.

70. Nagai K, Tamai H, Mukuta T, Morita T, Matsubayashi S, Kuma K, Nakagawa T. A follow-up study of 85 patients with Graves' disease in remission who developed undetectable serum thyroid-stimulating hormone concentrations using sensitive TSH assays. *Horm. Res.* 1991; 35(5): 185–9.

71. Biondi B, Bartalena L, Cooper DS, Hegedüs L, Laurberg P, Kahaly GJ. The 2015 European thyroid association guidelines on

diagnosis and treatment of endogenous subclinical hyperthyroidism. *Eur. Thyroid J.* 2015; 4(3): 149–63.

72. Hedley AJ, Young RE, Jones SJ, Alexander WD, Bewsher PD. Antithyroid drugs in the treatment of hyperthyroidism of Graves' disease: Long-term follow-up of 434 patients. *Clin. Endocrinol. (Oxf)* 1989; 31(2): 209–18.

73. Villagelin D, Romaldini JH, Santos RB, Milkos AB, Ward LS. Outcomes in relapsed Graves' disease patients following radioiodine or prolonged low dose of methimazole treatment. *Thyroid* 2015; 25(12): 1282–90.

74. Azizi F, Malboosbaf R. Long-term antithyroid drug treatment: A systematic review and meta-analysis. *Thyroid* 2017; 27(10): 1223–31.

75. Cooper DS. The side-effects of antithyroid drugs. *Endocrinologist* 1999; 9(6): 457–78.

76. Chivu RD, Chivu LI, Ion DA, Barbu C, Fica S. Allergic reactions to antithyroid drugs are associated with autoimmunity a retrospective case-control study. *Rev. Med. Chir. Soc. Med. Nat. Iasi* 2006; 110(4): 830–2.

77. Otsuka F, Noh JY, Chino T, Shimizu T, Mukasa K, Ito K, Ito K, Taniyama M. Hepatotoxicity and cutaneous reactions after antithyroid drug administration. *Clin. Endocrinol. (Oxf.)* 2012; 77(2): 310–5.

78. Tajiri J, Noguchi S, Murakami N. Usefulness of granulocyte count measurement four hours after injection of granulocyte colony-stimulating factor for detecting recovery from antithyroid drug-induced granulocytopenia. *Thyroid* 1997; 7(4): 575–8.

79. Salama A, Mueller-Eckhardt C. Immune-mediated blood cell dyscrasias related to drugs. *Semin. Hematol.* 1992; 29(1): 54–63.

80. Cheung CL, Sing CW, Tang CS, Cheng VK, Pirmohamed M, Choi CH, Hung CS, et al. HLA-b*38:02:01 predicts carbimazole/methimazole-induced agranulocytosis. *Clin. Pharmacol. Ther.* 2016; 99(5): 555–61.

81. Pearce SH. Spontaneous reporting of adverse reactions to carbimazole and propylthiouracil in the UK. *Clin. Endocrinol. (Oxf.)* 2004; 61(5): 589–94.

82. Nakamura H, Miyauchi A, Miyawaki N, Imagawa J. Analysis of 754 cases of antithyroid drug-induced agranulocytosis over 30 years in Japan. *J. Clin. Endocrinol. Metab.* 2013; 98(12): 4776–83.

83. Kobayashi S, Noh JY, Mukasa K, Kunii Y, Watanabe N, Matsumoto M, Ohye H, et al. Characteristics of agranulocytosis as an adverse effect of antithyroid drugs in the second or later course of treatment. *Thyroid* 2014; 24(5): 796–801.

84. Sheng WH, Hung CC, Chen YC, Fang CT, Hsieh SM, Chang SC, Hsieh WC. Antithyroid-drug-induced agranulocytosis complicated by life-threatening infections. *Q.J.M.* 1999; 92(8): 455–61.

85. Andersohn F, Konzen C, Garbe E. Systematic review: Agranulocytosis induced by nonchemotherapy drugs. *Ann. Intern. Med.* 2007; 146(9): 657–65.

86. Andrès E, Zimmer J, Mecili M, Weitten T, Alt M, Maloisel F. Clinical presentation and management of drug-induced agranulocytosis. *Expert Rev. Hematol.* 2011; 4(2): 143–51.

87. Julia A, Olona M, Bueno J, Revilla E, Rosselló J, Petit J, Morey M, et al. Drug-induced agranulocytosis: Prognostic factors in a series of 168 episodes. *Br. J. Haematol.* 1991; 79(3): 366–71.

88. Tajiri J, Noguchi S. Antithyroid drug-induced agranulocytosis: How has granulocyte colony-stimulating factor changed therapy? *Thyroid* 2005; 15(3): 292–7.

89. Fukata S, Kuma K, Sugawara M. Granulocyte colony-stimulating factor (G-CSF) does not improve recovery from antithyroid drug-induced agranulocytosis: A prospective study. *Thyroid* 1999; 9(1): 29–31.

90. Candoni A, De Marchi F, Vescini F, Mauro S, Rinaldi C, Piemonte M, Rabassi N, Dubbini MV, Fanin R. Graves' disease thyrotoxicosis and propylthiouracil related agranulocytosis successfully treated with therapeutic plasma exchange and G-CSF followed by total thyroidectomy. *Mediterr. J. Hematol. Infect. Dis.* 2017; 9(1): e2017058.

91. Balavoine AS, Glinoer D, Dubucquoi S, Wémeau JL. Antineutrophil cytoplasmic antibody-positive small-vessel vasculitis associated with antithyroid drug therapy: How significant is the clinical problem? *Thyroid* 2015; 25(12): 1273–81.

92. Guma M, Salinas I, Reverter JL, Roca J, Valls-Roc M, Juan M, Olivé A. Frequency of antineutrophil cytoplasmic antibody in Graves' disease patients treated with methimazole. *J. Clin. Endocrinol. Metab.* 2003; 88(5): 2141–6.

93. Shabtai R, Shapiro MS, Orenstein D, Taragan R, Shenkman L. The antithyroid arthritis syndrome reviewed. *Arthritis Rheum.* 1984; 27(2): 227–9.

94. Takaya K, Kimura N, Hiyoshi T. Antithyroid arthritis syndrome: A case report and review of the literature. *Intern. Med.* 2016; 55(24): 3627–33.

95. Heidari R, Niknahad H, Jamshidzadeh A, Abdoli N. Factors affecting drug-induced liver injury: Antithyroid drugs as instances. *Clin. Mol. Hepatol.* 2014; 20(3): 237–48.

96. Akmal A, Kung J. Propylthiouracil, and methimazole, and carbimazole-related hepatotoxicity. *Expert Opin. Drug Saf.* 2014; 13(10): 1397–406.

97. Hanson JS. Propylthiouracil and hepatitis. *Arch. Int. Med.* 1984; 144(5): 944–96.

98. Cooper DS, Rivkees SA. Putting propylthiouracil in perspective. *J. Clin. Endocrinol. Metab.* 2009; 94(6): 1881–2.

99. Williams KV, Nayak S, Becker D, Reyes J, Burmeister LA. Fifty years of experience with propylthiouracil-associated hepatotoxicity: What have we learned? *J. Clin. Endocrinol. Metab.* 1997; 82(6): 1727–33.

100. Rivkees SA, Szarfman A. Dissimilar hepatotoxicity profiles of propylthiouracil and methimazole in children. *J. Clin. Endocrinol. Metab.* 2010; 95(7): 3260–7.

101. Waseem M, Seshadri KG, Kabadi UM. Successful outcome with methimazole and lithium combination therapy for propylthiouracil-induced hepatotoxicity. *Endo. Prac.* 1998; 4: 197–200.

102. Okamura K, Sato K, Fujikawa M, Bandai S, Ikenoue H, Kitazono T. Remission after potassium iodide therapy in patients with Graves' hyperthyroidism exhibiting thionamide-associated side effects. *J. Clin. Endocrinol. Metab.* 2014; 99(11): 3995–4002.

103. Liaw YF, Huang MJ, Fan KD, Li KL, Wu SS, Chen TJ. Hepatic injury during propylthiouracil therapy in patients with hyperthyroidism. A cohort study. *Ann. Intern. Med.* 1993; 118(6): 424–8.

104. Huang MJ, Li KL, Wei JS, Wu SS, Fan KD, Liaw YF. Sequential liver and bone biochemical changes in hyperthyroidism: Prospective controlled follow-up study. *Am. J. Gastroenterol.* 1994; 89(7): 1071–6.

105. Niculescu DA, Dusceac R, Galoiu SA, Capatina CA, Poiana C. Serial changes of liver function tests before and during methimazole treatment in thyrotoxic patients. *Endocr. Pract.* 2016; 22(8): 974–9

106. Woeber KA. Methimazole-induced hepatotoxicity. *Endocr. Pract.* 2002; 8(3): 222–4.

107. Arab DM, Malatjalian DA, Rittmaster RS. Severe cholestatic jaundice in uncomplicated hyperthyroidism treated with methimazole. *J. Clin. Endocrinol. Metab.* 1995; 80(4): 1083–5.

108. Wang MT, Lee WJ, Huang TY, Chu CL, Hsieh CH. Antithyroid drug-related hepatotoxicity in hyperthyroidism patients: A population-based cohort study. *Br. J. Clin. Pharmacol.* 2014; 78(3): 619–29.

109. Yang J, Li LF, Xu Q, Zhang J, Weng WW, Zhu YJ, Dong MJ. Analysis of 90 cases of antithyroid drug-induced severe hepatotoxicity over 13 years in China. *Thyroid* 2015; 25(3): 278–83.

110. Geffner DL, Hershman JM. Beta-adrenergic blockade for the treatment of hyperthyroidism. *Am. J. Med.* 1992; 93(1): 61–8.

111. Cooper DS, Daniels GH, Ladenson PW, Ridgway EC. Hyperthyroxinemia in patients treated with high-dose propranolol. *Am. J. Med.* 1982; 73(6): 867–71.

112. Feely JS, Stevenson IH, Crooks J. Increased clearance of propranolol in thyrotoxicosis. *Ann. Intern. Med.* 1981; 94 (4 pt. 1): 472–4.

113. Roti E, Montermini M, Roti S, Gardini E, Robuschi G, Minelli R, Salvi M, et al. The effect of diltiazem, a calcium channel-blocking drug, on cardiac rate and rhythm in hyperthyroid patients. *Arch. Intern. Med.* 1988; 148(9): 1919–21.

114. Wood LC, Maloof F. Thyroid failure after potassium iodide treatment of diffuse toxic goiter. *Trans. Assoc. Am. Physicians* 1975; 88: 235–47.

115. Uchida T, Goto H, Kasai T, Komiya K, Takeno K, Abe H, Shigihara N, et al. Therapeutic effectiveness of potassium iodine in drug-naïve patients with Graves' disease: A single-center experience. *Endocrine* 2014; 47(2): 506–11.

116. Ross DS. Radioiodine therapy for hyper-thyroidism. *N. Engl. J. Med.* 2011; 364(6): 542–50.

117. Bonnema SJ, Hegedüs L. Radioiodine therapy in benign thyroid diseases: Effects, side effects, and factors affecting thera-peutic outcome. *Endocr. Rev.* 2012; 33(6): 920–80.

118. American Thyroid Association Taskforce On Radioiodine Safety, Sisson JC, Freitas J, McDougall IR, Dauer LT, Hurley JR, Brierley JD, et al. Radiation safety in the treatment of patients with thyroid diseases by radio-iodine [131]I: Practice recommendations of the American Thyroid Association. *Thyroid* 2011; 21(4): 335–46.

119. Berg GE, Michanek AM, Holmberg EC, Fink M. Iodine-131 treatment of hyperthy-roidism: Significance of effective half-life measurements. *J. Nucl. Med.* 1996; 37(2): 228–32.

120. Peters H, Fischer C, Bogner U, Reiners C, Schleusener H. Radioiodine therapy of Graves' hyperthyroidism: Standard vs. calculated [131]iodine activity. Results from a prospective, randomized, multicenter study. *Eur. J. Clin. Invest.* 1995; 25(3): 186–93.

121. Leslie WD, Ward L, Salamon EA, Ludwig S, Rowe RC, Cowden EA. A randomized comparison of radioiodine doses in Graves' hyperthyroidism. *J. Clin. Endocrinol. Metab.* 2003; 88(3): 978–83.

122. Uy HL, Reasner CA, Samuels MH. Pattern of recovery of the hypothalamic-pituitary-thyroid axis following radioactive iodine therapy in patients with Graves' disease. *Am. J. Med.* 1995; 99(2): 173–9.

123. Burch HB, Solomon BL, Cooper DS, Ferguson P, Walpert N, Howard R. The effect of antithyroid drug pretreatment on acute changes in thyroid hormone levels after (131)I ablation for Graves' disease. *J. Clin. Endocrinol. Metab.* 2001; 86(7): 3016–21.

124. Chiovato L, Fiore E, Vitti P, Rocchi R, Rago T, Dokic D, Latrofa F, et al. Outcome of thyroid function in Graves' patients treated with radioiodine: Role of thyroid-stimulating and thyrotropin-blocking antibodies and of radioiodine-induced thyroid damage. *J. Clin. Endocrinol. Metab.* 1998; 83(1): 40–6.

125. Andrade VA, Gross JL, Maia AL. Effect of methimazole pretreatment on serum thyroid hormone levels after radioactive treat-ment in Graves' hyperthyroidism. *J. Clin. Endocrinol. Metab.* 1999; 84(11): 4012–16.

126. Bonnema SJ, Bennedbaek FN, Veje A, Marving J, Hegedus L. Continuous methim-azole therapy and its effect on the cure rate of hyperthyroidism using radioactive iodine: An evaluation by a randomized trial. *J. Clin. Endocrinol. Metab.* 2006; 91(8): 2946–51.

127. Bonnema SJ, Bennedbaek FN, Veje A, Marving J, Hegedüs L. Continuous methim-azole therapy and its effect on the cure rate of hyperthyroidism using radioactive iodine: An evaluation by a randomized trial. *J. Clin. Endocrinol. Metab.* 2006; 91(8): 2946–51.

128. Walter MA, Christ-Crain M, Schindler C, Müller-Brand J, Müller B. Outcome of radio-iodine therapy without, on or 3 days off carbimazole: A prospective interventional three-group comparison. *Eur. J. Nucl. Med. Mol. Imaging* 2006; 33(6): 730–7.

129. Walter MA, Briel M, Christ-Crain M, Bonnema SJ, Connell J, Cooper DS, Bucher HC, Müller-Brand J, Müller B. Effects of antithyroid drugs on radioiodine treat-ment: Systematic review and meta-analysis of randomized controlled trials. *BMJ* 2007; 334(7592): 514.

130. Andrade VA, Gross JL, Maia AL. The effect of methimazole pretreatment on the effi-cacy of radioactive iodine therapy in Graves' hyperthyroidism: One-year follow-up of a prospective, randomized study. *J. Clin. Endocrinol. Metab.* 2001; 86(8): 3488–93.

131. Braga M, Walpert N, Burch HB, Solomon BL, Cooper DS. The effect of methimazole on cure rates after radioiodine treatment for Graves' hyperthyroidism: A randomized clinical trial. *Thyroid* 2002; 12(2): 135–9.

132. Tallstedt L, Lundell G, Torring O, Wallin G, Ljunggren JG, Blomgren H, Taube A. Occurrence of ophthalmopathy after

treatment for Graves' hyperthyroidism. The Thyroid Study Group. *N. Engl. J. Med.* 1992; 326(26): 1733–8.

133. Bartalena L, Marcocci C, Bogazzi F, Manetti L, Tanda ML, Dell'Unto E, Bruno-Bossio G, et al. Relation between therapy or hyperthyroidism and the course of Graves' ophthalmopathy. *N. Engl. J. Med.* 1998; 338(2): 73–8.

134. Perros P, Kendall-Taylor P, Neoh C, Frewin S, Dickinson J. A prospective study of the effects of radioiodine therapy for hyperthyroidism in patients with minimally active Graves' ophthalmopathy. *J. Clin. Endocrinol. Metab.* 2005; 90(9): 5321–3.

135. Shiber S, Stiebel-Kalish H, Shimon I, Grossman A, Robenshtok E. Glucocorticoid regimens for prevention of Graves' ophthalmopathy progression following radioiodine treatment: Systematic review and meta-analysis. *Thyroid* 2014; 24(10): 1515–23.

136. Tallstedt L, Lundell G, Blomgren H, Bring J. Does early administration of thyroxine reduce the development of Graves' ophthalmopathy after radioiodine treatment? *Eur. J. Endocrinol.* 1994; 130(5): 494–7.

137. Bartalena L, Marcocci C, Tanda ML, Manetti L, Dell'Unto E, Bartolomei MP, Nardi M, Martino E, Pinchera A. Cigarette smoking and treatment outcomes in Graves' ophthalmopathy. *Ann. Intern. Med.* 1998; 129(8): 632–5.

138. Träisk F, Tallstedt L, Abraham-Nordling M, Andersson T, Berg G, Calissendorff J, Hallengren B, et al. Thyroid-associated ophthalmopathy after treatment for Graves' hyperthyroidism with antithyroid drugs or iodine-131. *J. Clin. Endocrinol. Metab.* 2009; 94(10): 3700–7.

139. Ron E, Doody MM, Becker DV, Brill AB, Curtis RE, Goldman MB, Harris BS, et al. Cancer mortality following treatment for adult hyperthyroidism. Cooperative thyrotoxicosis therapy follow-up study group. *JAMA* 1998; 280(4): 347–55.

140. Franklyn JA, Maisonneuve P, Sheppard M, Betteridge J, Boyle P. Cancer incidence and mortality after radioiodine treatment for hyperthyroidism: A population-based cohort study. *Lancet* 1999; 353(9170): 2111–15.

141. Flynn RW, Macdonald TM, Jung RT, Morris AD, Leese GP. Mortality and vascular outcomes in patients treated for thyroid dysfunction. *J. Clin. Endocrinol. Metab.* 2006; 91(6): 2159–64.

142. Metso S, Auvinen A, Huhtala H, Salmi J, Oksala H, Jaatinen P. Increased cancer incidence after radioiodine treatment for hyperthyroidism. *Cancer* 2007; 109(10): 1972–9.

143. Ryödi E, Metso S, Jaatinen P, Huhtala H, Saaristo R, Välimäki M, Auvinen A. Cancer incidence and mortality in patients treated either With RAI or thyroidectomy for hyperthyroidism. *J. Clin. Endocrinol. Metab.* 2015; 100(10): 3710–17.

144. Sundaresh V, Brito JP, Wang Z, Prokop LJ, Stan MN, Murad MH, Bahn RS. Comparative effectiveness of therapies for Graves' hyperthyroidism: A systematic review and network meta-analysis. *J. Clin. Endocrinol. Metab.* 2013; 98(9): 3671–7.

145. Feroci F, Rettori M, Borrelli A, Coppola A, Castagnoli A, Perigli G, Cianchi F, Scatizzi M. A systematic review and meta-analysis of total thyroidectomy versus bilateral subtotal thyroidectomy for Graves' disease. *Surgery* 2014; 155(3): 529–40.

146. Adam MA, Thomas S, Youngwirth L, Hyslop T, Reed SD, Scheri RP, Roman SA, Sosa JA. Is there a minimum number of thyroidectomies a surgeon should perform to optimize patient outcomes? *Ann. Surg.* 2017; 265(2): 402–7.

147. Roher HD, Goretzki PE, Hellmann P, Witte J. Complications in thyroid surgery. Incidence and therapy. *Chirurg* 1999; 70(9): 999–1010.

148. Lennquist S, Jortso E, Anderberg BO, Smeds S. Beta blockers compared with antithyroid drugs as preoperative treatment in hyperthyroidism: Drug tolerance, complications, and postoperative thyroid function. *Surgery* 1985; 98(6): 1141–7.

149. Erbil Y, Ozluk Y, Giris M, Salmaslioglu A, Issever H, Barbaros U, Kapran Y, Ozarmağan S, Tezelman S. Effect of lugol solution on thyroid gland blood flow and microvessel density in the patients with Graves' disease. *J. Clin. Endocrinol. Metab.* 2007; 92(6): 2182–9.

150. Whalen G, Sullivan M, Maranda L, Quinlan R, Larkin A. Randomized trial of a short course of preoperative potassium iodide in patients undergoing thyroidectomy for Graves' disease. *Am. J. Surg.* 2017; 213(4): 805–9,

151. Randle RW, Bates MF, Long KL, Pitt SC, Schneider DF, Sippel RS. Impact of potassium iodide on thyroidectomy for Graves' disease: Implications for safety and operative difficulty. *Surgery* 2018; 163(1): 68–72.

152. Feely J, Crooks J, Forrest AL, Hamilton WF, Gunn A. Propranolol in the surgical treatment of hyperthyroidism, including severely thyrotoxic patients. *Br. J. Surg.* 1981; 68(12): 865–9.

153. Fischli S, Lucchini B, Müller W, Slahor L, Henzen C. Rapid preoperative blockage of thyroid hormone production/secretion in patients with Graves' disease. *Swiss Med. Wkly.* 2016;146: w14243.

154. Ha J, Jo K, Kang B, Kim MH, Lim DJ. Cholestyramine use for rapid reversion to euthyroid states in patients with thyrotoxicosis. *Endocrinol. Metab. (Seoul)* 2016; 31(3): 476–9.

155. Langley RW, Burch HB. Perioperative management of the thyrotoxic patient. *Endocrinol. Metab. Clin. North Am.* 2003; 32(2): 519–34.

156. Levetan C, Wartofsky L. A clinical guide to the management of Graves' disease with radioactive iodine. *Endocr. Pract.* 1995; 1(3): 205–12.

157. Patel NN, Abraham P, Buscombe J, Vanderpump MP. The cost effectiveness of treatment modalities for thyrotoxicosis in a U.K. center. *Thyroid* 2006; 16(6): 593–8.

158. Dietlein M, Moka D, Dederichs B, Hunsche E, Lauterbach KW, Schicha H. Cost-effectiveness analysis: Radioiodine or antithyroid medication in primary treatment of immune hyperthyroidism. *Nuklearmedizin* 1999; 38(1): 7–14.

159. Donovan PJ, McLeod DS, Little R, Gordon L. Cost-utility analysis comparing radioactive iodine, anti-thyroid drugs and total thyroidectomy for primary treatment of Graves' disease. *Eur. J. Endocrinol.* 2016; 175(6): 595–603.

160. Torring O, Tallstedt L, Wallin G, Lundell G, Ljunggren JG, Taube A, Sääf M, Hamberger B. Graves' hyperthyroidism: Treatment with antithyroid drugs, surgery, or radioiodine—A prospective, randomized study. Thyroid study group. *J. Clin. Endocrinol. Metab.* 1996; 81(8): 2986–93.

161. Hookham J, Truran P, Allahabadia A, Balasubramanian SP. Patients' perceptions and views of surgery and radioiodine ablation in the definitive management of Graves' disease. *Postgrad. Med. J.* 2017; 93(1099): 266–70.

162. Major BJ, Busuttil BE, Frauman AG. Graves' ophthalmopathy: Pathogenesis and clinical implications. *Aust. N. Z. J. Med.* 1998; 28(1): 39–45.

163. Dolman PJ. PJ. Evaluating Graves' orbitopathy. *Best Pract. Res. Clin. Endocrinol. Metab.* 2012; 26(3): 229–48.

164. Wiersinga WM. Quality of life in Graves' ophthalmopathy. *Best Pract. Res. Clin. Endocrinol. Metab.* 2012; 26(3): 359–70.

165. Bahn RS. Current insights into the pathogenesis of Graves' ophthalmopathy. *Horm. Metab. Res.* 2015; 47(10): 773–8.

166. Khong JJ, McNab AA, Ebeling PR, Craig JE, Selva D. Pathogenesis of thyroid eye disease: Review and update on molecular mechanisms. *Br. J. Ophthalmol.* 2016; 100(1): 142–50.

167. Smith TJ, Hegedüs L. Graves' disease. *N. Engl. J. Med.* 2016; 375(16): 1552–65.

168. Bahn RS. Graves' ophthalmopathy. *N. Engl. J. Med.* 2010; 362(8): 726–38.

169. Spitzweg C, Joba W, Hunt N, Heufelder AE. Analysis of human thyrotropin receptor gene expression and immunoreactivity in human orbital tissue. *Eur. J. Endocrinol.* 1997; 136(6): 599–607.

170. Fernando R, Atkins S, Raychaudhuri N, Lu Y, Li B, Douglas RS, Smith TJ. Human fibrocytes coexpress thyroglobulin and thyrotropin receptor. *Proc. Natl. Acad. Sci. U. S. A.* 2012;109(19): 7427–32.

171. Smith TJ, Hegedüs L, Douglas RS. Role of insulin-like growth factor-1 (IGF-1) pathway in the pathogenesis of Graves' orbitopathy. *Best Pract. Res. Clin. Endocrinol. Metab.* 2012; 26(3): 291–302.

172. Stan MN, Bahn RS. Risk factors for development or deterioration of Graves' ophthalmopathy. *Thyroid* 2010; 20(7): 777–83.

173. Hegedus L, Brix TH, Vestergaard P. Relationship between cigarette smoking and Graves' ophthalmopathy. *J. Endocrinol. Invest.* 2004; 27(3): 265–71.

174. Zang S, Ponto KA, Kahaly GJ. Clinical review: Intravenous glucocorticoids for Graves' orbitopathy: Efficacy and morbidity. *J. Clin. Endocrinol. Metab.* 2011; 96(2): 320–32.

175. Bartalena L, Krassas GE, Wiersinga W, Marcocci C, Salvi M, Daumerie C, Bournaud C, et al. Efficacy and safety of three different cumulative doses of intravenous methylprednisolone for moderate to severe and active Graves' orbitopathy. *J. Clin. Endocrinol. Metab.* 2012; 97(12): 4454–63.

176. Kahaly GJ, Pitz S, Hommel G, Dittmar M. Randomized, single blind trial of intravenous versus oral glucocorticoid monotherapy in Graves' orbitopathy. *J. Clin. Endocrinol. Metab.* 2005; 90(9): 5234–40.

177. Dolman PJ, Rath S. Orbital radiotherapy for thyroid eye disease. *Curr. Opin. Ophthalmol.* 2012; 23(5): 427–32.

178. Mourits MP, van Kempen-Harteveld ML, Garcia MB, Koppeschaar HP, Tick L, Terwee CB. Radiotherapy for Graves' orbitopathy: Randomized placebo-controlled study. *Lancet* 2000; 355(9214): 1505–9.

179. Gorman CA. Radiotherapy for Graves' ophthalmopathy: Results at one year. *Thyroid* 2002; 12(3): 251–5.

180. Bradley EA, Gower EW, Bradley DJ, Meyer DR, Cahill KV, Custer PL, Holck DE, Woog JJ. Orbital radiation for Graves ophthalmopathy: A report by the American Academy of Ophthalmology. *Ophthalmology* 2008; 115(2): 398–409.

181. Wei RL, Cheng JW, Cai JP. The use of orbital radiotherapy for Graves' ophthalmopathy: Quantitative review of the evidence. *Ophthalmologica* 2008; 222(1): 27–31.

182. Stiebel-Kalish H, Robenshtok E, Hasanreisoglu M, Ezrachi D, Shimon I, Leibovici L. Treatment modalities for Graves' ophthalmopathy: Systematic review and meta-analysis. *J. Clin. Endocrinol. Metab.* 2009; 94(8): 2708–16.

183. Wakelkamp IMMJ, Tan H, Saeed P, Schlingemann RO, Verbraak FD, Blank LE, Prummel MF, Wiersinga WM. Orbital irradiation for Graves' ophthalmopathy. Is it safe? A long-term follow-up study. *Ophthalmology* 2004; 111(8): 1557–62

184. Braun TL, Bhadkamkar MA, Jubbal KT, Weber AC, Marx DP. Orbital decompression for thyroid eye disease. *Semin. Plast. Surg.* 2017; 31(1): 40–5.

185. Marcocci C, Kahaly GJ, Krassas GE, Bartalena L, Prummel M, Stahl M, Altea MA, et al. Selenium and the course of mild Graves' orbitopathy. *N. Engl. J. Med.* 2011; 364(20): 1920–31.

186. Rotondo Dottore G, Leo M, Casini G, Latrofa F, Cestari L, Sellari-Franceschini S, Nardi M, et al. Antioxidant actions of selenium in orbital fibroblasts: A basis for the effects of selenium in Graves' orbitopathy. *Thyroid* 2017; 27(2): 271–8.

187. Dharmasena A. Selenium supplementation in thyroid associated ophthalmopathy: An update. *Int. J. Ophthalmol.* 2014; 7(2): 365–75.

188. Salvi M, Vannucchi G, Curro N, Campi I, Covelli D, Dazzi D, Simonetta S, et al. Efficacy of B-cell targeted therapy with rituximab in patients with active moderate to severe Graves' orbitopathy: A randomized controlled study. *J. Clin. Endocrinol. Metab.* 2015; 100(2): 422–31.

189. Stan MN, Garrity JA, Carranza Leon BG, Prabin T, Bradley EA, Bahn RS. Randomized controlled trial of rituximab in patients with Graves' orbitopathy. *J. Clin. Endocrinol. Metab.* 2015; 100(2): 432–41.

190. Stan MN, Salvi M. Management of endocrine disease: Rituximab therapy for Graves' orbitopathy—Lessons from randomized control trials. *Eur. J. Endocrinol.* 2017; 176(2): R101–R9.

191. Smith TJ, Kahaly GJ, Ezra DG, Fleming JC, Dailey RA, Tang RA, Harris GJ, et al. Teprotumumab for thyroid-associated ophthalmopathy. *N. Engl. J. Med.* 2017; 376(18): 1748–61.

192. Wiersinga WM. Advances in treatment of active, moderate-to-severe Graves' ophthalmopathy. *Lancet Diabetes Endocrinol.* 2017; 5(2): 134–42.

193. Rapoport B, McLachlan SM. The thyrotropin receptor in Graves' disease. *Thyroid* 2007; 17(10): 911–22.

194. Fatourechi V. Pretibial myxedema: Pathophysiology and treatment options. *Am. J. Clin. Dermatol.* 2005; 6(5): 295–309.

195. Fatourechi V. Thyroid dermopathy and acropachy. *Best Pract. Res. Clin. Endocrinol. Metab.* 2012; 26(4): 553–65

196. Noppen M, Velkeniers B, Steenssens L, Vanhaelst L. Beneficial effects of plasma-pheresis followed by immunosuppressive therapy in pretibial myxedema. *Acta Clin. Belg.* 1988; 43(5): 381–3.

197. Bartalena L, Fatourechi V. Extrathyroidal manifestations of Graves' disease: A 2014 update. *J. Endocrinol. Invest.* 2014; 37(8): 691–700.

198. Heyes C, Nolan R, Leahy M, Gebauer K. Treatment-resistant elephantiasic thyroid dermopathy responding to rituximab and plasmapheresis. *Australas. J. Dermatol.* 2012; 53(1): e1–e4.

199. Biondi B, Cooper DS. Subclinical hyperthy-roidism. *N. Engl. J. Med.* 2018;378:2411–2419.

200. Biondi B, Bartalena L, Cooper DS, Hegedus L, Laurberg P, Kahaly GJ. The 2015 European Thyroid Association guidelines on diagnosis and treatment of endogenous subclinical hyperthyroidism. *Eur. Thyroid J.* 2015; 4(3): 149–63.

201. Gammage MD, Parle JV, Holder RL, Roberts LM, Hobbs FD, Wilson S, Sheppard MC, Franklyn JA. Association between serum free thyroxine concentration and atrial fibrillation. *Arch. Intern. Med.* 2007; 167(9): 928–34.

202. Li D, Radulescu A, Shrestha RT, Root M, Karger AB, Killeen AA, Hodges JS, et al. Association of biotin ingestion with perfor-mance of hormone and nonhormone assays in healthy adults. *JAMA* 2017; 318(12): 1150–60.

203. Hollowell JG, Staehling NW, Flanders WD, Hannon WH, Gunter EW, Spencer CA, Braverman LE. Serum TSH, T(4), and thyroid antibodies in the United States popula-tion (1988 to 1994): National Health and Nutrition Examination Survey (NHANES III). *J. Clin. Endocrinol. Metab.* 2002; 87(2): 489–99.

204. Rosario PW, Carvalho M, Calsolari MR. Symptoms of thyrotoxicosis, bone metabo-lism and occult atrial fibrillation in older women with mild endogenous subclinical hyperthyroidism. *Clin. Endocrinol. (Oxf)* 2016; 85(1): 132–6.

205. Sgarbi JA, Villaca FG, Garbeline B, Villar HE, Romaldini JH. The effects of early antithy-roid therapy for endogenous subclinical hyperthyroidism on clinical and heart abnor-malities. *J. Clin. Endocrinol. Metab.* 2003; 88(4): 1672–7.

206. Carlé A, Andersen SL, Boelaert K, Laurberg P. Management of endocrine disease: Subclinical thyrotoxicosis: Prevalence, causes, and choice of therapy. *Eur. J. Endocrinol.* 2017; 176(6): R325–R37.

207. Sawin CT, Geller A, Wolf PA, Belanger AJ, Baker E, Bacharach P, Wilson PW, Benjamin EJ, D'Agostino RB. Low serum thyrotropin concentrations as a risk factor for atrial fibrillation in older persons. *N. Engl. J. Med.* 1994; 331(19): 1249–52.

208. Cappola AR, Fried LP, Arnold AM, Danese MD, Kuller LH, Burke GL, Tracy RP, Ladenson PW. Thyroid status, cardiovascu-lar risk, and mortality in older adults. *JAMA* 2006; 295(9): 1033–41.

209. Selmer C, Olesen JB, Hansen ML, Lindhardsen J, Olsen AM, Madsen JC, Faber J, et al. The spectrum of thyroid dis-ease and risk of new onset atrial fibrillation: A large population cohort study. *BMJ* 2012; 345: e7895.

210. Gencer B, Collet TH, Virgini V, Bauer DC, Gussekloo J, Cappola AR, Nanchen D, et al. Subclinical thyroid dysfunction and the risk of heart failure events: An individual participant data analysis from 6 prospective cohorts. *Circulation* 2012; 126(9): 1040–9.

211. Blum MR, Bauer DC, Collet TH, Fink HA, Cappola AR, da Costa BR, Wirth CD. Subclinical thyroid dysfunction and fracture risk: A meta-analysis. *J. Am. Med. Assoc.* 2015; 313(20): 2055–65.

212. Yang R, Yao L, Fang Y, Sun J, Guo T, Yang K, Tian L. The relationship between subclinical thyroid dysfunction and the risk of fracture or low bone mineral density: A systematic review and meta-analysis of cohort studies. *J. Bone Miner. Metab.* 2018; 36(2): 209–220.

213. Vadiveloo T, Donnan PT, Cochrane L, Leese GP. The thyroid epidemiology, audit, and research study (TEARS): The natural history of endogenous subclinical hyperthyroidism. *J. Clin. Endocrinol. Metab.* 2011; 96(1): E1–8.

214. Das G, Ojewuyi TA, Baglioni P, Geen J, Premawardhana LD, Okosieme OE. Serum thyrotrophin at baseline predicts the natural course of subclinical hyperthyroidism. *Clin. Endocrinol. (Oxf)* 2012; 77(1): 146–51.

215. Rosario PW. The natural history of subclinical hyperthyroidism in patients below the age of 65 years. *Clin. Endocrinol. (Oxf)* 2008; 68(3): 491–2.

216. Figge J, Leinung M, Goodman AD, Izquierdo R, Mydosh T, Gates S, Line B, Lee DW. The clinical evaluation of patients with subclinical hyperthyroidism and free triiodothyronine (free T3) toxicosis. *Am. J. Med.* 1994; 96(3): 229–34.

217. Meyerovitch J, Rotman-Pikielny P, Sherf M, Battat E, Levy Y, Surks MI. Serum thyrotropin measurements in the community: Five-year follow-up in a large network of primary care physicians. *Arch. Intern. Med.* 2007; 167(14): 1533–8.

218. Carlé A, Andersen SL, Boelaert K, Laurberg P. Management of endocrine disease: Subclinical thyrotoxicosis: Prevalence, causes and choice of therapy. *Eur. J. Endocrinol.* 2017; 176(6): R325–R37.

219. Mudde AH, Houben AJ, Nieuwenhuijzen Kruseman AC. Bone metabolism during anti-thyroid drug treatment of endogenous subclinical hyperthyroidism. *Clin. Endocrinol. (Oxf.)* 1994; 41(4): 421–4.

220. Faber J, Jensen I, Petersen L, Nygaard B, Hegedus L, Siersback-Nielsen K. Normalization of serum thyrotrophin by means of radioidoine treatment in subclinical hyperthyroidism: Effect on bone loss in postmenopausal women. *Clin. Endocrinol.* 1998; 48(3): 285–90.

221. Buscemi S, Verga S, Cottone S, Andronico G, D'Orio L, Mannino V, Panzavecchia D, Vitale F, Cerasola G. Favorable clinical heart and bone effects of anti-thyroid drug therapy in endogenous subclinical hyperthyroidism. *J. Endocrinol. Invest.* 2007; 30(3): 230–5.

222. Burch HB, Wartofsky L. Life-threatening thyrotoxicosis. Thyroid storm. *Endocrinol. Metab. Clin. North Am.* 1993; 22(2): 263–77.

223. Akamizu T, Satoh T, Isozaki O, Suzuki A, Wakino S, Iburi T, Tsuboi K, et al. Diagnostic criteria, clinical features, and incidence of thyroid storm based on nationwide surveys. *Thyroid* 2012; 22(7): 661–79.

224. Brooks MH, Waldstein SS, Bronsky D, Sterling K. Serum triiodothyronine concentration in thyroid storm. *J. Clin. Endocrinol. Metab.* 1975; 40(2): 339–41.

225. Sherman SI, Simonson L, Ladenson PW. Clinical and socioeconomic predispositions to complicated thyrotoxicosis: A predictable and preventable syndrome? *Am. J. Med.* 1996; 101(2): 192–8.

226. Nayak B, Burman K. Thyrotoxicosis and thyroid storm. *Endocrinol. Metab. Clin. North Am.* 2006; 35(4): 663–86.

227. Jongjaroenprasert W, Akarawut W, Chantasart D, Chailurkit L, Rajatanavin R. Rectal administration of propylthiouracil in hyperthyroid patients: Comparison of suspension enema and suppository form. *Thyroid* 2002; 12(7): 627–31.

228. Hodak SP, Huang C, Clarke D, Burman KD, Jonklaas J, Janicic-Kharic N. Intravenous methimazole in the treatment of refractory hyperthyroidism. *Thyroid* 2006; 16(7): 691–5.

229. Solomon BL, Wartofsky L, Burman KD. Adjunctive cholestyramine therapy for thyrotoxicosis. *Clin. Endocrinol. (Oxf.)* 1993; 38(1): 39–43.

230. Muller C, Perrin P, Faller B, Richter S, Chantrel F. Role of plasma exchange in the thyroid storm. *Ther. Apher. Dial.* 2011; 15(6): 522–31.

231. Delbridge L. Solitary thyroid nodule: Current management. *ANZ J. Surg* 2006; 76(5): 381–6.

232. Burman KD, Earll JM, Johnson MC, Wartofsky L. Clinical observations on the solitary autonomous thyroid nodule. *Arch. Intern. Med.* 1974; 134(5): 915–19.

233. Smith M, McHenry C, Jarosz H, Lawrence AM, Paloyan E. Carcinoma of the thyroid in patients with autonomous nodules. *Am. Surg.* 1988; 54(7): 448–9.

234. Yalla NM, Reynolds LR. Hürthle cell thyroid carcinoma presenting as a "hot" nodule. *Endocr. Pract.* 2011; 17(3): e68–72.

235. Krohn K, Paschke R. Somatic mutations in thyroid nodular disease. *Mol. Genet. Metab.* 2002; 75(3): 202–8.

236. Stanbury JB, Ermans AE, Bourdoux P, Todd C, Oken E, Tonglet R, Vidor G, Braverman LE, Medeiros-Neto G. Iodine-induced hyperthyroidism: Occurrence and epidemiology. *Thyroid* 1998; 8(1): 83–100.

237. Kornelius E, Chiou JY, Yang YS, Lo SC, Peng CH, Lai YR, Huang CN. Iodinated contrast media-induced thyroid dysfunction in euthyroid nodular goiter patients. *Thyroid* 2016; 26(8):1030–8.

238. Brian SR, Cheng DW, Goldberg PA. Unusual case of amiodarone-induced thyrotoxicosis: "Illicit" use of a technetium scan to diagnose a transiently toxic thyroid nodule. *Endocr. Pract.* 2007; 13(4): 413–6.

239. Blum M, Shenkman L, Hollander CS. The autonomous nodule of the thyroid: Correlation of patient age, nodule size, and functional status. *Am. J. Med. Sci.* 1975; 269(1): 43–50.

240. Goldstein R, Hart IR. Follow-up of solitary autonomous thyroid nodules treated with [131]I. *N. Engl. J. Med.* 1983; 309(24): 1473–6.

241. Ferrari C, Reschini E, Paracchi A. Treatment of the autonomous thyroid nodule: A review. *Eur. J. Endocrinol.* 1996; 135(4): 383–90.

242. Zakavi SR, Mousavi Z, Davachi B. Comparison of four different protocols of I-131 therapy for treating single toxic thyroid nodule. *Nucl. Med. Commun.* 2009; 30(2): 169–75.

243. Thomas CG, Jr., Croom RD. Current management of the patient with autonomously functioning nodular goiter. *Surg. Clin. North Am.* 1987; 67(2): 315–28.

244. Siegel RD, Lee SL. Toxic nodular goiter. Toxic adenoma and toxic multinodular goiter. *Endocrinol. Metab. Clin. North Am.* 1998; 27(1): 151–68.

245. Zingrillo M, Torlontano M, Ghiggi MR, Frusciante V, Varraso A, Liuzzi A, Trischitta V. Radioiodine and percutaneous ethanol injection in the treatment of large toxic thyroid nodule: A long-term study. *Thyroid* 2000; 10(11): 985–9.

246. Tarantino L, Francica G, Sordelli I, Sperlongano P, Parmeggiani D, Ripa C, Parmeggiani U. Percutaneous ethanol injection of hyperfunctioning thyroid nodules: Long-term follow-up in 125 patients. *AJR Am J Roentgenol* 2008; 190(3): 800–8.

247. Lippi F, Ferrari C, Manetti L, Rago T, Santini F, Monzani F, Bellitti P, et al. Treatment of solitary autonomous thyroid nodules by percutaneous ethanol injection: Results of an Italian multicenter study. The multicenter study group. *J. Clin. Endocrinol. Metab.* 1996; 81(9): 3261–4.

248. Tarantino L, Francica G, Sordelli I, Sperlongano P, Parmeggiani D, Ripa C, Parmeggiani U. Percutaneous ethanol injection of hyperfunctioning thyroid nodules: Long-term follow-up in 125 patients. *AJR Am J Roentgenol* 2008; 190(3): 800–8.

249. Ha EJ, Baek JH, Lee JH. The efficacy and complications of radiofrequency ablation of thyroid nodules. *Curr. Opin. Endocrinol. Diabetes Obes.* 2011; 18(5): 310–4.

250. Shahrzad MK. Laser thermal ablation of thyroid benign nodules. *J. Lasers Med. Sci.* 2015; 6(4): 151–6.

251. Ha EJ, Baek JH, Kim KW, Pyo J, Lee JH, Baek SH, Døssing H, Hegedüs L. Comparative efficacy of radiofrequency and laser ablation for the treatment of benign thyroid nodules: Systematic review including traditional pooling and Bayesian network meta-analysis. *J. Clin. Endocrinol. Metab.* 2015; 100(5): 1903–11.

252. Che Y, Jin S, Shi C, Wang L, Zhang X, Li Y, Baek JH. Treatment of benign thyroid nodules: Comparison of surgery with radiofrequency ablation. *AJNR Am J Neuroradiol* 2015; 36(7): 1321–5.

253. Korkusuz Y, Gröner D, Raczynski N, Relin O, Kingeter Y, Grünwald F, Happel C. Thermal ablation of thyroid nodules: Are radiofrequency ablation, microwave ablation and high intensity focused ultrasound equally safe and effective methods? *Eur. Radiol.* 2018; 28(3): 929–35.

254. Woeber KA. Iodine and thyroid disease. *Med. Clin. North Am.* 1991; 75(1): 169–78.

255. Tonacchera M, Chiovato L, Pinchera A, Agretti P, Fiore E, Cetani F, Rocchi R, et al. Hyperfunctioning thyroid nodules in toxic multinodular goiter share activating thyrotropin receptor mutations with solitary toxic adenoma. *J. Clin. Endocrinol. Metab.* 1998; 83(2): 492–8.

256. Gabriel EM, Bergert ER, Grant CS, van Heerden JA, Thompson GB, Morris JC. Germline polymorphism of codon 727 of human thyroid-stimulating hormone receptor is associated with toxic multinodular goiter. *J. Clin. Endocrinol. Metab.* 1999; 84(9): 3328–35.

257. Boi F, Loy M, Piga M, Serra A, Atzeni F, Mariotti S. The usefulness of conventional and echo colour Doppler sonography in the differential diagnosis of toxic multinodular goiters. *Eur. J. Endocrinol.* 2000; 143(3): 339–46.

258. Hurley DL, Gharib H. Evaluation and management of multinodular goiter. *Otolaryngol. Clin. North Am.* 1996; 29(4): 527–40.

259. Tarantini B, Ciuoli C, Di Cairano G, Guarino E, Mazzucato P, Montanaro A, Burroni L, Vattimo AG, Pacini F. Effectiveness of radioiodine (^{131}I) as definitive therapy in patients with autoimmune and non-autoimmune hyperthyroidism. *J. Endocrinol. Invest.* 2006; 29(7): 594–8.

260. Kyrilli A, Tang BN, Huyge V, Blocklet D, Goldman S, Corvilain B, Moreno-Reyes R. Thiamazole pretreatment lowers the ^{131}I activity needed to cure hyperthyroidism in patients with nodular goiter. *J. Clin. Endocrinol. Metab.* 2015; 100(6): 2261–7.

261. Ceccarelli C, Antonangeli L, Brozzi F, Bianchi F, Tonacchera M, Santini P, Mazzeo S, et al. Radioiodine ^{131}I treatment for large nodular goiter: Recombinant human thyrotropin allows the reduction of radioiodine ^{131}I activity to be administered in patients with low uptake. *Thyroid* 2011; 21(7): 759–64.

262. Romão R, Rubio IG, Tomimori EK, Camargo RY, Knobel M, Medeiros-Neto G. High prevalence of side effects after recombinant human thyrotropin-stimulated radioiodine treatment with 30 mCi in patients with multinodular goiter and subclinical/clinical hyperthyroidism. *Thyroid* 2009; 19(9): 945–51.

263. Franklyn JA, Daykin J, Holder R, Sheppard MC. Radioiodine therapy compared in patients with toxic nodular or Graves' hyperthyroidism. *Q.J.M.* 1995; 88(3): 175–80.

264. Erickson D, Gharib H, Li H, van Heerden JA. Treatment of patients with toxic multinodular goiter. *Thyroid* 1998; 8(4): 277–82.

265. Adam M, Thomas S, Youngwirth L, Hyslop T, Reed SD, Scheri RP, Roman SA, Sosa JA. Is there a minimum number of thyroidectomies a surgeon should perform to optimize patient outcomes. *Ann. Surg.* 2017; 265(2): 402–407.

266. Cirocchi R, Trastulli S, Randolph J, Guarino S, Di Rocco G, Arezzo A, D'Andrea V, et al. Total or near-total thyroidectomy versus subtotal thyroidectomy for multinodular non-toxic goiter in adults. *Cochrane Database Syst. Rev.* 2015; 8: CD01037.

3

Thyroiditis

ROBERT C. SMALLRIDGE AND VICTOR BERNET

Thyroiditis	81	Treatment	87
Chronic lymphocytic thyroiditis	81	Subacute thyroiditis	87
Treatment	82	Introduction	87
Silent thyroiditis (non-postpartum)	82	Epidemiology	87
Introduction	82	Pathophysiology	87
Epidemiology	83	Diagnosis	87
Pathophysiology	83	Treatment	88
Diagnosis	83	Riedel's thyroiditis	89
Treatment	84	Etiology	89
Postpartum thyroiditis	84	Pathophysiology	89
Introduction	84	Diagnosis	89
Epidemiology	84	Treatment	89
Pathophysiology	84	Radiation thyroiditis	89
Diagnosis	85	Introduction	89
Treatment	86	Epidemiology	90
Infectious/post-infectious thyroiditis	86	Pathophysiology	90
Introduction	86	Diagnosis	90
Epidemiology	86	Treatment	90
Pathophysiology	86	Trauma-induced thyroiditis	90
Diagnosis	86	References	90

THYROIDITIS

Thyroiditis is an inflammation of the thyroid gland, of which there are numerous causes, both non-infectious and infectious (Table 3.1). The most common cause is autoimmune (e.g., chronic lymphocytic thyroiditis or Hashimoto's disease).

Chronic lymphocytic thyroiditis

Chronic lymphocytic thyroiditis is one of the most common of all autoimmune disorders (1). In this condition, there is an enhanced presentation of thyroid antigens and a reduction in immune tolerance with an increase in Th-1 lymphocyte activity and destruction of thyroid follicles. The destruction results from several effects including cytokine-induced apoptosis and ICAM-1-mediated CD8 + cell-mediated cytotoxicity (2).

Clinically, almost all patients have antithyroid antibodies (Tabs) in their serum, most commonly antithyroid peroxidase (TPO-Ab) but also antithyroglobulin (TG-Ab). 10–20% of adults have detectable Tabs, with a greater prevalence in women and older individuals. Patients often have a small goiter and are asymptomatic with a normal serum

Table 3.1 Types of thyroiditis

Chronic Lymphocytic Thyroiditis
Silent Thyroiditis; Non-Postpartum
Postpartum
Infectious/Post-Infectious Thyroiditis
Acute Infectious
Subacute
Riedel's Thyroiditis
Radiation Thyroiditis
Trauma-Induced Thyroiditis
Drug-Induced Thyroiditis (see Chapter 5,
  "Drug-Induced Thyroid Dysfunction")

thyrotropin (TSH). The natural development, however, is progressive damage to the thyroid follicles with subsequent evolution to subclinical, then overt hypothyroidism. This progression may be slow, occurring over years (3), and the early symptoms (fatigue, weight gain) are often unrelated to thyroid dysfunction; thus, measuring TSH (and when elevated, a free T4) is an important component of evaluating a patient's symptoms. While Hashimoto's thyroiditis is almost always painless, there are occasional patients with pain, and so must be considered in the differential diagnosis of neck pain and a tender thyroid gland (4).

The etiology of Hashimoto's thyroiditis is multifactorial. It is estimated that genetic susceptibility contributes 70–80% toward the disorder. Specific contributors include HLA class II antigens, cytotoxic T-lymphocyte antigen-4 (CTLA-4), protein tyrosine phosphatase non-receptor type 22, cytokines (e.g., TNF-alpha; INF-alpha; IL-2), thyroglobulin and the vitamin D receptor on thyrocytes (1, 5, 6). Environmental factors contribute 20–30% toward the development of chronic thyroiditis. Many studies have confirmed an increase in thyroiditis in populations after iodine is introduced into their diet. Interestingly, while Graves' disease is aggravated by smoking, there is a decrease in TPO-Ab titer and hypothyroidism in smokers. Moderate alcohol ingestion also reduces the frequency of hypothyroidism; the effect is dose responsive and the mechanism is unknown (5, 6). Selenoproteins (iodothyronine deiodinases and glutathione peroxidases) are present in thyrocytes, and recent studies have examined the possible role of selenium (Se^{++}) in thyroid dysfunction. While low serum Se^{++} is associated with Hashimoto's thyroiditis, to date there are no consistent data

showing a benefit of Se^{++} supplementation on TPO-Ab level, and more trials are needed (7). An ongoing clinical trial is examining whether adding Se^{++} to L-T4 in patients with autoimmune thyroiditis improves quality of life or markers of immune activity, and if it will affect the dose of L-T4 needed (8). There is an association of low vitamin D levels with autoimmunity, and limited data show that vitamin D supplementation may reduce TPO-Ab titers in L-T4-treated patients with Hashimoto's thyroiditis (9). Stress has been shown to induce or aggravate Graves' hyperthyroidism, but limited data show no effect of stress on TPO-Ab levels or hypothyroidism. There are also endogenous factors contributing to the risk of chronic thyroiditis, including female sex and postpartum thyroiditis (see below). Fetal microchimerism, whereby fetal cells enter the maternal circulation, may also increase the mother's risk of developing autoimmune disorders (5).

TREATMENT

The presence of a thyroid antibody (usually TPO-Ab but also TG-Ab) does not, in itself, require therapy, but does increase the likelihood of developing hypothyroidism and, thus, patients' thyroid function should be monitored annually. A higher titer antibody generally predicts a more rapid progression to hypothyroidism. When TSH becomes persistently elevated, then treatment with L-thyroxine may be initiated and TSH restored to the normal range for euthyroid individuals.

Silent thyroiditis (non-postpartum)

INTRODUCTION

Silent or "painless" thyroiditis is a painless inflammation of the thyroid that produces a transient hyperthyroid state (10). The terms silent thyroiditis and painless thyroiditis are most commonly used to describe this condition. However, silent thyroiditis has also been called transient painless thyroiditis, painless thyroiditis with transient hyperthyroidism, painless subacute thyroiditis, atypical thyroiditis, occult subacute thyroiditis, lymphocytic thyroiditis, spontaneously resolving lymphocytic thyroiditis, and transient thyrotoxicosis with lymphocytic thyroiditis. Silent thyroiditis often occurs in the postpartum period and is then called postpartum thyroiditis.

EPIDEMIOLOGY

The incidence of painless thyroiditis was reported with increasing frequency in the late 1970s and early 1980s in the Great Lakes region of the United States and Canada. Silent thyroiditis has also been reported in South America, India, and Japan. However, it has been reported to be less frequent on the east and west coasts of the United States and in Europe and Argentina (11). Patients are usually between 30 and 60 years of age, but silent thyroiditis can occur in all age groups. There is a female-to-male predominance of approximately 1.5:1. There is an 11% chance that patients may have recurrent episodes of silent thyroiditis (12).

PATHOPHYSIOLOGY

In most cases, silent thyroiditis is an autoimmune disease and likely a variant of Hashimoto's thyroiditis. Histologically, silent thyroiditis is characterized by a lymphocytic infiltration of the thyroid, and it is sometimes associated with lymphoid follicles (13). It is associated with other autoimmune diseases, such as autoimmune adrenal insufficiency, lupus erythematosus, idiopathic thrombocytopenic purpura, and rheumatoid arthritis (14). Silent thyroiditis has been associated with HLA DR3, which suggests a genetic component to the disease (15). Thyroid autoantibodies are present in the serum in up to 50% of patients, which suggests an autoimmune process (10). No association with a viral infection has been found. However, the lack of antibodies in some patients and lack of clear female predominance suggests that silent thyroiditis may be a heterogeneous disorder.

DIAGNOSIS

Patients with silent thyroiditis present with symptoms and signs of thyrotoxicosis. The most common symptoms include palpitations, weight loss, nervousness, heat intolerance, and fatigue. The thyrotoxic phase may last from 1 to 12 months, but it usually lasts about 3 months. Approximately one-half of patients have a goiter, in which the thyroid is 1.5 to 3 times the normal size, diffusely enlarged, symmetric, firm, and nontender (10). The course of the disease typically follows three different phases. The first phase is characterized by thyrotoxicosis, and many, but not all patients will go on to develop hypothyroidism as a second stage of silent thyroiditis. Most patients then become euthyroid in the third stage, but permanent hypothyroidism may develop months to years later.

During the first phase of silent thyroiditis, the serum T4 and T3 levels are increased and serum TSH is decreased. The T4/T3 ratio is higher in silent thyroiditis than in Graves' disease, reflecting glandular hormonal stores. The radioactive iodine uptake is very low. Thyroglobulin levels are increased, which may be useful in distinguishing silent thyroiditis from factitious thyrotoxicosis. Serum thyroglobulin concentrations may remain slightly increased even one to two years after recovery of normal thyroid function (16). Thyroid autoantibody levels are increased approximately 30 to 50% of the time. However, approximately 50% of the positive antibody titers become negative within six months after thyroid recovery (10, 12). The white cell count is usually normal. The sedimentation rate is normal in 50% of cases, with only mild elevation in the remaining cases (17). Fine-needle aspiration (FNA) of the thyroid shows lymphocytic infiltration, but aspiration is rarely needed to make the diagnosis. Biopsies show that silent thyroiditis lacks some of the features of chronic lymphocytic thyroiditis, such as Hürthle cells and germinal centers (13).

Patients with silent thyroiditis have a low radioactive iodine uptake, which distinguishes it from states of high radioactive iodine uptake such as Graves' disease or toxic nodular goiter. Other imaging studies which discriminate between painless thyroiditis and Graves' disease include a low 99mTc-pertechnetate thyroid uptake and thyroid vascularity measured by color flow Doppler sonography (18). Silent thyroiditis, with its low radioactive iodine uptake, must be distinguished from iodine-induced thyrotoxicosis, excess thyroid hormone ingestion, and amiodarone-induced thyrotoxicosis (AIT). In addition, struma ovarii can cause a low radioactive iodine uptake over the thyroid, but in these cases, uptake over the ovarian tumor will be increased.

Thyroid hormone levels decrease during the hypothyroid phase and then return to normal during the recovery phase. TSH levels often rise transiently in the recovery phase. The radioactive iodine uptake may also rise transiently above the normal range during the recovery phase of silent thyroiditis.

TREATMENT

As silent thyroiditis usually presents with mild to moderate symptoms of thyrotoxicosis, treatment to relieve symptoms may not be necessary. For patients who are more than mildly symptomatic, beta-adrenergic blocking agents can be administered. Antithyroid drugs are not useful because destroying thyroid cells releases thyroid hormones, causing the thyrotoxic phase of silent thyroiditis. If severe thyrotoxicosis is present, corticosteroids can be administered to decrease the inflammatory process (17). Patients have rarely been treated with thyroidectomy when they have had frequent debilitating episodes of silent thyroiditis (17, 19). Once normal thyroid function returns with a normal or elevated radioiodine uptake, patients with recurrent episodes of silent thyroiditis may consider radioactive iodine ablation of the thyroid (20). The hypothyroid phase of silent thyroiditis usually does not need to be treated since it is usually quite mild, and most patients fully recover normal thyroid function, at least initially. However, if the hypothyroid stage is severe or prolonged, thyroxine can be administered for several months. Almost all patients recover normal thyroid function after an episode of silent thyroiditis, but since approximately 50% of patients with silent thyroiditis will ultimately develop hypothyroidism, thyroid function should be monitored yearly (17).

Postpartum thyroiditis

INTRODUCTION

Postpartum thyroiditis is a syndrome of thyroid dysfunction that occurs within the first year following parturition. Historically, an abnormal thyroid gland in the postpartum dates back almost two millennia, but the association of hypothyroid symptoms and response to thyroid therapy was first described in the mid-20th century (21). It is usually characterized by transient painless thyrotoxicosis with a low radioactive iodine uptake, often followed by a hypothyroid phase that is then followed by thyroid recovery. However, many postpartum thyroiditis patients ultimately develop permanent hypothyroidism within a few years (22–24).

EPIDEMIOLOGY

Postpartum thyroiditis has been reported in North America, South America, Europe, and Asia. An average prevalence figure of about 5–9% of postpartum women has been generally accepted (23, 25–28) with a range of 1.1–16.7% (29). The lower frequency of 1.1% in Asia may be related to variations in regional, dietary iodine intake or genetic differences in susceptibility (30). Approximately 10% of women in the general population have positive thyroid antibodies and approximately one-half of these patients develop postpartum thyroiditis. An increased incidence of postpartum thyroiditis (10–25%) is found among patients with type 1 diabetes mellitus as well as associations with other autoimmune disorders (e.g., systemic lupus erythematosus, multiple sclerosis, antipituitary antibodies) (31). Postpartum thyroid dysfunction has also been reported after pregnancy loss (24).

PATHOPHYSIOLOGY

Women who are prone to developing postpartum thyroiditis most likely have pre-existing, asymptomatic autoimmune thyroiditis. During pregnancy, the maternal immune system is partially suppressed, with a subsequent rebound in thyroid autoantibodies after delivery. Studies have shown that higher thyroid antibody levels are associated with a higher risk of thyroid dysfunction and clinical symptoms (32–35). Postpartum thyroiditis has also been related to HLA type. HLA-DR3, -DR4, and -DR5 are increased in patients with postpartum thyroiditis (36–39), consistent with an immune disorder. Biopsy specimens of thyroid tissue during postpartum thyroiditis have shown a lymphocytic infiltration (40). Smoking has been associated with postpartum thyroiditis in some (25, 41) but not all studies (28, 42, 43).

Several studies have shown postpartum thyroiditis to be associated with the presence of a goiter during pregnancy (26, 32, 44). One report using ultrasound showed a significant increase in thyroid volume between 8- and 20-weeks gestation in women who went on to develop postpartum thyroiditis (45). However, another prospective study using ultrasound found that thyroid size, before, during, or after pregnancy, was not a useful indicator for the development of postpartum thyroiditis (42). Therefore, even though postpartum thyroiditis may be associated with a goiter, the presence of a goiter is not a predictive indicator of postpartum thyroiditis.

DIAGNOSIS

Patients with postpartum thyroiditis may present with fatigue, palpitations, heat intolerance, nervousness, emotional liability, and other hyperthyroid symptoms. Many patients will have some enlargement of the thyroid. Postpartum thyroiditis is almost universally painless, although one case of painful disease has been reported (46). In postpartum thyroiditis, there is an absence of exophthalmos and, almost always, an increase in antithyroid antibody titers. Patients may present at a time when thyroid hormones levels are high, normal, or low. Since the thyrotoxic phase is a destructive type of thyroiditis, the 24-hour radioactive iodine uptake is low. However, radionuclide uptake measurements are usually not possible in postpartum women who are breast feeding.

Figure 3.1 shows the frequency of thyrotoxicosis, hypothyroidism, or both in postpartum thyroid dysfunction. The classical triphasic pattern of postpartum thyroiditis is mild thyrotoxicosis followed by transient hypothyroidism with subsequent thyroid recovery. This pattern of postpartum thyroiditis occurs in 25% of patients. The thyrotoxic phase usually presents one to six months postpartum. Frequently, a period of hypothyroidism develops over the next three to four months, followed by a return to normal thyroid

function. Some patients with postpartum thyroiditis only develop transient thyrotoxicosis without subsequent hypothyroidism. This can either take the form of thyroiditis-induced thyrotoxicosis in approximately 24% of patients or hyperthyroidism caused by Graves' disease in approximately 11% of patients. Some patients (40%) with postpartum thyroiditis present only with hypothyroidism (presumably the thyrotoxic phase was mild and not detected) that is followed by recovery of thyroid function (47). Figure 3.2 shows the possible stages of thyroid function in the natural history of postpartum thyroiditis. Ide et al., (48) reported that the thyrotoxic phase of postpartum thyroid disease occurred within 3 months of delivery in 86% of patients, while all cases of postpartum Graves' disease developed at 6.5 months or later. When the anti-TSH receptor antibody was positive, thyroid blood flow by Doppler ultrasonography was > 4% in all women with postpartum Graves' disease, while when the receptor antibody was negative, the thyroid blood flow was <4% in all patients with thyrotoxic postpartum thyroiditis.

All patients with postpartum thyroiditis should be monitored for the future development of thyroid failure. Approximately 20 to 64% of patients with transient thyroid disease postpartum develop hypothyroidism with long-term follow-up (33, 36, 37, 49, 50). Factors associated with the development of permanent hypothyroidism include higher titer of thyroid autoantibodies, greater severity of the hypothyroid phase of postpartum thyroiditis, and a previous history of spontaneous abortion (46, 49). Microsomal and thyroid peroxidase antibodies have been reported to have a sensitivity range of 0.45 to 0.89 and a specificity range of 0.9 to 0.98 (47).

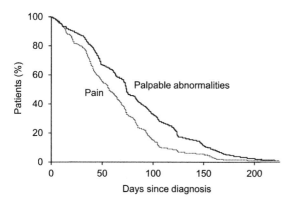

Figure 3.1 The graph correlates the time from the beginning of pain to the disappearance of pain and palpable abnormalities in 70 patients observed through the course of the disease. In all instances, pain and tenderness ceased first. The mean duration of pain was 65 days versus 84 days for palpable abnormalities. (From Nordyke RA, Gilbert FI, Jr., Lew C. *West J. Med.* 1991; 155(1): 61–3.)

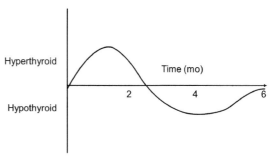

Figure 3.2 Natural history of subacute thyroiditis.

TREATMENT

Treatment of the thyrotoxic phase of postpartum thyroiditis is often not needed, since the symptoms are usually mild. Beta-adrenergic blocking drugs can be used in symptomatic patients, but should be used with caution in lactating women. The beta-adrenergic blocking drug can be tapered as the thyrotoxic phase resolves. If symptoms are mild and transient, then the hypothyroid phase can also be observed without treatment. If the hypothyroid stage is severe or prolonged, thyroxine should be administered for 6 to 12 months. After several months, the thyroid hormone can be tapered or withdrawn and the serum TSH measured to see if the patient remains euthyroid. Even if full thyroid recovery occurs, patients with a history of postpartum thyroiditis should be followed long-term for possible development of permanent hypothyroidism. Some experts prefer to keep women on thyroid hormone therapy until they are finished having children. Since postpartum thyroiditis can recur in up to 80% of subsequent pregnancies, future pregnancies should also be monitored (47). Negro et al. treated 85 euthyroid antibody–positive women in the first trimester of pregnancy with selenium, 200 g daily starting at 12-weeks gestation, versus placebo. Postpartum thyroiditis developed significantly less frequently in the women administered selenium than in women given placebo (28.6 vs. 48.6% p ≤ 0.01) (51). This study will require confirmation and determination of possible adverse effects before selenium therapy can be recommended. Many European countries, but not the United States, have dietary selenium intake deemed insufficient for optimal plasma glutathione peroxidase activity (52).

Infectious/post-infectious thyroiditis

Acute infectious

INTRODUCTION

Infectious thyroiditis is an inflammatory process caused by the invasion of the thyroid by bacteria, mycobacteria, fungi, protozoa, or flatworms. Infectious thyroiditis may rarely cause thyrotoxicosis.

EPIDEMIOLOGY

Infectious thyroiditis is a rare disorder. The thyroid is felt to be relatively resistant to infection because of its vascularity, its large concentration of iodine, the presence of hydrogen peroxide, and its encapsulation. Infectious thyroiditis may be more prevalent in the pediatric age group (53).

PATHOPHYSIOLOGY

Many different bacteria that can infect the thyroid, including *Streptococcus*, *Staphylococcus*, *Escherichia coli*, *Salmonella*, *Bacteroides*, *Pasteurella* and *Treponema pallidum*, *Mycobacterium tuberculosis* and several fungi, including *Coccidioides immitis*, *Aspergillus*, *Candida albicans* (54) and *Nocardia* spp., have been associated with thyroiditis (55). *Pneumocystis carinii* may also cause infectious thyroiditis. Patients who are immunocompromised or have acquired immunodeficiency syndrome are at particular risk for infectious thyroiditis.

Most often, this infection is caused by a direct extension of an internal fistulous tract between the pyriform sinus and the thyroid (56, 57). This tract is more common in children and may represent the course of migration of the ultimobranchial body from its embryonic origin in the fifth pharyngeal pouch. This extension tends to develop more commonly in the left thyroid lobe than in the right. However, infection in the thyroid may occur in a normal thyroid, multinodular goiter, or in a degenerating thyroid nodule as well. As noted above, immunocompromised patients may have a higher risk of infectious thyroiditis (58). Infectious thyroiditis with thyrotoxicosis has also been reported to occur after repeated FNA of a cystic thyroid nodule (59).

DIAGNOSIS

Patients with infectious thyroiditis usually present with pain and may have a swollen, hot, and tender thyroid (55). As a result, affected individuals may avoid extension of their neck due to pain, swallowing may be painful, and dysphagia may be present. They may also present with signs of infection in adjacent tissues, cervical lymphadenopathy, and systemic signs of fever and chills.

Laboratory data may include an increased white blood cell count and increased sedimentation rate. The patient may have increased thyroid hormone levels and present with symptoms of thyrotoxicosis, due to hormonal release from the thyroid (55). In one review, 12 out of 56 cases had laboratory data suggesting hyperthyroidism (60). However, most patients are biochemically euthyroid, and the radioactive iodine uptake will usually be normal. Thyroid ultrasound or computed tomography (CT) scan of the neck may show a local abscess that can be aspirated and cultured to make the diagnosis (61). A barium swallow can be obtained to evaluate for possible predisposing factors such as a fistulous tract between the pyriform sinus and the thyroid.

TREATMENT

Treatment depends on the identification of the organism causing the infection. Aspiration of the thyroid should be obtained with appropriate staining and culture of the material. Systemic antibiotics, which are tailored to the specific infectious agent, are administered (53). An abscess will require surgical exploration and drainage, and fistulae also require surgery or cauterization of the pyriform sinus to prevent recurrent infection (62–64).

Subacute thyroiditis

INTRODUCTION

Subacute thyroiditis is a painful, inflammatory thyroid condition associated with thyrotoxicosis. In the past, it has also been called granulomatous thyroiditis, giant cell thyroiditis, non-infectious thyroiditis, acute nonsuppurative thyroiditis, and de Quervain's thyroiditis.

EPIDEMIOLOGY

Subacute thyroiditis is not nearly as common as Graves' disease, but it is more common than silent thyroiditis if postpartum thyroiditis is excluded. It has been reported to occur at the rate of one in every five to eight cases of Graves' disease (65). In Olmsted County, Minnesota, subacute thyroiditis occurred at a rate of 4.9 cases per 100,000/yr (66), whereas the incidence of Graves' disease was 10/100,000/year in men and three times as frequent in women (67). Subacute thyroiditis has been reported in North America, Europe, Scandinavia, and Japan, but it is not often reported in the tropical and subtropical areas of the world. In Hawaii, subacute thyroiditis is seen at the same rate among Caucasians and Japanese, indicating a similar prevalence among these two races living in the same environment (68). It is not known whether the lack of occurrence in the tropical and subtropical areas is due to a lower actual frequency or

ascertainment bias. However, despite the possible geographic variation, subacute thyroiditis is recognized more frequently during the summer months (69, 70). Subacute thyroiditis has been reported in all age groups. It is most common in the third to sixth decades of life, and it is rare in children. Female patients outnumber male patients in a ratio of up to 6:1 (71).

PATHOPHYSIOLOGY

The cause of subacute thyroiditis is not known, but an infectious etiology is likely; for example, it tends to occur following an upper respiratory tract infection. Mumps, measles, influenza, common colds, adenovirus, Epstein-Barr virus, coxsackievirus, and cat-scratch disease have all been associated with subacute thyroiditis (72–76). Subacute thyroiditis (and recurrences) is associated with HLA-B35 approximately 72% of the time (77), suggesting a genetic susceptibility to antecedent viral infections. Subacute thyroiditis has been reported in twins and family members (78, 79). Infiltrative diseases, such as amyloid, have also been reported to cause a subacute thyroiditis–like clinical picture (80), and anaplastic thyroid cancer can rarely begin with painful, rapid thyroid enlargement known as "malignant pseudothyroiditis" (81). Thyroiditis induced by amiodarone can also occasionally present with a similar clinical picture.

The thyroid gland in subacute thyroiditis is enlarged and firm; it may adhere to adjacent tissues. Thyroid tissue obtained by FNA biopsy shows an inflammatory infiltrate of neutrophils, lymphocytes, histiocytes, and multinucleated giant cells (82, 83).

DIAGNOSIS

Patients with subacute thyroiditis usually present with an acute onset of malaise, feverishness, and pain in the region of the thyroid gland. The pain may radiate from the thyroid to the jaw and to the ears, or down to the anterior chest wall. Coughing, swallowing, turning the head, or wearing tight clothing around the neck can aggravate the discomfort. Approximately one-third to one-half of patients may present with unilateral thyroid pain, and one-third of patients can have migratory discomfort wherein the pain spreads from one thyroid lobe to the other, so-called "creeping thyroiditis." Approximately one-third of cases may present with diffuse pain in the thyroid (65, 76, 84). Some biopsy-proven cases of subacute thyroiditis have been reported to be painless (82, 85, 86).

Many patients may have systemic symptoms of malaise, myalgias, fever, and anorexia. As noted above, approximately 50% of patients have a history of an antecedent upper respiratory infection. Symptoms of thyrotoxicosis are also present in 50–60% of patients, and these may include heat intolerance, palpitations, tremor, and nervousness. Cases of subacute thyroiditis causing thyroid storm have been reported (87).

Physical examination shows an uncomfortable patient with a tender, enlarged, and firm thyroid gland. The process is often asymmetric, and lymphadenopathy is usually not present. Symptoms of thyrotoxicosis may last 4 to 10 weeks, but the inflammation with a painful, tender thyroid often lasts for eight weeks, and on rare occasions, up to one year. Pain and tenderness resolve first, followed by the resolution of the palpable thyroid abnormalities, as shown in Figure 3.3 (68). If the patient is not seen until late in the course of the disease and after pain resolves, the discovery of a thyroid nodule as the residual of lobar enlargement may lead to unnecessary surgery, unless an FNA is performed.

Laboratory evaluation shows increased serum levels of free thyroxine (FT4) and triiodothyronine (T3) due to follicular disruption, with the release of stored thyroid hormones and thyroglobulin into the systemic circulation. The T4/T3 ratio is typically higher than in Graves' disease, reflecting glandular hormone stores. Serum TSH level is suppressed (88). The white blood cell count is usually normal but may be moderately increased. The erythrocyte sedimentation rate is virtually always increased, often to as high or higher than 100 mm/hr (76, 84). C-reactive protein is also usually elevated in patients with untreated subacute thyroiditis (89). Thyroid autoantibodies are usually absent or present in low titer, and if present, they are usually transient. The 24-hour radioactive iodine uptake initially is very low but may rebound and become elevated during the subsequent hypothyroid stage of recovery.

As the course of subacute thyroiditis progresses, the serum concentration of thyroid hormones returns to normal. In more severe cases, transient hypothyroidism develops (90). Thyroid function usually returns to normal, but permanent hypothyroidism may occur in 15% of patients with extended follow-up. Patients treated with corticosteroid therapy may develop hypothyroidism more commonly than those not treated with corticosteroids (66). Recurrent bouts of subacute thyroiditis may occur in 4% of patients, 6 to 21 years after the initial episode (66). Figure 3.4 shows the typical phases of thyroid function during subacute thyroiditis.

TREATMENT

Nonsteroidal anti-inflammatory drugs (NSAIDs) or salicylates (2 g/day) are used initially to treat subacute thyroiditis (91). However, corticosteroids are used for more severe cases of pain or in patients not responding to NSAIDs, and result in rapid clinical improvement (92). Corticosteroids produce partial or near complete relief of pain and neck tenderness within 24 to 48 hours. If symptoms do not respond promptly, an alternate diagnosis, such as acute infectious thyroiditis, should be considered. Typically, prednisone in an initial dose of 40 mg/day is used for about a week, followed by a tapering dose of 10 mg/wk and withdrawal by four weeks. As the drug is tapered, exacerbation of pain may occur in approximately 20% of patients (71, 91). If this occurs, the dose can be increased and treatment continued for another month. A smaller dose of 15 mg prednisolone, tapered by 5 mg every two weeks, was also effective in most patients, although 20% required therapy for more than eight weeks (93). In extremely rare cases, neck pain and malaise may be prolonged. In these cases, thyroidectomy may be needed (94). Beta-adrenergic

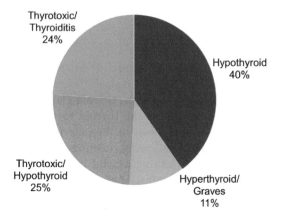

Figure 3.3 Frequency of hyperthyroidism, hypothyroidism, or both in postpartum thyroid dysfunction.

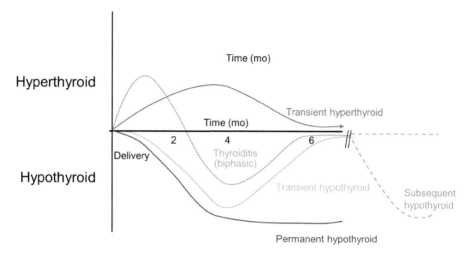

Figure 3.4 Natural history of postpartum thyroiditis.

antagonist drugs may be helpful in controlling symptoms of thyrotoxicosis. However, they are not usually needed because corticosteroids or NSAIDs usually alleviate thyrotoxicosis as well as the thyroid pain.

Riedel's thyroiditis

ETIOLOGY

Riedel's thyroiditis is an aggressive fibroinflammatory condition of uncertain etiology which involves the thyroid and tissues surrounding the thyroid gland. It should be distinguished from a fibrosing form of Hashimoto's thyroiditis, which is limited to the thyroid gland.

PATHOPHYSIOLOGY

Riedel's thyroiditis may be confined to the neck but may also be a component of an IgG-4 related systemic inflammatory disease (95–97). Thyroid tissue IgG-4, measured by immunohistochemistry, is detected in both Riedel's and Hashimoto's thyroiditis, with a trend for more staining detected in the former (97). Serum IgG-4 level was not elevated in two patients in which it was measured (98). In one series, 38% of patients had extracervical fibrotic processes (fibrosing mediastinitis or retroperitoneal, orbital, or pancreatic fibrosis) (98). Histologic criteria include (a) a fibroinflammatory process, (b) extension into surrounding tissues, (c) inflammatory cells (lymphocytes, eosinophils, plasma cells), (d) occlusive phlebitis, and (e) no neoplasm (99).

DIAGNOSIS

Patients with Riedel's thyroiditis may present with tracheal narrowing, dysphagia, vocal cord paralysis/hoarseness, or neck pain. Parathyroid involvement may lead to hypocalcemia from hypoparathyroidism. Imaging of the neck should include an ultrasound and possibly CT scan to determine if the carotid vessels, trachea, or esophagus is compromised. PET-CT may also be helpful in identifying extracervical tissue involvement (96).

TREATMENT

Surgery should be limited to a biopsy for diagnosis and possibly isthmusectomy to relieve constriction of the trachea, as blurred tissue planes make more extensive surgery risky. Initial systemic therapy has been with glucocorticoids. For some unresponsive patients, tamoxifen has been successful, perhaps through stimulating TGF-beta1 which inhibits the fibroblast growth factor and inflammation (96). Mycophenolate mofetil and prednisone have been used, as has rituximab (100). Given the rarity of this disease, and variable clinical course, no definitive therapy has been established.

Radiation thyroiditis

INTRODUCTION

Radioactive ^{131}I and external beam radiation are used to treat thyroid disease. Radiation thyroiditis with a thyrotoxic phase has been reported following radiation treatment with both forms of radiation therapy.

EPIDEMIOLOGY

Radiation thyroiditis from ^{131}I occurred in 5% and 16% of patients receiving either 30 mCi or 100 mCi, respectively, for ablation of residual normal thyroid tissue (101). Thyroiditis was more common with larger thyroid remnant uptake. Transient increases in T3 and T4 levels at about 10 days after therapy are seen in some hyperthyroid patients treated with radioactive iodine (102). Although clinically significant exacerbation of hyperthyroidism is usually not observed (103), painful radiation thyroiditis requiring anti-inflammatory drug therapy (104) as well as thyroid storm has been reported after radioiodine therapy (105). Local tenderness, difficulty swallowing, and hyperthyroidism may also occur after recombinant human TSH stimulated 131-Iodine therapy for multinodular goiter (106).

Radiation thyroiditis causing transient thyrotoxicosis has also been reported with external beam radiation. In a prospective study of external beam radiation directed to the neck for metastatic cancer treatment, 8 out of 22 patients developed a subnormal TSH after receiving 40 Gy of external beam radiation over two weeks. Levels of T4 and T3 tended to rise after 40 Gy of radiation, but the levels were not statistically different from the baseline (107). Several case reports of external beam radiation-induced overt thyrotoxicosis have been reported (108, 109).

PATHOPHYSIOLOGY

Radiation presumably causes a destructive thyroiditis with the release of preformed thyroid hormone into the bloodstream. The thyrotoxicosis is transient. The radiation dose that has been reported to cause external beam radiation-induced thyrotoxicosis varies between 37 and 50 Gy (108, 110). It is likely that the greater the external beam radiation dose, the more frequently thyrotoxic thyroiditis and subsequent hypothyroidism occur.

DIAGNOSIS

In radioactive iodine-induced thyroiditis, manifestations usually occur within 2 weeks after radioactive iodine is administered. Symptoms, if present, consist of neck and ear pain, dysphagia, thyroid tenderness, and/or transient symptoms of thyrotoxicosis. External beam radiation-induced thyrotoxic thyroiditis usually occurs within a few weeks of radiation exposure. It is characterized by increased serum levels of thyroid hormones and suppressed serum levels of TSH. Serum thyroid autoantibodies are typically negative. The 24-hour radioactive iodine uptake is low.

TREATMENT

Since the thyrotoxicosis from radiation thyroiditis is transient, observation may be all that is needed. Treatment with beta-adrenergic blocking agents can be used to control tachycardia and tremor. Patients with ^{131}I-induced thyrotoxic thyroiditis may have significant neck pain requiring treatment with corticosteroids (104). After patients are treated with external beam radiation therapy, they should be monitored long-term for the development of hypothyroidism.

Trauma-induced thyroiditis

Several reports of trauma-induced thyroiditis have been described, and this condition may be associated with thyrotoxicosis. Thyroid biopsy, parathyroid surgery, surgical trauma, and trauma induced by a seat belt have all been reported to cause thyrotoxicosis (111–113). The thyroid may be tender due to the trauma. The thyrotoxicosis is transient and associated with a low uptake of radioactive iodine.

REFERENCES

1. Lee HJ, Li CW, Hammerstad SS, Stefan M, Tomer Y. Immunogenetics of autoimmune thyroid diseases: A comprehensive review. *J. Autoimmun.* 2015; 64: 82–90.
2. Zaletel K, Gaberscek S. Hashimoto's thyroiditis: From genes to the disease. *Curr. Genomics* 2011; 12: 576–88.
3. Hutfless S, Matos P, Talor MV, Caturegli P, Rose NR. Significance of prediagnostic thyroid antibodies in women with autoimmune thyroid disease. *J. Clin. Endocrinol. Metab.* 2011; 96: E1466–71.
4. Mazza E, Quaglino F, Suriani A, Palestini N, Gottero C, Leli R, Taraglio S. Thyroidectomy for painful thyroiditis resistant to steroid treatment: Three new cases with review of the literature. *Case Rep. Endocrinol.* 2015; 2015: 138327.

5. Ajjan RA, Weetman AP. The pathogenesis of Hashimoto's thyroiditis: Further developments in our understanding. *Horm. Metab. Res.* 2015; 47: 702–10.

6. Wiersinga WM. Clinical relevance of environmental factors in the pathogenesis of autoimmune thyroid disease. *Endocrinol. Metab. (Seoul)* 2016; 31: 213–22.

7. van Zuuren EJ, Albusta AY, Fedorowicz Z, Carter B, Pijl H. Selenium supplementation for Hashimoto's thyroiditis. *Cochrane Database Syst. Rev.* 2013: CD010223: CD010223.

8. Winther KH, Watt T, Bjorner JB, Cramon P, Feldt-Rasmussen U, Gluud C, Gram J, et al. The chronic autoimmune thyroiditis quality of life selenium trial (CATALYST): Study protocol for a randomized controlled trial. *Trials* 2014; 15: 115.

9. Krysiak R, Kowalcze K, Okopien B. The effect of vitamin D on thyroid autoimmunity in non-lactating women with postpartum thyroiditis. *Eur. J. Clin. Nutr.* 2016; 70: 637–9.

10. Woolf PD. Transient painless thyroiditis with hyperthyroidism: A variant of lymphocytic thyroiditis? *Endocr. Rev.* 1980; 1: 411–20.

11. Schneeberg NG. Silent thyroiditis. *Arch. Intern. Med.* 1983; 143: 2214.

12. Nikolai TF, Coombs GJ, McKenzie AK. Lymphocytic thyroiditis with spontaneously resolving hyperthyroidism and subacute thyroiditis. Long-term follow-up. *Arch. Intern. Med.* 1981; 141: 1455–8.

13. Nikolai TF, Brosseau J, Kettrick MA, Roberts R, Beltaos E. Lymphocytic thyroiditis with spontaneously resolving hyperthyroidism (silent thyroiditis). *Arch. Intern. Med.* 1980; 140: 478–82.

14. Parker M, Klein I, Fishman LM, Levey GS. Silent thyrotoxic thyroiditis in association with chronic adrenocortical insufficiency. *Arch. Intern. Med.* 1980; 140: 1108–9.

15. Farid NR, Hawe BS, Walfish PG. Increased frequency of HLA-DR3 and 5 in the syndromes of painless thyroiditis with transient thyrotoxicosis: Evidence for an autoimmune aetiology. *Clin. Endocrinol. (Oxf.)* 1983; 19: 699–704.

16. Smallridge RC, De Keyser FM, Van Herle AJ, Butkus NE, Wartofsky L. Thyroid iodine content and serum thyroglobulin: Cues to the natural history of destruction-induced thyroiditis. *J. Clin. Endocrinol. Metab.* 1986; 62: 1213–9.

17. Nikolai TF, Coombs GJ, McKenzie AK, Miller RW, Weir GJ. Treatment of lymphocytic thyroiditis with spontaneously resolving hyperthyroidism (silent thyroiditis). *Arch. Intern. Med.* 1982; 142: 2281–3.

18. Uchida T, Suzuki R, Kasai T, Onose H, Komiya K, Goto H, Takeno K, et al. Cutoff value of thyroid uptake of (99m) Tc-pertechnetate to discriminate between Graves' disease and painless thyroiditis: A single center retrospective study. *Endocr. J.* 2016; 63: 143–9.

19. Gorman CA, Duick DS, Woolner LB, Wahner HW. Transient hyperthyroidism in patients with lymphocytic thyroiditis. *Mayo Clin. Proc.* 1978; 53: 359–65.

20. Mittra ES, McDougall IR. Recurrent silent thyroiditis: A report of four patients and review of the literature. *Thyroid* 2007; 17: 671–5.

21. Smallridge RC., Clark T. Sawin historical vignette: What do criminology, Harry Houdini, and King George V have in common with postpartum thyroid dysfunction? *Thyroid* 2014; 24: 1752–8.

22. Smallridge RC. Postpartum thyroid dysfunction: A frequently undiagnosed endocrine disorder. *Endocrinologist* 1996; 6: 44–50.

23. Stagnaro-Green A. Approach to the patient with postpartum thyroiditis. *J. Clin. Endocrinol. Metab.* 2012; 97: 334–42.

24. Alexander EK, Pearce EN, Brent GA, Brown RS, Chen H, Dosiou C, Grobman WA, et al. 2017 Guidelines of the American Thyroid Association for the diagnosis and management of thyroid disease during pregnancy and the postpartum. *Thyroid* 2017; 27: 315–89.

25. Fung HY, Kologlu M, Collison K, John R, Richards CJ, Hall R, McGregor AM. Postpartum thyroid dysfunction in Mid Glamorgan. *Br. Med. J. (Clin. Res. Ed.)* 1988; 296: 241–4.

26. Amino N, Mori H, Iwatani Y, Tanizawa O, Kawashima M, Tsuge I, Ibaragi K, Kumahara Y, Miyai K. High prevalence of transient postpartum thyrotoxicosis and hypothyroidism. *N. Engl. J. Med.* 1982; 306: 849–52.

27. Gerstein HC. How common is postpartum thyroiditis? A methodologic overview of the literature. *Arch. Intern. Med.* 1990; 150: 1397–400.

28. Jansson R, Bernander S, Karlsson A, Levin K, Nilsson G. Autoimmune thyroid dysfunction in the postpartum period. *J. Clin. Endocrinol. Metab.* 1984; 58: 681–7.

29. Nicholson WK, Robinson KA, Smallridge RC, Ladenson PW, Powe NR. Prevalence of postpartum thyroid dysfunction: A quantitative review. *Thyroid* 2006; 16: 573–82.

30. Rajatanavin R, Chailurkit LO, Tirarungsikul K, Chalayondeja W, Jittivanich U, Puapradit W. Postpartum thyroid dysfunction in Bangkok: A geographical variation in the prevalence. *Acta Endocrinol. (Copenh.)* 1990; 122: 283–7.

31. Di Bari F, Granese R, Le Donne M, Vita R, Benvenga S. Autoimmune abnormalities of postpartum thyroid diseases. *Front. Endocrinol. (Lausanne)* 2017; 8: 166.

32. Hayslip CC, Fein HG, O'Donnell VM, Friedman DS, Klein TA, Smallridge RC. The value of serum antimicrosomal antibody testing in screening for symptomatic postpartum thyroid dysfunction. *Am. J. Obstet. Gynecol.* 1988; 159: 203–9.

33. Solomon BL, Fein HG, Smallridge RC. Usefulness of antimicrosomal antibody titers in the diagnosis and treatment of postpartum thyroiditis. *J. Fam. Pract.* 1993; 36: 177–82.

34. Harris B, Othman S, Davies JA, Weppner GJ, Richards CJ, Newcombe RG, Lazarus JH, et al. Association between postpartum thyroid dysfunction and thyroid antibodies and depression. *BMJ* 1992; 305: 152–6.

35. Stagnaro-Green A, Roman SH, Cobin RH, el-Harazy E, Wallenstein S, Davies TF. A prospective study of lymphocyte-initiated immunosuppression in normal pregnancy: Evidence of a T-cell etiology for postpartum thyroid dysfunction. *J. Clin. Endocrinol. Metab.* 1992; 74: 645–53.

36. Tachi J, Amino N, Tamaki H, Aozasa M, Iwatani Y, Miyai K. Long term follow-up and HLA association in patients with postpartum hypothyroidism. *J. Clin. Endocrinol. Metab.* 1988; 66: 480–4.

37. Vargas MT, Briones-Urbina R, Gladman D, Papsin FR, Walfish PG. Antithyroid microsomal autoantibodies and HLA-DR5 are associated with postpartum thyroid dysfunction: Evidence supporting an autoimmune pathogenesis. *J. Clin. Endocrinol. Metab.* 1988; 67: 327–33.

38. Kologlu M, Fung H, Darke C, Richards CJ, Hall R, McGregor AM. Postpartum thyroid dysfunction and HLA status. *Eur. J. Clin. Invest.* 1990; 20: 56–60.

39. Jansson R, Safwenberg J, Dahlberg PA. Influence of the HLA-DR4 antigen and iodine status on the development of autoimmune postpartum thyroiditis. *J. Clin. Endocrinol. Metab.* 1985; 60: 168–73.

40. Nikolai TF, Turney SL, Roberts RC. Postpartum lymphocytic thyroiditis. Prevalence, clinical course, and long-term follow-up. *Arch. Intern. Med.* 1987; 147: 221–4.

41. Kuijpens JL, Pop VJ, Vader HL, Drexhage HA, Wiersinga WM. Prediction of postpartum thyroid dysfunction: Can it be improved? *Eur. J. Endocrinol.* 1998; 139: 36–43.

42. Rasmussen NG, Hornnes PJ, Hoier-Madsen M, Feldt-Rasmussen U, Hegedüs L. Thyroid size and function in healthy pregnant women with thyroid autoantibodies. Relation to development of postpartum thyroiditis. *Acta Endocrinol. (Copenh.)* 1990; 123: 395–401.

43. Lazarus JH, Hall R, Othman S, Parkes AB, Richards CJ, McCulloch B, Harris B. The clinical spectrum of postpartum thyroid disease. *QJM* 1996; 89: 429–35.

44. Lervang HH, Pryds O, Ostergaard Kristensen HP. Thyroid dysfunction after delivery: Incidence and clinical course. *Acta Med. Scand.* 1987; 222: 369–74.

45. Adams H, Jones MC, Othman S, Lazarus JH, Parkes AB, Hall R, Phillips DI, Richards CJ. The sonographic appearances in postpartum thyroiditis. *Clin. Radiol.* 1992; 45: 311–5.

46. Lazarus JH, Othman S. Review: Thyroid disease in relation to pregnancy. *Clin Endocrinol* 1991; 34: 91–8.

47. Smallridge RC. Postpartum thyroid disease: A model of immunologic dysfunction. *Clin. Appl. Immunol. Rev.* 2000; 1: 89–103.

48. Ide A, Amino N, Kang S, Yoshioka W, Kudo T, Nishihara E, Ito M, Nakamura H, Miyauchi A. Differentiation of postpartum Graves' thyrotoxicosis from postpartum destructive thyrotoxicosis using antithyrotropin receptor antibodies and thyroid blood flow. *Thyroid* 2014; 24: 1027–31.

49. Othman S, Phillips DIW, Parkes AB, Richards CJ, Harris B, Fung H, Darke C, et al. A long-term follow-up of postpartum thyroiditis. *Clin. Endocrinol. (Oxf.)* 1990; 32: 559–64.

50. Azizi F. The occurrence of permanent thyroid failure in patients with subclinical postpartum thyroiditis. *Eur. J. Endocrinol.* 2005; 153: 367–71.

51. Negro R, Greco G, Mangieri T, Pezzarossa A, Dazzi D, Hassan H. The influence of selenium supplementation on postpartum thyroid status in pregnant women with thyroid peroxidase autoantibodies. *J. Clin. Endocrinol. Metab.* 2007; 92: 1263–8.

52. Hu S, Rayman MP. Multiple nutritional factors and the risk of Hashimoto's thyroiditis. *Thyroid* 2017; 27: 597–610.

53. Brook I. Microbiology and management of acute suppurative thyroiditis in children. *Int. J. Pediatr. Otorhinolaryngol.* 2003; 67: 447–51.

54. Gandhi RT, Tollin SR, Seely EW. Diagnosis of Candida thyroiditis by fine needle aspiration. *J. Infect.* 1994; 28: 77–81.

55. Paes JE, Burman KD, Cohen J, Franklyn J, McHenry CR, Shoham S, Kloos RT. Acute bacterial suppurative thyroiditis: A clinical review and expert opinion. *Thyroid* 2010; 20: 247–55.

56. Hatabu H, Kasagi K, Yamamoto K, Iida Y, Misaki T, Hidaka A, Endo K, Konishi J. Acute suppurative thyroiditis associated with piriform sinus fistula: Sonographic findings. *AJR Am. J. Roentgenol.* 1990; 155: 845–7.

57. Miyauchi A, Matsuzuka F, Kuma K, Takai S. Piriform sinus fistula: An underlying abnormality common in patients with acute suppurative thyroiditis. *World J. Surg.* 1990; 14: 400–5.

58. Yu EH, Ko WC, Chuang YC, Wu TJ. Suppurative *Acinetobacter baumannii* thyroiditis with bacteremic pneumonia: Case report and review. *Clin. Infect. Dis.* 1998; 27: 1286–90.

59. Nishihara E, Miyauchi A, Matsuzuka F, Sasaki I, Ohye H, Kubota S, Fukata S, Amino N, Kuma K. Acute suppurative thyroiditis after fine-needle aspiration causing thyrotoxicosis. *Thyroid* 2005; 15: 1183–7.

60. Berger SA, Zonszein J, Villamena P, Mittman N. Infectious diseases of the thyroid gland. *Rev. Infect. Dis.* 1983; 5: 108–22.

61. Masuoka H, Miyauchi A, Tomoda C, Inoue H, Takamura Y, Ito Y, Kobayashi K, Miya A. Imaging studies in sixty patients with acute suppurative thyroiditis. *Thyroid* 2011; 21: 1075–80.

62. Parida PK, Gopalakrishnan S, Saxena SK. Pediatric recurrent acute suppurative thyroiditis of third branchial arch origin—Our experience in 17 cases. *Int. J. Pediatr. Otorhinolaryngol.* 2014; 78: 1953–7.

63. Zhang P, Tian X. Recurrent neck lesions secondary to pyriform sinus fistula. *Eur. Arch. Otorhinolaryngol.* 2016; 273: 735–9.

64. Sheng Q, Lv Z, Xiao X, Xu W, Liu J, Wu Y. Endoscopic-assisted surgery for pyriform sinus fistula in Chinese children: A 73-consecutive-case study. *J. Laparoendosc. Adv. Surg. Tech. A* 2016; 26: 70–4.

65. Woolner LB, McConahey WM, Beahrs OH. Granulomatous thyroiditis (de Quervain's thyroiditis). *J. Clin. Endocrinol. Metab.* 1957; 17: 1202–21.

66. Fatourechi V, Aniszewski JP, Fatourechi GZ, Atkinson EJ, Jacobsen SJ. Clinical features and outcome of subacute thyroiditis in an incidence cohort: Olmsted County, Minnesota, study. *J. Clin. Endocrinol. Metab.* 2003; 88: 2100–5.

67. Furszyfer J, Kurland LT, McConahey WM, Elveback LR. Graves' disease in Olmsted County, Minnesota, 1935 through 1967. *Mayo Clin. Proc.* 1970; 45: 636–44.

68. Nordyke RA, Gilbert FI, Jr., Lew C. Painful subacute thyroiditis in Hawaii. *West. J. Med.* 1991; 155: 61–3.

69. Martino E, Buratti L, Bartalena L, Mariotti S, Cupini C, Aghini-Lombardi F, Pinchera A. High prevalence of subacute thyroiditis during summer season in Italy. *J. Endocrinol. Invest.* 1987; 10: 321–3.

70. Saito S, Sakurada T, Yamamoto M, Yamaguchi T, Yoshida K. Subacute thyroiditis: Observations on 98 cases for the last 14 years. *Tohoku J. Exp. Med.* 1974; 113: 141–7.

71. Singer PA. Thyroiditis. Acute, subacute, and chronic. *Med. Clin. North Am.* 1991; 75: 61–77.

72. Hung W. Mumps thyroiditis and hypothyroidism. *J. Pediatr.* 1969; 74: 611–3.

73. Hintze G, Fortelius P, Railo J. Epidemic thyroiditis. *Acta Endocrinol. (Copenh.)* 1964; 45: 381–401.

74. Swann NH. Acute thyroiditis: Five cases associated with adenovirus infection. *Metabolism* 1964; 13: 908–10.

75. Shumway M, Davis PL. Cat-scratch thyroiditis treated with thyrotropic hormone. *J. Clin. Endocrinol. Metab.* 1954; 14: 742–3.

76. Volpe R, Johnston MW. Subacute thyroiditis: A disease commonly mistaken for pharyngitis. *Can. Med. Assoc. J.* 1957; 77: 297–307.

77. Nyulassy S, Hnilica P, Buc M, Guman M, Hirschová V, Stefanovic J. Subacute (de Quervain's) thyroiditis: Association with HLA-Bw35 antigen and abnormalities of the complement system, immunoglobulins and other serum proteins. *J. Clin. Endocrinol. Metab.* 1977; 45: 270–4.

78. Kramer AB, Roozendaal C, Dullaart RP. Familial occurrence of subacute thyroiditis associated with human leukocyte antigen-B35. *Thyroid* 2004; 14: 544–7.

79. Hamaguchi E, Nishimura Y, Kaneko S, Takamura T. Subacute thyroiditis developed in identical twins two years apart. *Endocr. J.* 2005; 52: 559–62.

80. Ikenoue H, Okamura K, Kuroda T, Sato K, Yoshinari M, Fujishima M. Thyroid amyloidosis with recurrent subacute thyroiditis-like syndrome. *J. Clin. Endocrinol. Metab.* 1988; 67: 41–5.

81. Alagol F, Tanakol R, Boztepe H, Kapran Y, Terzioglu T, Dizdaroglu F. Anaplastic thyroid cancer with transient thyrotoxicosis: Case report and literature review. *Thyroid* 1999; 9: 1029–32.

82. Sanders LR, Moreno AJ, Pittman DL, Jones JD, Spicer MJ, Tracy KP. Painless giant cell thyroiditis diagnosed by fine needle aspiration and associated with intense thyroidal uptake of gallium. *Am. J. Med.* 1986; 80: 971–5.

83. Shabb NS, Salti I. Subacute thyroiditis: Fine-needle aspiration cytology of 14 cases presenting with thyroid nodules. *Diagn. Cytopathol.* 2006; 34: 18–23.

84. Greene JN. Subacute thyroiditis. *Am. J. Med.* 1971; 51: 97–108.

85. Rotenberg Z, Weinberger I, Fuchs J, Maller S, Agmon J. Euthyroid atypical subacute thyroiditis simulating systemic or malignant disease. *Arch. Intern. Med.* 1986; 146: 105–7.

86. de Bruin TW, Riekhoff FP, de Boer JJ. An outbreak of thyrotoxicosis due to atypical subacute thyroiditis. *J. Clin. Endocrinol. Metab.* 1990; 70: 396–402.

87. Swinburne JL, Kreisman SH. A rare case of subacute thyroiditis causing thyroid storm. *Thyroid* 2007; 17: 73–6.

88. Weihl AC, Daniels GH, Ridgway EC, Maloof F. Thyroid function tests during the early phase of subacute thyroiditis. *J. Clin. Endocrinol. Metab.* 1977; 44: 1107–14.

89. Pearce EN, Bogazzi F, Martino E, Brogioni S, Pardini E, Pellegrini G, Parkes AB, et al. The prevalence of elevated serum C-reactive protein levels in inflammatory and noninflammatory thyroid disease. *Thyroid* 2003; 13: 643–8.

90. Larsen PR. Serum triiodothyronine, thyroxine, and thyrotropin during hyperthyroid, hypothyroid, and recovery phases of subacute nonsuppurative thyroiditis. *Metabolism* 1974; 23: 467–71.

91. Volpe R. The management of subacute (DeQuervain's) thyroiditis. *Thyroid* 1993; 3: 253–5.

92. Yamamoto M, Saito S, Sakurada T, Fukazawa H, Yoshida K, Kaise K, Kaise N, et al. Effect of prednisolone and salicylate on serum thyroglobulin level in patients with subacute thyroiditis. *Clin. Endocrinol. (Oxf.)* 1987; 27: 339–44.

93. Kubota S, Nishihara E, Kudo T, Ito M, Amino N, Miyauchi A. Initial treatment with 15 mg of prednisolone daily is sufficient for most patients with subacute thyroiditis in Japan. *Thyroid* 2013; 23: 269–72.

94. Duininck TM, van Heerden JA, Fatourechi V, Curlee KJ, Farley DR, Thompson GB, Grant CS, Lloyd RV. De Quervain's thyroiditis: Surgical experience. *Endocr. Pract.* 2002; 8: 255–8.

95. Dahlgren M, Khosroshahi A, Nielsen GP, Deshpande V, Stone JH. Riedel's thyroiditis and multifocal fibrosclerosis are part of the IgG4-related systemic disease spectrum. *Arthritis Care Res. (Hoboken)* 2010; 62: 1312–8.

96. Hennessey JV. Clinical review: Riedel's thyroiditis: A clinical review. *J. Clin. Endocrinol. Metab.* 2011; 96: 3031–41.

97. Stan MN, Sonawane V, Sebo TJ, Thapa P, Bahn RS. Riedel's thyroiditis association with IgG4-related disease. *Clin. Endocrinol. (Oxf.)* 2017; 86: 425–30.

98. Fatourechi MM, Hay ID, McIver B, Sebo TJ, Fatourechi V. Invasive fibrous thyroiditis (Riedel thyroiditis): The Mayo Clinic experience, 1976–2008. *Thyroid* 2011; 21: 765–72.

99. Papi G, LiVolsi VA. Current concepts on Riedel thyroiditis. *Am. J. Clin. Pathol.* 2004; 121;Suppl: S50–63.

100. Soh SB, Pham A, O'Hehir RE, Cherk M, Topliss DJ. Novel use of rituximab in a case of Riedel's thyroiditis refractory to glucocorticoids and tamoxifen. *J. Clin. Endocrinol. Metab.* 2013; 98: 3543–9.

101. Cherk MH, Kalff V, Yap KS, Bailey M, Topliss D, Kelly MJ. Incidence of radiation thyroiditis and thyroid remnant ablation success rates following 1110 MBq (30 mCi) and 3700 MBq (100 mCi) post-surgical ^{131}I ablation therapy for differentiated thyroid carcinoma. *Clin. Endocrinol. (Oxf.)* 2008; 69: 957–62.

102. Tamagna EI, Levine GA, Hershman JM. Thyroid-hormone concentrations after radioiodine therapy for hyperthyroidism. *J. Nucl. Med.* 1979; 20: 387–91.

103. Koornstra JJ, Kerstens MN, Hoving J, Visscher KJ, Schade JH, Gort HB, Leemhuis MP. Clinical and biochemical changes following ^{131}I therapy for hyperthyroidism in patients not pretreated with antithyroid drugs. *Neth. J. Med.* 1999; 55: 215–21.

104. Mizokami T, Hamada K, Maruta T, Higashi K, Tajiri J. Painful radiation thyroiditis after ^{131}I therapy for Graves' hyperthyroidism: Clinical features and ultrasonographic findings in five cases. *Eur. Thyroid J.* 2016; 5: 201–6.

105. Thebault C, Leurent G, Potier J, Bedossa M, Bonnet F. A case of thyroid storm following radioiodine therapy underlying usefulness of cardiac MRI. *Eur. J. Intern. Med.* 2009; 20: e136–7.

106. Romao R, Rubio IG, Tomimori EK, Camargo RY, Knobel M, Medeiros-Neto G. High prevalence of side effects after recombinant human thyrotropin-stimulated radioiodine treatment with 30 mCi in patients with multinodular goiter and subclinical/clinical hyperthyroidism. *Thyroid* 2009; 19: 945–51.

107. Nishiyama K, Kozuka T, Higashihara T, Miyauchi K, Okagawa K. Acute radiation thyroiditis. *Int. J. Radiat. Oncol. Biol. Phys.* 1996; 36: 1221–4.

108. Blitzer JB, Paolozzi FP, Gottlieb AJ, Zamkoff KW, Chung CT. Thyrotoxic thyroiditis after radiotherapy for Hodgkin's disease. *Arch. Intern. Med.* 1985; 145: 1734–5.

109. Aizawa T, Watanabe T, Suzuki N, Suzuki S, Miyamoto T, Ichikawa K, Oguchi M, Hashizume K. Radiation-induced painless thyrotoxic thyroiditis followed by hypothyroidism: A case report and literature review. *Thyroid* 1998; 8: 273–5.

110. Petersen M, Keeling CA, McDougall IR. Hyperthyroidism with low radioiodine uptake after head and neck irradiation for Hodgkin's disease. *J. Nucl. Med.* 1989; 30: 255–7.

111. Kobayashi A, Kuma K, Matsuzuka F, Hirai K, Fukata S, Sugawara M. Thyrotoxicosis after needle aspiration of thyroid cyst. *J. Clin. Endocrinol. Metab.* 1992; 75: 21–4.

112. Espiritu RP, Dean DS. Parathyroidectomy-induced thyroiditis. *Endocr. Pract.* 2010; 16: 656–9.

113. Leckie RG, Buckner AB, Bornemann M. Seat belt-related thyroiditis documented with thyroid Tc-99m pertechnetate scans. *Clin. Nucl. Med.* 1992; 17: 859–60.

4

Rare forms of hyperthyroidism*

NICOLE O. VIETOR AND HENRY B. BURCH

Thyrotropin (TSH)-induced hyperthyroidism 97
Thyroid hormone resistance 99
Struma ovarii 100
Trophoblastic tumors 101
Metastatic thyroid cancer 102
References 103

THYROTROPIN (TSH)-INDUCED HYPERTHYROIDISM

TSH-secreting pituitary adenomas are rare tumors that indicate an uncommon cause of hyperthyroidism. These tumors account for only 0.5–3% of all pituitary tumors with an annual incidence from a recent Swedish study of 0.15 per 1 million inhabitants and a prevalence of 2.8 per 1 million (1, 2).

The diagnosis of a TSH-secreting pituitary adenoma can present a challenge, and may be difficult to distinguish from thyroid hormone resistance (RTH). Differentiation of a TSH-secreting pituitary tumor from RTH is critical as the management of the two conditions is vastly different. According to the recently published American Thyroid Association clinical practice guidelines, the diagnosis should be based on (1) an inappropriately normal or elevated TSH level in the setting of elevated free T4 and/or total T3 concentrations, (2) a pituitary tumor detected on a CT or MRI scan, as the majority are macroadenomas, and (3) the absence of either a family history or genetic testing consistent with RTH (3). Once laboratory interference with the TSH or free T4 assay has been excluded, the measurement of alpha subunits, sex hormone-binding globulin, resting energy expenditure (when available), dynamic testing with thyrotropin-releasing hormone (TRH) stimulation testing (when available), and T3 suppression testing have been performed to make the diagnosis (Figure 4.1).

* The views expressed in this manuscript are those of the authors and do not reflect the official policy of the Department of the Army, the Department of Defense, the National Institutes of Health, or the United States Government. One or more authors are military service members or employees of the U.S. Government. This work was prepared as part of our official duties. Title 17 U.S.C. 105 provides the "Copyright protection under this title is not available for any work of the United States Government." Title 17 U.S.C. 101 defines a U.S. Government work as a work prepared by a military service member or employee of the U.S. Government as part of that person's official duties. We certify that all individuals who qualify as authors have been listed; each has participated in the conception and design of this work, the analysis of data (when applicable), the writing of the document, and/or the approval of the submission of this version; that the document represents valid work; that if we used information derived from another source, we obtained all necessary approvals to use it and made appropriate acknowledgments in the document; and that each takes public responsibility for it.Disclosure Summary: The authors have nothing to disclose.

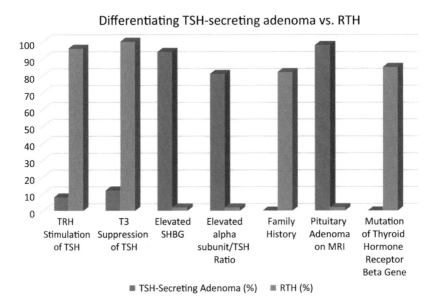

Figure 4.1 Differentiating TSH-secreting pituitary adenomas vs. thyroid hormone resistance (THR) (4, 5).

TSH-secreting adenomas usually have a disproportionate hypersecretion of the alpha subunit of glycoprotein hormones, leading to an elevated molar ratio of serum alpha subunit to TSH. The calculation of this ratio is performed by dividing the alpha-subunit concentration (ng/mL) by TSH (m/L) and multiplying by ten. A ratio of greater than one favors the diagnosis of TSH-secreting pituitary adenoma over RTH. Of note, measuring alpha subunits is not useful for this purpose in postmenopausal women due to the elevation in gonadotropins and concomitant elevation of alpha subunits. Elevated sex hormone-binding globulin, a thyroid hormone–dependent protein, elevated resting energy expenditure, a blunted TSH response to TRH administration, inability to completely suppress TSH secretion with T3 administration, as well as clinical evidence of thyrotoxicosis also support the diagnosis of a TSH-secreting pituitary adenoma (4, 6).

Pituitary surgery is currently recommended as the first line therapy for TSH-secreting adenomas (3). Surgical resection is a highly effective treatment with a remission (defined as total tumor removal and complete endocrinological remission) rate of 84% in a recent single-center study of 90 patients undergoing transsphenoidal resection (7). In this study, remission was achieved in 100% of patients with microadenomas, 81% of patients with macroadenomas, but only 38% of patients with cavernous sinus invasion (7). Another recent series from 2 tertiary referral centers reported the normalization of thyroid function in 75% of patients following pituitary surgery, including 65 patients undergoing a transsphenoidal approach, 1 patient with a macroadenoma and extrasellar extension undergoing a transcranial approach, and 2 patients who had a combined approach (8). Normalization of TSH hypersecretion and pituitary imaging occurred in this series in only 58% (8). Recurrence rates within 3 years following pituitary surgery are low (0–3%), as is the development of new pituitary hormone deficiencies (9–17%) in experienced hands (7, 8). Current clinical practice guidelines make a strong recommendation for referral to a high-volume pituitary surgeon (3). Patients should be made euthyroid with a short course of antithyroid drugs prior to surgery and thyroid targeted therapies such as radioactive iodine, thyroidectomy, or chronic use of antithyroid drugs, should be avoided, due to the theoretical concern of pituitary tumor growth.

The use of somatostatin analogs, dopamine agonists, and radiotherapy have also been studied as adjunctive therapies to surgical resection. Preoperative somatostatin analog (octreotide and lanreotide) therapy yields a > 50% reduction in TSH in the majority of patients (92%) and TSH normalization with the restoration of euthyroid state in 79–100% (4, 9–11). Bromocriptine appears to be less effective, however, with most patients failing to show a reduction in TSH secretion (4). Despite biochemical improvement with somatostatin analog therapy, preoperative medical therapy does not significantly improve surgical outcome, with tumor shrinkage in 38–52% of patients and negative imaging after surgery in only 57% (4, 8, 9). Radiation therapy successfully controls thyroid hypersecretion in 37% of patients within 2 years, but high rates (32%) of new pituitary deficiencies have been reported (8). Current clinical practice guidelines recommend treatment with octreotide and/or external beam radiation therapy only as a postoperative adjunctive therapy in patients with persistent central hyperthyroidism after pituitary surgery (3). Somatostatin analogs and radiation therapy can also be considered when surgery is contraindicated or, in the case of somatostatin analog therapy, if there is no visible pituitary tumor on MRI (3).

THYROID HORMONE RESISTANCE

Resistance to thyroid hormone (RTH) is a rare inherited disorder characterized by the reduced responsiveness of target tissues to thyroid hormone and can result in a wide range of clinical features from hypothyroidism to hyperthyroidism. RTH is the most common disease within the broader category of "impaired sensitivity to thyroid hormone" (12). The incidence of RTH has been reported to be 1 in 40,000 live births and occurs equally in males and females (13). More than 3000 cases have been described to date; a defect in the thyroid hormone receptor beta gene (RTH-beta) has been found in up to 85% of these individuals, with the majority having an autosomal dominant inheritance pattern (12, 14). Thyroid hormone receptors are transcription factors which mediate thyroid hormone action at the tissue level and, when defective, can lead to reduced tissue responsiveness to thyroid hormone (Figure 4.2). The pituitary thyrotrophs also exhibit resistance to thyroid hormone, leading to increased TSH secretion, which results in elevated T3 and T4 levels. The TSH secreted in RTH may have an increased sialic acid content and hence increased bioactivity (15), which leads to a goiter in many affected patients.

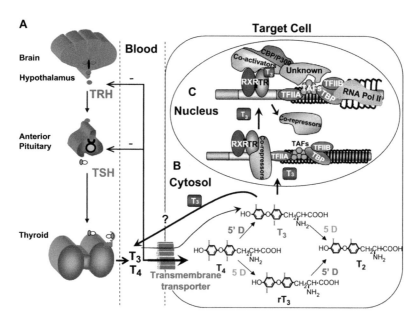

Figure 4.2 Regulation of thyroid hormone supply in the blood (A), intracellular metabolism (B), and genomic action (C). Reproduced with permission (5).

A broad range of clinical symptoms have been reported with RTH but most commonly patients present without severe clinical symptoms despite the abnormal thyroid function tests. Interestingly, clinical symptoms vary widely from patient to patient even within families who harbor the same mutation (16, 17). Due to varying tissue responsiveness to thyroid hormone, features of hyperthyroidism (hyperactivity, tachycardia) and hypothyroidism (delayed growth and bone age, learning disabilities) can be present. The most common clinical features are diffuse thyroid goiter (65–95%) and tachycardia (33–75%). However, emotional disturbance (60%), attention deficit disorder (40–60%), learning disability (30%), intellectual disability (38%), and sensorineural hearing loss (21%) have also been reported. Short stature, delayed bone age, and low body mass index can occur. Over half of patients experience recurrent ear and throat infections (18, 19). Frank hypothyroidism can be seen in patients inappropriately treated with thyroid ablative therapy in a misguided attempt to lower T4 and T3 levels.

The diagnosis of RTH should be considered when thyroid function tests reveal elevated T4 and T3 levels and a non-suppressed TSH. Due to very similar thyroid function test abnormalities, RTH must be distinguished from a TSH-producing adenoma. RTH patients exhibit normal alpha subunit and SHBG concentrations, an increase in TSH concentration in response to TRH administration, and a reduction in TSH concentration in response to T3 (4). In addition, patients with RTH often will have a positive family history, or positive genetic testing for THR-beta, and a negative pituitary MRI (Figure 4.1) (5). Approximately 15% of RTH patients are not found to have TRH-β mutation, due to either the presence of mutations in portions of the THR-β gene not tested or within other genes involved in mediating thyroid hormone action.

Currently, there are no available treatments to correct the underlying genetic defect in RTH. Fortunately, most of these patients do not need treatment, as endogenous thyroid hormone production increases to compensate for partial tissue resistance allowing for a normal metabolic state. Treatment is aimed at relieving symptoms; commonly, tachycardia and goiter. Beta-adrenergic blocking drugs are effective at treating tachycardia. Although large LT3 doses every other day have been reported to be effective in reducing goiter

size (20), this approach is generally not advised. Thyroidectomy is not recommended for goiter reduction as recurrence is common. Patients who have inappropriately undergone thyroidectomy or radioiodine ablation often require treatment with high doses of LT4, and TSH normalization is the goal of treatment. In children with RTH and diminished thyroid reserve due to prior ablative therapy (or Hashimoto's thyroiditis), LT4 dosing to return TSH secretion to the normal range is indicated and regular assessment of growth, bone maturation, and mental development should guide therapy. LT4 dose changes can occur every 6 weeks after clinical and laboratory assessment, to include, when available, metabolic rate, nitrogen balance, and serum SHBG. Development of a catabolic state indicates overtreatment (5). An increased risk of miscarriage and low birth weight in infants without the THR mutation who are born to mothers with RTH has been reported (21), as these fetuses have normal sensitivity to high maternal thyroid hormone levels, analogous to the situation with poorly controlled Graves' disease during pregnancy. It has been suggested that pregnant RTH women carrying healthy infants should be considered for antithyroid drug therapy if T4 levels exceed 20–50% above the upper limit of normal, although data in this area are limited (22). Finally, a case report from 1999 reported success with utilizing 3,5,3'-triiodothyroacetic acid for a pregnant female with RTH whose fetus also harbored the mutation (23).

STRUMA OVARII

Struma ovarii is a rare form of an ovarian teratoma. Teratomas are tumors composed of epithelial tissue and have been reported to contain elements of bone, teeth, hair, skin, or thyroid. Struma ovarii is defined as an ovarian teratoma composed of >50% thyroid tissue and represents an extremely rare form of hyperthyroidism, as only 5–10% of struma ovarii patients present with thyrotoxicosis (24, 25). More commonly, patients present with pelvic pain, abnormal uterine bleeding, and abdominal or pelvic masses (25, 26). Only about 200 cases of struma ovarii have been reported in the literature, and these lesions represent <1% of all ovarian neoplasms (24, 27). The diagnosis is often made postoperatively due to the low frequency of clinical thyrotoxicosis at initial presentation. However, struma ovarii should be considered in any thyrotoxic patient with a very low or absent radioactive iodine uptake in the thyroid gland. The differential diagnosis in this situation includes thyroiditis, factitious thyrotoxicosis, and iodine-induced hyperthyroidism. Struma ovarii can be differentiated from these conditions with the detection of a pelvic mass that concentrates radioactive iodine.

Benign struma ovarii should initially be managed with surgical resection following the preoperative normalization of thyroid hormone and beta blockade if thyrotoxicosis is present (3). However, 5–24% of these tumors may contain thyroid cancer (24, 25) and more extensive surgery with total abdominal hysterectomy, bilateral salpingo-oophorectomy, and lymph node sampling may be considered in patients presenting with extensive disease. Papillary cancer is the most commonly reported form of thyroid malignancy found in struma ovarii but follicular and insular carcinomas have also been reported (28). The optimal surgical approach is debated in the literature due to the potential consequences of extensive gynecologic surgery, such as loss of fertility.

Following gynecologic surgery, total thyroidectomy and radioactive iodine ablation are recommended for patients with high-risk disease, defined as a gross extraovarian extension of the tumor, large lesions (>4 cm), distant or peritoneal metastases, or the presence of a BRAF mutation or synchronous primary thyroid cancer (3, 29). A recent analysis of the National Cancer Institute's Surveillance, Epidemiology and End Results (SEER) database including 68 patients with struma ovarii, found that 6 out of 68 patients harbored papillary thyroid cancer in both the thyroid gland and the ovary (27). High-risk mutations such as BRAF and RAS have been detected in struma ovarii and may lead to more aggressive treatment (30, 31). After surgical resection of struma ovarii localized to the ovary, recurrence rates were 7.5% at 25 years with excellent survival (32). Recurrence rates of malignant struma ovarii have been reported to be up to 35% in those treated with tumor resection alone but 0% in those patients treated with adjuvant radioactive iodine (25). In general, adjuvant therapy with total thyroidectomy and radioactive iodine ablation should be performed in patients with high-risk malignant struma ovarii. Follow up with thyroglobulin levels and imaging has been proposed for long-term surveillance.

TROPHOBLASTIC TUMORS

Trophoblastic tumors including molar pregnancy, gestational trophoblastic neoplasias (which includes invasive mole and choriocarcinoma), and nonseminomatous germ-cell tumors can rarely cause hyperthyroidism due to the production of the glycoprotein hormone hCG. HCG, TSH, luteinizing hormone (LH), and follicle-stimulating hormone (FSH) are also glycoprotein hormones that have a common alpha subunit and distinct beta subunits (34). HCG has a low affinity for the TSH receptor, but in high concentration, as seen in trophoblastic tumors, it can activate the TSH receptor and cause hyperthyroidism. When hCG levels rise above 50,000 IU/L, the risk of hyperthyroidism increases, and once hCG levels reach >200,000 IU/L, 67% of patients exhibit a suppressed TSH and can present with overt thyrotoxicosis (35, 36).

Hydatidiform moles (HM), also called molar pregnancy, are the result of an aberrant fertilization and are characterized by abnormal chorionic villi with trophoblast hyperplasia due to the overexpression of paternal genes. In the United States, the incidence of HM is between 0.5–2.5 per 1,000 pregnancies, but is more common in Asian and Latin American countries. The risk increases in women >50 years and <15 years. HM are considered pre-malignant lesions with 3–5% developing into choriocarcinomas (37). These patients typically present with abnormal vaginal bleeding during pregnancy. Pelvic ultrasound is characteristic, with a vesicular pattern of multiple echoes, hollow areas within the placental mass, and no fetus (Figure 4.3). Rarely, patients can present with symptoms due to metastatic diseases, such as cough, dyspnea, hemoptysis, pleuritic pain due to lung metastases, or focal neurologic signs and convulsions with cerebral metastases. Increased thyroid function has been reported in up to 64% of patients with HM with 5% experiencing clinical hyperthyroidism. The exact prevalence of clinical hyperthyroidism in patients with choriocarcinoma is unknown, though many case reports have been published (37). Surgical uterine evacuation is the primary therapy for HM (3). Medial therapy for uterine evacuation is controversial and there is a paucity of data on the safety of this approach. Theoretical concerns include trophoblastic embolization to

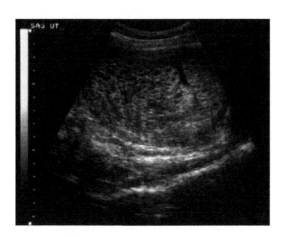

Figure 4.3 Pelvic ultrasound of a complete hydatidiform mole with a characteristic vesicular pattern of multiple echoes, holes within the placental mass, and no fetus. (Reproduced with permission Berkowitz R, Goldstein D. (40).)

the lungs or precipitation of metastatic disease with uterine contractions induced by medical therapy. Prophylactic chemotherapy with methotrexate or actinomycin D has been studied in patients with HM who are at high risk for development of GTN. A recent meta-analysis reported a reduction in progression to malignancy by 67% with prophylactic chemotherapy (38). Chemotherapy is the recommended treatment for GTN although there is no consensus on the optimal regimen. Commonly, methotrexate and actinomycin D are utilized (39). As recently reviewed, biweekly actinomycin-D given intravenously may be superior to weekly intramuscular methotrexate in patients with GTN and low-risk WHO scores, but not in patients classified as high-risk (40). The recent American Thyroid Association clinical practice guidelines recommend methimazole administration in addition to the treatment of the primary tumor for patients who present with hyperthyroidism (3).

Germ cell tumors in men have an annual incidence of 4.8 per 100,000 and account for 98% of all testicular cancers (41). Nonseminomatous tumors account for approximately half of the germ cell tumors and 20–40% produce hCG in high levels, often >50,000 IU per liter. Choriocarcinoma is the most aggressive form and is associated with the highest levels of hCG production (36). Therefore, patients presenting with a nonseminomatous germ cell tumor and overt thyrotoxicosis often

have widely metastatic disease at diagnosis. The primary treatment for stage I disease is surgical resection with radical orchiectomy. Loss of fertility is a concern with surgical management, so semen cryopreservation should be considered prior to orchiectomy. Further management with systemic chemotherapy, typically a cisplatin-based triplet regimen, is reserved for advanced stage disease. Prognosis is adversely affected by the presence or absence of a primary mediastinal tumor, elevated tumor markers (hCG) after orchiectomy, and nonpulmonary visceral metastases. With all three features, prognosis, unfortunately, is poor with only 50% long-term survival (36). Current practice guidelines advocate for antithyroid drugs given in conjunction with management of the primary tumor (3).

METASTATIC THYROID CANCER

Differentiated thyroid cancer (DTC) metastases can rarely produce excess thyroid hormone and result in hyperthyroidism. Fewer than 100 cases have been reported in the literature, most commonly arising from follicular carcinoma, although papillary carcinoma–causing hyperthyroidism has been reported (42). Recent case reports of five patients with metastatic follicular thyroid cancer revealed elevated levels of D1 and D2 mRNA in the tumors. These patients also were found to have clinical hyperthyroidism, elevated T3, and elevated T3 to T4 ratio (43, 44). This suggests that at least in some cases, the pathogenesis is due to the excessive conversion of T4 to T3 by tumor cells. In these cases, an elevated FT3 level or FT3/FT4 ratio greater than 3.5 can suggest the diagnosis (45). Although it is not routine practice to measure T3 levels following thyroid cancer treatment, it has been suggested that an occasional measurement of FT3 be performed in patients with massively metastatic follicular thyroid carcinoma under TSH-suppressive therapy, especially when the FT4 levels decrease on fixed doses of levothyroxine (45). An exogenous iodine load, such as following a CT scan, can also lead to hyperthyroidism in patients with functional metastatic differentiated thyroid cancer, similar to iodine-induced hyperthyroidism in the setting of multinodular goiter (46).

The prevalence of functioning metastatic DTC is unknown due to the rarity of the condition, but a recent case series of patients with massive metastatic follicular cancer reported 20% of patients exhibiting T3 thyrotoxicosis (45). Diagnosis is often difficult as patients with widely metastatic DTC are placed on high doses of LT4 in an effort to suppress TSH to undetectable levels. However, the diagnosis should be considered when reduction or withdrawal of thyroid hormone does not improve what was initially thought to be iatrogenic hyperthyroidism.

Treatment of hyperthyroidism due to metastatic DTC will include both beta blockers and antithyroid drugs to improve clinical and biochemical thyrotoxicosis, and treatment of the underlying metastatic disease according to current practice guidelines for the treatment of DTC, which includes surgical resection, radioiodine therapy, and, if needed, external beam radiation (29). It is critical to achieve a euthyroid state prior to surgical resection or radioactive iodine, as thyroid storm has been reported (47). Tyrosine-kinase inhibitors (TKI) have recently been approved by the Federal Drug Administration for the treatment of progressive radioiodine-refractory metastatic thyroid cancer, and may also be an option to control the hyperthyroidism associated with metastatic, progressive disease. A recent case report of two patients with metastatic follicular thyroid carcinoma with T3 thyrotoxicosis reported control of T3 overproduction with lenvatinib (48). Although further research is needed, TKI therapy may be considered in refractory cases.

REFERENCES

1. Beck-Peccoz P, Persani L, Mannavola D, Campi I. TSH-secreting adenomas. *Best Pract. Res. Clin. Endocrinol. Metab.* 2009;23(5):597–606.

2. Onnestam L, Berinder K, Burman P, et al. National incidence and prevalence of TSH-secreting pituitary adenomas in Sweden. *J. Clin. Endocinol. Metab.* 2013;98(2):626–635.

3. Ross DS, Burch HB, Cooper DS, et al. American Thyroid Association guidelines for diagnosis and management of hyperthyroidism and other causes of thyrotoxicosis. *Thyroid* 2016;26(10):1343–1421.

4. Beck-Peccoz P, Brucker-Davis F, Persani L, et al. Thyrotropin-secreting pituitary tumors. *Endocr. Rev.* 1996; 17(6):610–638.

5. Refetoff S, Dumitrescu A. Syndromes of reduced sensitivity to thyroid hormone: Genetic defects in hormone receptors, cell transporters, and deiodination. *Best Pract. Res. Clin. Endocrinol. Metab.* 2007;21(2):277–305.

6. Amlashi F, Tritos N. Thyrotropin-secreting pituitary adenomas: epidemiology, diagnosis, and management. *Endocrine* 2016;52(3):427–440.

7. Yamada S, Fukuhara N, Horiguchi K, et al. Clinicopathologial characteristics and therapeutic outcomes in thyrotropin-secreting pituitary adenomas: A single-center study of 90 cases. *J. Neurosurg.* 2014;121(6):1462–1473.

8. Malchiodi E, Profka E, Ferrante E, et al. Thyrotropin-secreting pituitary adenomas: Outcome of pituitary surgery and irradiation. *J. Clin. Endocrinol. Metab.* 2014;99(6):2069–2076.

9. Valdes Socin H, Chanson P, Delemer B, et al. The changing spectrum of TSH-secreting pituitary adenomas: Diagnosis and management in 43 patients. *Eur. J. Endocrinol.* 2003;148(4):433–442.

10. Rimareix F, Grunenwald S, Vezzosi D, et al. Primary medical treatment of thyrotropin-secreting pituitary adenomas by first-generation somatostatin analogs: A case study of seven patients. *Thyroid* 2015;25(8):877–881.

11. Van Varsseveld N, Bisschopt P, Biermasz N, et al. A long-term follow-up study of eighteen patients with thyrotropin-secreting pituitary adenomas. *Clin. Endocrinol.* 2014;80:395–402.

12. Refetoff S, Bassett J, Beck-Peccoz P, et al. Classification and proposed nomenclature for inherited defects of thyroid hormone action, cell transport, and metabolism. *Thyroid* 2014;24(3):407–409.

13. LaFranchi S, Snyder D, Sesser D, et al. Follow-up of newborns with elevated screening T4 concentrations. *J. Pediatr.* 2003;143(3):296–301.

14. Dumitrescu A Refetoff S. Impaired sensitivity to thyroid hormone: Defects of transport, metabolism and action (Chapter 58). In *Werner & Ingbar's The Thyroid: A Fundamental and Clinical Text.* Braverman LE and Cooper DS (eds.), Wolters Kluver/Lippincott, Williams & Wilkins Publications, Philadelphia, PA, 2013: 845–873.

15. Persani L, Borgato S, Romoli R, et al. Changes in the degree of sialylation of carbohydrate chains modify the biological properties of circulating thyrotropin isoforms in various physiological and pathological states. *J. Clin. Endocrinol. Metab.* 1998;83(7):2486–2492.

16. Weiss R, Weinberg M, Refetoff S. Identical mutations in unrelated families with generalized resistance to thyroid hormone occur in cytosine-guanine-rich areas of the thyroid hormone receptor beta gene: Analysis of 15 families. *J. Clin. Invest.* 1993;91(6):2408–2415.

17. Weiss R, Marocci C, Bruno-Bossio G, et al. Multiple genetic factors in the heterogeneity of thyroid hormone resistance. *J. Clin. Endocrinol. Metab.* 1993;76(1):257–259.

18. Brucker-Davis F, Skarulis M, Grace M, et al. Genetic and clinical features of 42 kindreds with resistance to thyroid hormone. *Ann. Intern. Med.* 1995;123(8):572–583.

19. Refetoff S, Weiss R, Usala S. The syndromes of resistance to thyroid hormone. *Endocr. Rev.* 1993;14(3):348–399.

20. Anselmo J Refetoff S. Regression of a large goiter in a patient with resistance to thyroid hormone by every other day treatment with triiodothyronine. *Thyroid* 2004;14(1):71–74.

21. Anselmo J, Cao D, Karrison T, et al. Fetal loss associated with excess thyroid hormone exposure. *JAMA* 2004;292(6):691–695.

22. Pappa T, Anselmo J, Mamanasiri S, et al. Prenatal diagnosis of resistance to thyroid hormone and its clinical implications. *J. Clin. Endocrinol. Metab.* 2017;102(10):3775–3782.

23. Asteria C, Rajanayagam O, Collingwood T, et al. Prenatal diagnosis of thyroid hormone resistance. *J. Clin. Endocrinol. Metab.* 1999;84(2):405–410.

24. Ross D. Syndromes of thyrotoxicosis with low radioactive iodine uptake. *Endocrinol. Metab. Clin. North Am.* 1998;27(1):169–185.

25. De Simone C, Lele S, Modesitt S. Malignant struma ovarii: A case report and analysis of cases reported in the literature with focus on survival and I131 therapy. *Gynecol. Oncol.* 2003;89(3):543–548.

26. Yoo S, Chang K, Lyu M, et al. Clinical characteristics of struma ovarii. *J. Gynecol. Oncol.* 2008;19(2):135–138.

27. Goffredo P, Sawka A, Pura J, et al. Malignant struma ovarii: A population-level analysis of a large series of 68 patients. *Thyroid* 2015;25(2):211–215.

28. Roth L, Talerman A. The enigma of struma ovarii. *Pathology* 2007;39(1):139–146.

29. Haugen B, Alexander E, Bible K, et al. 2015 American Thyroid Association management guidelines for adult patients with thyroid nodules and differentiated thyroid cancer: The American Association guidelines task force on thyroid nodules and differentiated thyroid cancer. Thyroid 2015;26(1): 1–133.

30. Wolff E, Hughes M, Merino M, et al. Expression of benign and malignant thyroid tissue in ovarian teratomas and the importance of multimodal management as illustrated by a BRAF-positive follicular variant of papillary thyroid cancer. Thyroid 2010;20(9):981–987.

31. Coyne C, Nikiforov Y. RAS mutation-positive follicular variant of papillary thyroid carcinoma arising in a struma ovarii. *Endocr. Pathol.* 2010;21(2):144–147.

32. Marti J, Clark V, Harper H, et al. Optimal surgical management of well-differentiated thyroid cancer arising in struma ovarii: A series of 4 patients and a review of 53 reported cases. *Thyroid* 2012;22(4):400–406.

33. Teale E, Gouldesbrough D, Peacey S. Graves' disease and coexisting struma ovarii: Struma expression of thyrotropin receptors and the presence of thyrotropin receptor stimulating antibodies. *Thyroid* 2006;16(8):791.

34. Jiang X, Dias J, He X. Structural biology of glycoprotein hormones and their receptors: Insights into signaling. *Mol. Cell Endocrinol.* 2014;382(1):424–451.

35. Lockwood C, Grenache D, Gronowski A. Serum human chorionic gonadotropin concentrations greater than 400,000 IU/L are invariably associated with suppressed serum thyrotropin concentrations. *Thyroid* 2009;19(8):863–868.

36. Pallais J, McInnis M, Saylor P, et al. Case 38–2015: A 21-year-old man with fatigue and weight loss. *N. Engl. J. Med.* 2015;373(24):2358–2368.

37. Hershman J. Physiological and pathological aspects of the effect of human chorionic gonadotropin on the thyroid. *Best Pract. Res. Clin. Endocrinol. Metab.* 2004;18(2):249–265.

38. Fu J, Fang F, Chen H, et al. Prophylactic chemotherapy for hydatidiform mole to prevent gestational trophoblastic neoplasia. *Cochrane Database Syst. Rev.* 2012;10:CD007289.

39. Lurain J. Trophoblastic disease I: Epidemiology, pathology, presentation and diagnosis of gestational trophoblastic disease, and management of hydatidiform mole. *Am. J. Obstet. Gynecol.* 2010;203(6):531–539.

40. Berkowitz R, Goldstein D. Current advances in the management of gestational trophoblastic disease. *Gynecol. Oncol.* 2013;128(1):3–5.

41. McGlynn K, Devesa S, Sigurdson A, et al. Trends in the incidence of testicular germ cell tumors in the United States. *Cancer* 2003;97(1):63–70.

42. Biyi A, Zaimi S, Doudouh A. Functioning metastases from thyroid papillary carcinoma in bone. *J. Nucl. Med. Technol.* 2016; 44(4):253–254.

43. Takano T, Miyauchi A, Ito Y, et al. Thyroxine to triiodothyronine hyperconversion thyrotoxicosis in patients with large metastases of follicular thyroid carcinoma. *Thyroid* 2006;16(6):615–618.

44. Kim B, Daniels G, Harrison B, et al. Overexpression of type 2 iodothyronine deiodinase in follicular carcinoma as a cause of low circulating free thyroxine levels. *J. Clin. Endocrinol. Metab.* 2003;88(2):594–598.

45. Miyauchi A, Takamura Y, Ito Y, et al. 3,5,3'-Triiodothyronine thyrotoxicosis due to increased conversion of administered levothyroxine in patients with massive metastatic follicular thyroid carcinoma. *J. Clin. Endocrinol. Metab.* 2008;93(6):2239–2242.

46. Lorberboym M, Mechanick JI. Accelerated thyrotoxicosis induced by iodinated contrast media in metastatic differentiated thyroid carcinoma. *J. Nucl. Med.* 1996;37(9):1532–1535.

47. Cerletty J, Listwan W. Hyperthyroidism due to functioning metastatic thyroid carcinoma. Precipitation of thyroid storm with therapeutic radioactive iodine. *JAMA* 1979;242(3):269–270.

48. Danilovic D, Camargo R, Casto G, et al. Rapid control of T3 thyrotoxicosis in patients with metastatic follicular thyroid cancer treated with lenvatinib. *Thyroid* 2015;25(11):1262–1264.

5

Drug-induced thyroid dysfunction

VICTOR BERNET AND ROBERT C. SMALLRIDGE

Iodine and iodine-containing products	111	Enhanced metabolic clearance of thyroid hormone	117
Lithium	113	Inhibition of thyroid hormone absorption and/or enterohepatic circulation	118
Cancer treatment–related drugs	114		
Immune system modulating–related drugs	115	Assay interference	118
Drugs impacting TSH synthesis or release	116	Thyrotoxicosis related to exogenous sources of thyroid hormone	118
Inhibition of T4 to T3 conversion	116		
Drugs impacting thyroxine-binding globulin levels or binding	117	Conclusion	119
		References	119

Drug-induced changes in thyroid hormone levels are frequently encountered in clinical practice and can make the interpretation of thyroid function test results very challenging. Thyroid function testing is a critical clinical tool for the assessment of a patient's thyroid status, and it is vital for the clinician to suspect the possibility of drug-related changes that could either cause or masquerade as thyroid dysfunction. Drugs can impact thyroid hormone economy at several points along its production, release, and metabolism.

There are multiple points in the process of thyroid hormonogenesis and metabolism where drugs and iodine-containing products can impact thyroid hormone (TH) levels and include: Iodine trapping and organification by thyrocytes, oxidation of iodine, iodination of tyrosine, thyroid hormone synthesis and release, thyroid hormone binding to binding proteins in the blood, conversion of T4 to T3 or reverse T3, and thyroid hormone absorption, including enterohepatic recirculation and metabolism of thyroid hormone products (1). Drugs can

also influence the hypothalamic-pituitary-thyroid axis thereby impacting thyrotropin releasing hormone (TRH) and thyroid stimulating hormone (TSH) production and/or secretion which then results in alterations in thyroid hormone production by the thyroid. Additionally, some drugs have been associated with increased risk for development of autoimmune thyroid disorders, resulting in the production of thyroid antibodies, such as antithyroid peroxidase and anti-thyroglobulin antibodies, impairing thyroid function, and antiTSH receptor antibodies which can stimulate or inhibit production of thyroid hormone.

The list of drugs impacting thyroid hormone economy continues to steadily grow, and includes newer drugs used for cancer-related treatments and those prescribed as immune system modulating agents (see Tables 5.1 and 5.2). In some cases, the effects on thyroid function are transient, in others, the impact is more prolonged, irrespective of whether the drug has been discontinued, and, often, serial monitoring of thyroid hormone levels will be indicated.

Table 5.1 Drug-related changes in thyroid function testing

Medication	TSH	T4	T3	TBG	TH clearance	Type 3 deiodination	TH displacement from binding proteins	TH absorption	Hypothyroidism	Thyrotoxicosis	Adjustment of TH dose
Bexarotene[a]	↓	↓	↓						* [b]		*
Corticosteroids	↓										
Dopamine	↓										
Octreotide	↓										
Metformin	↓[b]										
Iodine	↓↑	↓↑	↓↑							*	
Lithium	↓↑	↓↑	↓↑						*	*	*
Methimazole	↑	↓	↓						*		
Potassium perchlorate	↑	↓	↓						*		
Propylthiouracil	↑	↓	↓			→			*		
Ipodate/iopanoic acid	↓↑	↓↑	↓↑			→			*		
Propranolol_γ						→					
Androgen therapy				→							*
L-Asparaginase				→							*
Niacin				→							*
Estrogen				↑							*
5-Fluorouracil				↑							*
Heroin & Methadone				↑							*
Mitotane				↑				→			*
Raloxifene				↑							*
Tamoxifen				↑							*
Carbamazepine	NC	↓↔	↓↔		↑		↑				*
Phenytoin	NC	↓↔	↓↔		↑		↑				*
Phenobarbital					↑						*
Rifampin					↑						*

(Continued)

Table 5.1 (Continued) Drug-related changes in thyroid function testing

Medication	TSH	T4	T3	TBG	TH clearance	Type 3 deiodination	TH displacement from binding proteins	TH absorption	Hypothyroidism	Thyrotoxicosis	Adjustment of TH dose
Sertraline											*
Furosemide					↑						
Heparin	NC	↑	↑Э				←				
Salsalate (Acute)ᵉ	NC	→	→				←				
Salsalate (Chronic)ᶜ							←				
Salicylates (Acute)ᵉ	NC	NC	↓ᵍ				←				
Salicylates (Chronic)ᶜ	→		→								
Meclofenamate (Acute)ᵉ	NC	NC/↓ᵏ	↑								
Meclofenamate (Chronic)ᶜ	NC	NC	NC								
Aluminum hydroxide								→			*
Calcium								→			*
Resin-binders*								→			*
Iron								→			*
Proton pump inhibitors					*ҳ			→			*
Psyllium								→			*
Soybean oil								→			*
Sucralfate								→			*
Amiodarone	↓↑	↓↑	↓↑			→			*	*Φ	*
Biotin ¥	↓↑	↓↑	↓↑								

Legend: TH = Thyroid hormone; TBG = Thyroid-binding globulin; NC = no change from baseline; ↑ = Increase; ↓ = Decrease; ↑↓ May see increase or decrease; * = Effect seen; a - non-deiodinase-mediated peripheral degradation of TH. b = in patients on TH replacement; Э = Impacts FT4 and FT3 not TT4 or TT3; ς = Spurious low FT4 and FT3; c = 1 week Rx; e = single-dose; g = Drop in FT3 and FT3; k = ↓ in TT4 but FT4 remains stable; γ - propranolol dose >240 mg/day; h - Central hypothyroidism; Φ - Amiodarone induce thyrotoxicosis can be Type1 iodine induced and Type 2 destructive thyroiditis. ҳ - may ↑ TH clearance by enhanced activity of uridine diphosphate-glucuronosyl-transferase (UGT) enzymes; ¥ Biotin can impact TSH, T4, and T3 levels done in assays using a biotinylated method.

Table 5.2 Effect on thyroid parameters by anti-cancer and immune regulatory medications

Medication	Drug type	Thyrotoxicosis phase/destructive thyroiditis	Primary hypothyroidism	Adjustment TH dose	Immune dysregulation	Thyrotoxicosis	Hypophysitis/central hypothyroidism	Type 3 deiodination </β>
Axitinib	TKI		*	*				
Cabozantinib	TKI	*	*					
Cediranib	TKI		*					
Dasatinib	TKI	*	*	*				
Imatinib	TKI		*	*				* §
Lenvatinib	TKI		*					
Motesanib	TKI	*	*	*				* §
Nilotinib	TKI	*	*		*	*		
Pazopanib	TKI		*			*		
Sorefanib	TKI	*	*	*				
Sunitinib	TKI	*	*	*	*			* §
Vandetanib	TKI	*	*	*				* §
Ipilimumab	CTLA4	*	*		*		*	
Tremelimumab	CTLA4	*			*	*	*	
Alemtuzumab	PDL1	*	*		*	*		
Pembrolizumab	PD1	*		*	*	*		
Nivolumab	PD1	*	*		*	*	*	
Thalidomide	IMD	*	*		*	*		
Lenalidomide	IMD	*	*		*	*		
Interferon-α	CTK	*			*	*		
IL-2	CTK	*			*	*		

Legend: CTLA4 = Anti-cytotoxic T-lymphocyte antigen-4; PD-1 = Programmed death receptor-1; PD-L1 = Programmed death-ligand 1; TKI = Tyrosine kinase inhibitor; IMD = Immunomodulatory drug; CTK = Cytokine; § = Possible increased deiodinase-3 activity leading to increased T4 to rT3 conversion.

IODINE AND IODINE-CONTAINING PRODUCTS

Iodine is an essential component of thyroid hormone and patterns of dietary iodine intake have been related to predispositions for development of thyroid disorders. The recommended daily allowance for iodine intake is 150 mcg for adults, 220 mcg during pregnancy, and 290 mcg for lactating mothers, with toxicity being unlikely to occur until intake exceeds 1100 mcg/day (2). Supra-physiologic amounts of iodine are found in multiple products, including radiographic iodinated contrast media, nutritional supplements, foods (e.g., kelp), skin cleansers (iodine-containing disinfectants), and medications (e.g., amiodarone).

Acute exposure to excess iodine leads to the Wolff-Chaikoff effect, a transient decline in thyroid hormone synthesis from thyroid peroxidase inhibition, resulting in decreased sodium-iodine symporter (NIS) activity, followed by an "escape" from this phenomenon and the resumption of thyroid hormone production (3, 4). Thyrotoxicosis related to iodine exposure is also known as the Jod-Basedow (Jod is German for iodine) phenomenon and typically occurs in patients with underlying thyroid disorders such as nodular goiter, a state of chronic iodine deficiency, or dormant Graves' disease (5). Iodine-induced thyrotoxicosis may be either short-lived or chronic in nature (6).

Hypothyroidism can result from excess iodine exposure as there can be a failure to escape from the Wolff-Chaikoff effect. This is more commonly seen in patients with predisposing thyroid disorders such as Hashimoto's thyroiditis, postpartum thyroiditis, reduced thyroid gland reserve from previous surgery or prior ^{131}I treatment for Graves' disease, or medications like amiodarone or interferon-α (7, 8). In the case of iodine-induced hypothyroidism, the serum TSH level and TPO antibody titer are important parameters in clinical decision making. With TSH elevations ≥ 10 mU/L, the institution of thyroid hormone replacement should be considered, while patients with TSH levels between 5–10 mU/L can potentially be monitored, although thyroid hormone therapy may be prescribed if hypothyroid symptoms are present. The presence of TPO antibodies increases the risk for development of hypothyroidism and iodine exposure in patients with Hashimoto's thyroiditis appears to exacerbate risk for developing hypothyroidism (7). Iodine-induced hypothyroidism has been noted with iodine supplementation programs and may be transient in cases where the iodine exposure is limited or persistent if exposure is chronic in nature (9). Thyroid hormone replacement is indicated when hypothyroidism persists.

Radiographic iodinated contrast media used in various imaging studies like CT scans contain massive amounts of iodine (~320–370 mg/ml), providing ~2500–5000 mcg of bioavailable free iodine. With increased CT utilization in clinical practice, this is a common route of excess iodine exposure (10). Serum iodine levels typically remain above the normal range for 4–8 weeks. Studies report that renal excretion of iodine is initially elevated and then returns to pre-exposure levels at around 30–50 days post-exposure with patients >40 years of age taking longer to excrete the iodine load (11, 12).

Hyperthyroidism secondary to iodinated contrast exposure can result in either subclinical or overt thyrotoxicosis, and there are reports of thyroid storm as well. A retrospective case control study found that even individuals with no known underlying thyroid condition have a two- to threefold risk of developing hyperthyroidism or hypothyroidism following exposure. A large community-based cohort study found a 1.6- to 2-fold rise of post-iodine contrast associated hyperthyroidism compared to those without such an exposure (13). However, other studies have not confirmed such a marked increase in thyroid dysfunction in individuals after iodinated contrast exposure (14, 15).

Patients with iodine-induced hyperthyroidism have a suppressed serum TSH and either normal or elevated T4 and T3 levels. Urinary iodine, spot or 24-hour collection, can be used to document iodine excess. Nuclear medicine imaging may reveal faint or reduced thyroid uptake of iodine or technetium, and the radioactive iodine uptake will be reduced as well. Further iodine exposure should be avoided in cases of iodine-induced hyperthyroidism, as the thyrotoxicosis may resolve spontaneously provided that iodine exposure is limited. Therapy with β-blockers or antithyroid medications (e.g., methimazole) are appropriate management options in patients with significant symptoms of hyperthyroidism, especially those with a persistent thyrotoxic state, elderly patients, and those with underlying comorbidities, especially cardiovascular disease.

In patients with an underlying predisposition for developing hyperthyroidism, particularly those who also have conditions such as coronary artery disease or cardiac arrhythmias that can be exacerbated by thyrotoxicosis, prophylactic treatment with methimazole can be considered. Potassium perchlorate, which competitively blocks iodine uptake by cells thru NIS, can also be used but is not readily available in the United States (16). A study in euthyroid patients exhibiting thyroid autonomy found that treatment with either methimazole 20 mg/day or sodium perchlorate 900 mg/day, given for 14 days starting 1 day prior to an iodine load for coronary angiography, kept FT4 and FT3 at baseline levels and prevented TSH suppression while T4 and T3 levels rose and TSH dropped significantly within the reference range in control subjects. However, treatment did not fully prevent the development of subclinical hyperthyroidism as one case of mild thyrotoxicosis was noted in each treatment group and two in the control group (17).

[131]I-based imaging and treatments such as ^{131}I, ^{131}I-MIBG, or combined treatments agents such as ^{131}I-tositumomab (CD-20 antibody targeting lymphocytes) and [131]I- iobenguane (MIBG) targeting adrenergic tissues can lead to ^{131}I uptake by thyrocytes and resultant hypothyroidism from β-radiation-mediated destruction of thyroid tissue. ^{131}I-Tositumomab has been reported to be associated with a hypothyroidism rate of between 9–41% occurring between 6 and 24 months post exposure (18–20). [131]I- iobenguane used in the treatment of neuroendocrine tumors has been found to cause hypothyroidism in 12–64% of treated individuals (21). Thyrocyte uptake of the ^{131}I can be prevented by administration of non-radioactive iodine agents, such as the saturated solution of potassium iodide (SSKI) or Lugol solution, starting 24 hours prior and continuing until 2 weeks following exposure to ^{131}I-containing agents.

Amiodarone is very rich in iodine: a 100 mg dose contains 37 mg of organic iodine and releases approximately 3.7 mg of free iodine into the circulation daily. It is associated with thyroid dysfunction in ~15–20% of individuals receiving this therapy (22). Thyroid disorders encountered with amiodarone therapy include amiodarone-induced hypothyroidism as well as thyrotoxicosis (amiodarone-induced thyrotoxicosis [AIT]) types 1 and 2. Type 1 AIT consists of iodine-induced hyperthyroidism while type 2 AIT represents a destructive thyroiditis, with the latter being the more common (23).

Amiodarone-induced hypothyroidism (AIH) occurs more frequently in iodine-sufficient areas of the world and is more prevalent in women (24, 25). Amiodarone-induced hypothyroidism tends to develop earlier than AIT and patients typically have underlying thyroid abnormalities with many having thyroid autoantibodies (26). The combination of female sex and antithyroid antibodies substantially increases the risk of developing AIH (27). The large and persistent iodine exposure associated with amiodarone therapy leads to the Wolff-Chaikoff effect and, as previously discussed, the thyroid of a patient with Hashimoto's thyroiditis may not be able to escape from this inhibitory effect (26). Patients with AIH have been found to have a positive perchloride discharge test, which is consistent with a defect in organification of iodine (26). Additionally, iodine-induced thyrocyte damage may hasten the trend toward the development of hypothyroidism seen with chronic lymphocytic thyroiditis. Remission of amiodarone-associated hypothyroidism can occur and is more likely in patients with negative thyroid antibody status and who are without a history of thyroid abnormalities. The symptoms and laboratory changes noted with AIH are similar to those noted with spontaneous hypothyroidism. Patients with persistent hypothyroidism can be treated with T4-based thyroid hormone replacement with dose adjustments occurring about every 6 weeks until the TSH falls within the desired goal. As many patients receiving amiodarone have a significant underlying cardiac disease, TSH suppression from excess thyroid replacement should be avoided. Amiodarone can also inhibit T_4 5'-monodeiodination which is further discussed in a subsequent section about drugs which inhibit T4 to T3 conversion.

AIT is more common with iodine-deficiency and is more common in men (25). Type 1 AIT is typically associated with pre-existing thyroid disease, diffuse or nodular goiters, increased vascularity on color flow Doppler sonography (CFDS), and low or low-normal radioactive iodine uptake (RAIU), while AIT 2 typically occurs without a history of thyroid disease, when the thyroid gland is normal size or slightly enlarged, there is a quiescent vascularity pattern by CFDS, and RAIU is low or undetectable. The onset of AIT can occur soon after amiodarone initiation or, being stored in several body tissues and having a half-life of up to 100 days, can occur months following amiodarone withdrawal (22, 28). Following amiodarone initiation, the median onset for AIT Type 1 is 3.5 months and 30 months for Type 2 (29).

As many patients receiving amiodarone are typically older and tend to have serious underlying cardiac arrhythmias, the occurrence of AIT should be promptly addressed, as an increase in mortality can be seen, especially in individuals with concomitant left ventricular dysfunction (30). Type 1 AIT, which represents a form of iodine-induced hyperthyroidism, is best treated with methimazole. However, iodine-saturated thyroid glands may have a reduced response to these agents, and higher doses (e.g., 40–60 mg methimazole) may be required (22). There are reports of successfully utilizing potassium perchlorate (1 g/day or less) to decrease iodine uptake by the thyroid but this agent is not readily available in North America (31).

Type 2 AIT, a destructive form of thyroiditis due to a direct toxic effect of amiodarone on thyrocytes, may be monitored without therapy in mild cases and when amiodarone can be discontinued. However, most patients typically require treatment with glucocorticoids such as prednisone (32). Approximately 0.5–0.7 mg/kg body weight of prednisone per day is recommended with therapy being tapered over ~3 months; one study found at least half of patients achieved normal thyroid hormone levels within 4 weeks (33). Thionamide therapy alone has not been found to be useful in pure cases of AIT type 2 with 85% of individuals still having thyrotoxicosis at 6 weeks of therapy whereas only 24% of patients receiving prednisone remained thyrotoxic (34).

However, many cases of AIT appear to have a "mixed" form of thyrotoxicosis with a combination of destructive thyroiditis and increased hormone production by the thyroid. This circumstance may be suspected if thyrotoxicosis from apparent Type 1 AIT does not respond to antithyroid medications, or if Type 2 AIT does not respond promptly to a course of prednisone. In instances where a "mixed" etiology appears evident, combination therapy with prednisone and antithyroid medications has been found to be efficacious (24). Radioactive iodine ablation with ^{131}I can be considered in Type 1 AIT if the RAIU is elevated adequately (35). There are also reports describing the use of recombinant human TSH

(rhTSH) injections to raise iodine uptake to allow for ^{131}I ablation, but this process can be associated with clinically significant rhTSH-stimulated rises in serum thyroid hormone levels and related risks (36, 37). As many patients with AIT have severe cardiac disease, thyroidectomy may be warranted, although it is associated with increased perioperative risk (38).

LITHIUM

Lithium is known to impact thyroid physiology in several ways. Lithium-associated goiter was first reported in the late 1960s. Lithium can inhibit thyroid hormone secretion, which may lead to the development of hypothyroidism or goiter. This effect has been employed to control hyperthyroidism, although it is seldom used for this purpose (39). Lithium's impact on thyroid cellular function is thought to be related to the inhibition of TSH's effect on cyclic AMP-mediated cellular signaling, with associated downstream impact on the phosphoinositol pathway (40). Lithium may also impact the hypothalamic-pituitary axis. TSH elevations have been noted in patients receiving lithium, and an exaggerated rise in TSH levels with TRH stimulation has been reported in euthyroid bipolar subjects on lithium therapy (40, 41). One study reported 83% frequency of a transient rise of TSH from baseline on lithium therapy, suggesting that the hypothalamic-pituitary axis reaches a new set point, since the serum TSH then returns to the normal range at 12 months (42). As noted in rat studies, T3 nuclear binding in the brain may be impacted by lithium and reverse T3 (rT3) may rise in humans with lithium as well (43). A correlation with serum T3 levels and efficacy of treatment has been noted with lithium and it is hypothesized that lithium exerts at least some of its effects through alterations in T3 concentrations which then impact brain cell function (42).

The risk of hypothyroidism associated with lithium therapy is predicated on several underlying issues, including pre-existing autoimmune thyroid disease, gender predisposition, dietary iodine status, exposure to goitrogens, and duration of lithium therapy. There also appears to be an increased risk for development of lithium-related thyroid disorders with older age (44). Individuals receiving lithium who also have underlying autoimmune thyroid disease are at increased risk for developing hypothyroidism; an annual rate of 6.4% of those with positive thyroid antibodies have been found to require L-thyroxine therapy for hypothyroidism in comparison to only 0.8% for those without thyroid antibodies (45). An annual rate of hypothyroidism of 1.5% was reported in a study of 150 patients on lithium during 15 years of followup (46). Similar to the rate seen in the general population, lithium therapy is reported to have a 5:1 female:male ratio for development of hypothyroidism (45). The reported prevalence of hypothyroidism associated with lithium therapy ranges between 3.4 and 52% and appears to vary with the population being studied (45).

While lithium does not appear to stimulate the development of thyroid autoimmunity, it does appear to accelerate activity of pre-existing thyroiditis (47). Additionally, lithium and iodine have been found to act synergistically in the development of hypothyroidism (48). Based on these data, TSH, free T4, and thyroid antibody status should be checked prior to the initiation of lithium therapy and at least annually thereafter (49). More frequent testing can be considered in the face of a positive family history for thyroid disease, positive antibody titer, or other thyroid abnormalities such as a goiter or borderline TSH level.

Thyrotoxicosis has also been reported in the context of lithium therapy and typically occurs after years of treatment (50). Graves' disease, toxic multinodular goiter and various forms of thyroiditis (e.g., silent, granulomatous, and destructive thyroiditis without lymphocytic infiltration) have all been described with lithium-associated hyperthyroidism (51, 52). Lithium-associated thyrotoxicosis (2.7 cases per 1000 person-years) occurs more frequently than in the general population (0.8–1.2 cases per 1000 person-years) (50). While it remains to be confirmed that lithium stimulates the development of TSH receptor antibodies, in at least one study ~64% of individuals with lithium-related hyperthyroidism were identified as having autoimmune thyrotoxicosis (50). It remains unclear if there is a specific relation between lithium therapy and the development of thyroid eye disease (53, 54). Treatment options for lithium-associated thyrotoxicosis include standard therapies for hyperthyroidism, including antithyroid medications, ^{131}I ablation, and thyroidectomy plus beta-blockade to mitigate symptoms from thyrotoxicosis. In cases of destructive thyroiditis with severe thyrotoxicosis, glucocorticoids may be utilized.

CANCER TREATMENT-RELATED DRUGS

Numerous tyrosine kinase inhibitors (TKI) have been associated with the development of primary hypothyroidism, including axitinib, cediranib, dasatinib, imatinib, motesanib, nilotinib, sorafenib, and sunitinib (see Table 5.2) (55–57). TKIs have also been reported to worsen control of hypothyroidism in patients with primary hypothyroidism, including some who were post-thyroidectomy and on stable thyroid hormone therapy (58, 59).

There are several potential mechanisms that can explain the thyroid disorders encountered with TKI therapy. Destructive thyroiditis is suspected in some cases as thyrotoxicosis can lead to the development of hypothyroidism. The thyroid is a vascular gland and destructive thyroiditis may be induced by the reduction of blood flow secondary to the inhibition of angiogenic-related kinase pathways, for example, through effects on vascular-endothelial growth factor (VEGF) and platelet-derived growth factor (PDGFR) receptors. TKI-related reductions in serum free T4 and T3 levels have been noted in patients on TH replacement as well. Potential explanations include increased metabolism of TH through either increased non-deiodination clearance or a rise in type 3 deiodination activity that can be seen with certain TKIs, for example, sunitinib (59). In a group of euthyroid subjects being treated for gastrointestinal stromal tumors (GISTs) with sunitinib, 62% developed an abnormal TSH (TSH >20 mU/L in 21%; TSH >7 mU/L in 14%; TSH between 5–7 mU/L in 17% and also 10% with TSH <0.5 mU/L) (56). However, it must be noted that certain GIST tumors themselves can induce consumptive hypothyroidism by means of overexpression of deiodinase-3. As noted, a phase of thyrotoxicosis with suppressed TSH may precede the onset of TKI-induced hypothyroidism. As TKI-related thyroid dysfunction appears relatively common, it is recommended that TSH and free T4 be checked prior to the institution of TKI therapy then monitored monthly for several months and at 2–3-month intervals thereafter (55).

IMMUNE SYSTEM MODULATING-RELATED DRUGS

Pembrolizumab, a programmed death receptor-1 (PD-1) blocker, has been associated with the development of immune-related adverse events, including thyroid disease. In patients receiving at least one dose of pembrolizumab, 14% were noted to have a thyroid-related adverse event: Silent thyroiditis (54%) or hypothyroidism (23%), and a significant increase in levothyroxine dose requirement in three individuals previously on stable TH therapy (60). A positive TPO antibody titer was noted in 31% of the cases, and diffuse thyroid uptake of [18]fluorodeoxyglucose ([18]FDG) was reported in 64% of patients without any known thyroid malignancy with a median time of onset at 12 weeks. Increased [18]FDG uptake by the thyroid is well known to occur in patients with chronic lymphocytic thyroiditis (61). While the majority of patients did not develop anti-TPO antibodies or thyroid disease, those with a history of hypothyroidism or with positive antithyroid antibody status are at risk for recurrence or worsening of their underlying thyroid disorder (62).

Ipilimumab and tremelimumab are anti-cytotoxic T-lymphocyte-associated antigen 4 (CTLA-4) monoclonal antibodies which through CTLA-4 receptor blockade lead to anti-tumor activity by means of augmented T-cell activation (63). Ipilimumab is associated with endocrine immune-related adverse events, with a reported rate of hypophysitis between 0–17% and thyroiditis and/or hypothyroidism occurring in 1.5–9% (64–66).

Hypophysitis causing central adrenal insufficiency, hypogonadism, as well as hypothyroidism is also seen with these agents. If central adrenal insufficiency and hypothyroidism are diagnosed concomitantly, to avoid precipitation of adrenal crisis glucocorticoid therapy should be instituted prior to TH replacement. Long-term hormone replacement therapy is usually required as these pituitary axis defects rarely reverse (67). Tremelimumab-related Graves' hyperthyroidism and autoimmune hypothyroidism have also been reported (68, 69).

It is recommended that baseline TSH and free T4 levels be obtained prior to initiation of CTLA-4 monoclonal antibody therapy, and every 8–12 weeks thereafter during therapy. In patients receiving anti-PD-1 agents, one study found that 80% of the patients developing immune-related thyroid disease had baseline positive TPO antibody titers (70). The combined use of immune checkpoint inhibitors (CTLA-4, PD-1, and PD-L1) appears to increase the occurrence of thyroid-related adverse effects such as hypothyroidism, thyrotoxicosis, hypophysitis, and autoimmune thyroiditis (71).

The cytokine aldesleukin (IL-2), which stimulates natural killer cell and T-cell activity, thereby activating autoreactive lymphocytes, can lead to the development of autoimmune thyroiditis. Thyroid disorders are reported to occur in 10–50% of individuals receiving IL-2 with hypothyroidism, hyperthyroidism, and thyroiditis all having been noted (72, 73). The onset of hypothyroidism is typically between 4–17 weeks after IL-2 initiation and may resolve with cessation of therapy (74).

Drugs associated with the development of thyroid autoimmunity can also lead to thyroid dysfunction. Type I interferon (interferon-α) therapy used for the treatment of multiple sclerosis, chronic viral hepatitis, as well as some solid tumors and hematologic conditions has been associated with about a 6% prevalence of thyroid dysfunction (hypothyroidism 3.9% and thyrotoxicosis 2.3%) (75). The disease tends to be mild (e.g., subclinical) with ≥60% having spontaneous resolution whether interferon is continued or not. The development of thyroid disease is increased in females and individuals with underlying autoimmune thyroid disease. Thyroid function tests should be monitored during interferon therapy. Patients with positive anti-TPO or anti-thyroglobulin antibody titers are at risk for developing autoimmune thyroid disease, while those who are negative for both antibodies are at very low risk (76).

Alemtuzumab, a drug used for the treatment of multiple sclerosis, has been associated with an increased frequency of developing an autoimmune disease (22.2%) with thyroid disorders being the most common at 15.7% (77). The onset of autoimmune thyroid disease typically occurs within the first 12–18 months of treatment initiation, although cases after 5 years after exposure have been reported. Thyroid disease more commonly occurs in patients with a family history of autoimmune thyroid disease or a smoking history. TSH should be measured prior to initiation of therapy and then every 2–3 months during the treatment course.

Thalidomide and lenalidomide are agents with anti-tumor effects though mediated by immune destruction of tumor cells and have been used for the treatment of multiple myeloma, mantle cell lymphoma as well as erythema nodosum and lymphocytic skin infiltrations. In addition, these agents have antiangiogenic effects, can inhibit tumor growth, and can induce tumor cell apoptosis. Cases of hypothyroidism were first reported decades ago when thalidomide was first in use, and continue to be reported with its more recent resurgence in use. Thalidomide-related hypothyroidism appears to occur about 1–6 months following initiation (78). One study found that 20% of individuals with multiple myeloma receiving thalidomide developed a TSH >5 mU/L and ~7% had a TSH level spike >10 mU/L (79). Hypothyroidism appears to occur less frequently with lenalidomide at 5–10%, and a case of thyroiditis has also been reported (80). Thalidomide has also been associated with thyrotoxicosis and concomitant radiation exposure may play a role in the occurrence of autoimmune thyroid disease (81).

DRUGS IMPACTING TSH SYNTHESIS OR RELEASE

Drugs that can inhibit TSH secretion include dobutamine, dopamine, somatostatin analogs, glucocorticoids, metformin, and the retinoid X receptor ligand bexarotene (82–87). Dobutamine, dopamine, and high dose glucocorticoid therapy are used in critically ill patients and can confound the interpretation of thyroid function test (TFT) results in a population already predisposed to thyroid hormone changes related to the euthyroid sick syndrome. The suppressive effect of somatostatin analogs on thyrotropin-secreting pituitary cells has been successfully used to control inappropriate TSH secretion by TSH-secreting pituitary adenomas and while transient decreases in TSH can be noted with octreotide doses >100 mcg/day in individuals without such tumors, it does not appear to cause long-term suppression or hypothyroidism (88). Bexarotene, an antineoplastic agent used for the treatment of cutaneous T cell lymphoma, can cause severe central hypothyroidism by suppressing TSH secretion, an effect mediated through heterodimer formation between the retinoid X receptor and the T3 receptor in the nucleus of thyrotropes (87).

Metformin has also been reported to reduce TSH levels in patients with type 2 diabetes mellitus and chronic hypothyroidism on stable thyroid hormone replacement (89). A later meta-analysis found that initiation of metformin is associated with a reduction in TSH in patients with overt or subclinical hypothyroidism but no change was noted in euthyroid individuals receiving metformin (90). Metformin activates AMP-activated protein kinase (AMPK) and sirtuin 1 (SIRT1) which are involved in regulation of fatty acid oxidation, hepatic gluconeogenesis, and insulin sensitivity (91). Metformin has also been reported to retard the progression of various cancers, including thyroid cancer, and may influence iodine uptake via the sodium iodide symporter. Metformin appears to affect TSH secretion in various circumstances. An initial case series noted that four patients on stable L-thyroxine developed suppressed TSH levels after initiation of metformin therapy (89). A later meta-analysis noted a reduction in TSH in both individuals receiving L-thyroxine for active, overt hypothyroidism and also those with subclinical hypothyroidism not receiving L-thyroxine (90). Euthyroid patients not receiving L-thyroxine did not exhibit a change in TSH levels. The metformin doses needed to achieve this effect have been reported to be as low as metformin XR 500 mg daily, and the aforementioned meta-analysis reported dosing of 1500–1700 mg per day. The change in TSH-related to metformin is hypothesized to be related to cAMP-mediated inhibition of TRH at the level of the hypothalamus, and not due to a change in T4 levels, L-thyroxine absorption, bioavailability, or degradation (92).

As noted above, drugs associated with the development of hypophysitis, such as ipilimumab and tremelimumab, can also impact TSH secretion and cause secondary hypothyroidism (93, 94). Anti-TSH antibodies have been noted in patients with anti-CTLA-4-induced hypophysitis (95).

INHIBITION OF T4 TO T3 CONVERSION

Medications known to reduce T4 to T3 conversion include amiodarone, glucocorticoids, gallbladder dyes, such as ipodate and iopanoic acid and propranolol and nadolol in high doses, and propylthiouracil. Amiodarone inhibits T4 5′-monodeiodination which can lead to a rise in serum T4 and rT3, a concomitant decline in serum T3, and a secondary rise in serum TSH levels (96). These changes typically resolve within 3-6 months of initiation of therapy or with discontinuation of amiodarone. If the serum TSH remains elevated after more than 3–6 months, the patient can be considered to have amiodarone-induced hypothyroidism. If amiodarone needs to be continued, treatment with levothyroxine should be initiated, but levothyroxine doses needed to normalize serum TSH levels may be higher than expected due to inhibition of T4 to T3 conversion as previously discussed (97). The radiocontrast agents ipodate and iopanoic acid also inhibit T4 to T3 conversion, but are no longer available in the United States (98).

DRUGS IMPACTING THYROXINE-BINDING GLOBULIN LEVELS OR BINDING

In serum, T4 and T3 can be bound or free, with thyroxine-binding globulin (TBG) and thyroid-binding prealbumin (TBPA, transthyretin) being the primary binding proteins for T4; TBPA only binds T4 and not T3. Measured total T4 and T3 levels represent both the bound and the free T4 and T3 concentrations, respectively. TBG levels can be impacted by various medications. For example, estrogens, tamoxifen, raloxifene, 5-fluorouracil, heroin, and methadone have all been found to increase TBG levels whereas niacin, corticosteroids, L-asparaginase, and androgens can decrease TBG (99–108). In patients with an intact hypothalamic-pituitary-thyroid axis, the system will respond to changes in protein binding of T4 and T3 so that free T4 and free T3 levels remain in their reference ranges once there is time for equilibration. However, in patients dependent on thyroid hormone replacement therapy, an adjustment in thyroid hormone dosing (a decrease in thyroid hormone doses with lower TBG, and an increase in thyroid hormone doses with rising TBG) is necessary to avoid patients developing serum thyroid hormone levels outside of their reference ranges, causing iatrogenic thyrotoxicosis or hypothyroidism.

There are also medications that distort *in vitro* tests of thyroid function, with particular reference to estimates of serum free thyroxine (109). Displacement of thyroid hormone from serum-binding proteins has been noted with heparin, aspirin, carbamazepine, furosemide, phenytoin, and salsalate therapy (110–114). Non-esterified fatty acids (NEFA) in a concentration of >3 mmol/l can increase the displacement of T4 from TBG. In patients receiving heparin, lipoprotein lipase becomes mobilized *in vivo*, which during sample storage or incubation can lead to rising NEFA levels which stimulate disassociation of T4 and T3 from thyroid-binding proteins resulting in spuriously high results in FT4 and FT3 assays. Heparin does not appear to impact TSH measurements nor total T4 and T3 levels (115). Furosemide has been found to inhibit T4 binding and appears to impact measurement in free T4 assays which involve less sample dilutions than others (109). Phenytoin and carbamazepine can displace T4 and T3 from thyroid-binding proteins leading to an increase in free hormone concentrations and a concomitant decrease in total T4 and T3 levels. As FT4 and FT3 assays tend to yield spuriously low levels in these circumstances, TSH levels, which are not impacted, should be relied on to guide therapy (116). The impact of aspirin, salsalate, and nonsteroidal anti-inflammatory drugs (NSAIDs) vary by drug and length of exposure. A single-dose or 1 week of salsalate therapy was found to decrease both free and total T4 and T3 levels while TSH remained unchanged after a lone dose and decreased after 1 week while remaining in the normal range (112). In the same study, acute TH changes noted with aspirin included lower TT3 and FT3 with stable TT4 and FT4 and TSH levels; after 1 week TSH, TT4, TT3, and FT3 all dropped but FT4 remained stable. Testing with the NSAID meclofenamate revealed an acute rise in TT4, TT3, FT3 with no change in TSH and FT4 and stability in all these levels after 1 week.

ENHANCED METABOLIC CLEARANCE OF THYROID HORMONE

Increased metabolic clearance of thyroid hormones has been noted with several medications, including carbamazepine, phenobarbital, phenytoin, rifampin, and sertraline (114, 117–(119). Carbamazepine, phenobarbital, phenytoin, and rifampin all appear to increase hepatic metabolism of TH and can thereby impact TH dosing for hypothyroidism. There are reports of patients with hypothyroidism on stable TH therapy whom after initiation of sertraline require an increase of LT4 dosing (120). Therefore, adjustments in thyroid hormone therapy may be required in situations when sertraline is instituted or discontinued although one study did not observe this in the patient population they studied (121). Bexarotene, a selective RXRα agonist, has also been reported to decrease T4, T3, and reverse T3 levels in athyrotic patients on stable thyroid hormone replacement with L-T4 (122). This finding is felt to represent augmented non-deiodinase-mediated peripheral degradation of thyroid hormones.

INHIBITION OF THYROID HORMONE ABSORPTION AND/OR ENTEROHEPATIC CIRCULATION

The absorption of thyroid hormone from the stomach and small bowel, as well as reabsorption of thyroid hormone released in bile (a.k.a.enterohepatic circulation of thyroid hormone), can be impaired by numerous drugs (123). Bile acid sequestrants (e.g., cholestyramine, colestipol, and colesevelam) and calcium carbonate directly bind TH in the gut preventing its absorption but do not have adverse effects in euthyroid individuals not taking TH (124, 125). Raloxifene, a selective estrogen modulator, has been shown to impair TH absorption (mechanism unknown), as has the antibiotic ciprofloxacin (126, 127). Aluminum hydroxide is associated with a nonspecific inhibition of absorption of TH or complexes with TH , while ferrous sulfate and psyllium bind to TH. These along with sucralfate have been found to potentially interfere with gastrointestinal absorption of TH (128–130). T4 absorption testing has revealed reduced T4 absorption when TH is taken together with either sevelamer, lanthanum carbonate, or chromium (131, 132). Hypothyroid patients who take these compounds with their thyroid hormone may encounter reduced thyroid hormone absorption or enterohepatic reabsorption leading to inadequate hormonal levels and rise in TSH. Conversely, if the thyroid hormone dosing regimen was arrived at while taking these drugs and thyroxine together, and then the two drugs are subsequently dosed separately, iatrogenic thyrotoxicosis may occur due to improved thyroxine absorption. It is recommended that thyroid hormones be taken at least 3–4 hours before or after taking any of these products. Proton pump inhibitors (PPIs) can be associated with a rise in TSH and a decrease in TH levels in hypothyroid patients taking thyroid hormone (133). Adequate gastric acid is required for optimal TH absorption. PPIs reduce gastric acid production thereby negatively impacting TH absorption. PPIs may also increase clearance of TH by means of enhanced uridine diphosphate-glucuronosyl-transferase (UGT) enzymes (134).

ASSAY INTERFERENCE

More recently, it has become evident that biotin (vitamin B7), which is commonly used by individuals for various purported health benefits, can interfere with the accurate measurement of many substances, including thyroid hormones, TSH, thyroglobulin, and thyroid stimulating immunoglobulins if the assay method utilizes a streptavidin-biotin reporting system. This is most likely to occur in the presence of high levels of serum biotin, typically when consuming doses of biotin >5 mg/day. One report which tested several assays found that TSH may be lower, while T4 and T3 may be higher in individuals taking high doses of biotin for 7 days when compared with levels drawn at baseline or 7 days after cessation of biotin (135). Assays using other non-biotin-based methodologies are not affected by intake of biotin doses of up to 10 mg/day. All patients about to undergo thyroid function testing should be questioned for biotin use and advised to suspend it for 7 days prior to hormonal testing.

THYROTOXICOSIS RELATED TO EXOGENOUS SOURCES OF THYROID HORMONE

Individuals may become thyrotoxic when inadvertently or purposefully exposed to excess thyroid hormone. Patients may unintentionally receive excessive thyroid hormone doses for treatment of hypothyroidism, or deliberately for suppression of TSH in the context of thyroid cancer therapy.

Additionally, clinicians may encounter patients who have had thyroid hormone prescribed for non-thyroid conditions such as obesity, infertility, and depression. Thyrotoxicosis factitia typically refers to surreptitious consumption of thyroid hormone containing products, while accidental exposure can happen through unintentional poisoning in children, contamination by food such as hamburger or sausage in which the animal thyroid gland has been included, or when consuming over the counter (OTC) supplements containing T4 and/or T3 that may or may not listed as an ingredient (136, 137). There are reports of over-the-counter products having been found to contain supraphysiologic amounts of iodine or even active TH products. In one study on supplements marketed to improve thyroid health, 9 of 10 supplements were found to contain T3 (1.3–25.4 mcg/tablet) and 5 of 10 contained T4 (5.77–22.9 mcg/ tablet) and, if consumed at the recommended dose,5 supplements delivered T3 quantities of >10 mcg/day, and 4 delivered T4 quantities ranging between 8.57 to 91.6 mcg/day (138).

Patients with exogenous thyrotoxicosis can be expected to be found to have typical symptoms of thyrotoxicosis with the severity varying with the magnitude of exposure, a small or normal sized thyroid on physical exam, and suppressed serum TSH with elevated serum T4 and T3 levels if the compound contains T4 $\pm$ T3, or a lone elevation of serum T3 levels if only liothyronine has been ingested. Thyroglobulin serum levels are expected to be low in these instances as is radioactive iodine uptake (usually <5%) (139). In a case of surreptitious thyroid hormone ingestion or when the diagnosis is uncertain, fecal analysis for thyroxine could be considered (140).

While acute exposure to excess T4 can be fairly well tolerated, the elderly are at risk for adverse cardiovascular events, and there are reports of seizures principally in the pediatric population. More chronic exposure to excess thyroid hormone increases the risk of atrial fibrillation and can be associated with increased bone turnover, leading to osteopenia or osteoporosis (141, 142).

Management includes cessation of the TH-containing product or reduction of the prescribed thyroid hormone dose to achieve clinically appropriate serum TSH and thyroid hormone levels. With a half-life of 24 hours, T3 will be eliminated more quickly than T4, which has a half-life

of 1 week. Beta-blockers can be prescribed to mitigate cardiac symptoms and agents which inhibit T4 to T3 conversion (e.g., propranolol in doses >160 mg/day, glucocorticoids, and, where available, the radiographic contrast agents ipodate or iopanoic acid) can be utilized. Resin-binders, like cholestyramine, can reduce T4 and T3 reabsorption by blocking the enterohepatic circulation of thyroid hormones (143). Induced emesis, charcoal administration, and gastric lavage are also options which can be utilized in the context of thyroid hormone overdose or poisoning, and with plasmapheresis and exchange transfusion being an option for more severe cases (144, 145).

CONCLUSION

As evidenced by the discussion within this chapter, there are a large number of drugs that can impact thyroid hormone levels, due to the effects on various steps of thyroid hormone synthesis and metabolism, via effects on the immune system and direct toxicity to thyroid cells or by means of assay interference. One can expect this list to expand as newer agents enter clinical practice, especially with the anticipation of many more new TKIs in the future, a drug class already shown to be associated with major effects on thyroid gland integrity and thyroid hormone metabolism. When encountering patients with abnormal serum thyroid hormone and/or TSH levels, providers need to be vigilant about reviewing the patient's medication list, including OTC products, and consider potential drug effects as a cause for changes in thyroid hormone or thyroid antibody levels. Finally, drugs can cause artefactual changes in thyroid hormone levels due to assay interference that can mimic the effects of thyroid dysfunction, and, if not recognized, could lead to inappropriate therapy.

REFERENCES

1. Pittman CS, Chambers JB Jr, Read VH. The extrathyroidal conversion rate of thyroxine to triiodothyronine in normal man. *J. Clin. Invest.* 1971; 50(6): 1187–96.
2. World Health Organization. *Assessment of Iodine Deficiency Disorders and Monitoring Their Elimination: A Guide for Programme Managers*, 3rd edition. Geneva: World Health Organization, 2007.

3. Wolff J, Chaikoff IL. Plasma inorganic iodide as a homeostatic regulator of thyroid function. *J. Biol. Chem.* 1948; 174(2): 555–64.

4. Eng PH, Cardona GR, Fang SL, Previti M, Alex S, Carrasco N, Chin WW, Braverman LE. Escape from the Acute Wolff Chaikoff effect is associated with a decrease in thyroid sodium/iodide symporter messenger ribonucleic acid and protein. *Endocrinology* 1999; 140(8): 3404–10.

5. Roti E, Uberti ED. Iodine excess and hyperthyroidism. *Thyroid* 2001; 11(5): 493–500.

6. Leung AM, Braverman LE. Iodine-induced thyroid dysfunction. *Curr. Opin. Endocrinol. Diabetes Obes.* 2012; 19(5): 414–9.

7. Braverman LE, Ingbar SH, Vagenakis AG, Adams L, Maloof F. Enhanced susceptibility to iodide myxedema in patients with Hashimoto's disease. *J. Clin. Endocrinol. Metab.* 1971; 32(4): 515–21.

8. Braverman LE, Woeber KA, Ingbar SH. Induction of myxedema by iodide in patients euthyroid after radioiodine or surgical treatment of diffuse toxic goiter. *N. Engl. J. Med.* 1969; 281(15): 816–21.

9. Reinhardt W, Luster M, Rudorff KH, Heckmann C, Petrasch S, Lederbogen S, Haase R, et al. Effect of small doses of iodine on thyroid function in patients with Hashimoto's thyroiditis residing in an area of mild iodine deficiency. *Eur. J. Endocrinol.* 1998; 139(1): 23–8.

10. van der Molen AJ, Thomsen HS, Morcos SK, Contrast Media Safety Committee, European Society of Urogenital Radiology (ESUR). Effect of iodinated contrast media on thyroid function in adults. *Eur. Radiol.* 2004; 14(5): 902–7.

11. Nimmons GL, Funk GF, Graham MM, Pagedar NA. Urinary iodine excretion after contrast computed tomography scan: Implications for radioactive iodine use. *JAMA Otolaryngol. Head Neck Surg.* 2013; 139(5): 479–82.

12. Padovani RP, Kasamatsu TS, Nakabashi CCD, Camacho CP, Andreoni DM, Malouf EZ, Marone MM, Maciel RM, Biscolla RP. One month is sufficient for urinary iodine to return to its baseline value After the use of water-soluble iodinated contrast agents in post-thyroidectomy patients requiring radioiodine therapy. *Thyroid* 2012; 22(9): 926–30.

13. Rhee CM, Bhan I, Alexander EK, Brunelli SM. Association between iodinated contrast media exposure and incident hyperthyroidism and hypothyroidism. *Arch. Intern. Med.* 2012; 172(2): 153–9.

14. Marraccini P, Bianchi M, Bottoni A, Mazzarisi A, Coceani M, Molinaro S, Lorenzoni V, Landi P, Iervasi G. Prevalence of thyroid dysfunction and effect of contrast medium on thyroid metabolism in cardiac patients undergoing coronary angiography. *Acta Radiol.* 2013; 54(1): 42–7.

15. Koroscil TM, Pelletier PR, Slauson JW, Hennessey J. Short-term effects of coronary angiographic contrast agents on thyroid function. *Endocr. Pract.* 1997; 3(4): 219–21.

16. Arum SM, He X, Braverman LE. Excess iodine from an unexpected source. *N. Engl. J. Med.* 2009; 360(4): 424–6.

17. Nolte MR, Muller R, Siggelkow H, Emrich D, Hufner M. Prophylactic application of thyrostatic drugs during excessive iodine exposure in euthyroid patients with thyroid autonomy: A randomized study. *Eur. J. Endocrinol.* 1996; 134(3): 337–41.

18. Gopal AK, Rajendran JG, Gooley TA, Pagel JM, Fisher DR, Petersdorf SH, Maloney DG, Eary JF, Appelbaum FR, Press OW. High-dose [131I]tositumomab (anti-CD20) radioimmunotherapy and autologous hematopoietic stem-cell transplantation for adults > or = 60. years old with relapsed or refractory B-cell lymphoma. *J. Clin. Oncol.* 2007; 10(25(11)): 1396–402

19. Press OW, Unger JM, Braziel RM, Maloney DG, Miller TP, Leblanc M, Fisher RI, Southwest Oncology Group. Southwest Oncology Group. Phase II trial of CHOP chemotherapy followed by tositumomab/iodine I-131 tositumomab for previously untreated follicular non-Hodgkin's lymphoma: Five-year follow-up of Southwest Oncology Group Protocol S9911. *J. Clin. Oncol.* 2006; 24(25): 4143–9.

20. Kaminski MS, Tuck M, Estes J, Kolstad A, Ross CW, Zasadny K, Regan D, et al. ^{131}I-tositumomab therapy as initial treatment for follicular lymphoma. *N. Engl. J. Med.* 2005; 352(5): 441–9.

21. van Santen HM, de Kraker J, van Eck BL, de Vijlder JJ, Vulsma T. High incidence of thyroid dysfunction despite prophylaxis with potassium iodide during (131)I-meta-iodobenzylguanidine treatment in children with neuroblastoma. *Cancer*; 2002; 94(7): 2081–9.

22. Martino E, Bartalena L, Bogazzi F, Braverman LE. The effects of amiodarone on the thyroid. *Endocr. Rev.* 2001; 22(2): 240–54.

23. Bogazzi F, Bartalena L, Dell'Unto E, Tomisti L, Rossi G, Pepe P, Tanda ML, et al. Proportion of type 1 and type 2 amiodarone-induced thyrotoxicosis has changed over a 27-year period in Italy. *Clin Endocrinol* 2007; 67: 533–7.

24. Tanda ML, Piantanida E, Lai A, Liparulo L, Sassi L, Bogazzi F, Wiersinga WM, et al. Diagnosis and management of amiodarone-induced thyrotoxicosis: Similarities and differences between North American and European thyroidologists. *Clin. Endocrinol. (Oxf.)* 2008; 69(5): 812–8.

25. Diehl LA, Romaldini JH, Graf H, Bartalena L, Martino E, Albino CC, Wiersinga WM. Management of amiodarone-induced thyrotoxicosis in Latin America: An electronic survey. *Clin. Endocrinol. (Oxf.)* 2006; 65(4): 433–8.

26. Martino E, Aghini-Lombardi F, Mariotti S, Bartalena L, Lenziardi M, Ceccarelli C, Bambini G, et al. Amiodarone iodine-induced hypothyroidism: Risk factors and follow-up in 28 cases. *Clin. Endocrinol. (Oxf.)* 1987; 26(2): 227–37.

27. Trip MD, Wiersinga WM, Plomp TA. Incidence, predictability, and pathogenesis of amiodarone-induced thyrotoxicosis and hypothyroidism. *Am. J. Med.* 1991; 91(5): 507–11.

28. Kurt IH, Yigit T, Karademir BM. Atrial fibrillation due to late amiodarone-induced thyrotoxicosis. *Clin. Drug Invest.* 2008; 28(8): 527–31.

29. Tomisti L, Rossi G, Bartalena L, Martino E, Bogazzi F. The onset time of amiodarone-induced thyrotoxicosis (AIT) depends on AIT type. *Eur. J. Endocrinol.* 2014; 171(3): 363–8.

30. O'Sullivan AJ, Lewis M, Diamond T. Amiodarone-induced thyrotoxicosis: Left ventricular dysfunction is associated with increased mortality. *Eur. J. Endocrinol.* 2006; 154(4): 533–6.

31. Martino E, Aghini-Lombardi F, Mariotti S, Lenziardi M, Baschieri L, Braverman LE, Pinchera A. Treatment of amiodarone associated thyrotoxicosis by simultaneous administration of potassium perchlorate and methimazole. *J. Endocrinol. Invest.* 1986; 9(3): 201–7.

32. Vanderpump MP. Thyroid gland: Use of glucocorticoids in amiodarone-induced thyrotoxicosis. *Nat. Rev. Endocrinol.* 2009; 5(12): 650 –1.

33. Bogazzi F, Bartalena L, Tomisti L, Rossi G, Tanda ML, Dell'Unto E, Aghini-Lombardi F, Martino E. Glucocorticoid response in amiodarone-induced thyrotoxicosis resulting from destructive thyroiditis is predicted by thyroid volume and serum free thyroid hormone concentrations. *J. Clin. Endocrinol. Metab.* 2007; 92(2): 556 –62.

34. Bogazzi F, Tomisti L, Rossi G, Dell'Unto E, Pepe P, Bartalena L, Martino E. Glucocorticoids are preferable to thionamides as first-line treatment for amiodarone-induced thyrotoxicosis due to destructive thyroiditis: A matched retrospective cohort study. *J. Clin. Endocrinol. Metab.* 2009; 94(10): 3757–62.

35. Czarnywojtek A, Czepczynski R, Ruchala M, Wasko R, Zgorzalewicz-Stachowiak M, Szczepanek E, Zamyslowska H, et al. Radioiodine therapy in patients with amiodarone-induced thyrotoxicosis (AIT). *Neuro Endocrinol. Lett.* 2009; 30(2): 209 –14.

36. Albino CC, Paz-Filho G, Graf H. Recombinant human TSH as an adjuvant to radioiodine for the treatment of type 1 amiodarone induced thyrotoxicosis (AIT). *Clin. Endocrinol. (Oxf.)* 2009; 70(5): 810–1.

37. Bogazzi F, Tomisti L, Ceccarelli C, Martino E. Recombinant human TSH as an adjuvant to radioiodine for the treatment of type 1

amiodarone-induced thyrotoxicosis: A cautionary note. *Clin. Endocrinol. (Oxf.)* 2010; 72(1): 133–4.

38. Houghton SG, Farley DR, Brennan MD, van Heerden JA, Thompson GB, Grant CS. Surgical management of amiodarone-associated thyrotoxicosis: Mayo Clinic experience. *World J. Surg.* 2004; 28(11): 1083–7.

39. Spaulding SW, Burrow GN, Bermudez F, Himmelhoch JM. The inhibitory effect of lithium on thyroid hormone release in both euthyroid and thyrotoxic patients. *J. Clin. Endocrinol. Metab.* 1972; 35(6): 905–11.

40. Lazarus JH, John R, Bennie EH, Chalmers RJ, Crockett G. Lithium therapy and thyroid function a long-term study. *Psychol. Med.* 1981; 11(1): 85–92.

41. Lombardi G, Panza N, Biondi B, Di Lorenzo L, Lupoli G, Muscettola G, Carella C, Bellastella A. Effects of lithium treatment on hypothalamic-pituitary-thyroid axis: A longitudinal study. *J. Endocrinol. Invest.* 1993; 16(4): 259–63.

42. Baumgartner A, Vonstuckrad M, Mulleroerlinghausen B, Gräf KJ, Kürten I. The hypothalamic-pituitary-thyroid axis in patients maintained on lithium prophylaxis for years – High triiodothyronine serum concentrations are correlated to the prophylactic efficacy. *J. Affect. Disord.* 1995; 34(3): 211–8.

43. Bolaris S, Margarity M, Valcana T. Effects of LiCl on triiodothyronine (T3) binding to nuclei from rat cerebral hemispheres. *Biol. Psychiatry* 1995; 37(2): 106–11.

44. Kirov G, Tredget J, John R, Owen MJ, Lazarus JH. A cross-sectional and a prospective study of thyroid disorders in lithium-treated patients. *J. Affect. Disord.* 2005; 87(2–3): 313–7.

45. Lazarus JH. Lithium and thyroid. *Best Pract. Res. Clin. Endocrinol. Metab.* 2009 Dec; 23(6): 723–33.

46. Bocchetta A, Mossa P, Velluzzi F, Mariotti S, Zompo MD, Loviselli A. Ten-year follow-up of thyroid function in lithium patients. *J. Clin. Psychopharmacol.* 2001; 21(6): 594–8.

47. Bathge C, Blimentritt H, Berghofer A, Bschor T, Glenn T, Adli M, Schlattmann P, Bauer M, Finke R. Long term lithium and thyroid antibodies: A controlled study. *J. Psychiatry Neurosci.* 2005; 30: 423–7.

48. Shopsin B, Shenkman L, Blum M, Hollander CS. Iodine and lithium-induced hypothyroidism. Documentation of synergism. *Am. J. Med.* 1973; 55(5): 695–9.

49. McKnight RF, Adida M, Budge K, Stockton S, Goodwin GM, Geddes JR. Lithium toxicity profile: A systematic review and meta-analysis. *Lancet* 2012; 379(9817): 721–8.

50. Barclay ML, Brownlie BEW, Turner JG, Wells JE. Lithium associated thyrotoxicosis: A report of 14 cases, with statistical analysis of incidence. *Clin. Endocrinol. (Oxf)* 1994; 40(6): 759–64.

51. Mizukami Y, Michigishi T, Nonomura A, Nakamura S, Noguchi M, Takazakura E. Histological features of the thyroid gland in a patient with lithium induced thyrotoxicosis. *J. Clin. Pathol.* 1995; 48(6): 582–4.

52. Miller KK, Daniels GH. Association between lithium use and thyrotoxicosis caused by silent thyroiditis. *Clin. Endocrinol. (Oxf)* 2001; 55(4): 501–8.

53. Segal RL, Rosenblatt S, Eliasoph I. Endocrine exophthalmos during lithium therapy of manic depressive disease. *N. Engl. J. Med.* 1973; 289(3): 136–8.

54. Byrne AP, Delaney WJ. Regression of thyrotoxic ophthalmopathy following lithium withdrawal. *Can. J. Psychiatry* 1993; 38(10): 635–7.

55. Hamnvik OP, Larsen PR, Marqusee E. Thyroid dysfunction from antineoplastic agents. *J. Natl. Cancer Inst.* 2011; 103(21): 1572–87.

56. Desai J, Yassa L, Marqusee E, George S, Frates MC, Chen MH, Morgan JA, et al. Hypothyroidism after sunitinib treatment for patients with gastrointestinal stromal tumors. *Ann. Intern. Med.* 2006; 145(9): 660–4.

57. Schlumberger MJ, Elisei R, Bastholt L, Wirth LJ, Martins RG, Locati LD, Jarzab B, et al. Phase II study of safety and efficacy of motesanib in patients with progressive or symptomatic, advanced or metastatic medullary thyroid cancer. *J. Clin. Oncol.* 2009; 27(23): 3794–801.

58. de Groot JW, Zonnenberg BA, Plukker JT, van Der Graaf WT, Links TP. Imatinib induces hypothyroidism in patients receiving levothyroxine. *Clin. Pharmacol. Ther.* 2005; 78(4): 433–8.

59. Abdulrahman RM, Verloop H, Hoftijzer H, Verburg E, Hovens GC, Corssmit EP, Reiners C, et al. Sorafenib-induced hypothyroidism is associated with increased type 3 deiodination. *J. Clin. Endocrinol. Metab.* 2010; 95(8): 3758–62.

60. Delivanis DA, Gustafson MP, Bornschlegl S, Merten MM, Kottschade L, Withers S, Dietz AB, Ryder M. Pembrolizumab-induced thyroiditis: Comprehensive clinical review and insights into underlying involved mechanisms. *J. Clin. Endocrinol. Metab.* 2017; 102(8): 2770–80.

61. Karantanis D, Bogsrud TV, Wiseman GA, Mullan BP, Subramaniam RM, Nathan MA, Peller PJ, Bahn RS, Lowe VJ. Clinical significance of diffusely increased 18F-FDG uptake in the thyroid gland. *J. Nucl. Med.* 2007; 48(6): 896–901.

62. Osorio JC, Ni A, Chaft JE, Pollina R, Kasler MK, Stephens D, Rodriguez C, et al. Antibody-mediated thyroid dysfunction during T-cell checkpoint blockade in patients with nonsmall cell lung cancer. *Ann. Oncol.* 2017; 28(3): 583–9.

63. Ribas A, Camacho LH, Lopez-Berestein G, Pavlov D, Bulanhagui CA, Millham R, Comin-Anduix B, et al. Antitumor activity in melanoma and anti-self responses in a phase I trial with the anti-cytotoxic T lymphocyte-associated antigen 4 monoclonal antibodyCP-675,206. *J. Clin. Oncol.* 2005;23(35): 8968–77.

64. Ryder M, Callahan M, Postow MA, Wolchok J, Fagin JA. Endocrine-related adverse events following ipilimumab in patients with advanced melanoma: A comprehensive retrospective review from a single institution. *Endocr. Relat. Cancer* 2014; 21(2): 371–81.

65. Faje A. Immunotherapy and hypophysitis: Clinical presentation, treatment, and biologic insights. *Pituitary* 2016; 19(1): 82–92.

66. Orlov S, Salari F, Kashat L, Walfish PG. Induction of painless thyroiditis in patients receiving programmed death 1 receptor immunotherapy for metastatic malignancies. *J. Clin. Endocrinol. Metab.* 2015; 100(5): 1738–41.

67. Shaw SA, Camacho LH, McCutcheon IE, Waguespack SG. Transient hypophysitis after cytotoxic T lymphocyte-associated antigen 4 (CTLA4) blockade. *J. Clin. Endocrinol. Metab.* 2007; 92(4): 1201–2.

68. Gan EH, Mitchell AL, Plummer R, Pearce S, Perros P. Tremelimumab-induced Graves hyperthyroidism. *Eur. Thyroid J.* 2017 Jul;6 (3): 167–70.

69. Abdel-Rahman O, El Halawani H, Fouad M. Risk of endocrine complications in cancer patients treated with immune check point inhibitors: A meta-analysis. *Future Oncol.* 2016; 12(3): 413–25.

70. Osorio JC, Ni A, Chaft JE, Pollina R, Kasler MK, Stephens D, Rodriguez C, et al. Antibody-mediated thyroid dysfunction during T-cell checkpoint blockade in patients with non-small-cell lung cancer. *Ann. Oncol.* 2017; 28(3): 583–9.

71. Byun DJ, Wolchok JD, Rosenberg LM, Girotra M. Cancer immunotherapy – Immune checkpoint blockade and associated endocrinopathies. *Nat. Rev. Endocrinol.* 2017; 13(4): 195–207.

72. Vassilopoulou-Sellin R, Sella A, Dexeus FH, Theriault RL, Pololoff DA. Acute thyroid dysfunction (thyroiditis) after therapy with interleukin-2. *Horm. Metab. Res.* 1992; 24(9): 434–8.

73. Krouse RS, Royal RE, Heywood G, Weintraub BD, White DE, Steinberg SM, Rosenberg SA, Schwartzentruber DJ. Thyroid dysfunction in 281 patients with metastatic melanoma or renal carcinoma treated with interleukin-2 alone. *J. Immunother. Emphasis Tumor Immunol.* 1995; 18(4): 272–8.

74. Atkins MB, Mier JW, Parkinson DR, Gould JA, Berkman EM, Kaplan MM. Hypothyroidism after treatment with interleukin-2 and lymphokine-activated killer cells. *N. Engl. J. Med.* 1988; 318(24): 1557–63.

75. Monzani F, Caraccio N, Dardano A, Ferrannini E. Thyroid autoimmunity and dysfunction associated with type I interferon therapy. *Clin. Exp. Med.* 2004; 3(4): 199–210.

76. Carella C, Mazziotti G, Morisco F, Manganella G, Rotondi M, Tuccillo C, Sorvillo F, Caporaso N, Amato G. Long-term outcome of interferon-alpha-induced thyroid autoimmunity and prognostic influence of thyroid autoantibody pattern at the end of treatment. *J. Clin. Endocrinol. Metab.* 2001; 86(5): 1925–9.

77. Cossburn M, Pace AA, Jones J, Ali R, Ingram G, Baker K, Hirst C, et al. Autoimmune disease after alemtuzumab treatment for multiple sclerosis in a multi-center cohort. *Neurology* 2011; 77(6): 573–9.

78. Mellin GW, Katzenstein M. The saga of thalidomide. Neuropathy to embryopathy, with case reports of congenital anomalies. *N. Engl. J. Med.* 1962; 267: 1184–92.

79. Badros AZ, Siegel E, Bodenner D, Zangari M, Zeldis J, Barlogie B, Tricot G. Hypothyroidism in patients with multiple myeloma following treatment with thalidomide. *Am. J. Med.* 2002; 112(5): 412–3.

80. Stein EM, Rivera C. Transient thyroiditis after treatment with lenalidomide in a patient with metastatic renal cell carcinoma. *Thyroid* 2007; 17(7): 681–3.

81. Figaro MK, Clayton W Jr, Usoh C, Brown K, Kassim A, Lakhani VT, Jagasia S. Thyroid abnormalities in patients treated with lenalidomide for hematological malignancies: Results of a retrospective case review. *Am. J. Hematol.* 2011; 86(6): 467–70.

82. Boesgaard S, Hagen C, Hangaard J, Andersen AN, Eldrup E. Effect of dopamine and a dopamine D-1 receptor agonist on pulsatile thyrotropin secretion in normal women. *Clin Endocrinol* 1990; 32(4): 423–32.

83. Wilber JF, Utiger RD. The effect of glucocorticoids on thyrotropin secretion. *J. Clin. Invest.* 1969; 48(11): 2096–103.

84. Cooper DS, Klibanski A, Ridgway EC. Dopaminergic modulation of TSH and its subunits: In vivo and in vitro studies. *Clin. Endocrinol. (Oxf.)* 1983; 18(3): 265–75.

85. Agner T, Hagen C, Andersen AN, Djursing H. Increased dopaminergic activity inhibits basal and metoclopramide-stimulated prolactin and thyrotropin secretion. *J. Clin. Endocrinol. Metab.* 1986; 62(4): 778–82.

86. Davies RR, Miller M, Turner SJ, Goodship TH, Cook DB, Watson M, McGill A, et al. Effects of somatostatin analogue SMS 201–995 in normal man. *Clin. Endocrinol. (Oxf.)* 1986; 24(6): 665–74.

87. Sherman SI, Gopal J, Haugen BR, Chiu AC, Whaley K, Nowlakha P, Duvic M. Central hypothyroidism associated with retinoid X receptor-selective ligands. *N. Engl. J. Med.* 1999; 340(14): 1075–9.

88. Wémeau JL, Dewailly D, Leroy R, D'Herbomez M, Mazzuca M, Decoulx M, Jaquet P. Long term treatment with the somatostatin analog SMS 201–995 in a patient with a thyrotropin- and Growth Hormone-secreting pituitary adenoma. *J. Clin. Endocrinol. Metab.* 1988; 66(3): 636–9.

89. Vigersky RA, Filmore-Nassar A, Glass AR. Thyrotropin suppression by metformin. *J. Clin. Endocrinol. Metab.* 2006; 91(1): 225–7.

90. Lupoli R, Di Minno A, Tortora A, Ambrosino P, Lupoli GA, Di Minno MN. Effects of treatment with metformin on TSH levels: A meta-analysis of literature studies. *J. Clin. Endocrinol. Metab.* 2014; 99(1): E143–8.

91. Zhou G, Myers R, Li Y, Chen Y, Shen X, Fenyk-Melody J, Wu M, et al. Role of AMP-activated protein kinase in mechanism of metformin action. *J. Clin. Invest.* 2001; 108(8): 1167–74.

92. López M, Varela L, Vázquez MJ, Rodríguez-Cuenca S, González CR, Velagapudi VR, Morgan DA, et al. Hypothalamic AMPK and fatty acid metabolism mediate thyroid regulation of energy balance. *Nat. Med.* 2010; 16(9): 1001–8.

93. Wang PF, Chen Y, Song SY, Wang TJ, Ji WJ, Li SW, Liu N, Yan CX. Immune-related adverse events associated with anti-PD-1/PD-L1 treatment for malignancies: A meta-analysis. *Front. Pharmacol.* 2017; 8: 730.

94. Torino F, Barnabei A, Paragliola R, Baldelli R, Appetecchia M, Corsello SM. Thyroid dysfunction as an unintended side effect of anticancer drugs. *Thyroid* 2013; 23(11): 1345–66.

95. Iwama S, De Remigis A, Callahan MK, Slovin SF, Wolchok JD, Caturegli P. Pituitary expression of CTLA-4 mediates

hypophysitis secondary to administration of CTLA-4 blocking antibody. *Sci. Transl. Med.* 2014; 6(230): 230ra45.

96. Burger A, Dinichert D, Nicod P, Jenny M, Lemarchand-Béraud T, Vallotton MB. Effect of amiodarone on serum triiodothyronine, reverse triiodothyronine, thyroxin, and thyrotropin. A drug influencing peripheral metabolism of thyroid hormones. *J. Clin. Invest.* 1976; 58(2): 255–9.

97. Safran M, Fang SL, Bambini G, Pinchera A, Martino E, Braverman LE. Effects of amiodarone and desethylamiodarone on pituitary deiodinase activity and thyrotropin secretion in the rat. *Am. J. Med. Sci.* 1986; 292(3): 136–41.

98. Bürgi H, Wimpfheimer C, Burger A, Zaunbauer W, Rösler H, Lemarchand-Béraud T. Changes of circulating thyroxine, triiodothyronine and reverse triiodothyronine after radiographic contrast agents. *J. Clin. Endocrinol. Metab.* 1976; 43(6): 1203–10.

99. Arafah BM. Increased need for thyroxine in women with hypothyroidism during estrogen therapy. *N. Engl. J. Med.* 2001; 344(23): 1743–9.

100. Jensen IW. Oestrogen-like effect of tamoxifen on concentration of thyroxin-binding globulin. *Lancet* 1985; 2(8462): 1020–1.

101. Ceresini G, Morganti S, Rebecchi I, Bertone L, Ceda GP, Bacchi-Modena A, Sgarabotto M, et al. A one-year follow-up on the effects of raloxifene on thyroid function in postmenopausal women. *Menopause* 2004; 11(2): 176–9.

102. Ain KB, Refetoff S. Relationship of oligosaccharide modification to the cause of serum thyroxine-binding globulin excess. *J. Clin. Endocrinol. Metab.* 1988; 66(5): 1037–43.

103. Bastomsky CH, Dent RR, Tolis G. Elevated serum concentrations of thyroxine-binding globulin and caeruloplasmin in methadone-maintained patients. *Clin. Biochem.* 1977; 10(3): 124–6.

104. Chan V, Wang C, Yeung RT. Effects of heroin addiction on thyrotrophin, thyroid hormones and prolactin secretion in men. *Clin. Endocrinol. (Oxf.)* 1979; 10(6): 557–65.

105. Arafah BM. Decreased levothyroxine requirement in women with hypothyroidism during androgen therapy for breast cancer. *Ann. Intern. Med.* 1994; 121(4): 247–51.

106. Garnick MB, Larsen PR. Acute deficiency of thyroxine-binding globulin during L-asparaginase therapy. *N. Engl. J. Med.* 1979; 301(5): 252–3.

107. Cashin-Hemphill L, Spencer CA, Nicoloff JT, Blankenhorn DH, Nessim SA, Chin HP, Lee NA. Alterations in serum thyroid hormonal indices with colestipol-niacin therapy. *Ann. Intern. Med.* 1987; 107(3): 324–9.

108. Burr WA, Ramsden DB, Griffiths RS, Black EG, Hoffenberg R, Meinhold H, Wenzel KW. Effect of a single dose of dexamethasone on serum concentrations of thyroid hormones. *Lancet* 1976; 2(7976): 58–61.

109. Stockigt JR, Lim CF. Medications that distort in vitro tests of thyroid function, with particular reference to estimates of serum free thyroxine. *Best Pract. Res. Clin. Endocrinol. Metab.* 2009; 23(6): 753–67.

110. Schatz DL, Sheppard RH, Steiner G, Chandarlapaty CS, de Veber GA. Influence of heparin on serum free thyroxine. *J. Clin. Endocrinol. Metab.* 1969; 29(8): 1015–22.

111. Aanderud S, Myking OL, Strandjord RE. The influence of carbamazepine on thyroid hormones and thyroxine binding globulin in hypothyroid patients substituted with thyroxine. *Clin. Endocrinol. (Oxf.)* 1981; 15(3): 247–52.

112. Samuels MH, Pillote K, Asher D, Nelson JC. Variable effects of nonsteroidal antiinflammatory agents on thyroid test results. *J. Clin. Endocrinol. Metab.* 2003; 88(12): 5710–6.

113. Stockigt JR, Lim CF, Barlow JW, Wynne KN, Mohr VS, Topliss DJ, Hamblin PS, Sabto J. Interaction of furosemide with serum thyroxine-binding sites: In vivo and in vitro studies and comparison with other inhibitors. *J. Clin. Endocrinol. Metab.* 1985; 60(5): 1025–31.

114. Rootwelt K, Ganes T, Johannessen SI. Effect of carbamazepine, phenytoin and phenobarbitone on serum levels of thyroid hormones and thyrotropin in humans. *Scand. J. Clin. Lab. Invest.* 1978; 38(8): 731–6.

115. Stockigt JR, Lim CF. Medications that distort in vitro tests of thyroid function, with particular reference to estimates of serum free thyroxine. *Best Pract. Res. Clin. Endocrinol. Metab.* 2009; 23(6): 753–67.

116. Surks MI, DeFesi CR. Normal serum free thyroid hormone concentrations in patients treated with phenytoin or carbamazepine. A paradox resolved. *JAMA* 1996; 275(19): 1495–8.

117. Curran PG, DeGroot LJ. The effect of hepatic enzyme-inducing drugs on thyroid hormones and the thyroid gland. *Endocr. Rev.* 1991; 12(2): 135–50.

118. Finke C, Juge C, Goumaz M, Kaiser O, Davies R, Burger AG. Effects of rifampicin on the peripheral turnover kinetics of thyroid hormones in mice and in men. *J. Endocrinol. Invest.* 1987; 10(2): 157–62.

119. McCowen KC, Garber JR. Effect of SSRI antidepressants on L-thyroxine requirements. *Thyroid* 2010; 20(8): 937.

120. McCowen KC, Garber JR, Spark R. Elevated serum thyrotropin in thyroxine-treated patients with hypothyroidism given sertraline. *N. Engl. J. Med.* 1997; 337(14): 1010–1.

121. de Carvalho GA, Bahls SC, Boeving A, Graf H. Effects of selective serotonin reuptake inhibitors on thyroid function in depressed patients with primary hypothyroidism or normal thyroid function. *Thyroid* 2009; 19(7): 691–7.

122. Smit JW, Stokkel MP, Pereira AM, Romijn JA, Visser TJ. Bexarotene-induced hypothyroidism: Bexarotene stimulates the peripheral metabolism of thyroid hormones. *J. Clin. Endocrinol. Metab.* 2007; 92(7): 2496–9.

123. Surks MI, Sievert R. Drugs and thyroid function. *N. Engl. J. Med.* 1995; 333(25): 1688–94.

124. Witztum JL, Jacobs LS, Schonfeld G. Thyroid hormone and thyrotropin levels in patients placed on colestipol hydrochloride. *J. Clin. Endocrinol. Metab.* 1978; 46(5): 838–40.

125. Singh N, Weisler SL, Hershman JM. The acute effect of calcium carbonate on the intestinal absorption of levothyroxine. *Thyroid* 2001; 11(10): 967–71.

126. Siraj ES, Gupta MK, Reddy SS. Raloxifene causing malabsorption of levothyroxine. *Arch. Intern. Med.* 2003; 163(11): 1367–70.

127. Cooper JG, Harboe K, Frost SK, Skadberg Ø. Ciprofloxacin interacts with thyroid replacement therapy. *BMJ* 2005; 330(7498): 1002.

128. Liel Y, Sperber AD, Shany S. Nonspecific intestinal adsorption of levothyroxine by aluminum hydroxide. *Am. J. Med.* 1994 Oct; 97(4): 363–5

129. Campbell NR, Hasinoff BB, Stalts H, Rao B, Wong NC. Ferrous Sulfate reduces thyroxine efficacy in patients with hypothyroidism. *Ann. Intern. Med.* 1992; 117(12): 1010–3.

130. Campbell JA, Schmidt BA, Bantle JP. Sucralfate and the absorption of L-thyroxine. *Ann. Intern. Med.* 1994; 121(2): 152.

131. John-Kalarickal J, Pearlman G, Carlson HE. New medications which decrease levothyroxine absorption. *Thyroid* 2007; 17(8): 763–5.

132. Weitzman SP, Ginsburg KC, Carlson HE. Colesevelam hydrochloride and lanthanum carbonate interfere with the absorption of levothyroxine. *Thyroid* 2009; 19(1): 77–9.

133. Centanni M, Gargano L, Canettieri G, Viceconti N, Franchi A, Delle Fave G, Annibale B. Thyroxine in goiter, Helicobacter pylori infection, and chronic gastritis. *N. Engl. J. Med.* 2006; 354(17): 1787–95.

134. Sachmechi I, Reich DM, Aninyei M, Wibowo F, Gupta G, Kim PJ. Effect of proton pump inhibitors on serum thyroid-stimulating hormone level in euthyroid patients treated with levothyroxine for hypothyroidism. *Endocr. Pract.* 2007; 13(4): 345–9.

135. Li D, Radulescu A, Shrestha RT, Root M, Karger AB, Killeen AA, Hodges JS, et al. Association of biotin ingestion with performance of hormone and nonhormone assays in healthy adults. *JAMA* 2017; 318(12): 1150–60.

136. Bogazzi F, Bartalena L, Scarcello G, Campomori A, Rossi G, Martino E. The age of patients with thyrotoxicosis factitia in Italy from 1973 to 1996. *J. Endocrinol. Invest.* 1999; 22(2): 128–33.

137. Hedberg CW, Fishbein DB, Janssen RS, Meyers B, McMillen JM, MacDonald KL, White KE, et al. An outbreak of thyrotoxicosis caused by the consumption of bovine thyroid gland in ground beef. *N. Engl. J. Med.* 1987; 316(16): 993–8.

138. Kang GY, Parks JR, Fileta B, Chang A, Abdel-Rahim MM, Burch HB, Bernet VJ. Thyroxine and triiodothyronine content in commercially available thyroid health supplements. *Thyroid* 2013; 23(10): 1233–7.

139. Mariotti S, Martino E, Cupini C, Lari R, Giani C, Baschieri L, Pinchera A. Low serum thyroglobulin as a clue to the diagnosis of thyrotoxicosis factitia. *N. Engl. J. Med.* 1982; 307(7): 410–2.

140. Bouillon R, Verresen L, Staels F, Bex M, De Vos P, De Roo M. The measurement of fecal thyroxine in the diagnosis of thyrotoxicosis factitia. *Thyroid* 1993; 3(2): 101–3.

141. Shammas NW, Richeson JF, Pomerantz R. Myocardial dysfunction and necrosis after ingestion of thyroid hormone. *Am. Heart J.* 1994; 127(1): 232–4.

142. Gorman RL, Chamberlain JM, Rose SR, Oderda GM. Massive levothyroxine overdose: High anxiety–Low toxicity. *Pediatrics* 1988; 82(4): 666–9.

143. Shakir KM, Michaels RD, Hays JH, Potter BB. The use of bile acid sequestrants to lower serum thyroid hormones in iatrogenic hyperthyroidism. *Ann. Intern. Med.* 1993; 118(2): 112–3.

144. Jha S, Waghdhare S, Reddi R, Bhattacharya P. Thyroid storm due to inappropriate administration of a compounded thyroid hormone preparation successfully treated with plasmapheresis. *Thyroid* 2012; 22(12): 1283–6.

145. Cohen JH 3rd Ingbar SH, Braverman LE. Thyrotoxicosis due to ingestion of excess thyroid hormone. *Endocr. Rev.* 1989; 10(2): 113–24.

6

Hypothyroidism

MICHAEL T. MCDERMOTT

Introduction	129	Adrenal coverage	149
Classification and etiology	130	Coverage when patients are NPO for surgery, medical illness, or diagnostic procedures	149
Clinical manifestations	133		
Diagnosis	135		
Screening and case finding for hypothyroidism	138	Conditions that are not hypothyroidism but may appear to be thyroid conditions	149
Outcomes of untreated hypothyroidism	139		
Management/treatment	140	*Non-thyroidal illness (euthyroid sick syndrome)*	*149*
Treatment outcomes	143	*Steroid responsive encephalopathy associated with autoimmune thyroid disease (SREAAT) [formerly Hashimoto's encephalopathy]*	*149*
Recommendations regarding treatment for mild hypothyroidism	144		
Optimal TSH level on replacement therapy	*144*	*Wilson's low T3 syndrome*	*150*
Factors contributing to increased LT4 requirements	144	*Reverse T3 syndrome (reverse T3 dominance syndrome)*	*150*
Combination LT4/LT3 therapy	145	Myxedema coma	151
Persistent symptoms in patients on levothyroxine replacement therapy	147	References	153

INTRODUCTION

Hypothyroidism, at the most basic level, is a state of deficient thyroid hormone action in tissues that are dependent on thyroid hormone for normal function. While hypothyroidism is most often caused by the failure of the thyroid gland to produce sufficient amounts of thyroid hormone, other causes of thyroid hormone deficiency or defective thyroid hormone action are well recognized, and more will undoubtedly be identified in the future. Overt hypothyroidism, in which the serum levels of thyroid hormone are subnormal, is present in 0.3–3.7% of the US population and in 0.2–5.3% of Europeans (1, 2). Hypothyroidism increases in prevalence with age and is more common in women than men, in people with other autoimmune diseases, and in individuals with Down syndrome and Turner syndrome (1). Mild or subclinical hypothyroidism, defined later, is more common with the prevalence estimates of 3–15% (3).

Physiology of the Thyroid System: A Short Summary. A brief hypothalamic-pituitary-thyroid-peripheral tissue physiology that will set the stage for a discussion of the known and potential pathophysiological aberrations of this axis.

Regulation of thyroid function starts in the hypothalamus, which produces thyrotropin releasing hormone (TRH) in response to physiological feedback signals. TRH descends the pituitary stalk, binds to TRH receptors (TRH-R) on thyrotropes in the anterior pituitary gland, and stimulates the production and secretion of thyroid stimulating hormone (TSH), also known as thyrotropin. TSH is secreted into the circulation and travels to the thyroid gland where it binds to TSH receptors (TSH-R) on thyrocytes to stimulate the synthesis and secretion of two main thyroid hormones, thyroxine (T4) and triiodothyronine (T3), the former being predominantly a pro-hormone and the latter being the active form. In humans, the thyroid gland secretes about 100 mcg of T4 and 6 mcg of T3 daily into the circulation. The majority of the circulating T3 is made in the liver, where T4 is converted into T3 by removal of one iodine molecule by the enzyme, deiodinase 1 (D1); thus, approximately 26 mcg of T3 enters the circulation daily from the thyroid gland and liver (Figure 6.1). T4 and T3 are transported through the circulation bound to three main serum proteins, thyroxine-binding globulin (TBG), thyroxine-binding pre-albumin (TBPA, also known as transthyretin), and albumin. Protein bound T4 accounts for 99.98% of circulating T4 while only 0.02% is free; T3 is 99.70% protein bound and 0.30% free (Figure 6.2). Upon arrival at thyroid hormone dependent tissues, T4 enters cells and is converted into T3 by tissue-specific deiodinases, deiodinase 1 (discussed above), and deiodinase 2 (D2), present in the brain and pituitary gland. Other deiodinases, such as

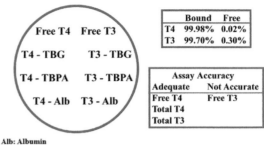

Alb: Albumin
TBG: Thyroxine Binding Globulin
TBPA: Thyroxine Binding Prealbumin (Transthyretin)

Figure 6.2 Protein-bound and free T4 and T3 in the circulation. Thyroxine (T4) and triiodothyronine (T3) circulate in the bloodstream bound to three main serum proteins, thyroxine-binding globulin (TBG), thyroxine-binding prealbumin (TBPA), and albumin. Protein-bound T4 accounts for 99.98% of circulating T4 while only 0.02% is free; T3 is 99.70% protein-bound and 0.30% free.

deiodinase 3 (D3), present in the brain and placenta, deactivate thyroid hormones by converting T4 to reverse T3 (RT3) and T3 into diiodothyronine (D2) (Figure 6.3). Deiodinase enzymes are subject to feedback regulation by circulating and tissue thyroid hormone levels through a process of ubiquitination and de-ubiquitination (4).

Uptake of T3 into the brain is dependent on organic anion transporter P1C1 (OATP1C1), which transports T4 across the blood brain barrier, and monocarboxylate transporter 8 (MCT8), which transports T3 across nerve cell membranes into neurons. Once inside cells, T3 binds to a thyroid hormone receptor (TR). T3 bound to TR associates with a cofactor, the retinoid X receptor (RXR) along DNA regulatory elements to stimulate or suppress the expression of thyroid hormone responsive genes. Thyroid hormone–regulated messenger RNA is then translated into proteins, some of which then undergo post-translational modifications before mediating the ultimate tissue effects of thyroid hormone (5). Theoretically genetic or epigenetic alterations at any of these steps could result in deficient thyroid hormone action at the tissue level.

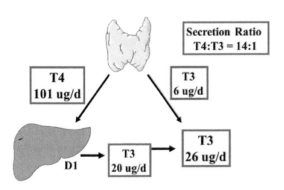

Figure 6.1 Thyroidal and extra-thyroidal production of thyroid hormones. The thyroid gland synthesizes and secretes two main thyroid hormones, thyroxine (T4) and triiodothyronine (T3). In humans, the thyroid gland secretes about 101 mcg of T4 and 6 mcg of T3 daily into the circulation. The majority of the circulating T3 is made in the liver, where T4 is converted into T3 by the removal of one iodine molecule by the enzyme, deiodinase 1 (D1); thus approximately 26 mcg of T3 enters the circulation daily from the thyroid gland and liver.

CLASSIFICATION AND ETIOLOGY

Primary hypothyroidism refers to thyroid hormone deficiency due to disease or disorders of the thyroid gland itself. The causes of primary

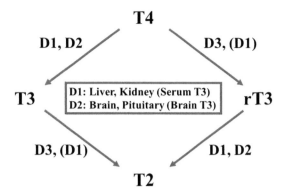

T4

D1, D2   D3, (D1)

T3   D1: Liver, Kidney (Serum T3)   rT3
      D2: Brain, Pituitary (Brain T3)

D3, (D1)   D1, D2

T2

Figure 6.3 Thyroid hormone metabolism by deiodinases. Thyroxine (T4) is the predominant thyroid hormone produced by the thyroid gland but it is a pro-hormone. Deiodinase enzymes, which remove iodine molecules, are present throughout the body to ensure that each tissue receives the exact amount of triiodothyronine (T3), the active hormone, that's required for its individual needs. Deiodinase 1 (D1) is present in the liver and kidneys, where it converts T4 into T3, generating the majority of the T3 in the circulation. Deiodinase 2 (D2) is present in the brain and is responsible for providing T3 for the brain and pituitary gland. Deiodinase 3 (D3), which is most abundant in the brain and placenta, converts T4 into reverse triiodothyronine (rT3), which has a 100 fold lower affinity for T3 receptors compared to T3. D1 also converts T4 into rT3 and rT3 into diiodothyronine (T2), but its affinity for T4 is much higher. T3 and RT3 are eventually deiodinated to T2, considered to be an inactive metabolite. Therefore, in humans, the thyroid gland functions mainly to produce a sufficient supply of the circulating pro-hormone T4 and deiodinases then provide appropriate intracellular T3 concentrations by regulating local T4 to T3 conversion in a highly tissue-specific manner.

hypothyroidism are shown in Table 6.1. The most common etiology of primary hypothyroidism in adults is chronic lymphocytic thyroiditis (Hashimoto's thyroiditis), a genetically based chronic inflammatory condition that leads to the gradual but progressive destruction of the thyroid gland, rendering it unable to make sufficient amounts of thyroid hormone to meet the needs of peripheral tissues. Hashimoto's thyroiditis is considered to be the most common of all autoimmune diseases. A genetic predisposition clearly plays a dominant role in the development of this disease, but environmental factors may also have

an important influence. For example, nutritional factors that have been linked to a higher risk for developing Hashimoto's thyroiditis include iodine excess, selenium deficiency, and possibly deficiencies of iron and vitamin D (6). Furthermore, selenium supplementation has been shown to reduce thyroid autoantibody titers in patients with this condition, although there has been no indication that selenium can reverse or prevent progression of thyroid dysfunction (7).

Primary hypothyroidism also commonly results from iatrogenic causes such as thyroidectomy and radioiodine (I-131) ablation treatment for hyperthyroidism or thyroid cancer. Post-surgical hypothyroidism virtually always occurs following a total thyroidectomy or adequately performed near-total thyroidectomy, but only develops in 56–64% of patients after a hemi-thyroidectomy or thyroid lobectomy and many of these experience only mild and transient hypothyroidism (8, 9). Factors that best predict the development of post-surgical hypothyroidism include the presence of underlying Hashimoto's thyroiditis and preoperative serum TSH levels > 2.0 mU/L; among those who develop mild postoperative hypothyroidism, progression to permanent hypothyroidism is best predicted by age > 46 years and preoperative serum TSH > 2.6 mU/L (8). Post-ablative hypothyroidism following I-131 treatment occurs in ~80% of patients with Graves' disease, ~55% of those with toxic multinodular goiter, and ~8% with a toxic solidary adenoma (1).

Severe iodine deficiency causes hypothyroidism by depriving the thyroid gland of iodine, the vital substrate for thyroid hormone synthesis. Iodine excess, especially when occurring suddenly, causes hypothyroidism by suppressing thyroid hormone secretion (Wolff-Chaikoff effect). Hypothyroidism can also occur transiently (usual duration of 3–6 months) during the recovery phases of the three main types of destructive thyroiditis: postpartum thyroiditis, silent (or painless) thyroiditis, and subacute thyroiditis. Thyroid dysfunction, including a high incidence of hypothyroidism, also occurs more frequently in patients with congenital thyroid hemiagenesis (10).

Numerous medications can impair thyroid function, causing primary hypothyroidism; the most notable of these are amiodarone, lithium, alpha interferon, and tyrosine kinase or multikinase inhibitors. Hypothyroidism, hyperthyroidism,

Table 6.1 Classification and etiology of hypothyroidism

1. Primary Hypothyroidism
   a. Chronic Lymphocytic Thyroiditis (Hashimoto's Disease)
   b. Iatrogenic Hypothyroidism
      i. Thyroidectomy
      ii. Radiation damage
         1 Radioiodine (I-131) ablation
         2 Radiation therapy for non-thyroid cancer
      iii. Medications
         1. Lithium
         2. Amiodarone
         3. Alpha interferon
         4. Tyrosine kinase inhibitors
         5. Check point inhibitors (ipilimumab, nivolumab)
         6. Anti-tuberculosis drugs (second line)
         7. Thalidomide and pomalidomide (used to treat multiple myeloma)
   c. Transient Thyroiditis
      i. Postpartum thyroiditis
      ii. Silent (painless) thyroiditis
      iii. Subacute (dequervain's) thyroiditis
      ilv. Palpation thyroiditis (e.G., After parathyroidectomy)
   d. Iodine Disorders
      i. Iodine deficiency (severe)
      ii. Iodine excess (severe)
   e. Infiltrative Disease
      i. Sarcoidosis
      ii. Malignancy (lymphoma, metastatic non-thyroid cancer)
   f. Congenital Hypothyroidism
      i. Genetic disorders of thyroid development
      ii. Genetic disorders of thyroid hormone synthesis
2. Central Hypothyroidism
   a. Hypothalamic-Pituitary Disorders
      i. Tumors
      ii. Surgical removal
      iii. Radiation therapy
      iv. Trauma (traumatic brain injury)
      v. Hemorrhage/Infarction (apoplexy, Sheehan's syndrome)
      vi. Infiltrative disorders (sarcoidosis, TB, hemochromatosis, histiocytosis X)
      vii. Medications (dopamine, opioids, glucocorticoids, somatostatin analogs, mitotane, bexarotene)
3. Peripheral Hypothyroidism
   a. Consumptive Hypothyroidism (deiodinase 3 expressing tumors)
   b. Thyroid Hormone Resistance Syndromes (TRβ, TRα, MCT8, SecisBP2 mutations)*

Adapted from (1).
TRβ = Thyroid Hormone Receptor Beta
TRα = Thyroid Hormone Receptor Alpha
MCT8 = Monocarboxylate Transporter 8
SecisBP2 = Selenoprotein Synthesis Proteins

and/or thyroiditis with transient or permanent hypothyroidism following an initial hyperthyroid phase, have all been well documented in patients being treated with tyrosine kinase and multikinase inhibitors (11), with alemtuzumab (an anti-CD52 monoclonal antibody) (12), and with immune checkpoint inhibitors such as ipilimumab, a monoclonal antibody directed against cytotoxic T-lymphocyte associated protein 4 (CTLA-4) and nivolumab, a monoclonal antibody inhibitor of the programmed cell death-1 (PD-1) receptor protein (13). Significant hypothyroidism with nivolumab has been reported to occur within 3–4 weeks of starting this medication (13) (see Chapter 5, "Drug-Induced Thyroid Dysfunction").

Central hypothyroidism (also known as secondary hypothyroidism) most often results from diseases or disorders of the hypothalamus or the pituitary gland that impair TRH production, TSH production, or both (1, 14). The most common conditions in this category are tumors, surgery, radiation, hemorrhage, infections, infiltrative disorders, and trauma affecting the hypothalamus or pituitary gland. Medications that have been shown to suppress TRH or TSH production include opioids, glucocorticoids, somatostatin analogs, mitotane, and bexarotene; use of these medications may cause central hypothyroidism. Metformin has also been reported to suppress TSH secretion and may interfere with thyroid test interpretation, but as of yet has not been implicated in causing *de novo* central hypothyroidism. The causes of central hypothyroidism are listed in Table 6.1.

Peripheral hypothyroidism refers to disorders where thyroid hormone may be produced and secreted normally but then fails to have normal effects on peripheral tissues. Two examples of this are consumptive hypothyroidism and thyroid hormone resistance syndromes. Consumptive hypothyroidism has been reported to occur in certain tumor types, most notably hepatic hemangiomas that express a high level of D3 that rapidly deactivates of T3 to T2, resulting in markedly deficient circulating T3 levels (15). Thyroid hormone resistance syndromes are a group of genetic disorders that cause deactivating mutations of the transport protein MCT8 or one of the TR isoforms (TRα or TRβ) (16). See Table 6.1 for these and other rare causes of hypothyroidism.

Hypothyroidism is also classified accordingly into three degrees of severity, although thyroid

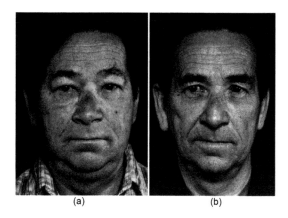

(a)   (b)

Figure 6.4 Facial changes with therapy of hypothyroidism. Primary hypothyroidism before (a) and after (b) treatment with levothyroxine. (From Smith TJ, et al. *Endocrine Reviews* 1989;10:366. Copyright 1989, The Endocrine Society.)

failure clearly exists on a continuous spectrum of severity. Mild hypothyroidism is defined biochemically as the presence of an elevated serum TSH level in the presence of a free T4 level that is still within the reference range; this condition is also known as subclinical hypothyroidism but the author prefers the term mild hypothyroidism because the condition may have clinical manifestations in some circumstances. Overt hypothyroidism is characterized by an elevated serum TSH and a free T4 level that is below the reference range (Figure 6.4). Myxedema coma (decompensated hypothyroidism) is a life-threatening form of severe hypothyroidism. The clinical manifestations, diagnosis, and management of mild hypothyroidism and overt hypothyroidism will be covered in the next sections and decompensated hypothyroidism (myxedema coma) will be discussed at the end.

CLINICAL MANIFESTATIONS

Clinical manifestations of hypothyroidism result from deficient thyroid hormone action at the tissue level. The "classic" features are shown in Table 6.2 (17, 18). These and other symptoms caused by hypothyroidism, however, are mostly nonspecific. Similar symptoms may also occur with numerous other conditions unrelated to the thyroid system. While symptoms tend to increase in number and severity with increasing severity of the thyroid hormone deficiency, they may be minimal or

Table 6.2 Common clinical manifestations of hypothyroidism

Symptom/Sign	Frequency	Symptom/Sign	Frequency
Adapted from (17)			
Dry skin	76%	Paresthesia	52%
Cold intolerance	64%	Cold skin	50%
Coarse skin	60%	Constipation	48%
Puffy eyelids	60%	Slow movements	36%
Decreased sweating	54%	Hoarseness	34%
Weight gain	54%	Impaired learning	22%
Adapted from (18)			
Fatigue	81%	Palpitations	35%
Dry skin	63%	Restlessness	33%
Shortness of breath	51%	Hair loss	30%
Mood lability	46%	Dysphagia	29%
Constipation	39%	Wheezing	27%
Globus sensation	36%	Vertigo	24%

Laboratory: Hyponatremia, macrocytic anemia, creatine phosphokinase (CPK) elevation, prolactin elevation, hyperlipidemia (increased total cholesterol, LDL, HDL, triglycerides and lipoprotein (a)) (21).

absent in some patients with biochemically significant disease and can be numerous in patients with only mild disease.

A 1997 study detailed the most common current clinical manifestations of overt hypothyroidism (17). A subsequent Danish case control study reported somewhat different findings; evaluating 140 subjects with overt hypothyroidism (mean TSH 54.5 mU/L), the authors identified 13 symptoms as being most suggestive of hypothyroidism: fatigue (81% of cases), dry skin (63%), shortness of breath (51%), mood lability (46%), constipation (39%), globus sensation (36%), palpitations (35%), restlessness (33%), hair loss (30%), difficulty swallowing (29%), wheezing (27%), vertigo (24%), and anterior neck pain (16%). However, there was considerable overlap with symptoms experienced by euthyroid controls; hypothyroid patients reported a mean of five symptoms and euthyroid controls reported a mean of two symptoms, but an equal proportion of both groups reported having three of these symptoms (18). This same group also reported that symptoms were a more reliable indicator of thyroid deficiency in men and younger patients and less reliable in women and the elderly (19, 20). Elderly persons with hypothyroidism generally experience fewer classic symptoms and signs; prominent features in this age group include fatigue and weakness (1, 20).

Some signs of thyroid disease or hypothyroidism, such as the presence of a goiter, a thyroidectomy scar, and a delayed relaxation phase of the deep tendon reflexes can be somewhat more informative. However, most of the "classical" signs of hypothyroidism are also nonspecific and subtle or often not present. A typical example of the facial features of severe hypothyroidism is shown in Figure 6.4.

General laboratory abnormalities, although certainly not diagnostic, can also give clues to the presence of hypothyroidism; these include hyponatremia, macrocytic anemia, and elevated creatine phosphokinase (CPK) levels. Hypothyroidism has also been well documented to cause mixed hyperlipidemia with elevation of all major lipids and lipoproteins [total cholesterol, LDL, HDL, Triglycerides, and Lp (a)] (21). Obstructive sleep apnea has been reported to occur in 30% of patients with overt hypothyroidism (22). Decreased volume of the hippocampus has been found on functional brain imaging in adults with hypothyroidism; no specific symptoms were reported in this study, but this same group previously reported that reduced hippocampal volume can be associated with impaired visuo-spatial memory (23). And notably, hypothyroid patients are more frequently diagnosed with psychiatric disorders and treated with antidepressants, anxiolytics, and antipsychotic medications (24). Table 6.2 lists most of the common clinical features of overt hypothyroidism (17, 18, 21).

Various survey instruments have been developed to provide a more objective method for the detection and analysis of hypothyroid symptoms by clinicians and investigators (25–27). The presence of these same symptoms in numerous other clinical conditions and even in patients with no demonstrable disease leaves the clinical utility of these tools uncertain and they have not been widely adopted in clinical practice.

Acute severe hypothyroidism occurs when patients have their levothyroxine therapy withdrawn in preparation for radionuclide imaging or treatment for thyroid cancer. This special situation has been shown to cause reversible depression, decreased fine motor performance, slowed reaction times and decreased processing speed (28), abnormal brain functional connectivity on functional MRI imaging, and acutely diminished quality of life (29).

Mild hypothyroidism may not cause any symptoms or may similarly be associated with a variety of nonspecific symptoms that are common in the general population. A 2013 cross-sectional Dutch study of 942 subjects with TSH values of 4.1–9.9 mU/L, 70 subjects with TSH levels >10 mU/L and 8,334 euthyroid controls, reported that health related quality of life (HR-QOL) scores were not reduced in either group of hypothyroid patients compared to euthyroid controls (30). The effects of mild thyroid failure on cognitive function remain controversial due to conflicting results generated from numerous studies (31–35) but, if present, appear to be minimal.

Impaired left ventricular dynamics (36) and slowing of VO2 kinetics at the onset and following submaximal exercise (37) have both been reported in subjects with mild thyroid failure. However, overall functional capacity has been found to not be diminished in mildly hypothyroid elderly patients (38). Atherogenic lipoprotein profiles are evident even with mild hypothyroidism (39–41) and tend to improve with thyroid hormone therapy (39,40). Non-alcoholic fatty liver disease, cancer mortality, arthritis, kidney dysfunction, and diabetes have all been reported to be associated with hypothyroidism, but causality is not proven in these disease association studies (1–3).

Patients with central hypothyroidism may also have symptoms and signs of the hypothalamic-pituitary disorder that underlies this type of hypothyroidism. These may include features of mass effect, excess or deficiency of other hormones, infection, or inflammation (14). Patients with peripheral forms of hypothyroidism may have manifestations of an underlying hepatic hemangioma or syndromic features associated with the mutations causing thyroid

hormone resistance (15) (see Chapter 4, "Rare Forms of Hyperthyroidism").

DIAGNOSIS

Measurement of the serum TSH level is the most sensitive and accurate test for detecting primary hypothyroidism. The exquisite control exerted by the hypothalamic-pituitary unit over the thyroid system results in a log-linear relationship between serum TSH levels and serum free T4 levels, such that small decreases in serum free T4 concentrations result in large increments in the serum TSH level (Figure 6.5). High TSH levels, therefore, almost always signal the presence of primary hypothyroidism and normal TSH levels almost always indicate intact thyroid gland function. When interpreting serum TSH levels, it should be kept in mind that serum TSH levels have a diurnal pattern with

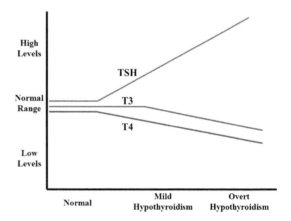

Figure 6.5 Hormone changes during primary hypothyroidism development. When the thyroid gland begins to fail, serum T4 levels decline. Because of the log-linear relationship between T4 and TSH, small decrements of T4 still within the reference range result in significant increases in TSH production by the pituitary gland. Mild hypothyroidism is therefore characterized by a serum TSH level that is mildly to moderately elevated while the serum total T4 and free T4 levels remain within the reference range; T3 levels usually change little, if any, at this stage. As thyroid failure progresses, the T4 levels drop below the normal range and the TSH levels increase further. Overt hypothyroidism is defined by a frankly elevated serum TSH with T4 levels that are below the reference range; T3 levels decline also but often remain within the reference range until hypothyroidism is severe.

the highest levels occurring in the late afternoon and evening (1). Furthermore, serum TSH levels increase with age in individuals with and without evidence of thyroid disease (Figure 6.6) (42), suggesting that age-specific reference ranges for TSH should be used, although age-specific reference ranges are not usually shown on laboratory reports.

If the serum TSH level is elevated above the reference range, the serum TSH measurement should be repeated at least once and a serum free T4 should then be ordered to further assess the severity of the hypothyroidism. An elevated serum TSH in association with a free T4 that is below the reference range defines overt hypothyroidism. A more modest TSH elevation in association with a free T4 value that is still within the reference range defines

mild hypothyroidism (subclinical hypothyroidism) (Figure 6.5); nearly 75% of patients with mild hypothyroidism have serum TSH levels less than 10 mU/L. There is no indication, under most circumstances, to measure either a serum total T3 or free T3 in hypothyroid patients since serum T3 levels are relatively preserved through the activation of deiodinases under hypothyroid conditions and offer no additional information regarding the severity of the hypothyroidism over that given by the TSH and free T4 values. A recommended testing scheme for hypothyroidism is shown in Table 6.3.

Serum TSH levels can occasionally be falsely elevated or suppressed, resulting in a mistaken diagnosis of hypothyroidism or hyperthyroidism. Biotin is used as a reagent in many hormone

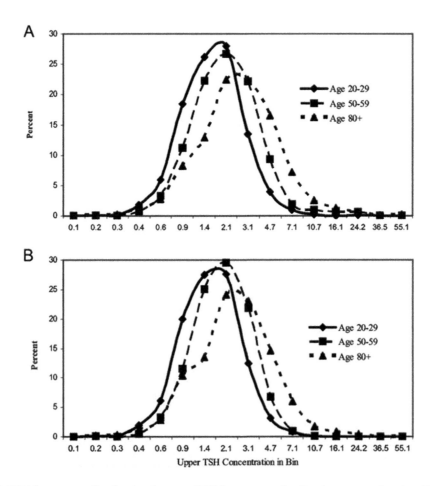

Figure 6.6 TSH frequency distribution by age. TSH frequency distribution curves for the disease free population (panel A) and the reference population (panel B) for people age 20–29 years old, 50–59 years old, and >80 years old, showing a progressive rightward shift with age (42).

Table 6.3 Diagnostic evaluation of hypothyroidism

Primary Hypothyroidism Suspected (symptoms and/or goiter)
   Measure TSH
   If TSH elevated:
      Recheck TSH and measure free T4
      Consider ordering anti-TPO antibodies
Central Hypothyroidism Suspected (Headaches, Visual Abnormalities, Known Pituitary Disease)
   Measure TSH and free T4
   If TSH low or low normal and free T4 low:
      Consider pituitary imaging
      Assess other pituitary functions

assays, including those for TSH and free T4. When patients take biotin supplements, commonly used for cosmetic skin, nail, and hair conditions, thyroid disorders can be erroneously diagnosed, depending on the assay techniques used (43). This situation can be resolved by asking patients to repeat their thyroid testing after at least two days of abstinence from the biotin supplements. Macro-TSH is another, though far less common, cause of falsely elevated serum TSH levels. Macro-TSH refers to large molecular complexes of TSH bound to anti-TSH autoantibodies, most commonly in the context of autoimmune disease. These complexes interfere with accurate TSH measurement, resulting in anomalous TSH elevations in the presence of normal free T4 levels. Macro-TSH can be detected by gel filtration chromatography or polyethylene glycol (PEG) precipitation (44). Heterophile anti-mouse antibodies occur most often in lab workers, farm workers, and homeless individuals, but can develop in anyone; these antibodies can also falsely elevate serum TSH levels. Conditions in which elevated serum TSH levels do not reflect primary hypothyroidism, and may therefore cause diagnostic confusion, are listed in Table 6.4.

Measurement of anti-thyroperoxidase antibodies (anti-TPO) and anti-thyroglobulin antibodies (anti-Tg) in hypothyroid subjects is a controversial topic. Antibody measurement is not recommended by the current clinical practice guidelines of the American Association of Clinical Endocrinologists (AACE) and the American Thyroid Association (ATA) (45) because adults with hypothyroidism not due to an iatrogenic cause or medications (Table 6.1) almost always have chronic lymphocytic thyroiditis and therefore testing offers little additional information and does not usually affect treatment decisions. However, some providers find it beneficial to demonstrate to their patients that their hypothyroidism has an autoimmune etiology; this may also facilitate a discussion about the increased risk of developing other autoimmune disorders for which increased vigilance may be useful. Patients with mild hypothyroidism who have positive anti-TPO antibodies have a two- to threefold higher risk of progression to overt hypothyroidism than do antibody negative individuals (cumulative risk over 9 years, 59% vs. 23%) (3).

Thyroid sonography often shows a hypoechogenic pattern in the thyroid parenchyma in patients with chronic lymphocytic thyroiditis (1) but thyroid imaging is not generally indicated in the evaluation of hypothyroidism. Sonography is recommended, however, if one or more nodules are palpable on physical examination or have been identified incidentally by other imaging studies.

Central hypothyroidism is more difficult to diagnose. The diagnosis is suggested by the presence of free T4 levels that are below or at the low end of the reference range in association with serum TSH levels that are similarly low or low normal and the presence of symptoms consistent with hypothyroidism, especially in a patient with known hypothalamic or pituitary disease (1, 14). Sometimes serum TSH levels may be normal or slightly elevated, but in these cases, TSH has been shown to have reduced bioactivity due to abnormal glycosylation (1). If a diagnosis of central hypothyroidism is made in someone with no prior history of hypothalamic-pituitary disease, dedicated hypothalamic-pituitary imaging and testing for other pituitary hormone abnormalities should be performed.

Table 6.4 Causes of elevated serum TSH not due to primary hypothyroidism

1. Assay interference
  a. Biotin use
  b. Macro-TSH
  c. Heterophile antibodies
2. Normal aging (TSH can be above the reference range in persons > 70 years)
3. Recovery from nonthyroidal illness
4. TSH-producing pituitary tumor
5. Thyroid hormone resistance syndromes
6. Familial TSH resistance (mostly due to inactivating mutations in the TSH receptor gene)

Peripheral hypothyroidism is rare, and there is no general agreement on when and how to initiate investigations for these conditions. However, the presence of very high serum TSH levels in association with normal free T4 levels may prompt one to measure serum total T3; a very low serum T3 in these circumstances should lead to imaging for deiodinase expressing tumors causing "consumptive hypothyroidism," starting with the liver. Tumors producing this syndrome are typically hemangiomas, hemangioblastomas, and gastrointestinal tumors (15). The identification of thyroid hormone resistance syndromes is beyond the scope of this chapter but is discussed in detail elsewhere in this book (see Chapter 4, "Rare Forms of Hyperthyroidism").

SCREENING AND CASE FINDING FOR HYPOTHYROIDISM

Current recommendations for screening for hypothyroidism vary greatly across organizations because of insufficient evidence that identifying and treating asymptomatic mild hypothyroidism is beneficial (1). The American Thyroid Association (ATA) and the American Association of Clinical Endocrinologists (AACE) (45), the Latin American Thyroid Society (LATS) (46), the United States Preventive Services Task Force (USPSTF) (47), and the UK Royal College of Physicians (1, 45) have all published recommendations based on their assessments of the best available evidence (Table 6.5).

Case finding, which means testing patients with suggestive symptoms or who are at increased risk for the development of hypothyroidism (presence of a goiter, personal history of autoimmune disease, positive family history of autoimmune thyroid disease) is, in contrast to screening, widely recommended to be done at the discretion of the on-site provider (45–47). Recommendations for thyroid testing in pregnancy are covered elsewhere in this book (see Chapter 12, "Thyroid Disease and Pregnancy").

Table 6.5 Recommendations for screening for thyroid disease (1, 45–47)

Organization	Recommendations – Who to screen
American Thyroid Association	Women and men >35 years old, every 5 years
American Association of Clinical Endocrinologists	Older patients, especially women
American Academy of Family Physicians	Patients ≥60 years old
American College of Physicians	Women >50 years old with an incidental finding suggestive of symptomatic thyroid disease
Latin American Thyroid Society	Women of fertile age and over, especially >60 years old
Royal College of Physicians, UK	Screening not justified in adults
US Preventive Services Task Force	Insufficient evidence for or against screening

OUTCOMES OF UNTREATED HYPOTHYROIDISM

There are no known studies describing the long-term consequences of untreated overt hypothyroidism, since patients are usually symptomatic and require treatment for symptom control. However, there have been reports that even treated hypothyroidism might be associated with increased mortality rates. A 30-year Danish observational cohort study analyzed data from 3,587 individuals and 682 twins with hypothyroidism who were identified through a national registry based on having had at least 2 dispensed prescriptions for thyroid hormone (with exclusion for previous hyperthyroidism, thyroid cancer, central hypothyroidism, and congenital hypothyroidism); they were matched 1:4 with euthyroid controls. An excess mortality rate of just over 50% (HR 1.52; 95% CI: 1.41–1.65) was reported but with attenuation of this effect when co-morbidities (Charlson score) were taken into account. Mortality was increased among discordant dizygotic twin pairs (HR 1.61; 95% CI: 1.00–2.58) but not among discordant monozygotic twin pairs (HR 1.06; 95% CI: 0.55–2.55). The authors concluded that there is excess mortality of about 50% among hypothyroid patients, an effect that is partly explained by co-morbid conditions but also influenced by genetic confounding (48). A large prospective study of 75,076 women (age: 20–89) was conducted over a 28-year period to determine cause-specific mortality from thyroid disease. Women with hypothyroidism were found to have an increased mortality risk for diabetes mellitus (HR 1.58; 95% CI: 1.03–2.41) and cerebrovascular disease (HR 1.45; 95% CI: 1.01–2.08) but not for other causes (49).

While data on the long-term consequences of overt thyroid failure are lacking, there have been numerous longitudinal observational studies of patients with untreated mild ("subclinical") hypothyroidism. A meta-analysis of 11 prospective cohort studies involving over 55,000 subjects examined the risk of fatal and non-fatal coronary heart disease (CHD) events associated with mild hypothyroidism. The authors reported an increasing risk of all CHD events with increasing baseline serum TSH levels, although statistical significance was found only for those with serum TSH levels in the 10.0–19.9 mU/L range (HR 1.89; 95% confidence interval 1.28–2.80) (3). A literature review

in 2013 concluded that current evidence supports mild hypothyroidism being a risk factor for cardiovascular disease in younger patients (<60 years of age) but the risk is less evident after age 65, particularly in those with TSH values <10 mU/L (50).

A retrospective cohort analysis of the Taiwan National Health Insurance Research Database over a 10-year period compared 1,165 subjects with newly diagnosed Hashimoto's thyroiditis and 4,660 euthyroid controls without the disorder and reported an increased risk for developing coronary heart disease (CHD) in patients with Hashimoto's thyroiditis (HR 1.44; 95% CI: 1.05–1.99), but the risk was significant only in women and only in those less than 49 years of age. Interestingly, the risk was reduced in those subjects who were treated with LT4 replacement (HR 0.84; 95% CI: 0.47–1.52) (51). The Women's Health Initiative study found no evidence that mild hypothyroidism is associated with incident myocardial infarctions in elderly postmenopausal women without known coronary artery disease (52). Similarly, the Cardiovascular Health Study of 679 mildly hypothyroid patients >65 years old reported no increased risk of coronary heart disease, heart failure, or cardiovascular death (53). Cardiovascular risks do not appear to be correlated with the presence or absence of anti-TPO antibodies (54). The Atherosclerosis Risk in Communities Study group measured thyroid function at baseline (1990–1992) and evaluated the impact of thyroid function on cardiovascular risk factors and cardiovascular events over a 20-year period in 11,359 subjects. They reported a mild and progressive TSH level dependent association with hyperlipidemia but found no effect on cardiovascular outcomes (55).

An evaluation of mortality in the Third National Health and Nutrition Examination Survey (NHANES) analyzed the effects of pre-existing congestive heart failure (CHF) and race using data from 749 hypothyroid patients, 691 of whom had mild hypothyroidism, and from 14,130 euthyroid controls. Mild hypothyroidism was associated with a higher mortality risk than euthyroidism in subjects with CHF (HR 1.44; 95% CI: 1.01–2.06) but not those without CHF (HR 0.97; 95% CI: 0.85–1.11) and in black subjects (HR 1.44; 95% CI: 1.03–2.03) but not in non-black participants (HR 0.95; 95% CI: 0.83–1.08) (56).

Investigating the effects of age, a 2015 analysis of the Clalit Health Medical Organization data base evaluated 1,956 subjects who were at least 65 years old and who had mild hypothyroidism. During a 10 year follow-up period, these elderly patients had a significantly increased early mortality rate which was found to correlate with the degree of TSH elevation (57).

Evidence for stroke risk is inconsistent with conflicting data from two recent studies. One group reported no evidence of an increased risk for ischemic stroke among otherwise healthy postmenopausal women with mild hypothyroidism (58). Conversely, another group reported that mild hypothyroidism conferred a significantly increased risk of fatal strokes (59).

Overall, therefore, existing published evidence suggests that mild hypothyroidism is a risk factor for coronary heart disease, congestive heart failure, and increased mortality. The findings have been most apparent in younger patients (<65 years of age) and in those with serum TSH levels >10 mU/L. Some (1, 3), but not all (57), studies examining older patients (>65 years old) have suggested that these risks may be minimal or absent in the older population, including the "oldest of the old" (1, 3), especially when TSH levels are only mildly elevated (<10 mU/L). Indeed, mild elevations in TSH may be associated with a functional advantage in the elderly (60).

Mild hypothyroidism progresses to overt hypothyroidism at a rate of approximately 2–6% per year (3). The risk for progression is higher in patients with positive anti-TPO antibodies (2–3 times higher) and in those with higher serum TSH and lower free T4 values (3). It is noteworthy that up to 46% of patients with TSH values that are elevated but less than 7 mU/L will show normalization of the TSH in the subsequent two-year period if untreated (3).

MANAGEMENT/TREATMENT

Treatment of hypothyroidism involves thyroid hormone replacement in quantities sufficient to relieve symptoms and return serum TSH levels into the normal range. Levothyroxine (LT4) monotherapy is the most commonly used form of thyroid hormone replacement; this is based on the premise that the thyroid gland makes predominantly T4 and a small amount of T3, while most of the T3 in the body comes from conversion of T4 into T3 by deiodinase enzymes in the liver and various other organs throughout the body. Most hypothyroid patients have a satisfactory resolution of symptoms with adequate LT4 therapy.

Thyroid hormone preparations that are currently available are listed in Table 6.6. Thyroxine (T4) itself is not well absorbed from the gastrointestinal tract but synthetic LT4, the sodium salt made by replacing a hydrogen ion with sodium, is very well absorbed (~75%). The molecular structures of T4 and LT4 are shown in Figure 6.7; they are identical aside from the sodium substitution for enhanced absorption and are therefore considered bioidentical (61). LT4 is rapidly absorbed in the duodenum and has a half-life of 5–7 days; upon initiation of LT4 or a change in LT4 dosage, a new steady state is reached in approximately 5–6 weeks. Oral liquid LT4 preparations have been shown to have enhanced and less variable absorption compared to LT4 tablets in hypothyroid patients, including those with issues that interfere with absorption such as gastrointestinal diseases and the concomitant use of proton-pump inhibitor medications (62–64).

Synthetic LT3 preparations are similarly identical to the T3 produced by the human thyroid gland. Desiccated thyroid extract (DTE) preparations are made by drying and powdering animal thyroid glands. The most common forms of DTE come from porcine thyroid glands. DTE products

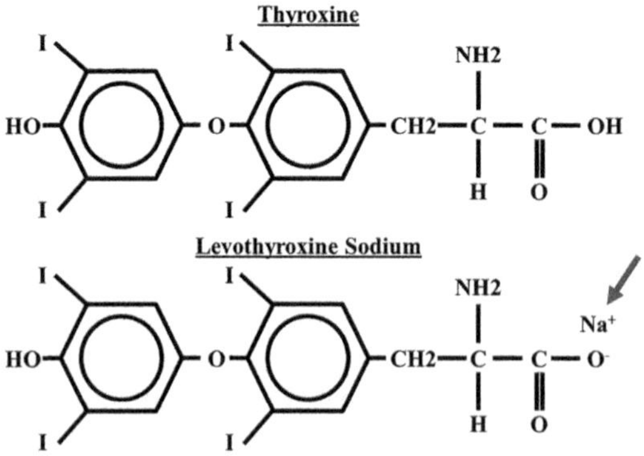

Figure 6.7 Molecular Structures of Thyroxine and Levothyroxine Sodium. Thyroxine (T4) is not well absorbed from the gastrointestinal tract but synthetic levothyroxine sodium (LT4), the sodium salt made by replacing a hydrogen ion with sodium, is well absorbed. The molecular structures of T4 and LT4 are shown. The structures are identical aside from the sodium substitution in LT4 which allows for enhanced intestinal absorption.

consist of about 80% T4 and 20% T3 (approximately a 4:1 ratio of T4 to T3). The T4 to T3 ratio may vary somewhat in DTE products, depending on the brand and manufacturing process (61).

Current clinical practice guidelines recommend LT4 as the initial treatment of choice because of its proven efficacy in symptom relief, long-term experience with its benefits, favorable side effect profile, good gastrointestinal absorption, ease of administration, long serum half-life, and low cost (45, 65, 66). LT4 should be taken orally with water one hour before or four hours after a meal and separated by at least four hours from supplements containing iron, calcium, or soy. Alternatively, it can be taken at bedtime, 2–3 hours after the last meal (1). If a patient misses a daily dose, two doses can be taken together the next day and then the usual daily dose resumed. If two daily doses are missed, we instruct the patient to take two doses together two days consecutively and then resume the usual daily dose. If three or more doses are missed, we instruct the patient to take two doses together on three consecutive days and then resume the usual daily dose.

Treatment of overt hypothyroidism (Table 6.7) can be initiated with a full LT4 replacement dose (1.6 mcg/kg) if the patient is young and known to be or likely to be free of coronary heart disease. LT4 doses tend to be higher in patients following a thyroidectomy (1). Serum TSH should then be checked about 6 weeks later and the dose adjusted, if needed, to maintain the serum TSH value within the reference range. Overt hypothyroidism in patients with known or probable coronary heart disease and in the elderly (>age 65–70 years) is best managed with a "start low, go slow" approach by initiating an LT4 dose of 25–50 mcg daily and increasing the dose by 25 mcg increments every 4–8 weeks while monitoring symptoms and serum TSH values until TSH levels are in the target range. Treatment of mild hypothyroidism, if recommended (Table 6.8), is usually initiated with LT4 25–50 mcg daily and a TSH recheck in about six weeks with subsequent dosage adjustments made

Table 6.6 Thyroid hormone preparations for treatment of hypothyroidism

Generic Name	Content	Trade Name	Form
Levothyroxine	LT4	Generic	Pill
Levothyroxine	LT4	Synthroid	Pill
Levothyroxine	LT4	Levothroid	Pill
Levothyroxine	LT4	Unithroid	Pill
Levothyroxine	LT4	Tirosint	Gel Cap
Levothyroxine	LT4		Liquid (not available in the US)
Liothyronine	LT3	Generic	Pill
Liothyronine	LT3	Cytomel	Pill
Liothyronine	LT3		Extended Release
Desiccated Thyroid Extract	T4/T3	Armour	Pill
Desiccated Thyroid Extract	T4/T3	Westhroid	Pill
Desiccated Thyroid Extract	T4/T3	Naturethroid	Pill

Table 6.7 Treatment of overt hypothyroidism

Young Patient (<Age 60 years), No Known Cardiovascular Disease:
    Levothyroxine, full replacement dose: 1.6 mcg/kg (0.8 mcg/lb) daily
    Recheck TSH in 6–8 weeks
    Adjust dose as needed to relieve symptoms and keep TSH in reference range
Older Patient (>Age 60 years), Known/Suspected Cardiovascular Disease:
    Levothyroxine, low dose: 12.5–50 mcg daily
    Titrate dose up in 12.5–25 mcg increments every 4–8 weeks
    Monitor TSH every 6–8 weeks
    Adjust dose as needed to relieve symptoms and keep TSH in reference range

Table 6.8 Recommendations regarding which patients should be considered for treatment of mild hypothyroidism (3, 45, 65, 66)

American Thyroid Association (2012/2014) TSH ≤10 mU/L: Consider treatment based on individual factors. TSH >10 mU/L: Consider treatment because of increased CVD and CHF risk. **European Thyroid Association (2013)** Age <65–70 years TSH <10 mU/L: Consider treatment based on symptoms. TSH ≥10 mU/L: Treatment is recommended. Age >70 years TSH <10 mU/L: Follow carefully without treatment. TSH ≥10 mU/L: Consider treatment based on symptoms.

Table 6.9 Treatment of mild hypothyroidism

Age <70 Years Old and/or Significant Symptoms:
  Levothyroxine 25–50 mcg daily
  Recheck TSH in 6–8 weeks
  Adjust dose as needed to relieve symptoms and keep TSH in reference range
Age ≥70 Years Old:
  Take into account the presence or absence of hypothyroid symptoms, the presence of a goiter, the degree of TSH elevation, TPO antibody status and the presence or absence of cardiovascular risk factors, coronary heart disease and congestive heart failure. Mild elevations in serum TSH may be normal for older persons.

to maintain serum TSH levels within the reference range (Table 6.9).

While an LT4 dose requirement of 1.6 mcg/kg per day is commonly suggested as the initial dose for patients who have overt hypothyroidism and are under 60 years of age, there may be considerable variability in actual dose requirements depending on the cause of hypothyroidism, body weight, and the age of the patient. A 2014 report of levothyroxine dose requirements following thyroidectomy for benign thyroid disease retrospectively evaluated 92 adults following thyroidectomy and found significant variability based mainly on body weight and age. They evaluated a BMI- and age-related nomogram for initial LT4 dose estimation and found that it produced a euthyroid result at first follow-up in 68% of patients compared to 41% of patients who were initiated with traditional dose estimates. They proposed their BMI/age nomogram as a tool to more accurately estimate initial postoperative LT4 dose requirements (67). Another study specifically evaluating obese female patients after thyroidectomy similarly found significant dose requirement variability when the dose estimate was based on weight alone and suggested a starting LT4 dose in obese post-thyroidectomy patients of either 125 mcg daily or 2.3 mcg/kg/day of ideal body weight (IBW) with subsequent adjustment as needed (68).

US Pharmacopoeia (USP) standards require that LT4 preparations be accurate to within 5% of their stated content throughout their shelf-life. Using a name brand LT4 preparation or a generic preparation consistently from the same manufacturer is the best way to reduce dosage variability and variable thyroid hormone levels. When generic preparations are prescribed, dosage consistency cannot be guaranteed if the medication manufacturer is changed periodically. Therefore, in situations where consistency is critical (pregnancy, old age, thyroid cancer), it is best to recommend name brand preparations or use of the same generic manufacturer for all prescription renewals. For patients who have some residual thyroid function, such as those with mild hypothyroidism, and for those for whom dosage consistency is less critical, the use of generic preparations is reasonable and less expensive.

A 2013 survey of members of the Endocrine Society, the American Thyroid Association, and the American Association of Clinical Endocrinologists found that the majority of members favor the use of LT4 alone as the initial treatment for hypothyroidism and most employ age-specific TSH targets to assess the adequacy of thyroid hormone therapy (69). The preference for higher TSH targets in the elderly was echoed in a 2015 survey study of members of the American College of Physicians, the American Academy of Family Practice, and the Endocrine Society (70) and is consistent with current clinical practice guidelines for the treatment of hypothyroidism in the elderly (65).

TREATMENT OUTCOMES

Treatment of patients with overt hypothyroidism results in the rapid resolution of most hypothyroid symptoms in the majority of patients. Since weight gain is often a feature of hypothyroidism, it would be anticipated that weight loss would ensue once thyroid hormone replacement has been initiated. It is somewhat surprising therefore that published research has not shown this to occur (71). Multiple observational studies have reported minimal or no weight loss after the institution of thyroid hormone therapy for hypothyroidism; weight loss that did occur in two studies was attributed mainly to the resolution of edema or to the loss of lean mass (71).

Randomized controlled trials evaluating long-term outcomes have not been conducted because nearly all patients with overt hypothyroidism are symptomatic and it would be unethical to have a chronically placebo treated-control group. Several small randomized controlled trials have been conducted to evaluate the effects of LT4 therapy on symptoms in patients with mild hypothyroidism. These studies did not demonstrate consistent effects on symptoms such as tiredness, memory, or quality of life; however, subjects in the studies mostly had very mild hypothyroidism and baseline serum TSH levels <10 mU/L (3). There was a suggestion that patients with TSH values >12 mU/L may have experienced some significant symptomatic benefit (3).

Stott et al., in the Thyroid Hormone Replacement for Untreated Older Adults with Subclinical Hypothyroidism (TRUST) Study, conducted a large randomized controlled trial of LT4

replacement in elderly patients with mild hypothyroidism (72). They randomized 737 subjects, age 65 and older (mean age: 74.4 years) with TSH levels of 4.99–19.99 mU/L (mean TSH: 6.40 +/– 2.01 mU/L) to receive LT4 (N = 368) or placebo (N = 369) for one year. In the LT4 group, TSH decreased to the mid-normal range (mean TSH: 3.63 mU/L) while in the placebo group TSH remained mildly elevated (mean TSH: 5.48 mU/L). They reported no difference in either of the two primary outcomes (Thyroid Symptom Score and Tiredness Score) and observed no differences in any of the secondary outcome measures (blood pressure, body mass index, waist circumference, grip strength, hyperthyroid symptoms). Of note, baseline TSH levels in these subjects were only mildly elevated and baseline symptoms in the hypothyroid subjects did not differ significantly from euthyroid controls (72).

Overall these studies indicate that symptomatic improvement is unlikely to occur in patients with mild hypothyroidism who have minimal symptoms and only slight elevations in serum TSH at baseline but that there may be noticeable benefit in patients with more prominent symptoms and when serum TSH levels are above 10–12 mU/L (3).

Observational studies, as noted above, have suggested that mild hypothyroidism is associated with a significantly increased risk of adverse cardiovascular events and mortality, especially in patients <65 years of age. Surrogate markers of cardiovascular health such as hypertension, hypercholesterolemia, atherogenic lipoprotein profiles, and coagulation abnormalities tend to improve or resolve with LT4 treatment (39, 40) and it has been assumed that these changes should logically translate into substantial cardiovascular and mortality benefits, but this has not been definitively demonstrated. Interestingly, there is evidence suggesting that these traditional cardiovascular risk factors may not underlie the development of cardiovascular disease observed in subjects with mild hypothyroidism (3).

Observational studies in which subjects were started on LT4 therapy at the discretion of their on-site providers have suggested that LT4 therapy may significantly lower the risk of ischemic heart disease events and congestive heart failure, although the benefit has appeared to be limited to individuals under 70 years of age (51, 73). Notably, there have been no long-term randomized controlled trials that have evaluated the effects of LT4 therapy on cardiovascular outcomes and death in mildly hypothyroid patients, and therefore the efficacy of this intervention on long-term cardiovascular outcomes remains unproven and conjectural (3).

RECOMMENDATIONS REGARDING TREATMENT FOR MILD HYPOTHYROIDISM

This imperfect evidence base has led to some general guidelines for providers for making individualized, patient-specific decisions regarding the treatment of mild hypothyroidism. Treatment should be strongly considered for patients <70 years old if the serum TSH level is >10 mU/L. Treatment decisions should be more individualized if the patient is >70 years old and/or has a serum TSH level <10 mU/L, taking into account the presence or absence of hypothyroid symptoms, the presence of a goiter, the degree of TSH elevation, TPO antibody status, desire for pregnancy, and the presence or absence of cardiovascular risk factors, coronary heart disease, and congestive heart failure. If symptomatic benefit is not apparent within 3–6 months or if there are significant side effects, treatment should be discontinued. If a decision is made not to treat, monitoring of symptoms and the serum TSH value should be done every 6–12 months, and treatment then initiated if suggestive symptoms develop or worsen or the TSH rises above 10 mU/L (3, 45, 65, 66).

Optimal TSH level on replacement therapy

The reference range for TSH levels in the US population in many labs is 0.45–4.5 mU/L. However, the TSH distribution for the population does not follow a normal distribution, resulting in a mean serum TSH of approximately 1.5–1.7 mU/L. This has led many practitioners to target a TSH value in the lower end of the reference range for patients on LT4 therapy. Research findings in this area have thus far been inconsistent. Clinical symptoms and cognitive function have been reported to not differ among patients with TSH levels on LT4 therapy prospectively targeted at the lower, middle, or upper end of the TSH reference range (34, 35). However, following a thyroidectomy, biomarkers of peripheral thyroid hormone action

have been reported to be closest to preoperative values only when TSH levels are maintained in the 0.03–0.3 mU/L range (74).

Investigations in elderly patients (>age 65–70) have suggested, in contrast, that TSH levels in the upper end or slightly above the population reference range may be associated with longevity and that mild hypothyroidism in elderly patients, including the "oldest of the old," appears to have no adverse effects on coronary heart disease mortality or overall mortality and may even have a beneficial effect (60). Current clinical practice guidelines therefore state that evidence does not support targeting specific TSH values within the normal reference range in most patients and that it may be reasonable to raise the TSH target to 4.0–6.0 mU/L in patients above age 70–80 years old (65).

FACTORS CONTRIBUTING TO INCREASED LT4 REQUIREMENTS

LT4 dose requirements may change over time. In patients with mild hypothyroidism, this can be due to progressive failure of the thyroid gland resulting in increased dependence on exogenous thyroid hormone as endogenous thyroid function declines. The most common cause of increasing LT4 dose requirements in patients with overt hypothyroidism is non-adherence to the prescribed LT4 regimen (75, 76). Documented causes of increasing LT4 dose requirements are listed in Table 6.10. Medications that can alter thyroid hormone dose requirements are shown in Table 6.11. Mechanisms by which medications may alter thyroid hormone dose requirements include decreased levothyroxine absorption from the intestines, alterations of thyroid hormone binding to serum proteins, increased thyroid hormone metabolism, and

Table 6.10 Causes of persistently elevated or rising serum TSH levels on thyroid hormone replacement

Non-Adherence
Pharmacy Error
Change of Brands
Malabsorption
Medications
Pregnancy
Assay Interference (Heterophile Antibodies, Biotin)

Table 6.11 Medications that may alter thyroid hormone dose requirements

1. Decrease Thyroid Hormone Absorption from GI Tract
   a. Iron
   b. Calcium
   c. Proton Pump Inhibitors
   d. Antacids
   e. Sucralfate
   f. Bile Acid Resins
   g. Orlistat
   h. Sevelamer
2. Alter Thyroid Hormone Binding by Serum Proteins
   a. Estrogens
3. Increase Thyroid Hormone Metabolism
   a. Anti-Epileptic Medications
   b. Anti-Tuberculosis Medications
   c. Sertraline (+/−)
4. Amiodarone (blocks T4 to T3 conversion in the pituitary gland)

Adapted from (1).

reduced T4 to T3 conversion in the pituitary gland (amiodarone).

Non-adherence to LT4 therapy is best managed by education about the importance of taking medications as directed by the provider and with tips on how to remember to take thyroid medication at the same time every day. Despite these measures, some patients continue to present challenges regarding medication adherence. One effective (albeit extreme) approach to this that can be appropriate in some situations is to have a patient take all 7 of their doses for the coming week on one day per week or take 3–4 tablets twice a week, under direct observation by a health care worker, family member, or guardian. With both regimens, TSH levels have been reported to remain stable throughout the inter-dose period and there has been no demonstrated short-term toxicity with this approach (65).

Overtreatment with LT4 should be carefully avoided. LT4 doses high enough to suppress the serum TSH level often cause symptoms of thyroid hormone excess, such as anxiety, fatigue, heat intolerance, excess sweating, palpitations, tremors, and insomnia. Moreover, chronic thyroid hormone excess poses a significantly increased risk in elderly and postmenopausal patients for the development of atrial fibrillation and osteoporosis, respectively,

regardless of whether the thyroid hormone excess is caused by endogenous hyperthyroidism or exogenous LT4 administration (77). Among patients with hypothyroidism, an excess risk of developing major osteoporotic fractures has been found to be related to the cumulative duration of time they spent with low serum TSH levels (78).

Despite the known risks, overtreatment with LT4 is fairly common, being reported in 6–10% of patients in recent reports (79, 80). A retrospective cohort study using the United Kingdom Clinical Practice Research Datalink reported that among 52,298 hypothyroid subjects on thyroid hormone replacement therapy, 5.8% had serum TSH levels <0.1 mU/L (79). Among 1,450 participants in the Baltimore Longitudinal Study of Aging who were being prescribed levothyroxine replacement therapy, 9.6% had suppressed serum TSH levels and for 1/3 of these, overtreatment persisted for at least 2 years (80).

COMBINATION LT4/LT3 THERAPY

Although thyroid hormone replacement relieves symptoms for most hypothyroid patients, both clinical experience and published literature indicate that some patients have persistent symptoms despite apparently adequate therapy (24, 25, 34, 35, 61, 76, 81–83). Abnormally low resting energy expenditure (REE) has also been shown to persist with LT4 replacement in doses sufficient to maintain serum TSH levels within the population reference range (84, 85). Furthermore, LT4-treated patients typically have higher free T4 levels, lower free T3 levels, and lower free T3/T4 ratios compared to euthyroid individuals with similar serum TSH levels (86, 87). In the NHANES cohort, LT4-treated hypothyroid subjects had higher body weights than controls despite higher levels of exercise and similar caloric intakes, and also tended to use anti-depressant medications more often (87). This has caused investigators and clinicians to question whether traditional LT4 therapy is truly physiological and is the most appropriate therapy for all patients (83, 87). The concept and practice of treating select patients with a combination of LT4 and LT3 have emerged as a topic of significant interest.

Multiple randomized controlled trials evaluating the efficacy of combination LT4 and LT3 therapy compared to LT4 therapy alone have been published since 1999. Symptomatic benefits and a preference for combination LT4/LT3 therapy were demonstrated in some of these reports. However, the majority of the investigations reported no subjective or objective benefits from combination therapy (1). Most studies were small and of short duration, assessed nonspecific symptoms, and did not specifically target patients who had persistent symptoms on LT4 therapy, leaving investigators unconvinced of efficacy but uncertain about whether adequate studies had been done (1). The largest study to date, consisting of over 600 subjects followed for one year, was similarly unable to demonstrate efficacy (1). However, in a follow-up study, this group genotyped over 500 of their original subjects and identified a polymorphism of the D2 enzyme, Thr92Ala, in 16% of the cohort. Subjects with this D2 polymorphism were shown to have more symptoms at baseline and to have statistically significant improvement in symptoms on combination LT4/LT3 therapy (88); the authors postulated that this relatively common deiodinase 2 variation might be causally related to poorer psychological wellbeing and a better response to combination LT4/LT3 therapy (88). In contrast, a previous study reported that the Thr92Ala polymorphism of D2 was not associated with impaired well-being or neurocognitive functioning or with a preference for combined LT4/LT3 treatment (89).

The clinical consequences of the Thr92Ala polymorphism on D2 function are not entirely clear. Investigators have suggested that D2 activity might be reduced, causing decreased T4 to T3 conversion in the brain under hypothyroid conditions. The D2 enzyme is normally ubiquitinated with subsequent proteolysis in the presence of high T4 concentrations, whereas its proteolytic degradation is prevented by deubiquitination when the prevailing T4 supply is low. However, the Thr92Ala substitution is located in the D2 instability loop that is closely linked to ubiquitination and may somehow impair D2 rescue under hypothyroid conditions, resulting in greater dependence on circulating T3 levels to maintain an adequate T3 supply to the brain. The Thr92Ala polymorphism, as well as an Ala92Ala polymorphism of D2, have more recently been shown to be associated with reduced serum T3 and reduced intracellular T3 concentrations in thyroidectomized patients replaced with LT4 alone (90). Clinical genetic testing to determine in advance who may and who may not benefit from this therapy (pharmacogenetics) is not currently available.

If and when combination LT4/LT3 therapy is utilized, it is suggested that it be administered in an approximate LT4 to LT3 ratio of 14:1 to 10:1 to come close to the human physiological T4 to T3 secretion ratio of 14:1. Because LT3 has a much shorter half-life than LT4, clinicians often administer it in 2 doses approximately 8–12 hours apart. Many clinicians, but not all, recommend that patients on combination LT4/LT3 have their TSH levels measured in the morning before taking either LT4 or LT3 because of the rise in serum T3 that occurs in the first few hours after LT3 is ingested. Serum TSH levels in these patients, as with those on LT4 monotherapy, should be maintained within the reference range to avoid the toxicities and complications of chronic thyroid hormone excess.

An older approach to combination T4/T3 therapy is the use of DTE. Currently the only DTE preparations are made from porcine thyroid glands. Patients who avoid pork products for religious or other reasons should be made aware of the source of DTE products. Because the hormones in DTE are not synthetic, some individuals consider them to be "natural" thyroid hormone. However, porcine thyroid glands and porcine thyroid physiology are not the same as their human counterparts. In contrast to the T4/T3 molar ratio of approximately 14:1 secreted physiologically by the human thyroid gland, porcine thyroid glands produce T4 and T3 in a T4/T3 ratio of about 4:1. Therefore desiccated porcine thyroid glands contain a much higher concentration of T3 than do human thyroid glands. When administered orally, these preparations result in an abrupt rise in serum T3 levels, often transiently into the supraphysiological range. This could potentially cause short-term or even long-term complications known to occur with thyroid hormone excess. Compounded thyroid products from compounding pharmacies are another source available to patients who wish to access combination T4/T3 products. However, due to variability and lack of standardization, the use of compounded thyroid hormone products cannot be recommended (65).

A short-term randomized controlled trial evaluated 70 LT4 treated hypothyroid patients who were randomized to 16 weeks of treatment with either DTE or continued LT4. TSH levels were similar in the two groups although DTE-treated patients had lower serum-free T4 levels and higher total T3 levels during the treatment period. Symptoms were not different between the groups, but the DTE group lost a small amount of weight and 48.6% of subjects expressed a preference for DTE while 18.6% preferred LT4; there were no adverse events reported in either group (91). A 2017 mail survey study of frequent thyroid hormone prescribers conducted by members of the American Thyroid Association, the American Association of Clinical Endocrinologists, and the Endocrine Society revealed a high incidence of reported adverse events in patients taking DTE, although there was no comparator group of patients on LT4 alone (92). There are no published studies that have adequately evaluated the long-term efficacy or safety of DTE or of compounded thyroid hormone products.

Treatment with LT3 alone is not recommended because this approach is clearly not physiologic. Administration of once daily LT3 is associated with significant excursions of serum total T3 and free T3 (93). Sustained release LT3 preparations, though not yet available as FDA approved preparations in the US, may provide a smoother serum T3 profile and may be more suitable for future studies of combination T4/T3 therapy.

Current evidence from these multiple randomized controlled trials, literature reviews, and meta-analyses, therefore, generally conclude that the existing data do not support the generalized use of combination LT4/LT3 for treating hypothyroid patients. Clinical practice guidelines of the American Thyroid Association, American Association of Clinical Endocrinologists, and the European Thyroid Association state that there is no consistently strong evidence for the superiority of LT4/LT3 combination therapy over LT4 alone and recommend against routine use of combination LT4/LT3 therapy (45, 65, 66, 94). They also recommend against using DTE, citing potential safety concerns regarding the transient supra-physiological T3 levels that occur with DTE and the paucity of long-term safety outcome data (45, 65). Nonetheless, these organizations and other experts in the field acknowledge that some patients prefer treatment with combined LT4/LT3 or DTE, and that individualized approaches are reasonable to use in patients who have persistent symptoms on adequate doses of LT4 provided that

these therapies are used safely with maintenance of serum TSH levels within the reference range (45, 65, 76).

PERSISTENT SYMPTOMS IN PATIENTS ON LEVOTHYROXINE REPLACEMENT THERAPY

Numerous studies have shown that, despite adequate LT4 treatment maintaining TSH values within the reference range, a significant number of patients continue to experience symptoms consistent with thyroid hormone deficiency (24, 25, 34, 35, 61, 76, 81–83). A survey was conducted by the American Thyroid Association of 12,000 hypothyroid patients (95% female) who were currently being treated with thyroid hormone replacement therapy and responded to the survey; 60% were taking LT4 alone, 25% were taking combination LT4/LT3, and 10% were taking DTE or a compounded thyroid hormone preparation. The mean satisfaction score for treatment effects among respondents was 5 on a visual analog scale of 1–10. The most common reasons for dissatisfaction included fatigue/low energy (75%), body weight issues (70%), memory problems (55%), mood problems (45%), and other issues (35%). The mean score for satisfaction with their doctor was 5–6 and for their belief that the doctor was knowledgeable was also 5–6 on the 1–10 visual analog scale. Among these 12,000 respondents, 10–45% had changed doctors 1–4 times and 10% had changed doctors 5–10 times over thyroid management issues (82).

Persistent symptoms in hypothyroid patients who appear to be adequately treated according to lab test results have posed a dilemma for countless clinicians who care for hypothyroid patients. The discerning clinician should consider multiple possibilities: The current thyroid hormone dose may not be optimal, or the thyroid regimen may not be physiological for that individual patient. The patient could possibly have a hypothalamic or pituitary disorder, rendering the serum TSH an unreliable test. There could also be a subtle, or possibly not yet identifiable, genetic, epigenetic, or other acquired disorder somewhere within the thyroid hormone regulatory or response system for which tests are not readily accessible or not yet available. Studies have suggested that chronic lymphocytic thyroiditis may possibly cause symptoms that are independent of thyroid hormone levels

(95). Furthermore, multiple other autoimmune conditions are known to occur more commonly in patients with chronic lymphocytic thyroiditis (96, 97), further adding to the complexity of symptom management. Subtle or overt hypoparathyroidism may also be present if the patient's hypothyroidism is post-surgical or post-ablative and this could be a source of symptoms if not adequately managed. Alternatively, the symptoms may not be thyroid-related or endocrine-related at all (98). Some potential causes of persistent symptoms suggestive of thyroid hormone deficiency in adequately treated hypothyroid patients are listed in Table 6.12. Table 6.13 shows the autoimmune disorders that occur more commonly in patients with Hashimoto's thyroiditis (96, 97).

Satisfactory outcomes for these patients require a skillful and compassionate approach. Listening attentively to the patient's residual symptoms and concerns without interruption will help set the stage for progress. It is often useful then to explain briefly to the patient, in understandable language,

Table 6.12 Possible causes of persistent symptoms in patients treated for hypothyroidism

Inadequate LT4 Dose
Lifestyle Measures Suboptimal
Unhealthy Diet
Lack of Exercise
Inadequate Sleep
Excess Stress
Coexisting Disease
Chronic Fatigue Syndrome
Fibromyalgia
Sleep Apnea
Climacteric Syndrome
Iron Deficiency
Vitamin D Deficiency
Vitamin B12 Deficiency
Other Autoimmune Disease
Other Medical Illness
Kidney, Liver, Heart, Lung, Blood
Viral and Post-Viral Syndromes
Psychiatric Illness (especially depression)
Substance Abuse
Deiodinase 2 Polymorphism
Thr92Ala Polymorphism
Other Subtle Disorder of Thyroid Regulation or Action

Adapted from (97).

Table 6.13 Autoimmune diseases that occur with increased frequency in patients with chronic lymphocytic thyroiditis (495 subjects) (95)

Autoimmune condition	Women	Men
Rheumatoid Arthritis	4.7%	1.5%
Vitamin B12 Deficiency	4.5%	0%
Adrenal Insufficiency	1.2%	3%
Celiac Disease	1.2%	0%
Multiple Sclerosis	0.7%	1.5%
Inflammatory Bowel Disease	0.7%	1.5%
Systemic Lupus Erythematosus	0.7%	0%

pertinent aspects of thyroid physiology and how and why we use the tests we order. An acknowledgement that everything is not known about thyroid function and that there could be conditions, yet to be identified, for which we currently do not have diagnostic tests is often helpful. It is important for the patient to understand also that symptoms that are frequently experienced by hypothyroid patients are nonspecific and could be due to other conditions unrelated to the thyroid system (98). In addition to a good history and physical examination, one could then offer additional testing for other endocrine related and metabolic conditions, such as diabetes mellitus, calcium abnormalities, adrenal disorders, hypogonadism, sleep apnea, celiac disease, vitamin D deficiency, vitamin B12 deficiency, and depression, and explain that additional general medical testing may be more efficiently done by their primary care provider.

Management advice may include lifestyle measures, starting with a well-balanced diet, regular exercise, adequate sleep, and stress reduction. Treatment of other endocrine-related and metabolic disorders uncovered during the evaluation can be discussed or implemented. Contributing non-endocrine medical and psychiatric conditions can be discussed but are often more appropriately managed by primary care providers and other specialists.

Some, but not all, endocrinologists and primary care providers will also consider a trial of combination LT4/LT3 or DTE therapy as discussed above. Though current clinical practice guidelines do not recommend either combination LT4/LT3 or DTE as routine therapy, it is reasonable to consider these regimens in patients who have not responded well to LT4 monotherapy or who express a strong preference for these therapies, as long as they are given safely with careful attention to maintaining the serum TSH within the reference range to avoid the known toxicities of excess thyroid hormone administration (45, 65, 66, 76, 82).

ADRENAL COVERAGE

Patients with primary hypothyroidism due to chronic lymphocytic thyroiditis have an increased likelihood of having coexisting primary adrenal insufficiency, and patients with central hypothyroidism have an increased risk of also having central adrenal insufficiency. The initiation of LT4 therapy for treatment of hypothyroidism increases the metabolic clearance rate of cortisol, which results in a compensatory increase in adrenal cortisol production in individuals with an intact hypothalamic-pituitary-adrenal axis. However, patients with compromised hypothalamic-pituitary-adrenal function may be unable to adequately compensate. Consequently, precipitation of an adrenal crisis is a well-documented, though uncommon, result of initiating LT4 therapy. With this precaution in mind, some experts recommend ruling out adrenal insufficiency in the appropriate clinical setting, for example, in ill hospitalized patients when there is any indication or suspicion that coexisting primary or central adrenal insufficiency may be present.

COVERAGE WHEN PATIENTS ARE NPO FOR SURGERY, MEDICAL ILLNESS, OR DIAGNOSTIC PROCEDURES

Hypothyroid patients on nothing by mouth (NPO) status for surgery, medical illness, or preparation for a gastrointestinal endoscopic procedure, may not be able to take oral LT4 for one or more days. Intravenous LT4 is available but is very expensive. Since the half-life of LT4 is 5 days, there is little change in serum thyroid hormone levels when a patient is NPO for 1–2 days, and therefore there is no need for intravenous LT4 to be administered when patients are NPO for up to two or even 3 days. When a patient will be NPO for longer than this, intravenous LT4 can be given as a single daily bolus; the usual dose of intravenous LT4 is about 75% of the patient's usual oral dose (65).

CONDITIONS THAT ARE NOT HYPOTHYROIDISM BUT MAY APPEAR TO BE THYROID CONDITIONS

Non-thyroidal illness (euthyroid sick syndrome)

Non-Thyroidal Illness (NTI; also known as Euthyroid Sick Syndrome) refers to a cluster of abnormalities of circulating thyroid hormone and TSH levels that occur in patients who have non-thyroidal illnesses. This condition is covered elsewhere in this text and will therefore only be mentioned here for completeness. Systemic illnesses initially result in inhibition of deiodinase 1, resulting in reduced T4 to T3 conversion, which lowers serum T3 levels. With more severe illness, cytokine-induced reductions in TRH and TSH secretion can result in reduced serum TSH and free T4 levels. In the midst of a severe non-thyroidal illness, a patient may therefore have reduced serum levels of TSH and free T4 and markedly low levels of T3. This situation may cause diagnostic confusion with central hypothyroidism. Upon recovery from the non-thyroidal illness, TSH levels rise and transiently become mildly elevated into a range consistent with mild primary hypothyroidism. These thyroid hormone alterations are considered by many authorities to be compensatory changes in thyroid hormone economy that may be beneficial for recovery from the non-thyroidal illness. Furthermore, thyroid hormone therapy has not been shown to be beneficial. A very careful evaluation is usually needed to distinguish the NTI changes from actual thyroid disease and to avoid unnecessary and potentially harmful treatment. Whenever possible, it is best to avoid starting thyroid hormone therapy and to repeat the thyroid testing in the outpatient setting after the patient has recovered from their NTI (99, 100).

Steroid responsive encephalopathy associated with autoimmune thyroid disease (SREAAT) [formerly Hashimoto's encephalopathy]

Steroid Responsive Encephalopathy Associated with Autoimmune Thyroid Disease (SREAAT) is an acute encephalopathy of unknown cause that typically presents with symptoms of impaired mental status, somnolence, multiple stroke-like episodes, and seizures (101, 102). Because many affected patients have been found to have positive antithyroid antibodies in the serum and also in the cerebrospinal fluid (CSF), it was initially believed that these antibodies might play a pathophysiological role in causing the encephalopathy, possibly by promoting an antibody-mediated cerebritis; the condition was therefore termed "Hashimoto's Encephalopathy." However, it remains unclear if there is a pathogenic role for these antibodies in this condition. Reported cases have been hypothyroid, euthyroid, or even hyperthyroid, and treatment of hypothyroid patients with thyroid hormone replacement has produced no beneficial effects on the encephalopathy. Moreover, a substantial number of patients have experienced significant improvement following a course of intravenous or oral glucocorticoid therapy. Because the encephalopathy does not appear to be related to thyroid antibodies or to thyroid dysfunction but does respond well to glucocorticoid therapy, the term "Hashimoto's Encephalopathy" fell out of favor and the condition has become more accurately referred to as steroid-responsive encephalopathy associated with autoimmune thyroid disease (SREAAT) (101, 102).

Wilson's low T3 syndrome

Wilson's low T3 syndrome is an untested and unproven notion that has been proposed and promoted in books and on the internet without any substantiating scientific investigation. The purported pathophysiological basis of the condition is an unexplained but usually reversible reduction in the ability of a person to convert T4 into T3 with resultant deficiency of the active thyroid hormone. Underlying factors thought to precipitate or contribute to the impaired T4 to T3 conversion include family or job-related stress and Scottish, Irish, Russian, or Native American heritage. A diagnosis of Wilson's low T3 syndrome is said to be made by the finding of a low axillary body temperature but not by testing TSH or thyroid hormone levels. The proposed treatment is a program of progressively increasing doses of LT3, often to very high doses, until the axillary temperature returns to normal and other symptoms begin to resolve, after which the LT3 therapy can often be discontinued. There is no scientific evidence to prove the existence of this condition or to demonstrate the efficacy and safety of the proposed treatment. The American Thyroid

Association (ATA) leadership denounced the practice of diagnosing and treating Wilson's syndrome in a strong public document (ATA statement, May 24, 2005): The American Thyroid Association has found no scientific evidence supporting the existence of Wilson's syndrome. The theory proposed to explain this condition is at odds with established facts about thyroid hormone. Diagnostic criteria for Wilson's syndrome are imprecise and could lead to misdiagnosis of many other conditions. The T3 therapy advocated for Wilson's syndrome has never been evaluated objectively in a properly designed scientific study. Furthermore, administration of T3 can produce high concentrations of T3 in the blood, subjecting patients to new symptoms and potentially harmful effects on the heart and bones. At least one death has been reported in patients taking high doses of T3 for this syndrome (103). The ATA supports efforts to learn more about the causes of somatic symptoms that affect many individuals, to test rigorously the idea that some as yet unidentified abnormality in thyroid hormone action might account for even a small subset of these symptoms, and to pursue properly designed clinical trials to assess the effectiveness of lifestyle, dietary, and pharmacological treatments for these common ailments. However, unsupported claims, such as those made for Wilson's syndrome, do nothing to further these aims.

Reverse T3 syndrome (reverse T3 dominance syndrome)

The reverse T3 syndrome, also referred to as the reverse T3 dominance syndrome, is another untested and unproven notion that is a variation of the same theme with an additional pathophysiological twist. It is proposed that, for various reasons, some patients develop reduced ability to convert T4 into T3, with resultant increased T4 conversion to reverse T3 (RT3). It is suggested that the high RT3 levels compete for occupancy of tissue T3 receptors and thereby further decrease T3 action at the tissue levels. The proposed remedy is to take LT3 supplements. Like Wilson's syndrome, there is no scientific evidence to prove the existence of this condition or to support the efficacy or safety of LT3 therapy in these individuals. Furthermore, it has been well demonstrated that T3 has over 100 times the affinity for the T3 receptor as does RT3 (104), making it highly unlikely that elevated RT3

Table 6.14 Myxedema coma – clinical feature scoring system 1 (105)

Feature	Score	Feature	Score
Temperature		Cardiovascular	
Over 35°C	0	HR > 60	0
32–35°C	10	HR 50–59	10
Under 32°C	20	HR 40–49	20
Central Nervous System Symptoms		HR < 40	30
Absent	0	Other EKG Changes	10
Somnolent/Lethargic	10	Pericardial/Pleural Effusion	10
Obtunded	15	Pulmonary Edema	15
Stupor	20	Cardiomegaly	15
Coma/Seizures	30	Hypotension	20
Gastrointestinal		Metabolic Disorders	
Anorexia/Pain/Constipation	5	Hyponatremia	10
Decreased Motility	15	Hypoglycemia	10
Paralytic Ileus	20	Hypoxemia	10
Precipitating Event		Hypercarbia	10
Present	10	Decreased GFR	10

Precipitating Events for Myxedema Coma
Cold Exposure
Infection
Stroke
Myocardial Infarction
Pulmonary Embolism
Diabetic Ketoacidosis
Medications (CNS Suppressant)
Myxedema Coma Score Interpretation

Score	Myxedema Coma
24 or Under	Unlikely
25–59	Suggestive
60 or Over	Likely

levels have any antagonistic effect on tissue T3 action.

MYXEDEMA COMA

Myxedema coma, also known as decompensated hypothyroidism, is a life-threatening condition characterized by an exaggeration of the manifestations of hypothyroidism. Myxedema coma originally had a mortality rate of 100%. Today the outlook is much improved for appropriately treated patients with mortality rates in recent studies varying from 0 to 45% (1, 105).

Myxedema coma usually occurs in elderly patients who have inadequately treated or untreated hypothyroidism and a superimposed precipitating event. Important events include prolonged cold exposure, infection, trauma, surgery, myocardial infarction, congestive heart failure, pulmonary embolism, stroke, respiratory failure, gastrointestinal bleeding, and administration of various drugs, particularly those that have a depressive effect on the central nervous system (1, 105–107).

Hypothermia, bradycardia, and hypoventilation are common. Blood pressure, although generally reduced, is more variable. Pericardial, pleural, and peritoneal effusions are often found. An ileus is frequently present and acute urinary retention may be seen. Central nervous system manifestations include seizures, stupor, and coma. Deep

Table 6.15 Myxedema coma – clinical feature scoring system 2 (106)

Feature	Score
Glasgow Coma Scale	
0–10	4
11–13	3
14	2
15	0
TSH	
Over 30	2
15–30	1
Free T4 Low	1
Hypothermia	1
Bradycardia	1
Precipitating Event	1
Score Interpretation	

Score	Category	Recommendation
8–10	Most Likely	Treat
5–7	Likely	Treat if No Other Plausible Cause
Under 5	Unlikely	Consider Other Diagnoses

tendon reflexes are absent or exhibit a delayed relaxation phase. Typical hypothyroid skin and hair changes are often apparent. A goiter, although frequently absent, is a helpful finding. A thyroidectomy scar may also be an important clue.

Serum T4 (total and free T4) and T3 (total and free T3) are usually very low, and the TSH is significantly elevated. Other frequent abnormalities include anemia, hyponatremia, hypoglycemia, and elevated serum levels of cholesterol and creatine kinase (CK). Arterial blood gases often reveal carbon dioxide retention and hypoxemia. The electrocardiogram often shows sinus bradycardia, various types and degrees of heart block, low voltage, and T-wave flattening.

The diagnosis must be made on clinical grounds on the basis of the findings described earlier. There have been two proposed Myxedema Coma Scoring Systems that have been published to facilitate making an accurate diagnosis (106, 107) (Tables 6.14 and 6.15).

The initial goal of treatment is to rapidly replace the depleted thyroid hormone pool. The normal total body pool of T4 is about 1000 mcg (500 mcg in the thyroid, 500 mcg in the rest of the body). LT4, LT3, or both may be used to treat this emergency condition. Due to the rarity of the condition,

Table 6.16 Treatment of myxedema coma (65, 107)

Thyroid Hormone Replacement (Rapid)(see text)
  Levothyroxine 200–300 mcg IV over 5 minutes, then
  Levothyroxine 50–100 mcg daily PO or IV
  Triiodothyronine 5–10 mcg IV every 6–12 hours
Glucocorticoid Therapy (Stress Doses for 2 Days)
  Hydrocortisone 200 mg daily, or
  Methylprednisolone 40 mg daily, or
  Prednisone 50 mg daily, or
  Dexamethasone 7.5 mg daily
Support Circulation, Oxygenation, and Ventilation
  IV Fluids
  Oxygen
  Mechanical Ventilation (if needed)
  Passive Rewarming (if severely hypothermic)
Treat Precipitating Cause (critically important)

there are no randomized trials comparing different thyroid hormone replacement regimens. The best regimen remains undetermined, but the author and colleagues at our institution favor a loading dose (bolus) of intravenous LT4, 300–500 mcg on day one, followed by intravenous LT4 (75% of the calculated oral dose) daily. Some experts recommend administering IV LT3 in doses of 5 mcg every 4–6 hours if there is no clinical response to IV LT4 after several days. Some experts recommend combination LT4 and LT3 therapy from the start, using a lower dose of IV LT4 (200–300 mcg) and a loading dose of 10 mcg of LT3, followed by IV LT4 100 mcg IV per day plus LT3 10 mcg every 8–12 hours (65, 108). The theoretical advantages of LT3 therapy are that it is the active thyroid hormone, and that it crosses the blood brain barrier better than LT4. Other measures of immediate and equal importance are to administer stress doses of glucocorticoids, to support vital functions and oxygenation, to enable passive rewarming of the hypothermic patient, and to treat any identified precipitating conditions. A summary of the treatment of myxedema coma is outlined in Table 6.16.

REFERENCES

1. Chaker L, Bianco AC, Jonklass J, Peeters RP. Hypothyroidism. *Lancet* 2017; 390(10101):1550–62.
2. Garmendia Madariaga A, Santos Palacios S, Guillén-Grima F, Galofré JC. The incidence and prevalence of thyroid dysfunction in Europe: A meta-analysis. *J. Clin. Endocrinol. Metab.* 2014; 99(3):923–31.
3. Peeters RP. Subclinical hypothyroidism. *N. Engl. J. Med.* 2017; 376(26):2556–65.
4. Gereben B, McAninch EA, Ribeiro MO, Bianco AC. Scope and limitations of iodothyronine deiodinases in hypothyroidism. *Nat. Rev. Endocrinol.* 2015; 11(11):642–52.
5. Mendoza A, Hollenberg AN. New insights into thyroid hormone action. *Pharmacol. Ther.* 2017; 173:135–45.
6. Hu S, Rayman MP. Multiple nutritional factors and the risk of Hashimoto's thyroiditis. *Thyroid* 2017; 27(5):597–610.
7. Wichman J, Winther KH, Bonnema SJ, Hegedus L. Selenium supplementation significantly reduces thyroid autoantibody levels in patients with chronic autoimmune thyroiditis: A systematic review and meta-analysis. *Thyroid* 2016; 26(12):1681–92.
8. Ahn D, Sohn JH, Jeon JH. Hypothyroidism following hemithyroidectomy: Incidence, risk factors, and clinical characteristics. *J. Clin. Endocrinol. Metab.* 2016; 101(4):1429–36.
9. Park S, Jeon MJ, Song E, Oh HS, Kim M, Kwon H, Kim TY, et al. Clinical features of early and late postoperative hypothyroidism after lobectomy. *J. Clin. Endocrinol. Metab.* 2017; 102(4):1317–24.
10. Szczepanek-Parulska E, Zybek-Kocik A, Wartofsky L, Ruchala M. Thyroid hemiagenesis: Incidence, clinical significance, and genetic background. *J. Clin. Endocrinol. Metab.* 2017; 102(9):3124–37.
11. Morganstein DL, Lai Z, Spain L, Diem S, Levine D, Mace C, Gore M, Larkin J. Thyroid abnormalities following the use of cytotoxic T-lymphocyte antigen 4 and programmed cell death receptor protein-1 inhibitors in the treatment of melanoma. *Clin. Endocrinol. (Oxf.)* 2017; 86(4):614–20.
12. Daniels GH, Vladic A, Brinar V, Zavalishin I, Valente W, Oyuela P, Palmer J, Margolin DH, Hollenstein J. Alemtuzumab related thyroid dysfunction in a phase 2 trial of patients with relapsing-remitting multiple sclerosis. *J. Clin. Endocrinol. Metab.* 2014; 99(1):80–9.
13. O'Malley G, Lee HJ, Parekh S, Galsky MD, Smith CB, Friedlander P, Yanagisawa RT, Gallagher EJ. Rapid evolution of thyroid dysfunction in patients treated with Nivolumab. *Endocr. Pract.* 2017; 23(10):1223–31.
14. Grunenwald S, Caron P. Central hypothyroidism in adults: Better understanding for better care. *Pituitary* 2015; 18(1):169–75.
15. Aw DKL, Sinha RA, Tan HC, Loh LM, Salvatore D, Yen PM. Studies of molecular mechanisms associated with increased deiodinase 3 expression in a case of consumptive hypothyroidism. *J. Clin. Endocrinol. Metab.* 2014; 99(11):3965–71.
16. Dumitrescu AM, Refetoff S. The syndromes of reduced sensitivity to thyroid hormone. *Biochim. Biophys. Acta* 2013; 1830(7):3987–4003.
17. Zulewski HK, Muller B, Exer P, Miserez AR, Staub JJ. Estimation of tissue hypothyroidism by a new clinical score: Evaluation of patients with various grades of hypothyroidism and controls. *J. Clin. Endocrinol. Metab.* 1997; 82(3):771–6.

18. Carle A, Pedersen IB, Knudsen N, Perrild H, Ovesen L, Laurberg P. Hypothyroid symptoms and the likelihood of overt thyroid failure: A population-based case-control study. *Eur. J. Endocrinol.* 2014; 171(5):593–602.

19. Carle A, Bulow Pedersen IB, Knudsen N, Perrild H, Ovesen L, Laurberg P. Gender differences in symptoms of hypothyroidism: A population-based DanThyr study. *Clin. Endocrinol. (Oxf.)* 2015; 83(5):717–25.

20. Carle A, Pederson IB, Knudsen N, Perrild H, Ovesen L, Andersen S, Laurberg P. Hypothyroid symptoms fail to predict thyroid insufficiency in old people: A population-based case-control study. *Am. J. Med.* 2016; 129(10):1082–92.

21. Duntas LH. Thyroid disease and lipids. *Thyroid* 2002; 12(4):287–93.

22. Sorensen JR, Winther KH, Bonnema SJ, Godballe C, Hegedus L. Respiratory manifestations of hypothyroidism: A systematic review. *Thyroid* 2016; 26(11):1519–27.

23. Cooke GE, Mullally S, Correia N, O'Mara SM, Gibney J. Hippocampal volume is decreased in adults with hypothyroidism. *Thyroid* 2014; 24(3):433–40.

24. Thvilum M, Brandt F, Almind D, Christensen K, Brix TH, Hegedüs L. Increased psychiatric morbidity before and after the diagnosis of hypothyroidism: A nationwide register study. *Thyroid* 2014; 24(5):802–8.

25. Quinque EM, Villinger A, Kratzsch J, Karger S. Patient-reported outcomes in adequately treated hypothyroidism – Insights from the German versions of ThyQoL, ThySRQ and ThyTSQ. *Health Qual. Life Outcomes* 2013; 11:68.

26. Watt T, Cramon P, Hegedus L, Bjorner JB, Bonnema SJ, Rasmussen ÅK, Feldt-Rasmussen U, Groenvold M. The thyroid-related quality of life measure ThyPRO has good responsiveness and ability to detect relevant treatment effects. *J. Clin. Endocrinol. Metab.* 2014; 99(10):3708–17.

27. Watt T, Bjorner JB, Groenvold M, Cramon P, Winther KH, Hegedüs L, Bonnema SJ, et al. Development of a short version of the thyroid-related patient-reported outcome ThyPRO. *Thyroid* 2015; 25(10):1069–79

28. Smith CD, Grondin R, LeMaster W, Martin B, Gold BT, Ain KB. Reversible cognitive, motor, and driving impairments in severe hypothyroidism. *Thyroid* 2015; 25(1):28–36.

29. Shin YW, Choi YM, Kim HS, Kim DJ, Jo HJ, O'Donnell BF, Jang EK, et al. Diminished quality of life and increased brain functional connectivity in patients with hypothyroidism after total thyroidectomy. *Thyroid* 2016; 26(5):641–9.

30. Klaver EI, van Loon HCM, Stienstra R, Links TP, Keers JC, Kema IP, Kobold AC, van der Klauw MM, Wolffenbuttel BH. Thyroid hormone status and health-related quality of life in the LifeLines Cohort Study. *Thyroid* 2013; 23(9):1066–73.

31. Pasqualetti G, Pagano G, Rengo G, Ferrara N, Monzani F. Subclinical hypothyroidism and cognitive impairment: Systematic review and meta-analysis. *J. Clin. Endocrinol. Metab.* 2015; 100(11):4240–48.

32. Rieben C, Segna D, da Costa BR, Collet TH, Chaker L, Aubert CE, Baumgartner C, et al. Subclinical thyroid dysfunction and the risk of cognitive decline: A meta-analysis of prospective cohort studies. *J. Clin. Endocrinol. Metab.* 2016; 101(12):4945–54.

33. Chaker L, Wolters FJ, Bos D, Korevaar TI, Hofman A, van der Lugt A, Koudstaal PJ, et al. Thyroid function and the risk of dementia: The Rotterdam study. *Neurology* 2016; 87(16):1688–95.

34. Samuels MH, Kolobova I, Smeraglio A, Peters D, Janowsky JS, Schuff KG. The effects of levothyroxine replacement or suppressive therapy on health status, mood, and cognition. *J. Clin. Endocrinol. Metab.* 2014; 99(3):843–51.

35. Samuels MH, Kolobova I, Smeraglio A, Niederhausen M, Janowsky JS, Schuff KG. Effect of thyroid function variations within the laboratory reference range on health status, mood, and cognition in levothyroxine-treated subjects. *Thyroid* 2016; 26(9):1173–84.

36. Tadic M, Ilic S, Kostic N, Caparevic Z, Celic V. Subclinical hypothyroidism and left ventricular mechanics: A three-dimensional speckle tracking study. *J. Clin. Endocrinol. Metab.* 2014; 99(1):307–14.

37. Werneck FZ, Coelho EF, de Lima JRP, Laterza MC, Barral MM, Teixeira Pde F, Vaisman M. Pulmonary oxygen

uptake kinetics during exercise in subclinical hypothyroidism. *Thyroid* 2014; 24(6):931–8.

38. Virgini VS, Wijsman LW, Rodondi N, Bauer DC, Kearney PM, Gussekloo J, den Elzen WP, et al. Subclinical thyroid dysfunction and functional capacity among elderly. *Thyroid* 2014; 24(2):208–14.

39. Brenta G, Berg G, Miksztowicz V, Lopez G, Lucero D, Faingold C, Murakami M, et al. Atherogenic lipoproteins in subclinical hypothyroidism and their relationship with hepatic lipase activity: Response to replacement treatment with levothyroxine. *Thyroid* 2016; 26(3):365–72.

40. Zhao M, Liu L, Wang F, Yuan Z, Zhang X, Xu C, Song Y, et al. A worthy finding: Decrease in total cholesterol and low-density lipoprotein cholesterol in treated mild subclinical hypothyroidism. *Thyroid* 2016; 26(8):1019–29.

41. McGowan A, Widdowson WM, O'Regan A, Young IS, Boran G, McEneny J, Gibney J. Postprandial studies uncover differing effects on HDL particles of overt and subclinical hypothyroidism. *Thyroid* 2016; 26(3):356–64.

42. Surks MI, Hollowell JG. Age-specific distribution of serum thyrotropin and Antithyroid antibodies in the US population: Implications for the prevalence of subclinical hypothyroidism. *J. Clin. Endocrinol. Metab.* 2007; 92(12):4575–82.

43. Li D, Radulescu A, Shrestha RT, Root M, Karger AB, Killeen AA, Hodges JS, et al. Association of biotin ingestion with performance of hormone and non-hormone assays in healthy adults. *JAMA* 2017; 318(12):1150–60.

44. Hattori N, Ishihara T, Yamagami K, Shimatsu A. Macro TSH in patients with subclinical hypothyroidism. *Clin. Endocrinol. (Oxf.)* 2015; 83(6):923–30.

45. Garber JR, Cobin RH, Gharib H, Hennessey JV, Klein I, Mechanick JI, Pessah-Pollack R, et al., for the American Association of Clinical Endocrinologists and American Thyroid Association Task Force on Hypothyroidism in Adults Study Groups. Clinical practice guidelines for hypothyroidism in adults; cosponsored by the American Association of Clinical Endocrinologists and the American Thyroid Association. *Endocr. Pract.* 2012; 18(6):988–1028.

46. Brenta G, Vaisman M, Sgarbi JA, Bergoglio LM, Andrada NC, Bravo PP, Orlandi AM, Graf H, Task Force on Hypothyroidism of the Latin American Thyroid Society (LATS) for the Task Force on Hypothyroidism of the Latin American Thyroid. Clinical practice guidelines for the management of hypothyroidism. *Arq. Bras. Endocrinol. Metab.* 2013; 57(4):265–91.

47. LeFevre ML, the US Preventative Services Task Force. Screening for thyroid dysfunction: US Preventative Services Task Force recommendation statement. *Ann. Intern. Med.* 2015; 162(9):641–50.

48. Thvilum M, Brandt F, Almind D, Christensen K, Hegedus L, Brix TH. Excess mortality in patients diagnosed with hypothyroidism: A nationwide cohort study of singletons and twins. *J. Clin. Endocrinol. Metab.* 2013; 98(3):1069–75.

49. Journy NMY, Bernier MO, Doody MM, Alexander BH, Linet MS, Kitahara CM. Hyperthyroidism, hypothyroidism, and cause-specific mortality in a large cohort of women. *Thyroid* 2017; 27(8):1001–10.

50. Pasqualetti G, Tognini S, Polini A, Caraccio N, Monzani F. Is subclinical hypothyroidism a cardiovascular risk factor in the elderly? *J. Clin. Endocrinol. Metab.* 2013; 98(6):2256–66.

51. Chen WH, Chen YK, Lin CL, Yeh JH, Kao CH. Hashimoto's thyroiditis, risk of coronary heart disease, and L-thyroxine treatment: A nationwide cohort study. *J. Clin. Endocrinol. Metab.* 2015; 100(1):109–14.

52. LeGrys VA, Funk MJ, Lorenz CE, Giri A, Jackson RD, Manson JE, Schectman R, et al. Subclinical hypothyroidism and risk for incident myocardial infarction among postmenopausal women. *J. Clin. Endocrinol. Metab.* 2013; 98(6):2308–17.

53. Hyland KA, Arnold AM, Lee JS, Cappola AR. Persistent subclinical hypothyroidism and cardiovascular risk in the elderly: The Cardiovascular Health Study. *J. Clin. Endocrinol. Metab.* 2013; 98(2):533–40.

54. Collet TH, Bauer DC, Cappola AR, Asvold BO, Weiler S, Vittinghoff E, Gussekloo J,

et al. for the Thyroid Studies Collaboration. Thyroid antibody status, subclinical hypothyroidism, and the risk of coronary heart disease: An individual participant data analysis. *J. Clin. Endocrinol. Metab.* 2014; 99(9):3353–62.

55. Martin SS, Daya N, Lutsey PL, Matsushita K, Fretz A, McEvoy JW, Blumenthal RS, et al. Thyroid function, cardiovascular risk factors, and incident atherosclerosis risk in communities (ARIC) study. *J. Clin. Endocrinol. Metab.* 2017; 102(9):3306–15.

56. Rhee CM, Curhan GC, Alexander EK, Bhan I, Brunelli SM. Subclinical hypothyroidism and survival: The effects of heart failure and race. *J. Clin. Endocrinol. Metab.* 2013; 98(6):2326–36.

57. Grossman A, Weiss A, Koren-Morag N, Shimon I, Beloosesky Y, Meyerovitch J. Subclinical thyroid disease and mortality in the elderly: A retrospective cohort study. *Am. J. Med.* 2016; 129(4):423–30.

58. Giri A, Edwards TL, LeGrys VA, Lorenz CE, Funk MJ, Schectman R, Heiss G, Robinson JG, Hartmann KE. Subclinical hypothyroidism and risk for incident ischemic stroke among postmenopausal women. *Thyroid* 2014; 24(8):1210–17.

59. Chaker L, Baumgartner C, den Elzen WP, Ikram MA, Blum MR, Collet TH, Bakker SJ, et al. Subclinical hypothyroidism and the risk of stroke events and fatal stroke: An individual participant data analysis. *J. Clin. Endocrinol. Metab.* 2015; 100(6):2181–91.

60. Simonsick EM, Newman AB, Ferrucci L, Satterfield S, Harris TB, Rodondi N, Bauer DC, Health ABC Study. Subclinical hypothyroidism and functional mobility in older adults. *Arch. Intern. Med.* 2009; 169(21):2011–7.

61. Santoro N, Braunstein GD, Butts CL, Martin KA, McDermott M, Pinkerton JV. Compounded bioidentical hormones in endocrinology practice: An Endocrine Society scientific statement. *J. Clin. Endocrinol. Metab.* 2016; 101(4):1318–43.

62. Negro R, Valcavi R, Agrimi D, Toulis KA. Levothyroxine liquid solution versus tablet for replacement in hypothyroid patients. *Endocr. Pract.* 2014; 20(9):901–6.

63. Bruncato D, Scorsone A, Saura G, Ferrara L, Di Noto A, Aiello V, Fleres M, Provenzano V. Comparison of TSH levels with liquid formulation versus tablet formulations of levothyroxine in the treatment of adult hypothyroidism. *Endocr. Pract.* 2014; 20(7):657–62.

64. Vita R, Saraceno G, Trimarchi F, Benvenga S. Switching levothyroxine from the tablet to the oral solution formulation corrects the impaired absorption of levothyroxine induced by proton-pump inhibitors. *J. Clin. Endocrinol. Metab.* 2014; 99(12):4481–6.

65. Jonklaas J, Bianco AC, Bauer AJ, Burman KD, Cappola AR, Celi FS, Cooper DS, et al. for the American Thyroid Association Task Force on Thyroid Hormone Replacement. Guidelines for the treatment of hypothyroidism: Prepared by the American Thyroid Association Task Force on thyroid hormone replacement. *Thyroid* 2014; 24(12):1670–751.

66. Pearce SH, Brabant G, Duntas LH, Monzani F, Peeters RP, Razvi S, Wemeau JL. 2013 ETA guideline: Management of subclinical hypothyroidism. *Eur. Thyroid J.* 2013; 2(4):215–28.

67. Di Donna V, Santoro MG, de Waure C, Ricciato MP, Paragliola RM, Pontecorvi A, Corsello SM. A new strategy to estimate levothyroxine requirement after total thyroidectomy for benign thyroid disease. *Thyroid* 2014; 24(12):1759–64.

68. Glymph K, Gosmanov AR. Levothyroxine replacement in obese hypothyroid females after total thyroidectomy. *Endocr. Pract.* 2016; 22(1):22–9.

69. Burch HB, Burman KD, Cooper DS, Hennessey JV. A 2013 survey of clinical practice patterns in the management of primary hypothyroidism. *J. Clin. Endocrinol. Metab.* 2014; 99(6):2077–85.

70. Papaleontiou M, Gay BL, Esfandiari NH, Hawley ST, Haymart MR. The impact of age in the management of hypothyroidism: Results of a nationwide survey. *Endocr. Pract.* 2016; 22(6):708–15.

71. Lee SY, Braverman LE, Pearce EN. Changes in body weight after treatment of primary hypothyroidism with levothyroxine. *Endocr. Pract.* 2014; 20(11):1122–8.

72. Stott DJ, Rodondi N, Kearney PM, Ford I, Westendorp RGJ, Mooijaart SP, Sattar N, et al. Thyroid hormone therapy for older adults with subclinical hypothyroidism. *N. Engl. J. Med.* 2017; 376(26):2534–44.

73. Razvi S, Weaver JU, Butler TJ, Pearce SH. Levothyroxine treatment of subclinical hypothyroidism, fatal and nonfatal cardiovascular events, and mortality. *Arch. Intern. Med.* 2012; 172(10):811–7.

74. Ito M, Miyauchi A, Hisakado M, Yoshioka W, Ide A, Kudo T, Nishihara E, et al. Biochemical markers reflecting thyroid function in athyreotic patients on levothyroxine monotherapy. *Thyroid* 2017; 27(4):484–90.

75. Robertson HMA, Narayanaswamy AKP, Pereira O, Copland SA, Herriot R, McKinlay AW, Bevan JS, Abraham P. Factors contributing to high levothyroxine doses in primary hypothyroidism: An interventional audit of a large community database. *Thyroid* 2014; 24(12):1765–71.

76. Biondi B, Wartofsky L. Treatment with thyroid hormone. *Endocr. Rev.* 2014; 35(3):433–512.

77. Blum MR, Bauer DC, Collet TH, Fink HA, Cappola AR, da Costa BR, Wirth CD, et al. Subclinical thyroid dysfunction and fracture risk: A meta-analysis. *JAMA* 2015; 313(20):2055–65.

78. Abrahamsen B, Jorgensen HL, Laulund AS, Nybo M, Bauer DC, Brix TH, Hegedüs L. The excess risk of major osteoporotic fractures is driven by cumulative hyperthyroid as opposed to hypothyroid time: An observational register-based time-resolved cohort analysis. *J. Bone Miner. Res.* 2015; 30(5):898–905.

79. Taylor PN, Iqbal A, Minassian C, Sayers A, Draman MS, Greenwood R, Hamilton W, et al. Falling threshold for treatment of borderline elevated thyrotropin levels – Balancing benefits and risks: Evidence from a large community based study. *JAMA Intern. Med.* 2014; 174(1):32–9.

80. Mammen JS, McGready J, Oxman R, Chia CW, Ladenson PW, Simonsick EM. Thyroid hormone therapy and the risk of thyrotoxicosis in community-resident older adults: Findings from the Baltimore Longitudinal Study of Aging. *Thyroid* 2015; 25(9):979–86.

81. Winther KH, Cramon P, Watt T, Bjorner JB, Ekholm O, Feldt-Rasmussen U, Groenvold M, et al. Disease-specific as well as generic quality of life is widely impacted in autoimmune hypothyroidism and improves during the first six months of levothyroxine therapy. *PLoS ONE* 2016; 11(6):e0156925

82. Peterson SJ, Cappola AR, Castro MR, et al. An online survey of hypothyroid patients demonstrates prominent dissatisfaction. *Thyroid* 2018; 28(6):707–721.

83. McAninch EA, Bianco AC. The history and future treatment of hypothyroidism. *Ann. Intern. Med.* 2016; 164(1):50–6.

84. Samuels MH, Kolobova I, Smeraglio A, Peters D, Purnell JQ, Schuff KG. Effects of levothyroxine replacement or suppressive therapy on energy expenditure and body composition. *Thyroid* 2016; 26(3):347–55.

85. Samuels MH, Kolobova I, Antosik M, Niederhausen M, Purnell JQ, Schuff KG. Thyroid function variation in the normal range, energy expenditure, and body composition in L-T4-Treated subjects. *J. Clin. Endocrinol. Metab.* 2017; 102(7):2533–42.

86. Ito M, Miyauchi A, Kang S, Hisakado M, Yoshioka W, Ide A, Kudo T, et al. Effect of the presence of remnant thyroid tissue on the serum thyroid hormone balance in thyroidectomized patients. *Eur. J. Endocrinol.* 2015; 173(3):333–40.

87. Peterson SJ, McAninch EA, Bianco AC. Is a normal TSH synonymous with "Euthyroidism" in levothyroxine monotherapy? *J. Clin. Endocrinol. Metab.* 2016; 101(12):4964–73.

88. Panicker V, Saravanan P, Vaidya B, Evans J, Hattersley AT, Frayling TM, Dayan CM. Common variation of in the DIO_2 gene predicts baseline psychological well-being and response to combination thyroxine plus triiodothyronine therapy in hypothyroid patients. *J. Clin. Endocrinol. Metab.* 2009; 94(5):1623–9.

89. Appelhof BC, Peeters RP, Wiersinga WM, Visser TJ, Wekking EM, Huyser J, Schene AH, et al. Polymorphisms in type 2 deiodinase are not associated with well-being, neurocognitive functioning, and preference for combined thyroxine/3,5,3'-triiodothyronine

therapy. *J. Clin. Endocrinol. Metab.* 2005; 90(11):6296–9.

90. Castagna MG, Dentice M, Cantara S, Ambrosio R, Maino F, Porcelli T, Marzocchi C, et al. DIO_2 Thr92Ala reduced deiodinase-2 activity and serum T3 levels in thyroid deficient patients. *J. Clin. Endocrinol. Metab.* 2017; 102(5):1623–30.

91. Hoang TD, Olsen CH, Mai VQ, Clyde PW, Shakir MK. Desiccated thyroid extract compared with levothyroxine in the treatment of hypothyroidism: A randomized, double-blind, crossover study. *J. Clin. Endocrinol. Metab.* 2013; 98(5):1982–90.

92. Shresta RT, Malabanan A, Haugen BR, Levy EG, Hennessey JV. Adverse event reporting in patients treated with thyroid hormone extract. *Endocr. Pract.* 2017; 23(5):566–75.

93. Jonklaas J, Burman KD. Daily administration of short-acting liothyronine is associated with significant triiodothyronine excursions and fails to alter thyroid-responsive parameters. *Thyroid* 2016; 26(6):770–8.

94. Wiersinga WM, Duntas L, Fadeyev V, Nygaard B, Vanderpump MPJ. 2012 ETA Guidelines: The use of L-T4 + L-T3 in the treatment of hypothyroidism. *Eur. Thyroid J.* 2012; 1(2):55–71.

95. Ott J, Promberger R, Kober F, Neuhold N, Tea M, Huber JC, Hermann M. Hashimoto's thyroiditis affects symptom load and quality of life unrelated to hypothyroidism: A prospective case-control study in women undergoing thyroidectomy for benign goiter. *Thyroid* 2011; 21(2):161–7.

96. Boelaert K, Newby PR, Simmonds MJ, Holder RL, Carr-Smith JD, Heward JM, Manji N, et al. Prevalence and relative risk of other autoimmune diseases in subjects with autoimmune thyroid disease. *Am. J. Med.* 2010; 123(2):183.e1–9.

97. Roy A, Laszkowska M, Sundstrom J, Lebwohl B, Green PH, Kämpe O, Ludvigsson JF. Prevalence of celiac disease in patients with autoimmune thyroid disease: A meta-analysis. *Thyroid* 2016; 26(7):880–90.

98. Guglielmi R, Frasoldati A, Zini M, Grimaldi F, Gharib H, Garber JR, Papini E. Italian Association of Clinical Endocrinologists Statement-Replacement Therapy for Primary Hypothyroidism: A brief guide for clinical practice. *Endocr. Pract.* 2016; 22(11):1319–26.

99. Van den Berghe G. Non-thyroidal illnesses in the ICU: A syndrome with different faces. *Thyroid* 2014; 24(10):1456–65.

100. Boonen E, Van den Berghe G. Endocrine responses to critical illness: Novel insights and therapeutic implications. *J. Clin. Endocrinol. Metab.* 2014; 99(5):1569–82.

101. Menon V, Subramanian K, Thamizh JS. Psychiatric presentations heralding Hashimoto's encephalopathy: A systematic review and analysis of cases reported in literature. *J. Neurosci. Rural Pract.* 2017; 8(2):261–7.

102. Zhou JY, Xu B, Lopes J, Blamoun J, Li L. Hashimoto encephalopathy: Literature review. *Acta Neurol. Scand.* 2017; 135(3):285–90.

103. https://en.wikipedia.org/wiki/Wilson%27s_temperature_syndrome.

104. Schuster LD, Schwartz HL, Oppenheimer JH. Nuclear receptors for 3,5,3'-triiodothyronine in human liver and kidney: Characterization, quantitation. *J. Clin. Endocrinol. Metab.* 1979; 48(4):627–32.

105. Beynon J, Akhtar S, Kearney T. Predictors of outcome in myxedema coma. *Crit. Care* 2008; 12(1):111.

106. Popoveniuc G, Chandra T, Sud A, Sharma M, Blackman MR, Burman KD, Mete M, Desale S, Wartofsky L. A diagnostic scoring system for myxedema coma. *Endocr. Pract.* 2014; 20(8):808–17.

107. Chiong YV, Brammerlin E, Mariash CN. Development of an objective tool for the diagnosis of myxedema coma. *Transl. Res.* 2015; 166(3):233–43.

108. Klubo-Gwiezdzinska J, Wartofsky L. Thyroid emergencies. *Med. Clin. North Am.* 2012; 96(2):385–403.

7

Thyroid nodules and multinodular goiter

POORANI N. GOUNDAN AND STEPHANIE L. LEE

Introduction	159	Ultrasonography	163
Prevalence	159	Thyroid scintigraphy	167
Pathogenesis	160	Other imaging modalities	169
History and examination	161	Fine needle biopsy and cytology	170
Laboratory testing	162	Management and follow-up	173
Imaging	163	References	175

INTRODUCTION

A nontoxic goiter is a uniform or asymmetric enlargement of the thyroid gland that is not associated with hypo- or hyperthyroidism and is also not a result of inflammation or neoplasia. A thyroid nodule is a discrete lesion within the thyroid caused by an excess proliferation of cells compared to the surrounding normal thyroid parenchyma. Thyroid nodules are a common clinical problem that may be discovered due to symptoms observed by patients, identified on physical examination, or incidentally noted on imaging studies performed for unrelated reasons.

The widespread use of high-resolution ultrasound (US) and fine needle biopsy (FNB) and, more recently, the introduction of molecular testing used in conjunction with cytology has markedly improved the evaluation and management of thyroid nodules. These advances in technology, however, have not been without unexpected and sometimes undesirable consequences. Increased sensitivity of current imaging equipment, for example, has resulted in the frequent discovery of subclinical nodules and papillary microcarcinomas in the thyroid gland, often

creating difficult management decisions for both the clinician and the patient.

This chapter on nodular thyroid disease includes a discussion on the prevalence and pathogenesis of thyroid nodules. The clinical evaluation, including laboratory tests, a review of the uses and limitations of US, thyroid scanning, and FNB with molecular testing will be reviewed. Finally, the long-term management of benign solitary nodules and multinodular glands will be outlined. The clinical management of nodular thyroid disease includes recommendations from recent practice management guidelines by the American Thyroid Association (2015) (1), the American Association of Clinical Endocrinologists, the American College of Endocrinology in collaboration with the Associazione Medici Endocrinologi (2016) (2), the European Thyroid Association (2017) (3, 4) and the American College of Radiology (ACR) (5).

PREVALENCE

The incidence of goiter, either due to iodine deficiency or environmental goitrogens, varies with the geographic region examined. Iodine deficiency is the most common worldwide etiology of goiter. Denmark, a region marked by mild to moderate iodine-deficiency, has a goiter prevalence of 15 to 23% (6). In contrast, in Great Britain, an area with adequate iodine intake, nonendemic or sporadic goiter affects 5% of the adult population (7). Iodine deficiency had been a frequent cause of goiter in the United States in the early 20th century, but with the iodinization of salt, the incidence of goiter decreased. There has been a concern that a re-emergence of iodine deficiency goiter would occur with the declining American dietary iodine intake; results from the NHANES I (1971–1974) and NHANES III (1988–1994) studies showed a decrease in median urinary iodine concentration from 320 mcg/L to 145 mcg/L. More recently, however, the levels have stabilized with a median urinary iodine concentration of 168 mcg/L and 164 mcg/L in the NHANES 2001–2002 and 2007–2008 evaluations, respectively (8). Although from a public health point of view, the median iodine intake of adults is adequate compared to the recommended intake of 150 mcg/day by the WHO, a significant proportion of the population will have a mildly insufficient iodine intake, which may contribute to goiter and nodule formation.

Solitary palpable thyroid nodules are found in 4 to 7% of the adult population in North America, 6.4% in women and 1.5% in men from 30 to 59 years of age. The prevalence of nodules increases with age, especially in women and in persons exposed to ionizing radiation in infancy or childhood. The data provided by the Framingham study showed that a new nodule developed in 1.3% of the cohort over a 15-year period, suggesting an incidence of palpable nodules of 0.1% per year with an estimated 10% lifetime expectancy of palpable nodule development (9).

The prevalence of palpable nodules, however, substantially underestimates the clinical problem. In an autopsy series, Mortensen and colleagues reported that in patients whose glands appeared clinically normal, one or more thyroid nodules were detected in approximately 50% (10). Furthermore, 35% of the glands had nodules measuring greater than 2 cm that had not been detected on physical exam. More recently, US data support these early autopsy studies. In an unselected population, the prevalence of nodules on US has been demonstrated to be nearly 20% in a Finnish cohort and 67% in a population in California (11, 12).

Most thyroid nodules are benign. Studies to estimate the rate of cancer in nodules are biased by the selection of those cases that are sent for surgery. When reviewing cases sent for surgery without prior biopsy, 6.5% of nodules were found to have cancer in a community hospital in North Carolina (13). Similarly, in 2,300 patients with solitary cold nodules who were evaluated using FNB, 391 underwent surgery that revealed 28% of the surgical specimens and 5% of the total nodules were malignant (14). The frequency of malignancy in patients with single nodules and patients with multinodular glands are similar. In a study of 5,637 patients, Belfiore and colleagues reported thyroid cancer in 4.1% of solitary nodules versus 4.7% of multinodular glands (15). A separate study showed that cancer rates were similar for patients with thyroid glands with one nodule and with two or more nodules (14.8% vs. 14.9%, respectively). In individual nodules selected for biopsy, however, the rate of malignancy was 14.8% when the nodule was solitary and 8.1% for nodules in glands with multiple nodules (16). Therefore, while the overall risk for malignancy in glands with solitary and multiple nodules may be the same, the risk for malignancy for a solitary nodule is higher than an individual nodule in a multinodular goiter.

PATHOGENESIS

It was initially suggested by David Marine, and later by Selwyn Taylor, that nodular goiters were the result of TSH simulation in the setting of iodine deficiency resulting initially in a diffuse parenchymal hyperplasia. They theorized that when periods of hyperplasia are intermittently interrupted by "resting" phases of reduced follicular cell growth with iodine repletion there is increased colloid storage. Alternating between phases of growth and rest, therefore, results in multinodular goiter formation (17). Other than iodine deficiency, there are other goitrogens that may also cause a subclinical or clinical elevation in TSH including soy beans, cassava, sorghum, cruciferous vegetables (such as cabbage), and seaweed/kelp (i.e., iodine excess). It is important to emphasize, however, that the exact role of TSH as a thyroid growth factor in the development of goiter remains controversial (18). Non-TSH related growth factors also have been identified. Insulin-like growth factor-1 (IGF-1) has been associated with thyroid stimulation and synergism with TSH to cause thyroid follicular growth. The elevated IGF-1 levels seen in patients with acromegaly are associated with a high rate of thyroid disorders, including goiter and nodules (19). In rodents, exposure to glucagon-like peptide-1 (GLP-1) agonists exhibits calcitonin (C)-cell effects including c-cell carcinomas. On the other hand, cell lines originating from human C-cells that are exposed to high dose GLP-1 do not demonstrate an increase in calcitonin secretion. Further, in human clinical trials there has been no demonstrable elevation in calcitonin levels nor the development of a medullary thyroid carcinoma derived from C-cells (20).

Thyroid nodules are caused by both the monoclonal and polyclonal expansion of cells. This was demonstrated when 9 multinodular glands were examined, a total of 16 monoclonal and 9 polyclonal nodules were found. One third of the glands contained exclusively monoclonal or polyclonal nodules. One third of the glands, however, contained both polyclonal and monoclonal nodules (21). Mutations including those of oncogenes and tumor suppressor genes, either sporadic or familial, are thought to play a role in the monoclonal expansion of cells seen in various different types of nodules. Activating mutations of the TSH receptor gene and Gs-alpha gene mutations can lead to the activation of adenylyl cyclase that is linked with cell proliferation and thyroid hormone production (22, 23). With the exception of a few genetic mutations (*BRAF V600E* with or without *TERT* mutation), there are no oncogenic markers exclusively associated with either benign or cancerous nodules. Rather, there is a broad overlap between the genetic alterations (mutations, fusions and, gene overexpression) between benign and malignant disease. The *RET/PTC* rearrangement has been associated with thyroid cancer occurring following radiation exposure. *RET/PTC 3* was characteristically associated with solid and invasive thyroid cancer following the Chernobyl nuclear accident. With time, *RET/PTC 3* rearrangement has declined in parallel with an increase in the *RET/PTC 1* subtype among *RET/PTC*-positive tumors (24).

Several genetic defects have been linked to congenital goiters and genetic predisposition is suggested by association in familial and twin studies. Genes associated with goiter formation include those that are involved in thyroid hormone syntheses, such as the thyroglobulin, thyroid peroxidase gene, sodium-iodide symporter, pendrin (Pendred syndrome), TSH receptor, and iodotyrosine deiodinase genes. There are several loci that have been associated with familial goiter, including MNG1 on chromosome 14q31, MNG2 on Xp22, and loci on chromosomes 2q, 3p, 7q, and 8p (25).

An increased prevalence of thyroid disease may be present in patients with inherited genetic syndromes including Cowden syndrome, Werner syndrome, familial adenomatous polyposis, multiple endocrine neoplasia type 2 (MEN type 2), and Carney complex (26). Cowden syndrome, a condition associated with *PTEN* gene mutations, is associated with a family history of cancer (including breast, uterine) and skin or tongue hamartomas. Cowden syndrome has an increased likelihood of benign and malignant thyroid disease. The risk of thyroid cancer is approximately 10% (27). Carney complex, associated with a mutation in the type 1 alpha regulatory subunit gene (*PRKAR1A*), is associated with thyroid nodules in up to 60 to 70% of patients but with malignant disease in less than 10% of patients (28). Familial adenomatous polyposis, associated with ACP gene mutations, has an incidence of thyroid cancer of up to 12% of patients. This syndrome is often associated with the cribriform variant of papillary thyroid cancer (29, 30). There is nearly 100% penetrance for the development of medullary thyroid cancer (MTC) in patients with MEN type 2 syndromes in which mutations of the RET proto-oncogene occurs. MEN2A is also associated with pheochromocytoma and primary hyperparathyroidism. MEN2B, on the other hand, is not associated with primary hyperparathyroidism. Most cases of MTC are sporadic and only 25% are familial. (see Chapter 9, "Medullary Thyroid Carcinoma in Medical Management of Thyroid Disease").

HISTORY AND EXAMINATION

Thyroid nodules may be asymptomatic and may come to attention either following careful palpation of the neck or an incidental finding on an imaging study. Alternatively, local compressive symptoms may be the reason for presentation.

History can provide clues for cancer risk assessment in nodules. The likelihood of harboring benign nodules increases with age, especially in women. The risk of cancer in a nodule is higher in men compared to women (8 vs 4%) (15). Thyroid cancer incidence is higher in younger

Table 7.1 US characteristics of thyroid nodules and risk for thyroid cancer (45–49)

Nodule characteristic	Sensitivity	Specificity	PPV
Hypoechogenicity	68–87%	43–81%	11–61%
Marked hypoechogenicity (similar to strap muscle)	27–41%	92–97%	68–80%
Solid consistency	89–91%	33–58%	26–39%
Microcalcification	36–59%	86–98%	39–85%
Macrocalcification	2–10%	96–98%	25–65%
Irregular/microlobulated margins	48–84%	83–92%	30–81%
Taller than wide configuration on transverse view	32–56%	91–93%	67–77%

patients (22.9%) compared with older patients (12.6%); the relative risk of malignancy decreases between ages 20 and 60 by 2.2% per year (31). There is an increased risk of thyroid cancer in patients with a history of head or neck radiation treatment. Up to 33% of nodules in patients with a history of head and neck radiation therapy are malignant (32–34).

Patients may present with symptoms such as a lump or swelling in the neck, hoarseness of voice, neck pressure or pain, cough, dyspnea, or dysphagia. History of the rapid growth of a nodule or cervical lymph node can give clues to the presence of a poorly differentiated or anaplastic thyroid cancer or a lymphoma. Very rapid growth over days, however, is usually due to cystic or hemorrhagic degeneration of a pre-existing thyroid nodule.

On physical examination, the characteristics of thyroid nodules, including location, consistency, dimensions, and number, need to be carefully recorded. Physical findings suggestive of malignancy include a hard, nontender nodule, fixation to adjacent tissue, and the presence of suspicious regional lymphadenopathy. It should be emphasized, however, that history and physical examination are often insufficient for diagnosing thyroid cancer in most patients.

LABORATORY TESTING

Serum TSH should be measured in all patients with a thyroid nodule by using a sensitive, third-generation assay. If TSH levels are lower than the reference range, this may warrant a thyroid scan to determine if the thyroid nodule is functional. A normal TSH does not, however, rule out the presence of an autonomous nodule (35). When

TSH levels were reviewed in 368 patients with known autonomous nodules from a relatively iodine-deficient area, 71% of the subjects had normal TSH levels. In this cohort, thyroid scans were performed in all patients during the work up of thyroid nodules, a practice that is no longer part of the routine evaluation of nodules. Routine measurement of serum thyroglobulin is not recommended (1, 2).

Currently, the issue of routine measurement of serum calcitonin in patients with thyroid nodules is controversial. The prevalence of MTC in patients with thyroid nodules ranges from 0.5 to 1.3% (36, 37). Measurement of calcitonin may lead to earlier detection of MTC because FNB cannot always distinguish between a MTC and a thyroid follicular lesion. Thus, calcitonin measurement may detect unsuspected MTC. For this reason, some experts recommend that serum calcitonin should be performed routinely in all patients with thyroid nodules. It is suggested that if basal calcitonin levels exceed 10 pg/mL, pentagastrin stimulation should be performed, and if peak calcitonin levels exceed 100 pg/mL, the risk of malignancy is sufficiently high that thyroidectomy is recommended (38). However, in the United States, routine calcitonin measurement is not endorsed in American practice guidelines because of the reduced specificity of unstimulated calcitonin levels (1, 2). False elevations of basal calcitonin may be seen in Hashimoto's thyroiditis, smokers, and those with renal impairment. Pentagastrin stimulation helps distinguish the falsely elevated levels from true malignancy. It is important to note, however, that pentagastrin is currently not available in the United States and most clinicians do not perform the alternate stimulation test with calcium infusion, limiting the specificity of calcitonin measurement. Additionally, there are concerns about the cost-effectiveness of calcitonin as a screening test, although in 2008 an investigator suggested that the routine use of calcitonin measurement in the evaluation of thyroid nodules appeared to be cost effective in the United States when compared to the measurement of TSH, colonoscopy, and mammography screening (39).

IMAGING

Ultrasonography

US is the primary imaging modality recommended to confirm the presence of a nodule, to document the presence of other more clinically significant nodules, to identify suspicious sonographic features in nodules, and to document the presence of abnormal regional adenopathy. Studies show poor concordance between physical examination and US findings (11, 40, 41). When a single nodule was detected by palpation, US showed that 48% of the glands contained more than one nodule; the majority (72%) of these newly detected nodules were less than 1 cm in diameter (40). Another study demonstrated that out of 169 subjects with abnormal thyroid glands on physical examination, there were corresponding nodules in 32% of the subjects on high-resolution US (41).

High-resolution US uses frequencies between 10 and 15 MHz, which enables examination of thyroid parenchyma and characterization of thyroid nodule features and volume. US enables risk stratification of thyroid nodules in a cost-effective way without exposure to ionizing radiation. It is, however, operator- and instrument-dependent, as high interobserver variability has been reported, especially for certain features such as nodule margins, volume, and presence of microcalcifications (42–44).

Careful documentation of the sonographic features should be recorded for each nodule, including, echogenicity, vascularity, margins, presence of calcifications, and size. Individually, these characteristics have varying sensitivity and specificity (Table 7.1). The classic high-risk sonographic features for cancer include a solid composition and the presence of microcalcifications, hypoechogenicity, irregular (infiltrative, undulating, lobulated) margins, and taller-than-wide configuration. Intranodular macrocalcification when present along with microcalcifications, but not necessarily when present alone, is associated with an increased risk of cancer. The presence of an interrupted peripheral calcification is also a high-risk feature, especially when seen with extranodular soft tissue growth beyond the calcification.

The features of follicular thyroid cancers differ compared to that of papillary thyroid cancers. Follicular thyroid cancer tends to be iso- or hyperechoic and is more likely to be associated with intranodular vascularity. Follicular lesions are less likely to harbor microcalcifications and are more likely to have a regular halo than papillary tumors (45, 50, 51).

Thyroid lymphomas are usually significantly hypoechoic and may be difficult to differentiate from a hypoechoic gland due to chronic thyroiditis. Thyroid lymphomas tend to be unilateral and relatively avascular by Doppler flow which may help distinguish it from a chronic thyroiditis (Figure 7.1).

Medullary thyroid cancer is generally hypoechoic and may be associated with intranodular calcification. The sonographic pattern overlaps with that seen in PTC. These tumors have a high likelihood of associated suspicious adenopathy.

It is equally important to be able to identify features of benign nodules to avoid unnecessary biopsies. A nodule with a spongiform appearance is defined as more than 50% of the nodule occupied by microcytic spaces. These lesions and purely cystic nodules are highly likely to be benign (1) and do not require biopsy unless there are clinical indications such as growth (Figure 7.2).

US of the thyroid gland is not complete without a visualization of the central and lateral neck nodes. An abnormal lymph node with metastatic disease is characterized by a rounded appearance (AP: longitudinal dimensions >0.5), presence of microcalcification, cystic appearance, and/or peripheral vascularity. The use of anatomic landmarks to identify the central and lateral compartments of the neck will ensure accurate localization for longitudinal observation of growth or development of abnormal sonographic characteristics and communication with surgeons regarding the location of abnormal lymph nodes if surgery is required. Level I compartment nodes include the submental and submandibular nodes. Levels II, III, and IV represent the area from superior to inferior that is bordered by the lateral edge of the carotid sheath medially and the lateral edge of the sternocleidomastoid muscle laterally. The carotid sheath contains the common carotid artery and the

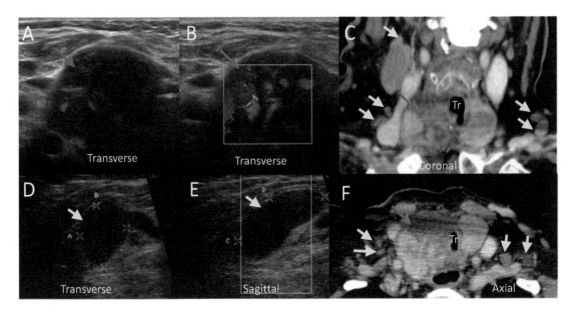

Figure 7.1 Large Cell Thyroid Lymphoma. Patient presented with dyspnea with a large hypoechoic thyroid, multiple enlarged cervical nodes, tracheal narrowing. Open biopsy was consistent with large cell thyroid lymphoma with metastatic nodes. **(A)** US transverse right lobe. **(B)** US transverse right lobe with Doppler. **(C)** CT coronal neck with enlarged heterogeneous thyroid with multiple small abnormal nodes. **(D)** Enlarged right level III nodes, transverse. **(E)** Enlarged right level III node, sagittal with Doppler. **(F)** CT axial neck showing more lymphoma involvement of the right lobe compared to the left lobe with tracheal deviation to the left and tracheal narrowing. Thyroid lymphoma (red arrows). Abnormal rounded lymph nodes (yellow arrows). Trachea (Tr).

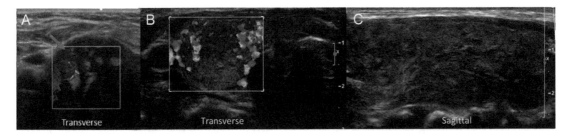

Figure 7.2 Lymphoma **(A)** compared to Hashimoto's thyroiditis **(B,C)**. The sonographic appearance of chronic thyroiditis and lymphoma have varying extent of hypoechoic echogenicity and heterogeneity but lymphoma tends not to be vascular by Doppler.

internal jugular vein. Level V is the area posterior to the lateral edge of the sternocleidomastoid muscle, also known as the posterior triangle. Level VI, which contains the thyroid gland, is bordered superiorly by the hyoid bone, inferiorly by the brachiocephalic artery, and laterally on either side by the medial edge of the carotid sheath. Inferior to the sternal notch are the level VII nodes (52).

Various organizations and investigators have proposed methods of risk stratification of thyroid nodules based on grayscale US characteristics through either pattern recognition or by developing a scoring system utilizing individual sonographic features (1, 2, 5, 53, 54). Most of these classification systems use a combination of nodule size and risk of cancer to determine whether a nodule should be considered for biopsy (Table 7.4). The American Thyroid Association, in their recent 2015 guidelines, recommends a five-tier stratification system based on US characteristics and patterns (Figure 7.3).

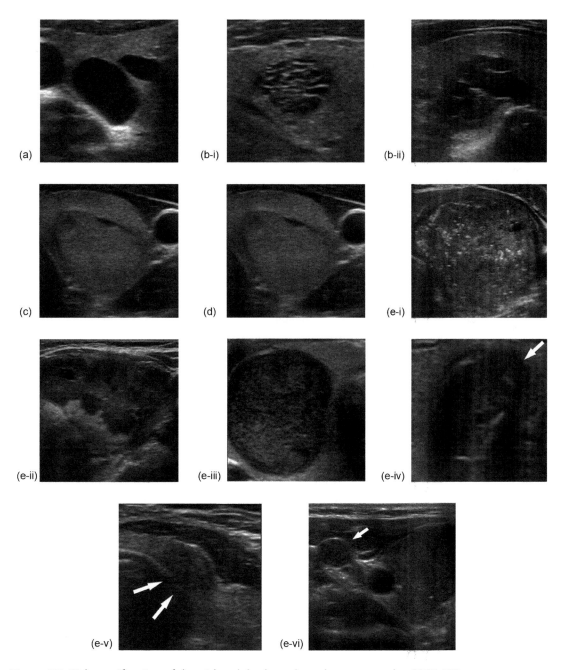

Figure 7.3 Risk stratification of thyroid nodules based on ultrasonography: 2015 ATA management guidelines for thyroid nodules and differentiated thyroid cancer (1). (a) Benign: Cystic nodule. (b) Very low suspicion: (i) Spongiform nodule and (ii) Partially cystic nodule with no suspicious features. (c) Low suspicion: Isoechoic nodule with regular margins. (d) Intermediate suspicion: Hypoechoic nodule. (e) High suspicion: Hypoechoic nodule with (1) Microcalcification, (2) Infiltrative/irregular margins, (3) Taller than wide configuration, (4) Rim calcification with small extrusion of soft tissue, (5) Evidence of extrathyroidal extension, and (6) Abnormal lymphadenopathy.

Table 7.2 Estimated malignancy risk based on ultrasound sonographic patterns and risk stratification system (1, 2, 53, 54, 58)

ATA 2015	AACE/ACE 2016	K-TIRADS	TIRADS – Russ
Benign 0%			TR 2: 0%
Very low suspicion < 3%	Low risk <1%	TR 2: Cystic <1% Spongiform <3%	TR 3: 0.25%
Low suspicion 5–10%	Intermediate risk 5–15%	TR 3: Low suspicion 3–15%	TR 4a: 6%
Intermediate suspicion 10–20%		TR 4: Intermediate suspicion 15–50%	
High suspicion >70–90%	High risk 50–90%		TR 4b: 69%
		TR 5: High suspicion >60%	TR 5: 100%

Table 7.3 A. ACR-TIRADSs thyroid grading system, B. ACR-TIRADS decision system (5)

A. Composition*	Echogenicity	Shape	Margin	Echogenic foci
Cystic 0	Anechoic 0	Wider than tall 0	Smooth 0	None 0
Spongiform 0	Hyper/isoechoic 1	Taller than wide 3	Ill-defined 0	Comet-tails 0
Mixed 1	Hypoechoic 2		Lobulated/ irregular 2	Macro 1
Solid 1	Very hypoechoic 3		ETE 3	Peripheral/rim 2
				Punctate 3
B. Points	**TIRADS Score**	**Classification**	**FNB**	**Follow-up US interval****
0	TR1	Benign	No FNB	Not required
2	TR2	Not suspicious	No FNB	Not required
3	TR3	Mildly suspicious	≥2.5 cm	If ≥1.5 cm, at years 1, 3, and 5
4–6	TR4	Moderately suspicious	≥1.5 cm	If ≥1 cm, at years 1, 2, 3, and 5
≥7	TR5	Highly suspicious	≥1.0 cm	If ≥0.5 cm, annually for 5 years

Summation of points from each column in panel A determines the TI-RADS score in panel B.
*Assign 2 points if the composition cannot be determined due to calcification. ETE is extrathyroidal extension.
**The follow-up intervals in this table are to detect uncommon cancer with a low-risk appearance (TR1, TR2) or false negative FNB but continued monitoring may be considered for nodule/goiter growth.

Using their recommendations, a biopsy should be considered for a hypoechoic nodule with or without additional high-risk features if >1 cm in maximal diameter and for an isoechoic nodule if >1.5 cm. When multiple nodules are found in a multinodular goiter, the nodule with the higher risk features should be selected for biopsy. When the nodular goiter contains multiple nodules with similar sonographic appearance, the largest nodule can be selected for biopsy. If a thyroid nodule is associated with an abnormal lymph node, the lymph node should be aspirated with or without biopsy of the nodule.

Thyroid Imaging Reporting and Data Systems (TIRADS) was originally developed in 2009 by Horvath and colleagues, with the concept of providing standardized reporting of nodule features while also directing future decisions on nodule evaluation and management, similar to the BIRADS classification for mammography findings (55). Subsequent iterations of this system have been proposed including by Kwak and colleagues, Russ and colleagues (French system), and the American College of Radiology (ACR) (5, 53, 56). In the ACR-TIRADS, for example, the scoring system assigns a numerical value for each US characteristic including composition (solid, cystic, mixed), echogenicity, shape, margins, and presence of echogenic foci. The associated score then dictates the size threshold for FNA and determines the interval for follow up if the FNA is benign (Table 7.3). The system developed by Russ et al. has the option of incorporating data on nodule stiffness from elastography measurements along with the grayscale US characteristics to stratify the cancer risk of individual nodules (57).

Thyroid scintigraphy

With increasing use of US and FNB in the diagnosis of thyroid nodules, the role of thyroid scintigraphy has declined. Indications for radioisotope scanning are to determine the functionality of a single nodule or nodules in a multinodular gland, to differentiate between Graves' disease and subacute thyroiditis, and to identify ectopic thyroid tissue (sublingual thyroid, mediastinal goiter, or struma ovarii) (Figures 7.4 and 7.5). Specifically,

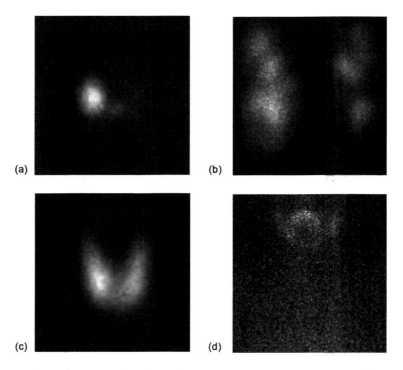

(a) (b) (c) (d)

Figure 7.4 Nuclear thyroid scintigraphy: The radionuclide scan may show several different patterns of function. The normal thyroid has a bi-lobed shape. Each lobe is located in a paratracheal position connected by an isthmus that crosses the trachea anteriorly at or just below the level of the cricoid cartilage. In a healthy subject, the radioisotope signal appears homogeneously distributed. Characteristically, salivary glands quantitatively have approximately the same amount of isotope trapping as the thyroid when visualized with ^{99m}Tc. Whereas, the salivary glands are not visualized with ^{123}I because images are obtained 6 to 24 hours later after the isotope has cleared from the salivary glands. (a) An autonomous hyperfunctioning (hot) nodule is characterized by focal increased uptake of isotope with reduced uptake in the rest of the thyroid gland to varying degrees due to suppression of endogenous serum TSH. (b) In an MNG, a pattern of inhomogeneous, irregular, or patchy uptake of functioning and nonfunctioning areas may be seen. The area of low uptake corresponds to a 'cold' nodule on ultrasound. (c) In Graves' disease, an enlarged gland has intense, diffuse, and homogeneous uptake occurs. (d) In subacute thyroiditis, there is low uptake throughout the thyroid gland when imaged during the hyperthyroid phase. Trapping can been seen in saliva/secretions in the nasopharynx.

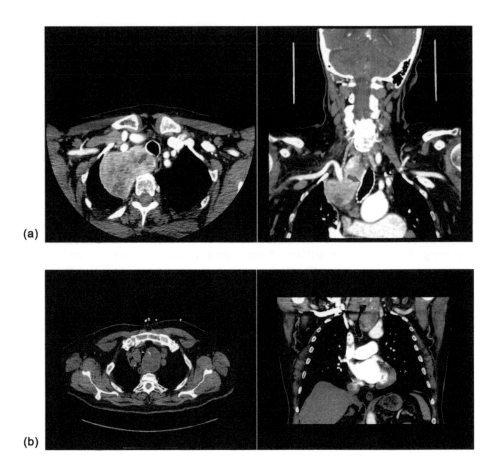

(a)

(b)

Figure 7.5 Nuclear scintigraphy and CT imaging of a mediastinal goiter: A 65-year-old male with an anterior mediastinal mass found on imaging. Further evaluation showed the lesion was iodine avid and consistent with a mediastinal goiter on **(a)** I123 thyroid scan and **(b)** fused SPECT/CT images. (SPECT = single-photon emission computed tomography.)

if a patient with a thyroid nodule has suppressed serum TSH levels, the next recommended step is a thyroid scan to determine whether the nodule is functional (1, 2). The AACE thyroid nodule guidelines also suggest that a thyroid scan may be considered in multinodular goiters, particularly in iodine deficient areas and independent of TSH levels, to detect functional autonomy (2). A nuclear thyroid scan may be helpful to exclude autonomous nodules from consideration of biopsy in the presence of multiple nodules meeting criteria for FNB based on US characteristics.

A gamma scintillation camera with a pinhole collimator is generally used for thyroid scanning; it has replaced the rectilinear scanner. The most commonly used radioisotope is radioiodine (^{123}I); technetium (^{99m}Tc) is used less frequently. Both isotopes are transported into thyroid follicular cells via the sodium-iodide symporter, but only iodine is organified and covalently attached to thyroglobulin and incorporated into hormone production. Because ^{99m}Tc is trapped but not organified, a nodule may appear functional (hot) on pertechnetate imaging and nonfunctional (cold) on ^{123}I imaging. In one study of 140 patients with hot or warm nodules on pertechnetate imaging, radioiodine scintigraphy revealed that 5% demonstrated no uptake in these nodules (59). Of these nodules, five were benign, one was a follicular carcinoma, and one was a papillary cancer with metastasis. For this reason, some caution against the use of ^{99m}Tc rather than ^{123}I for thyroid scintigraphy to avoid missing malignancy, while others feel the clinical implications are less significant (60).

The likelihood of carcinoma in cold thyroid nodules varies from approximately 5 to 15% (61–63). A

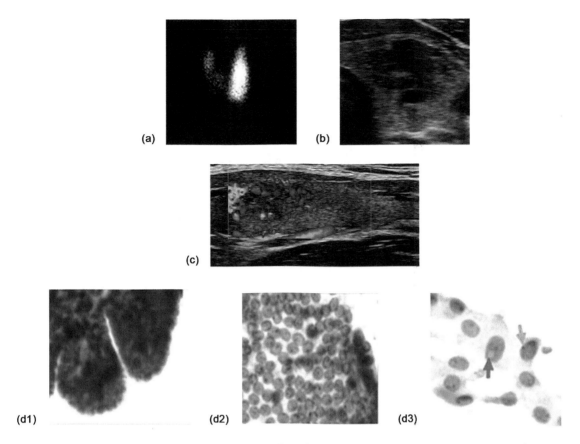

Figure 7.6 Autonomous thyroid nodule and papillary thyroid cancer: (a) Thyroid gland with a left side hyperfunctioning nodule on scintigraphy which on (b,c) Ultrasound showed a left side hypoechoic partially cystic nodule with irregular borders and increased nodular vascularity. (d) FNB cytology and subsequent surgical pathology confirmed the diagnosis of papillary thyroid cancer.

"hot nodule" has radioactive iodine uptake that is visibly higher in the nodule compared to the surrounding normal thyroid parenchyma. An autonomously functioning nodule is rarely malignant (62, 64); biopsy of scintigraphically "hot" nodules is usually not warranted. This is not true if there are concerning high-risk characteristics for cancer identified on US (Figure 7.6), as cases of thyroid cancer in functioning or hot nodules have been seen (65–67). However, most nodules are cold, and only 5 to 10% of palpable nodules are autonomous, highlighting the importance of correlating thyroid scintigraphy with thyroid US findings while making a management decision. Thyroid cancer in nodules with Graves' disease can be more aggressive and demonstrate a higher risk for multifocality, local invasion, and local and distant metastasis compared to those with autonomous thyroid nodules (68).

The aggressive disease has also been associated with toxic nodules, however (69).

Other imaging modalities

Magnetic resonance imaging or computed tomography is used occasionally to evaluate the size and extent of an MNG (Figure 7.7). These imaging techniques can be particularly helpful when evaluating substernal goiters and defining the relationship of the goiter to surrounding structures, especially to exclude tracheal compression. Neither technique separates benign from malignant thyroid nodules, and because of their relatively high cost, they are used less frequently than US (1, 2).

While the 18-FDG-PET scan is not recommended for the evaluation of a thyroid nodule,

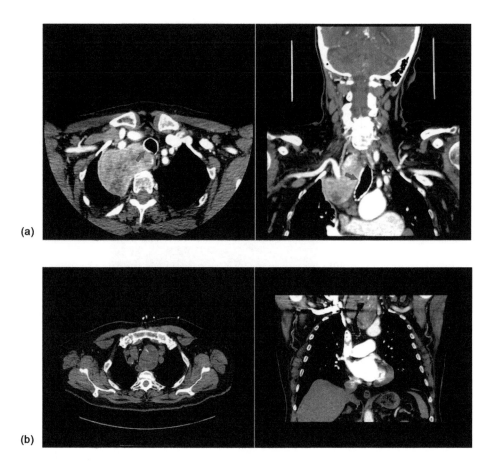

Figure 7.7 CT scan of goiter with mediastinal extension: **(a)** 70-year-old female with goiter with retrosternal extension causing tracheal deviation to the left without tracheal narrowing. **(b)** 71-year-old male with goiter with retrosternal extension with tracheal deviation and critical narrowing.

focal increased uptake in a thyroid nodule can indicate an increased risk of thyroid cancer. A meta-analysis of 1,051 cases of focal uptake on PET scan showed a 35% risk of thyroid malignancy compared to a 4% risk of malignancy in cases with diffuse uptake (70).

FINE NEEDLE BIOPSY AND CYTOLOGY

Fine needle biopsy (FNB) – now clearly considered the most accurate test for the evaluation of thyroid nodules – has emerged as safe and cost-effective.

Biopsies may be performed with direct palpation for solitary solid thyroid nodules, or as is now becoming standard, with US guidance. Ultrasound-guided FNB (US-FNB) biopsy should be considered for patients with small, impalpable, or partially cystic nodules, or those with previously insufficient cytology, especially when located inferiorly or posteriorly within the thyroid. There are many acceptable techniques for thyroid fine needle biopsy. Typically, 25- to 27-gauge needles are preferred to obtain specimens that are less bloody without compromising on cellularity (71). Excess blood in the biopsy specimen may obscure visualization of the follicular cells. Studies comparing capillary action (non-aspiration) and aspiration techniques have provided conflicting results with some showing no difference in non-diagnostic rates and some showing advantages of particular techniques (72–76). One study suggested, but did not show statistical significance, that the quality of the sample obtained when capillary action was used may be superior (76). It is best left up to the operator to determine the choice of biopsy technique based on experience and comfort level.

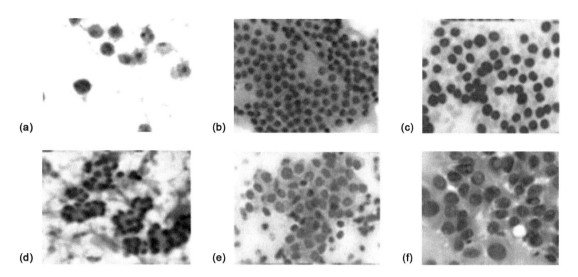

Figure 7.8 Bethesda categorization of thyroid cytology. (a) Bethesda 1: Nondiagnostic smear with scant follicular cells and histiocytes. (b) Bethesda II: Benign macrofollicles forming a flat sheet of cells. (c) Bethesda III: Atypia of undetermined significance/follicular lesion of undetermined significance–lesions with mild nuclear atypia or oncocytic changes; lesions with mixed microfollicles and macrofollicles. (d) Bethesda IV–predominantly microfollicular lesions. (e) Bethesda V: Suspicious for maglignancy - with some features suggestive of cancer. (f) Bethesda VI: Malignancy–definitive features of papillary thyroid cancer including nuclear atypia with a ground glass appearance, intranuclear cytoplasmic inclusions, nuclear clefts and grooves, and psammoma bodies.

Results of FNB can be categorized into four basic diagnostic groups: benign (negative), clinically suspicious (indeterminate), malignant (positive), and unsatisfactory (insufficient follicular cells or nondiagnostic). Classification systems have been devised to facilitate communication between cytopathologist, endocrinologist, and surgeons, and to help assign a risk of malignancy based on the diagnostic category. A commonly used classification of cytological findings, particularly in the United States, is the Bethesda system (77, 78).

The Bethesda classification system assigns the thyroid cytology into 6 categories, I–VI (Figure 7.8). In a meta-analysis of 25,445 thyroid FNB using the Bethesda system, the rate of assignment of a particular category varied considerably between investigators (Table 7.4) (79). The most common cytodiagnosis is that of adenomatoid (or "colloid") or benign thyroid nodule (Bethesda II). The colloid nodule shows abundant colloid, normal follicular cells, and some foam cells. Other benign diagnoses include cystic lesions (usually adenomatoid nodules with cystic degeneration), lymphocytic thyroiditis, and subacute (granulomatous, DeQuervain's) thyroiditis. The indeterminate category consists of specimens with features that are suggestive of but not diagnostic for malignancy. Atypia of undetermined significance (AUS) or follicular lesion of undetermined significance (FLUS) is used to describe the presence of focal or mild cytological atypia and/or architectural atypia. It is suggested that this category should be limited to 7% or less of the total biopsies (57). Follicular neoplasm or suspicious for follicular neoplasm (Bethesda IV) includes cases with high cellularity with follicular cells grouped in microfollicular or trabecular arrangements and scant colloid. Lesions classified as suspicious for malignancy (Bethesda V) or diagnostic for malignancy (Bethesda VI) hold the highest risk for malignancy. Hypocellular smears, which account for 5 to 15% of specimens, are considered nondiagnostic or unsatisfactory (Bethesda I). Most cytologists consider a satisfactory smear to contain at least 6 clusters of well-preserved cells, and each group must be composed of at least 10 cells from separate aspirates. Unsatisfactory smears usually result from poor biopsy technique, cystic lesions yielding fluid and foam cells, vascular lesions yielding too much blood, excessive air-drying, or poor smear preparation.

The risk of malignancy in each cytologic category will vary between institutions. When outlined by the State of the Science conference, it was estimated that the malignancy risk associated with the indeterminate categories of Bethesda III, IV, and V lesions would be 5 to 15%, 15 to 30%, and 60 to 75%, respectively (78). However, published data from various institutions shows the risk can range from 6 to 48% in Bethesda III, 14 to 49% in Bethesda IV, and 42 to 90% in Bethesda V nodules (80, 81). A wide range of malignancy risk in each Bethesda category is partly due to inter-observer variability in cytology diagnosis among cytopathologists, particularly for indeterminate cytologic categories (82, 83). More precise malignancy risk estimates than what is provided solely by these cytologic categories are needed for counseling patients and determining the optimal management plan. Awareness of an institution's malignancy rates for each category can help clarify the risk for indeterminate nodules and better guide the decision-making process.

FNB without molecular testing has a sensitivity of 65 to 98% (mean, 83%), a specificity of 72 to 100% (mean, 92%), and a diagnostic accuracy of 85 to 100% (mean, 95%). The predictive value of a cytological result that is positive or suspicious for malignancy is 75% (range, 50–96%). The false-negative rate may be as low as 1% and as high as 11% (mean, 5%), and false-positive rates range from 0% to 7% (mean, 5%) (84, 85). Recently, an expert panel proposed the reclassification of certain tumors as premalignant lesions, in other words, noninvasive follicular thyroid neoplasm with papillary-like nuclear features (NIFTP) (86). This change, as reflected in the newest version of the Bethesda classification system, would modify the expected risk of malignancy in each cytologic

category, particularly for Bethesda III, IV, and V (87–89) (Table 7.4).

Currently, there is a move toward incorporating the use of adjunctive genetic testing for indeterminate cytology results – Bethesda III and IV nodules (Table 7.4). Given the already high pre-test probability for cancer in lesions in the Bethesda V (suspicious for malignancy) category, molecular testing is generally not indicated. The Cancer Genome Atlas provided a comprehensive characterization of genetic alterations in papillary thyroid cancer (90). It classified papillary cancers based on the genetic mutation, associated downstream signaling pathways, and histopathologic characteristics into two categories—"*BRAF V600E*-like" and "*RAS*-like" tumors. Similarly, the genetic landscape of other thyroid cancers — medullary and poorly differentiated cancer — has been studied. Follicular adenomas and carcinomas, which are clonal expansions, have been associated with mutations in the *RAS* proto-oncogenes and *PAX8-PPAR gamma 1* fusion. Other mutations including *PTEN*, *RET* proto-oncogene (can be seen with radiation), and *THADA* are seen. Mutations and gene rearrangements leading to activation of the *MAPK* pathway can be seen in papillary thyroid cancers. These include *NTRK1* and *RET* proto-oncogene rearrangements, activating the mutation of *BRAF* and *RAS* and *RAS*-like genes. *TERT* mutations, when associated with other mutations such as *BRAF V600E,* are associated with more aggressive thyroid malignancy (91).

Molecular testing utilizes different techniques to risk stratify thyroid nodules with indeterminate cytology – detection of gene mutation/gene fusion products, analysis of gene expression

Table 7.4 Bethesda classification of thyroid nodule cytology (78, 79, 87–89)

Cytologic category	Percentage of cases – overall (range)	Risk of malignancy	Risk of malignancy (if NIFTP not considered malignancy)
Bethesda I	12.9 (1.8–23.6)	5–10%	5–10%
Bethesda II	59.3 (39–73.8)	0–3%	0–3%
Bethesda III	9.6 (3–27.2)	10–30%	6–18%
Bethesda IV	10.1 (1.2–25.3)	25–40%	10–40%
Bethesda V	2.7 (1.4–6.3)	50–75%	45–60%
Bethesda VI	5.4 (2–16.2)	97–99%	94–96%

Table 7.5 Performance characteristics of commercially available molecular testing for thyroid nodules with indeterminate cytology (92–95)

Molecular test	Cytology	Sensitivity	Specificity	Negative predictive value	Positive predictive value
Afirma	Bethesda III	90%	53%	95%	38%
Afirma	Bethesda IV	90%	49%	94%	37%
ThyroSeq	Bethesda III	91%	92%	97%	77%
ThyroSeq	Bethesda IV	90%	93%	96%	83%
ThyGenX + ThyraMIR	Bethesda III	94%	80%	97%	68%
ThyGenX + ThyraMIR	Bethesda IV	82%	91%	91%	82%

profiles, or detection microRNA markers. In the United States, the commercially available tests generally have better negative predictive values (NPV) of more than 90%, but variable positive predictive values (PPV) ranging from 38 to 83% (92–96) (Table 7.5).

ThyroSeq v.2 utilizes gene expression analysis and in a single-institution study showed a NPV of 96% and PPV of nearly 80% for the identification of thyroid cancer (93). It was initially considered a "rule in" test to detect thyroid cancer. However, a subsequent single-institution analysis demonstrated a lower PPV of 42% but with a NPV of 91%. Though, it is important to note that not all patients went to surgery, limiting the analysis of NPV and PPV (97). A new iteration of the test (ThyroSeq v.3) has incorporated additional gene mutations, deletions, and insertions, as well as gene copy number analysis to improve the sensitivity for the detection of malignancy. The test also sought to improve the categorization of Hürthle cell lesions, a notoriously challenging class of nodules. Initial analysis of the performance of Thyroseq v.3 at a single center reported a NPV of 97% and 98% for nodules with Bethesda III and IV cytology, respectively (98). The results of a multicenter, blinded, prospective study are pending.

Another commonly used test, initially called Afirma GEC (gene expression classifier), utilized a machine-trained algorithm to analyze patterns of gene expression and categorize nodules as either "benign" or "suspicious." A multicenter validation study found that this test is associated with a low PPV of 38% but an NPV of 95%, making it a good test to "rule out" malignancy (94). There were

concerns regarding the low benign-call rate with this test; some centers found a high percentage of nodules were assigned a "suspicious" expression pattern but ultimately had a low malignancy rate on surgical pathology. To improve the specificity of the test, the Gene Sequencing Classifier (GSC) was created; it employed a new computer-trained classifier utilizing RNA next generation sequencing and machine learning. In unpublished reports, the GSC assay increased the PPV while maintaining a high NPV.

The most commonly used commercially available molecular tests, ThyroSeq v.3 and Afirma GSC, are recommended only for Bethesda III and IV nodules. Their high NPV allows them to serve as "rule out" tests, avoiding unnecessary surgery in those nodules with a low likelihood of malignancy. Both ThyroSeq v3 and GSC will show whether a nodule contains the high-risk mutation, *BRAF V600E*, indicating a papillary thyroid carcinoma, but will also detect calcitonin and parathyroid hormone expression to preoperatively identify medullary thyroid carcinoma or a parathyroid adenoma, respectively. There are no direct comparisons of the performance of these tests yet. Side-by-side evaluation of these tests utilizing the existing studies are limited by differing malignancy rates at various institutions and small sample sizes (Table 7.5).

MANAGEMENT AND FOLLOW-UP

The management of thyroid nodules in a gland with a single nodule or a multinodular goiter depends on the etiology. There are three main reasons for which intervention is indicated: (a)

Either a suspicion for or definite diagnosis of cancer based on US characteristics, FNB, and molecular testing, (b) a nodule or nodular goiter causing local compressive symptoms or a nodule that is increasing in size over time, or (c) a toxic nodule or toxic multinodular goiter with thyroid hormone levels that warrant treatment. Any management decision must take into consideration the age of the patient and coexisting co-morbidities.

Thyroid nodules that are highly suspicious for thyroid cancer require a lobectomy or total thyroidectomy for diagnostic purposes. The management of nodules with a definitive diagnosis of cancer ranges from observation for small apparent low risk cancers, lobectomy for small tumors without evidence of invasion or nodal metastases, to total thyroidectomy with adjunctive treatment such as radioactive iodine therapy for higher risk cancers. Autonomously functioning nodules associated with hyperthyroidism may be treated with surgery, radioactive iodine therapy, or antithyroid drugs.

Surgical intervention may be considered for growing nodules or large nodules causing compressive symptoms, that is, hoarseness of voice, dysphagia, or dyspnea. The presence of tracheal narrowing, more importantly than deviation, should be sought in patients with large retrosternal goiters and dyspnea (1, 99).

Benign thyroid nodules can be observed conservatively. A retrospective study of 854 nodules followed over a mean of 4 years after an initial benign biopsy, demonstrated that only 30% of the nodules grew (more than 50% change in volume). Among the 172 nodules with initially benign cytology that did demonstrate an increase in size, only one nodule (0.6%) was found to be malignant. Overall, 10 malignant nodules were detected in the entire cohort and 8 of them had suspicious US features. Rosario and colleagues also demonstrated that initial or acquired suspicious US features rather than growth in nodule size following a benign biopsy was a higher risk for cancer (17.4% vs. 1.3%) (100).

For a nodule with a benign FNA cytology, the American Thyroid Association recommends repeating the US for nodules with high suspicion pattern in 1 year (1). In practice, many providers consider earlier repeat US and, potentially, repeat FNB for such high-risk nodules. Those nodules with low- to intermediate-suspicion US patterns and previous benign cytology should undergo repeat imaging in 1–2 years (1). Nodules with very low suspicion patterns (cystic and spongiform nodules) and nodules with two benign biopsies may not require additional surveillance US. The AACE guidelines recommend a follow up US at a 1-year interval, then, if stable, at a 2-year interval (2). The ACR TIRADS recommends repeating US at 1, 3, and 5 years for lower risk TR3 nodules and annual US for higher risk TR5 nodules for up to 5 years when the nodules do not meet the criteria for biopsy (5). Further monitoring can be stopped if there is no significant change in the size of the nodule. Significant growth is defined by the ATA (1) as a greater than 50% increase in nodule volume or more than 20% change in nodule diameter with a minimum of 2 mm growth in two or more dimensions. Since benign nodules may also grow, continued monitoring may be considered to assess for enlargement and the development of local compressive symptoms.

If an initial biopsy yields a nondiagnostic result, a repeat biopsy is recommended. A repeat biopsy with US guidance, especially for nodules without a predominantly cystic component, will be diagnostic in 60 to 80% of the cases (101–103). Overall, the frequency of malignancy in nodules with nondiagnostic biopsies is 2–4% (79, 104–106). However, if these nodules have high-risk US features (microcalcification, irregular margins, taller than wide configuration, or hypoechogenicity), the risk of malignancy may be as high as 25% (106). Previously, it was recommended to wait at least 3 months before repeating an US to avoid false positive results due to biopsy-induced reactive changes (107). Subsequent studies have not demonstrated a need to wait for repeat FNB; a shorter wait period before repeat aspiration attempts may be appropriate particularly for nodules with suspicious US features (108, 109).

Cystic nodules that are large and symptomatic may be aspirated for symptom control. In 60 to 90% of patients, there will be a recurrence of cystic fluid accumulation (110, 111). In such cases, a lobectomy or percutaneous ethanol injection (PEI) may be considered. The success rate of treating cystic nodules with PEI is 75 to 85% (112, 113). Radioactive iodine (RAI) therapy for obstructive goiter is an alternative to surgical therapy. The use of low-dose recombinant human TSH in preparation for RAI therapy can overcome issues of low isotope uptake in inactive areas of the gland (114, 115). Potential side effects, however, include a transient thyrotoxicosis, painful thyroiditis, thyroid swelling, and compression of the trachea.

TSH suppression therapy for benign nodules is no longer recommended. Only 30% will respond to this therapy with, at best, a modest reduction in gland size. Achieving the volume reduction requires suppressive dosing of thyroid hormone; the unwanted cardiovascular effects of suppressive therapy outweigh the potential benefit of volume reduction (99).

REFERENCES

1. Haugen BR, Alexander EK, Bible KC, et al. 2015 American Thyroid Association Management Guidelines for adult patients with thyroid nodules and differentiated thyroid cancer: The American thyroid association guidelines task force on thyroid nodules and differentiated thyroid cancer. *Thyroid* 2016;26(1):1–133.

2. Gharib H, Papini E, Garber JR, et al. American Association of Clincal Endocrinologists, American College of Endocrinology, and Associazione Medici Endocrinologi medical guidelines for clinical practice for the diagnosis and management of thyroid nodules – 2016 update. *Endocr. Pract.* 2016;22(5):622–39.

3. Paschke R, Cantara S, Crescenzi A, et al. European Thyroid Association Guidelines regarding thyroid nodule molecular fine-needle aspiration cytology diagnostics. *Eur. Thyroid J.* 2017;6(3):115–29.

4. Russ G, Bonnema SJ, Erdogan MF, et al L. European Thyroid Association Guidelines for ultrasound malignancy risk stratification of thyroid nodules in adults: The EU-TIRADS. *Eur. Thyroid J.* 2017;6(5):225–37.

5. Tessler FN, Middleton WD, Grant EG, et al. ACR thyroid imaging, reporting and data system (TI-RADS): White paper of the ACR TI-RADS committee. *J. Am. Coll. Radiol.* 2017;14(5):587–95.

6. Knudsen N, Perrild H, Christiansen E, et al. Thyroid structure and size and two-year follow-up of solitary cold thyroid nodules in an unselected population with borderline iodine deficiency. *Eur. J. Endocrinol.* 2000;142(3):224–30.

7. Tunbridge WM, Evered DC, Hall R, et al. The spectrum of thyroid disease in a community: The Whickham survey. *Clin. Endocrinol. (Oxf.)* 1977;7(6):481–93.

8. Caldwell KL, Makhmudov A, Ely E, et al. Iodine status of the U.S. population, National Health and Nutrition Examination Survey, 2005–2006 and 2007–2008. *Thyroid* 2011;21(4):419–27.

9. Vander JB, Gaston EA, Dawber TR. The significance of nontoxic thyroid nodules. Final report of a 15-year study of the incidence of thyroid malignancy. *Ann. Intern. Med.* 1968;69(3):537–40.

10. Mortensen J, Woolner LB, Bennett WA. Gross and microscopic findings in clinically normal thyroid glands. *J. Clin. Endocrinol. Metab.* 1955;15(10):1270–80.

11. Ezzat S, Sarti DA, Cain DR, Braunstein GD. Thyroid incidentalomas. Prevalence by palpation and ultrasonography. *Arch. Intern. Med.* 1994;154(16):1838–40.

12. Brander A, Viikinkoski P, Nickels J, Kivisaari L. Thyroid gland: US screening in a random adult population. *Radiology* 1991;181(3):683–7.

13. Werk EE, Vernon BM, Gonzalez JJ, et al. Cancer in thyroid nodules. A community hospital survey. *Arch. Intern. Med.* 1984;144(3):474–6.

14. Belfiore A, Giuffrida D, La Rosa GL, et al. High frequency of cancer in cold thyroid nodules occurring at young age. *Acta Endocrinol.* 1989;121(2):197–202.

15. Belfiore A, La Rosa GL, La Porta GA, et al. Cancer risk in patients with cold thyroid nodules: Relevance of iodine intake, sex, age, and multinodularity. *Am. J. Med.* 1992;93(4):363–9.

16. Frates MC, Benson CB, Doubilet PM, et al. Prevalence and distribution of carcinoma in patients with solitary and multiple thyroid nodules on sonography. *J. Clin. Endocrinol. Metab.* 2006;91(9):3411–7.

17. Taylor MS. Physiologic considerations in the genesis and management of nodular goiter. *Am. J. Med.* 1956;20(5):698–709.

18. Derwahl M, Broecker M, Kraiem Z. Thyrotropin may not be the dominant growth factor in benign and malignant

thyroid tumors. *J. Clin. Endocirnol. Metab.* 1999;84(3):829–34.

19. Dąbrowska AM, Tarach JS, Kurowska M, Nowakowski A. Thyroid diseases in patients with acromegaly. *Arch. Med. Sci.* 2014;10(4):837–45.

20. Hegedüs L, Moses AC, Zdravkovic M, et al. GLP-1 and calcitonin concentration in humans: Lack of evidence of calcitonin release from sequential screening in over 5000 subjects with type 2 diabetes or nondiabetic obese subjects treated with the human GLP-1 analog, liraglutide. *J. Clin. Endocrinol. Metab.* 2011;96(3):853–60.

21. Kopp P, Kimura ET, Aeschimann S, et al. Polyclonal and monoclonal thyroid nodules coexist within human multinodular goiters. *J. Clin. Endocrinol. Metab.* 1994;79(1):134–9.

22. Porcellini A, Ruggiano G, Pannain S, et al. Mutations of thyrotropin receptor isolated from thyroid autonomous functioning adenomas confer TSH-independent growth to thyroid cells. *Oncogene* 1997;15(7):781–9.

23. O'Sullivan C, Barton CM, Staddon SL, et al. Activating point mutations of the gsp oncogene in human thyroid adenomas. *Mol. Carcinog.* 1991;4(5):345–9.

24. Romei C, Elisei R. RET/PTC translocations and clinico-pathological features in human papillary thyroid carcinoma. *Front. Endocrinol.* 2012;3(3):54.

25. Böttcher Y, Eszlinger M, Tönjes A, Paschke R. The genetics of euthyroid familial goiter. *Trends Endocrinol. Metab.* 2005;16(7):314–9.

26. Richards ML. Familial syndromes associated with thyroid cancer in the era of personalized medicine. *Thyroid* 2010;20(7):707–13.

27. Dotto J, Nosé V. Familial thyroid carcinoma: A diagnostic algorithm. *Adv. Anat. Pathol.* 2008;15(6):332–49.

28. Stratakis CA, Courcoutsakis NA, Abati A, et al. Thyroid gland abnormalities in patients with the syndrome of spotty skin pigmentation, myxomas, endocrine overactivity, and schwannomas (carney complex). *J. Clin. Endocrinol. Metab.* 1997;82(7):2037–43.

29. Herraiz M, Barbesino G, Faquin W, et al. Prevalence of thyroid cancer in familial adenomatous polyposis syndrome and the role of screening ultrasound examinations. *Clin. Gastroenterol. Hepatol.* 2007;5(3):367–73.

30. Cetta F, Montalto G, Gori M, Curia MC, Cama A, Olschwang S. Germline mutations of the APC gene in patients with familial adenomatous polyposis-associated thyroid carcinoma: Results from a European Cooperative Study. *J. Clin. Endocrinol. Metab.* 2000;85(1):286–92.

31. Kwong N, Medici M, Angell TE, et al. The influence of patient age on thyroid nodule formation, multinodularity, and thyroid cancer risk. *J. Clin. Endocrinol. Metab.* 2015;100(12):4434–40.

32. Cerletty JM, Guansing AR, Engbring NH, et al. Radiation-related thyroid carcinoma. *Arch. Surg.* 1978;113(9):1072–6.

33. Favus MJ, Schneider AB, Stachura ME, et al. Thyroid cancer occurring as a late consequence of head-and-neck irradiation. Evaluation of 1056 patients. *N. Engl. J. Med.* 1976;294(19):1019–25.

34. Schneider AB, Shore-Freedman E, Ryo UY, et al. Radiation-induced tumors of the head and neck following childhood irradiation. Prospective studies. *Medicine* 1985;64(1):1–15.

35. Chami R, Moreno-Reyes R, Corvilain B. TSH measurement is not an appropriate screening test for autonomous functioning thyroid nodules: A retrospective study of 368 patients. *Eur. J. Endocrinol.* 2014;170(4):593–9.

36. Pacini F, Fontanelli M, Fugazzola L, et al. Routine measurement of serum calcitonin in nodular thyroid diseases allows the preoperative diagnosis of unsuspected sporadic medullary thyroid carcinoma. *J. Clin. Endocrinol. Metab.* 1994;78(4):826–9.

37. Niccoli P, Wion-Barbot N, Caron P, et al. Interest of routine measurement of serum calcitonin: study in a large series of thyroidectomized patients. The French Medullary Study Group. *J. Clin. Endocrinol. Metab.* 1997;82(2):338–41.

38. Costante G, Meringolo D, Durante C, et al. Predictive value of serum calcitonin levels for preoperative diagnosis of medullary thyroid carcinoma in a cohort of 5817 consecutive patients with thyroid nodules. *J. Clin. Endocrinol. Metab.* 2007;92(2):450–5.

39. Cheung K, Roman SA, Wang TS, et al. Calcitonin measurement in the evaluation of thyroid nodules in the United

States: A cost-effectiveness and decision analysis. *J. Clin. Endocrinol. Metab.* 2008;93(6):2173–80.

40. Tan GH, Gharib H, Reading CC. Solitary thyroid nodule. Comparison between palpation and ultrasonography. *Arch. Intern. Med.* 1995;155(22):2418–23.

41. Wiest PW, Hartshorne MF, Inskip PD, et al. Thyroid palpation versus high-resolution thyroid ultrasonography in the detection of nodules. *J. Ultrasound Med.* 1998;17(8):487–96.

42. Wienke JR, Chong WK, Fielding JR, et al. Sonographic features of benign thyroid nodules: Interobserver reliability and overlap with malignancy. *J. Ultrasound Med.* 2003;22(10):1027–31.

43. Lee HJ, Yoon DY, Seo YL, et al. Intraobserver and interobserver variability in ultrasound measurements of thyroid nodules. *J. Ultrasound Med.* 2018;37(1):173–8.

44. Brauer VFH, Eder P, Miehle K, et al. Interobserver variation for ultrasound determination of thyroid nodule volumes. *Thyroid* 2005;15(10):1169–75.

45. Papini E, Guglielmi R, Bianchini A, et al. Risk of malignancy in nonpalpable thyroid nodules: Predictive value of ultrasound and color-doppler features. *J. Clin. Endocrinol. Metab.* 2002;87(5):1941–6.

46. Kim EK, Park CS, Chung WY, et al. New sonographic criteria for recommending fine-needle aspiration biopsy of nonpalpable solid nodules of the thyroid. *Am. J. Roentgenol.* 2002;178(3):687–91.

47. Moon W-J, Jung SL, Lee JH, et al. Benign and malignant thyroid nodules: US differentiation—Multicenter retrospective study. *Radiology* 2008;247(3):762–70.

48. Nam SY, Roh J-L, Kim JS, Lee JH, Choi S-H, Kim SY. Focal uptake of (18) F-fluorodeoxyglucose by thyroid in patients with nonthyroidal head and neck cancers. *Clin. Endocrinol.* 2007;67(1):135–9.

49. Ahn SS, Kim E-K, Kang DR, et al. Biopsy of thyroid nodules: Comparison of three sets of guidelines. *Am. J. Roentgenol.* 2010;194(1):31–7.

50. Brito JP, Gionfriddo MR, Al Nofal A, et al. The accuracy of thyroid nodule ultrasound to predict thyroid cancer: Systematic review

and meta-analysis. *J. Clin. Endocrinol. Metab.* 2014;99(4):1253–63.

51. Jeh S, Jung SL, Kim BS, Lee YS. Evaluating the degree of conformity of papillary carcinoma and follicular carcinoma to the reported ultrasonographic findings of malignant thyroid tumor. *Korean J. Radiol.* 2007;8(3):192.

52. Robbins KT, Shaha AR, Medina JE, et al. Consensus statement on the classification and terminology of neck dissection. *Arch. Otolaryngol. Head Neck Surg.* 2008;134(5):536–8.

53. Russ G. Risk stratification of thyroid nodules on ultrasonography with the French TI-RADS: Description and reflections. *Ultrasonography* 2016;35(1):25–38.

54. Kwak JY, Jung I, Baek JH, et al. Image reporting and characterization system for ultrasound features of thyroid nodules: Multicentric Korean Retrospective Study. *Korean J. Radiol.* 2013;14(1):110.

55. Horvath E, Majlis S, Rossi R, et al. An ultrasonogram reporting system for thyroid nodules stratifying cancer risk for clinical management. *J. Clin. Endocrinol. Metab.* 2009;94(5):1748–51.

56. Kwak JY, Han KH, Yoon JH, et al. Thyroid imaging reporting and data system for US features of nodules: A step in establishing better stratification of cancer risk. *Radiology* 2011;260(3):892–9.

57. Russ G, Royer B, Bigorgne C, et al. Prospective evaluation of thyroid imaging reporting and data system on 4550 nodules with and without elastography. *Eur. J. Endocrinol.* 2013;168(5):649–55.

58. Na DG, Baek JH, Sung JY, et al. Thyroid imaging reporting and data system risk stratification of thyroid nodules: Categorization based on solidity and echogenicity. *Thyroid* 2016;26(4):562–72.

59. Reschini E, Ferrari C, Castellani M, et al. The trapping-only nodules of the thyroid gland: Prevalence study. *Thyroid* 2006;16(8):757–62.

60. Dige-Petersen H, Kroon S, Vadstrup S, et al. A comparison of 99Tc and 123I scintigraphy in nodular thyroid disorders. *Eur. J. Nucl. Med.* 1978;3(1):1–4.

61. Gharib H. Changing concepts in the diagnosis and management of thyroid nodules. *Endocrinol. Metab. Clin. North Am.* 1997;26(4):777–800.

62. Cases JA, Surks MI. The changing role of scintigraphy in the evaluation of thyroid nodules. *Semin. Nucl. Med.* 2000;30(2):81–7.

63. Burch HB. Evaluation and management of the solid thyroid nodule. *Endocrinol. Metab. Clin. North Am.* 1995;24(4):663–710.

64. Hamburger JI. Evolution of toxicity in solitary nontoxic autonomously functioning thyroid nodules. *J. Clin. Endocrinol. Metab.* 1980;50(6):1089–93.

65. Abdel-Razzak M, Christie JH. Thyroid carcinoma in an autonomously functioning nodule. *J. Nucl. Med.* 1979;20(9):1001–2.

66. Miller JM. Re: Thyroid carcinoma in an autonomously functioning nodule. *J. Nucl. Med.* 1980;21(3):296–7.

67. Hoving J, Piers DA, Vermey A, Oosterhuis JW. Carcinoma in hyperfunctioning thyroid nodule in recurrent hyperthyroidism. *Eur. J. Nucl. Med.* 1981;6(3):131–2.

68. Belfiore A, Garofalo MR, Guiffrida D, et al. Increased aggressiveness of thyroid cancer in patients with Graves' disease. *J. Clin. Endocrinol. Metab.* 1990;70(4):830–5.

69. Hayes FJ, Sheahan K, Heffernan A, McKenna TJ. Aggressive thyroid cancer associated with toxic nodular goitre. *Eur. J. Endocrinol.* 1996;134(3):366–70.

70. Soelberg KK, Bonnema SJ, Brix TH, Hegedüs L. Risk of malignancy in thyroid incidentalomas detected by ^{18}F-fluorodeoxyglucose positron emission tomography: A systematic review. *Thyroid* 2012;22(9):918–25.

71. Cibas ES. Fine-needle aspiration in the work-up of thyroid nodules. *Otolaryngol. Clin. North Am.* 2010;43(2):257–71.

72. Zhou JQ, Zhang JW, Zhan WW, et al. Comparison of fine-needle aspiration and fine-needle capillary sampling of thyroid nodules: A prospective study with emphasis on the influence of nodule size. *Cancer Cytopathol.* 2014;122(4):266–73.

73. Tublin ME, Martin JA, Rollin LJ, et al. Ultrasound-guided fine-needle aspiration versus fine-needle capillary sampling biopsy of thyroid nodules: Does technique matter? *J. Ultrasound Med.* 2007;26(12):1697–701.

74. Buzdugă CM, Găleşanu C, Vulpoi C, et al. Thyroid fine-needle biopsy: Aspiration versus capillary. *Rev. Med. Chir. Soc. Med. Nat. Iasi.* 2015;119(1):45–50.

75. Romitelli F, Di Stasio E, Santoro C, et al. A comparative study of fine needle aspiration and fine needle non-aspiration biopsy on suspected thyroid nodules. *Endocr. Pathol.* 2009;20(2):108–13.

76. Mair S, Dunbar F, Becker PJ, Du Plessis W. Fine needle cytology—Is aspiration suction necessary? A study of 100 masses in various sites. *Acta Cytol.* 1989;33(6):809–13.

77. Baloch ZW, Cibas ES, Clark DP, et al. The National Cancer Institute thyroid fine needle aspiration state of the science conference: A summation. *Cytojournal* 2008;5(1):6.

78. Cibas ES, Ali SZ. The Bethesda system for reporting thyroid cytopathology. *Thyroid* 2009;19(11):1159–65.

79. Bongiovanni M, Spitale A, Faquin WC, et al. The Bethesda system for reporting thyroid cytopathology: A meta-analysis. *Acta Cytol.* 2012;56(4):333–9.

80. Wang CC, Friedman L, Kennedy GC, et al. A large multicenter correlation study of thyroid nodule cytopathology and histopathology. *Thyroid* 2011;21(3):243–51.

81. Valderrabano P, McIver B. Evaluation and Management of indeterminate thyroid nodules: The revolution of risk stratification beyond cytologic diagnosis. *Cancer Control* 2017;24(5):1–14.

82. Yang J, Schnadig V, Logrono R, Wasserman PG. Fine-needle aspiration of thyroid nodules: A study of 4703 patients with histologic and clinical correlations. *Cancer* 2007;111(5):306–15.

83. Walts AE, Bose S, Fan X, et al. A simplified Bethesda system for reporting thyroid cytopathology using only four categories improves intra- and interobserver diagnostic agreement and provides non-overlapping estimates of malignancy risks. *Diagn. Cytopathol.* 2012;40(S1):E62–8.

84. Gharib H. Fine-needle aspiration biopsy of thyroid nodules: Advantages, limitations, and effect. *Mayo Clin. Proc.* 1994;69(1):44–9.

85. Gharib H, Goellner JR. Fine-needle aspiration biopsy of the thyroid: An appraisal. *Ann. Intern. Med.* 1993;118(4):282–9.

86. Nikiforov YE, Seethala RR, Tallini G, et al. Nomenclature revision for encapsulated follicular variant of papillary thyroid carcinoma. *JAMA Oncol.* 2016;2(8):1023–9.

87. Strickland KC, Howitt BE, Marqusee E, et al. The impact of noninvasive follicular variant of papillary thyroid carcinoma on rates of malignancy for fine-needle aspiration diagnostic categories. *Thyroid* 2015;25(9):987–92.

88. Faquin WC, Wong LQ, Afrogheh AH, et al. Impact of reclassifying noninvasive follicular variant of papillary thyroid carcinoma on the risk of malignancy in The Bethesda System for Reporting Thyroid Cytopathology. *Cancer Cytopathol.* 2016;124(3):181–7.

89. Cibas ES, Ali SZ. The 2017 Bethesda system for reporting thyroid cytopathology. *Thyroid* 2017;27(11):1341–6.

90. Agrawal N, Akbani R, Aksoy BA, et al. Integrated genomic characterization of papillary thyroid carcinoma. *Cell* 2014;159(3):676–90.

91. Nikiforov YE. Role of molecular markers in thyroid nodule management: Then and now. *Endocr. Pract.* 2017;23(8):979–88.

92. Nikiforov YE, Carty SE, Chiosea SI, et al. Highly accurate diagnosis of cancer in thyroid nodules with follicular neoplasm/suspicious for a follicular neoplasm cytology by ThyroSeq v2 next-generation sequencing assay. *Cancer* 2014;120(23):3627–34.

93. Nikiforov YE, Carty SE, Chiosea SI, et al. Impact of the multi-gene ThyroSeq next-generation sequencing assay on cancer diagnosis in thyroid nodules with atypia of undetermined significance/follicular lesion of undetermined significance cytology. *Thyroid* 2015;25(11):1217–23.

94. Alexander EK, Kennedy GC, Baloch ZW, et al. Preoperative diagnosis of benign thyroid nodules with indeterminate cytology. *N. Engl. J. Med.* 2012;367(8):705–15.

95. Labourier E, Shifrin A, Busseniers AE, et al. Molecular testing for miRNA, mRNA, and DNA on fine-needle aspiration improves the preoperative diagnosis of thyroid nodules with indeterminate cytology. *J. Clin. Endocrinol. Metab.* 2015;100(7):2743–50.

96. Lithwick-Yanai G, Dromi N, Shtabsky A, et al. Multicentre validation of a microRNA-based assay for diagnosing indeterminate thyroid nodules utilising fine needle aspirate smears. *J. Clin. Pathol.* 2017;70(6):500–7.

97. Valderrabano P, Khazai L, Leon ME, et al. Evaluation of ThyroSeq v2 performance in thyroid nodules with indeterminate cytology. *Endocr. Relat. Cancer* 2017;24(3):127–36.

98. Steward DL, Carty SE, Sippe RS, et al. Clinical validation of ThyroSeq v3 performance in thyroid nodules with indeterminate cytology: A prospective blinded multi-institutional validation study. *Thyroid* 2017;(27)S1: A-168.

99. Knobel M. Which Is the ideal treatment for benign diffuse and multinodular non-toxic goiters? *Front. Endocrinol. (Lausanne)* 2016;7:48.

100. Rosário PW, Purisch S. Ultrasonographic characteristics as a criterion for repeat cytology in benign thyroid nodules. *Arq. Bras. Endocrinol. Metabol.* 2010;54(1):52–5.

101. Alexander EK, Heering JP, Benson CB, et al. Assessment of nondiagnostic ultrasound-guided fine needle aspirations of thyroid nodules. *J. Clin. Endocrinol. Metab.* 2002;87(11):4924–7.

102. Orija I, Piñeyro M, Biscotti C, et al. Value of repeating a nondiagnostic thyroid fine-needle aspiration biopsy. *Endocr. Pract.* 2007;13(7):735–42.

103. Choi YS, Hong SW, Kwak JY, et al. Clinical and ultrasonographic findings affecting nondiagnostic results upon the second fine needle aspiration for thyroid nodules. *Ann. Surg. Oncol.* 2012;19(7):2304–9.

104. Theoharis CGA, Schofield KM, Hammers L, et al. The Bethesda thyroid fine-needle aspiration classification system: Year 1 at an academic institution. *Thyroid* 2009;19(11):1215–23.

105. Luu MH, Fischer AH, Pisharodi L, Owens CL. Improved preoperative definitive diagnosis of papillary thyroid carcinoma in FNAs prepared with both ThinPrep and conventional

smears compared with FNAs prepared with ThinPrep alone. *Cancer Cytopathol.* 2011;119(1):68–73.

106. Moon HJ, Kwak JY, Choi YS, Kim E-K. How to manage thyroid nodules with two consecutive non-diagnostic results on ultrasonography-guided fine-needle aspiration. *World J. Surg.* 2012;36(3):586–92.

107. Layfield LJ, Abrams J, Cochand-Priollet B, et al. Post-thyroid FNA testing and treatment options: A synopsis of the National Cancer Institute Thyroid Fine Needle Aspiration State of the Science Conference. *Diagn. Cytopathol.* 2008;36(6):442–8.

108. Singh RS, Wang HH. Timing of repeat thyroid fine-needle aspiration in the management of thyroid nodules. *Acta Cytol.* 2011;55(6):544–8.

109. Lubitz CC, Nagarkatti SS, Faquin WC, et al. Diagnostic yield of nondiagnostic thyroid nodules is not altered by timing of repeat biopsy. *Thyroid* 2012;22(6):590–4.

110. Bennedbæk FN, Hegedüs L. Treatment of recurrent thyroid cysts with ethanol: A randomized double-blind controlled trial. *J. Clin. Endocrinol. Metab.* 2003;88(12):5773–7.

111. Valcavi R, Frasoldati A. Ultrasound-guided percutaneous ethanol injection therapy in thyroid cystic nodules. *Endocr. Pract.* 2004;10(3):269–75.

112. Antonelli A, Campatelli A, Vito A, et al. Comparison between ethanol sclerotherapy and emptying with injection of saline in treatment of thyroid cysts. *Clin. Investig.* 1994;72(12):971–4.

113. Verde G, Papini E, Pacella CM, et al. Ultrasound guided percutaneous ethanol injection in the treatment of cystic thyroid nodules. *Clin. Endocrinol.* 1994;41(6):719–24.

114. Huysmans DA, Nieuwlaat W-A, Erdtsieck RJ, et al. Administration of a single low dose of recombinant human thyrotropin significantly enhances thyroid radioiodide uptake in nontoxic nodular goiter. *J. Clin. Endocrinol. Metab.* 2000;85(10):3592–6.

115. Nielsen VE, Bonnema SJ, Hegedüs L. Effects of 0.9 mg recombinant human thyrotropin on thyroid size and function in normal subjects: A randomized, double-blind, cross-over trial. *J. Clin. Endocrinol. Metab.* 2004;89(5):2242–7.

8

Differentiated thyroid carcinoma

CAROLYN MAXWELL AND JENNIFER A. SIPOS

Introduction	182	Initial risk assessment	195
Epidemiology	182	Risk stratification based upon the	
Oncogenesis	183	patient's clinical status after initial	
BRAF	183	therapy	195
TERT	184	Serum thyroglobulin in initial risk	
RAS	184	assessment	196
Risk factors for the development of thyroid		Imaging in initial risk assessment	197
carcinoma	185	Thyroid hormone therapy	197
Tumor histology	186	Levothyroxine (T4) suppression of TSH	197
Papillary thyroid carcinoma	186	Radioiodine (^{131}I) therapy	198
Papillary microcarcinoma	186	Goals of therapy	198
Papillary cancer within a thyroglossal duct	187	Decision to use ^{131}I therapy	199
Follicular variant papillary carcinoma		Preparation for ^{131}I therapy	200
(FVPTC)	188	Diagnostic whole-body ^{131}I scan and the	
Noninvasive follicular neoplasm with		stunning effect	201
papillary-like nuclear features (NIFTP)	188	Determining the appropriate ^{131}I	
Tall cell variant of PTC	188	administered activity	201
Columnar cell variant of PTC	189	Thyroid remnant ablation	201
Diffuse sclerosing variant of PTC	189	^{131}I adjuvant therapy	201
Hobnail variant of PTC	189	Treatment of residual, recurrent, or	
Follicular thyroid carcinoma	189	metastatic carcinoma with ^{131}I	201
Hürthle cell carcinoma (HCC)	190	Posttreatment scans	202
Tumor staging systems and prognostic		Complications of ^{131}I	202
scoring systems	191	Immediate complications	202
Factors influencing prognosis and affecting		Long-term complications	203
outcome	191	Leukemia and second primary	
Treatment of papillary and follicular thyroid		malignancy	203
carcinomas	192	Therapies for advanced thyroid cancer	203
Preoperative imaging	192	External beam radiation therapy (EBRT)	203
Surgery	192	Thermoablation	204
Lymph node dissection	194	Long-term follow-up and monitoring	205
Completion thyroidectomy	194	Thyroglobulin monitoring	205
Surgical complications	194	Imaging	205
Thyroidectomy during pregnancy	194	Response to therapy	207

Excellent response to therapy 207
Biochemical incomplete response to
  therapy—Elevated Tg and negative
  imaging 207

Structural incomplete response to
  therapy—Recurrent or metastatic
  disease 207
References 209

INTRODUCTION

Thyroid carcinoma comprises a spectrum of malignancies ranging from rarely lethal, slow-growing neoplasms to among the most aggressive cancers to afflict humanity. Differentiated thyroid cancers (those which are derived from follicular cells, including papillary, follicular, and Hürthle cell types) are typically associated with excellent survival rates. The goals of patient management are to minimize morbidity and mortality from cancer (tumor recurrence, metastases, and death) as well as from therapy [surgery, hypothyroidism, iodine-131 (^{131}I) therapy, thyroid-stimulating hormone (TSH) suppression] while still achieving a favorable outcome. And although staging systems predict outcome reasonably well, they remain inexact. Thus, while the majority of patients can be reassured that they are likely to do well, this outcome cannot be absolutely guaranteed. It is increasingly recognized that additional features not captured by traditional staging play an important role in predicting outcomes for individual patients. Consequently, the treatment paradigms for patients with differentiated thyroid cancer are rapidly shifting. This chapter will outline how to utilize prognostic features to determine the individual management strategy in patients with differentiated thyroid carcinoma.

EPIDEMIOLOGY

Thyroid cancer is the fifth most common malignancy in women and the eleventh most common cancer overall (1). Papillary thyroid carcinoma (PTC) accounts for approximately 80% of all thyroid carcinomas in the United States (1) (Table 8.1). Approximately 56,870 new cases of thyroid cancer and 2,010 disease-specific deaths occur each year in the United States (1). Thyroid cancer is nearly three times more common in women than in men. It may occur at any age but is most commonly diagnosed in adults aged 45–54 years old (1). Thyroid cancer death rates overall are <2% but vary significantly among the various types of thyroid cancer (2) (Table 8.1).

Data from the National Cancer Institute's Surveillance, Epidemiology, and End Results (SEER) program, demonstrate that the incidence of thyroid cancer steadily increased over the past three decades, increasing from a rate of 4.8 per 100,000 in 1975 to 15.0 per 100,000 in 2014, although more recently this rate has levelled off, with a rate ranging from 13.9 to 15.0 per 100,000 from 2009–2017 (3). The increasing incidence is attributable to papillary cancers; rates of diagnosis of other histologic types of thyroid cancer are stable (4). It is widely believed that much of the increased incidence is attributable to overdiagnosis, likely due to the widespread availability of radiology procedures unrelated to the thyroid, including CT scans, MRI, carotid Doppler, and FDG-PET scans. Such imaging leads to the discovery of "incidental" tumors that otherwise may have remained undetected. This theory is supported by data from autopsy studies which reveal papillary microcarcinomas in as many as 5–15% of cases, a prevalence that is 1000-fold higher than what is clinically diagnosed (5). Further evidence in support of the overdiagnosis theory is that the

Table 8.1 Incidence and survival rates of thyroid cancer

Cancer type	Frequency (%)	10-Year relative survival (%)	
		Females	Males
Papillary	81	99	99
Follicular	10	93	90
Hürthle	3.6	76	76
Medullary	3.2	87	68
Anaplastic	1.7	12	14

From Gilliland et al. 1997 (297) and Hundahl 1998 (142).

increased incidence of thyroid cancer is largely due to small tumors, 49% measuring <1 cm, and 87% measuring 2 cm or less (6), and that mortality has remained stable or improved slightly during this timeframe (7). More recent analysis of SEER data between 1974–2013, however, finds that alongside the rising incidence of small tumors, there has also been an increase in incidence rates of tumors of all sizes, including advanced stage papillary thyroid cancers larger than 5 cm. This suggests that the increased incidence over the past three decades is not solely attributable to an overdiagnosis bias (8).

Oncogenesis

The MAPK (mitogen-activated protein kinase) pathway is an intracellular signaling cascade that is initiated on the cell surface by binding of a signaling molecule to a transmembrane receptor, leading to phosphorylation of various downstream proteins and ultimately resulting in changes in cellular activity such as growth, proliferation, and apoptosis (see Figure 8.1). Oncogenic mutations in one of these signaling components alter the normal feedback control of these activities, resulting in constitutive activation of growth and proliferation or inhibition of apoptosis. The MAPK pathway is activated in the majority of thyroid cancers, either through a mutation in *RAS* or *BRAF* or a gene rearrangement in *RET/PTC* or *NTRK* (see Table 8.2). These mutations are almost always mutually exclusive, suggesting

that activation of one component of the pathway is sufficient to drive malignant transformation (9). Detection of these mutations may be used for preoperative identification of malignancy on FNA (see Chapter 7, "Thyroid Nodules and Multinodular Goiter"). Additionally, the identification of particular mutations is being increasingly used to prognosticate patients with thyroid cancer (see the section on Factors Influencing Prognosis). Drugs that target kinases in the MAP kinase pathway are important components of treatment in patients with progressive radioiodine-refractory disease.

BRAF

BRAF is a serine/threonine kinase in the MAPK-signaling pathway. When activated, it regulates cell differentiation, proliferation, and survival. The *BRAF V600E* pathogenic variant is the most common oncogene in sporadic PTC in adults (10); the incidence varies with the geographical location of the population, with reports ranging from 36 to 69% (11). *BRAF V600E* has been associated with tumors with more aggressive features such as lymph node metastases, extrathyroidal extension, and higher rates of recurrence (12), and in one study was a strong predictor of age-associated mortality in patients with PTC (13). Such findings have produced significant interest in the prognostic utility of a *BRAF* mutation; however, studies attempting to establish whether *BRAF* serves as an independent predictor of recurrence risk have

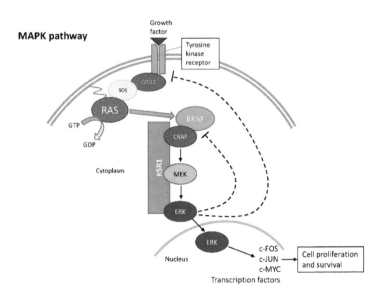

Figure 8.1 The MAPK cell signaling pathway.

Table 8.2 Common oncogenic mutations and their relative frequency

Cancer type	Mutations	Relative frequency (%)
PTC	BRAF	30–70
	RET/PTC	20
	RAS	10
	NTRK3	1–2
FTC	RAS (K, N, and H subtypes)	45
	PAX8/PPARγ	25
	PIK3CA	10–30
HCC	TP53	40
	PTEN	25
	RAS	20
	TERT	13
	MEN1	4

Derived from data in the following references: Chindris 2012 (277); Wei 2016 (301); Kasaian 2015 (299); Ganly 2013 (300).

produced mixed results (12, 14–17). Because *BRAF* is often associated with higher-risk clinico-pathologic features, it is yet to be determined what portion of poorer outcomes seen with *BRAF* mutation is attributable to the mutation itself apart from the pathological features (18). Further, the majority of new thyroid cancer diagnoses are considered to be low-risk tumors with an excellent prognosis (19), yet a large proportion of these tumors will harbor a *BRAF* mutation (11). Indeed, the majority of patients with a *BRAF* mutation will have an excellent outcome. Therefore, the high prevalence of *BRAF* limits its specificity as a prognostic variable (18), though it remains an active area of clinical interest and research.

TERT

Telomerase reverse transcriptase (*TERT*) promoter mutations are newly described in thyroid cancers (20, 21). The normal function of these enzymes and associated proteins is to add tandem repeats of the TTAGGG sequence to the end of chromosomes and maintain chromosomal integrity and genome stability (22). Highly expressed in germ line and stem cells, telomerase is considerably less expressed or even repressed in somatic cells (23). Loss of telomeres in somatic cells during cell division results in cells entering senescence (23). Reactivation of telomerase in somatic cells leads to immortalization by way of proliferation without restriction and inactivation of replicative senescence (24).

A 2014 study suggested that the presence of a *TERT* mutation was associated with a more aggressive clinical course (25), but subsequent studies were unable to confirm these results (26–28). However, a recent meta-analysis of 11 studies found that *TERT* promoter mutations rarely occur alone; they are most often found accompanying a *BRAF* mutation (29). The presence of both *BRAF* and *TERT* mutations is associated with a more aggressive clinical course (29) and higher mortality rates (30). Further study is needed to determine if a *TERT* mutation can be targeted with pharmacologic therapy.

RAS

The *RAS* oncogenes regulate two signaling pathways in the development of thyroid cancer, the MAP kinase cascade and the PI3K/Akt pathway (11). Activating mutations in its three proto-oncogenes—*HRAS*, *NRAS*, and *KRAS*—may be seen in benign follicular adenomas or malignant thyroid lesions. Mutations in *RAS* genes are most commonly seen in follicular tumors, with up to 45% of follicular thyroid carcinoma (FTC) and follicular variant of papillary thyroid carcinoma (FVPTC) harboring such pathogenic variants. Up to 20% of poorly differentiated and anaplastic carcinomas may also reveal one of these oncogenes (31). Recent data have helped define the clinical significance of *RAS* mutations, showing that differentiated cancers harboring *RAS* mutations have an excellent prognosis

(31, 32) and that cytologically benign, *RAS*-positive thyroid nodules have long-term stability when serially examined sonographically (33).

Risk factors for the development of thyroid carcinoma

A small group of nonmedullary thyroid cancers appear to be inherited, most of which are PTC. So-called "familial nonmedullary thyroid cancer (FNMTC)" is inherited as an autosomal dominant trait with incomplete penetrance and variable expressivity. It does not appear to be inherited at a single locus for the majority of families, but rather is due to multiple low penetrance alleles and environmental factors (34). The definition of FNMTC is inconsistent across studies; consequently, the frequency of this condition is unclear, but likely represents less than 5% of DTC cases. The identification of two first-degree relatives with thyroid cancer is estimated to have a 40–60% risk of representing sporadic disease, whereas the presence of three affected first-degree relatives imparts a 96% probability of an inherited condition (35). The phenotype of FNMTC and whether it is characterized by an earlier age of onset with a more aggressive disease course is controversial (36–39). The studies are limited by small sample sizes and variable definitions of inherited disease.

Given the rising incidence of thyroid cancer, there is great interest in potential environmental etiologic factors. Exposure to ionizing radiation during childhood is the best understood cause of papillary, and less commonly, follicular thyroid carcinoma. Treatment of benign conditions of the head and neck, such as acne, tonsillitis, and sinusitis, with radiation therapy was commonplace in the 1940s and 1950s. Fortunately, such treatments are no longer used, but their carcinogenic effects are still seen more than 60 years later (40). Other identified sources of radiation exposure include targeted irradiation of childhood head and neck cancers and exposure to fallout from nuclear testing and nuclear accidents (41).

While radiation exposure increases the risk of developing thyroid cancer, outcomes for these patients do not appear to differ significantly from thyroid cancer patients without radiation exposure (42). A study of 116 patients with a history of thyroid cancer and head and neck radiotherapy found no difference in disease specific survival or recurrence free survival when compared to 3,509 patients with differentiated thyroid cancer and no radiation history (43).

Although radiation exposure is a well-defined risk factor for the development of thyroid cancer, it is not sufficient to explain the rising incidence of thyroid cancers. The identification of somatic mutations associated with radiation exposure, namely *RET/PTC* rearrangements, have been declining over time. In contrast, there is a larger proportion of nonradiation-induced point mutations in *BRAF* and *RAS* identified in tumor tissues, suggesting another etiology as a potential driver of the increased incidence of thyroid cancer (44–46).

Thyroid cancer incidence began to rise in the mid-1970s; there was a similar inflection point in the rate of obesity in the US just a few years prior. The rising slopes of these two incidence curves are now nearly parallel (47). Several studies have revealed a higher risk of thyroid cancer in obese patients compared to their normal-weight peers (48, 49). The mechanism responsible for this potential association is unclear but is likely multifactorial. Leptin, an adipokine secreted by adipose tissue, interacts with several key factors involved in carcinogenesis including stimulation of angiogenesis, cell proliferation, and suppression of anti-inflammatory cytokines (50). Additionally, serum TSH levels are directly proportional to BMI (51). Higher-serum TSH is associated with a higher risk of malignancy in thyroid nodules (52) and more advanced disease stage at presentation (53). Other potential etiologies that have been investigated include insulin resistance (54), iodine deficiency (55), and IGF-I (56). Cigarette smoking has been linked to a reduced risk of developing thyroid cancer (57). In industrialized countries, the prevalence of smoking has declined (58), leading some to posit that the removal of this 'protective effect' could be contributing to the rise in thyroid cancer incidence (48). Additionally, endocrine-disrupting chemicals, namely polybromylated diphenyl ethers (PBDEs), which are highly prevalent in our environment as flame retardants, have a very long biological half-life and a chemical structure bearing a striking similarity to thyroxine, present an enticing culprit, but a direct role in the development of thyroid nodules or malignancy has not yet been proven (59).

TUMOR HISTOLOGY

Tumor histology is a major determinant of outcome, generally being best with PTC, intermediate with FTC, and worst with Hürthle cell thyroid carcinoma (HCC). There are numerous histologic subtypes of differentiated thyroid cancer.

Papillary thyroid carcinoma

Papillary thyroid carcinoma (PTC) is typically an unencapsulated invasive tumor with ill-defined margins. In approximately 10% of cases, the thyroid capsule is penetrated by a tumor that may invade surrounding tissues, while another 10% are fully encapsulated (60, 61). Most PTCs have a typical microscopic appearance with complex, branching papillae, and a fibrovascular core covered by a single layer of tumor cells (Figure 8.2a). The cellular features of PTC distinguish it from other tumors, permitting an accurate diagnosis by fine needle aspiration (FNA) cytology. The large cells contain pink to amphophilic finely granular cytoplasm and large pale nuclei with pseudoinclusions, sometimes called "orphan Annie eye" nuclei (Figure 8.2b), and nuclear grooves that identify it as PTC. Psammoma bodies—the "ghosts" of infarcted papillae that are virtually pathognomonic of PTC—are calcified, concentric lamellated spheres.

Multiple tumor foci are found in 32–39% of thyroidectomy specimens (62, 63). A recent large multicenter study and analysis of the SEER database found that tumor multifocality was not an independent predictor of poor prognosis in patients with PTC (64). Most tumors demonstrating multifocality have microscopic disease in the additional loci. An analysis of the impact of macroscopic multifocal disease revealed these tumors are still associated with a low risk of recurrence in the absence of bulky nodal involvement or gross extrathyroidal extension (ETE) (65).

Papillary tumors have a high likelihood of metastatic nodal disease, the frequency of which varies with the extent of surgical resection and degree of pathologic interrogation of surgical specimens (see Figure 8.2e). Lymph node metastases are found in almost half the cases at the time of diagnosis (66), while even more—up to 85% in some studies—have microscopic nodal metastases found on more careful histological study (67). The number and size of lymph node metastases increase as the primary tumor size enlarges beyond 5 mm (68). When the isthmus or both lobes are involved with tumor, nodal metastases are often bilateral or extend into the mediastinum, with the most common site being the lower paratracheal area (level VI) (69, 70). The prognostic importance of lymph node metastases is highly dependent upon the number of nodes involved, with one paper citing a 4% recurrence rate with <5 metastatic nodes as compared to 19% in patients with >5 metastatic nodes. The size of metastatic focus within the node also impacts the prognostic significance; all nodal foci measuring <2 mm imparts a risk of recurrence of 5% or less (71). Extranodal extension, wherein a tumor penetrates the lymph node capsule and invades the soft tissues, is associated with up to 15–30% recurrence rates (72, 73). The presence of clinically evident nodal involvement (sonographically abnormal or intraoperatively identified), as opposed to only pathological detection, is associated with a 14–42% risk of recurrent disease (74–77).

Less than 5% of patients with PTC have distant metastases at the time of diagnosis and another 5% develop them over the next two or three decades (66). Patients with more aggressive histologic subtypes (discussed below) may have a higher likelihood of distant spread. Although rare, distant metastases may be seen even in cases of papillary microcarcinoma (78). The lung is the most common site of distant metastasis and is the most common disease-specific cause of death from PTC. The presence of distant metastases worsens the prognosis, but patient age at diagnosis, primary tumor histology, location of the metastatic disease, tumor burden, and iodine avidity of the metastatic deposits have independent effects on predicting outcomes (79–83).

PAPILLARY MICROCARCINOMA

Papillary thyroid microcarcinoma (PTMC) is defined as a tumor ≤1.0 cm in diameter that is usually not palpable. PTMC may be found incidentally during surgery for benign thyroid disease or may be identified sonographically. A number of long-term observational studies of PTMC report low rates of growth and lymph node metastases (84, 85). Based on these data, there have been calls to reconsider surgery as the standard initial management of PTMC in select cases (18, 86). Still, not all PTMCs are innocuous; as many as 69% of cases have lymph node metastases with prophylactic neck dissections, and up to 2.8% have distant metastases and up to

0.5% may die of their disease (78, 87). Male gender, age <45 years, tumor size >5 mm, and tumor multifocality have all been identified as risk factors for lymph node metastases in PTMC (78, 88, 89).

PAPILLARY CANCER WITHIN A THYROGLOSSAL DUCT

PTC within a thyroglossal duct is a rare occurrence but is usually small (1 cm) and follows a benign course (90). Surgical resection of the thyroglossal duct via the Sistrunk procedure is the mainstay of treatment (91, 92). Some studies have found up to a 60% prevalence of intrathyroidal cancer in patients with thyroglossal duct cancer, so it is important to pursue careful sonographic examination of the thyroid when thyroglossal duct PTC is found (93). Thyroidectomy may be indicated if primary thyroid cancer is found or cannot be ruled out. Still, PTC

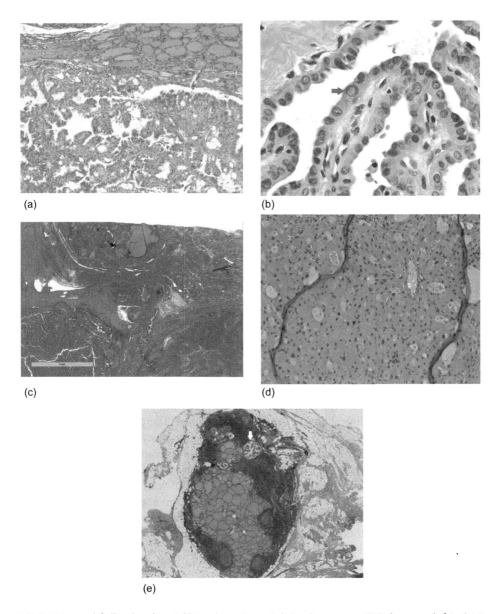

(a)

(b)

(c)

(d)

(e)

Figure 8.2 (a) Normal follicular thyroid histology (top right) adjacent to PTC (bottom left). (b) Arrow denotes a nuclear inclusion in high power view of PTC. (c) HCC with capsular invasion. (d) High-power view of HCC with fused follicles. (e) Metastatic lymph node with thyroid follicles, arrow denotes papillary structures.

within a thyroglossal duct is almost always small and associated with low recurrence rates, and mortality rates are quite low (94).

FOLLICULAR VARIANT PAPILLARY CARCINOMA (FVPTC)

"Classic" histology comprises 55 to 65% of all PTC cases and FVPTC approximately 20 to 40% (95). Opinions differ concerning the exact diagnostic criteria for FVPTC, resulting in the wide range of prevalence rates among studies. The diagnosis of FVPTC depends upon the presence of a micro-follicular, rather than a papillary structure, as well as the nuclear features of PTC. A major diagnostic feature of FVPTC, according to the original description, is that the microfollicular structure must involve the entire tumor (96); however, some find this too restrictive and make the diagnosis of FVPTC when 80% of the tumor contains micro-follicles (95). This variability in reported incidence rates of FVPTC is likely due to the fact that 40 (97) to 80% (95) of classic PTCs show areas of follicle formation. The importance of this distinction is purely academic, however, as the clinical outcomes and behaviors of FVPTC and classic PTC are the same (95, 97, 98).

NONINVASIVE FOLLICULAR NEOPLASM WITH PAPILLARY-LIKE NUCLEAR FEATURES (NIFTP)

Encapsulated follicular variant papillary cancers (eFVPTC) have a very indolent clinical course. Those tumors that show no evidence of invasion have a behavior that is consistent with a non-cancerous lesion, similar to a follicular adenoma (99). In contrast, invasive FVPTC has a clinical course similar to that seen in the classic variant of PTC. Molecular profiles also confirm a distinction between the invasive and noninvasive tumors. The noninvasive FVPTC tumors have a molecular signature akin to follicular adenomas, whereas invasive FVPTCs harbor mutations similar to that seen in PTC (11). To prevent over-treatment of the indolent, noninvasive tumors, an international, multidisciplinary group was convened to perform a clinicopathologic survey of 268 cases of FVPTC and examine the long-term outcomes (100). The authors compared the clinical course of 138 noninvasive lesions with that of 130 invasive tumors. After a median follow-up of 13 years, all of the patients with noninvasive tumors were alive without evidence of residual or recurrent

disease. In contrast, the invasive eFVPTC group had two deaths due to disease, five patients developed distant metastases, seven cases were identified with persistent/recurrent disease, and five patients had biochemical evidence of persistent disease during 3.5 years of follow up. The conclusion of this analysis was that a change in nomenclature for the non-invasive tumors from carcinoma was warranted; the group defined these tumors instead as "noninvasive follicular neoplasms with papillary-like nuclear features" or NIFTP (100). The diagnostic criteria include a well-demarcated tumor that is distinct from the normal thyroid parenchyma. There should be no evidence of tumor invasion into the surrounding normal thyroid tissue or tumor capsule (when present). Likewise, there should be no perineural or angiolymphatic invasion or extrathyroidal extension. The tumor must show a follicular architecture, with no well-formed papillary structures within the tumor (101). The presence of a psammoma body, or infarcted papilla, is an exclusion for the diagnosis of NIFTP. The nuclear features are those seen in papillary carcinoma, but typically are subtler and may be diffuse or patchy in distribution (100).

A task force from the American Thyroid Association (ATA) created a position paper in light of this proposed change in nomenclature. The group, consisting mainly of authors of the 2015 ATA Guidelines on the Management of Thyroid Nodules and Cancer (18), re-examined the literature and the outcomes of patients with noninvasive eFVPTC (102). The task force concluded that it was reasonable to drop the carcinoma designation and reclassify these lesions as a noncancer, as these tumors have a very low potential for recurrence after surgical removal. The task force recommended no further treatment beyond surgical removal; lobectomy is sufficient therapy. Because of a lack of follow up data on these patients, the optimal strategy for follow-up is unclear; the task force recommends that "occasional monitoring with serum thyroglobulin and neck ultrasound can be considered," though it is not mandatory (102).

TALL CELL VARIANT OF PTC

Tall cell variant (TCV) of PTC is a more aggressive histologic variant that is defined by cells that are three times as tall as they are wide, constituting at least 30–50% of the tumor. It accounts for approximately 1–10% of all PTCs (103, 104). Compared with classic variant PTC, tall cell variant PTCs tend to be diagnosed in older patients, are larger, and are more often associated with invasion into local soft tissues and with distant metastases (105). TCV often expresses the p53 oncogene, BRAF mutation, *RET/PTC* gene rearrangement, or *NTRK1* mutation (9, 106). Tall cell variant PTC metastases often lack or lose ^{131}I uptake, and mortality is higher compared to the classic variant of PTC, with 81.9% versus 97.8% 5-year disease specific survival, respectively (103, 104, 107).

COLUMNAR CELL VARIANT OF PTC

Columnar variant tumors are a rare subtype of papillary cancer that contain a predominance of rectangular cells with clear cytoplasm and frequently lack nuclear grooves or intranuclear inclusions (108). Histologically, these tumors vary from encapsulated to infiltrative (109). In unencapsulated tumors, distant metastases are very common and are typically unresponsive to ^{131}I therapy, resulting in a high mortality rate (110). Those tumors that are encapsulated may follow a more indolent clinical course, however (109). *BRAF* mutations may be seen in approximately one-third of columnar cell variant tumors, a rate similar to that seen in the classic variant (110).

DIFFUSE SCLEROSING VARIANT OF PTC

Diffuse sclerosing variants of PTC are characterized by diffuse involvement of the thyroid gland with extensive squamous metaplasia, fibrosis, calcification and abundant lymphocytic infiltration. The background thyroid shows chronic lymphocytic thyroiditis (111). These tumors are more likely to be seen in children and young adults, with a prevalence of 0.7–6.6% (109). In a recent meta-analysis, these tumors were associated with a higher rate of vascular invasion, extrathyroidal extension, lymph node metastasis, and distant metastasis, and were more likely to recur compared to classic PTCs (111). These tumors have been described in children exposed to radiation after the Chernobyl accident (112). The molecular profile of these tumors is varied; however, RET/PTC rearrangements and *BRAF* mutations are the most commonly seen alterations (104).

HOBNAIL VARIANT OF PTC

Hobnail variant tumors are moderately differentiated but characterized by a more aggressive clinical course (113, 114). These tumors are identified on cytology by their predominance of comet-like or bulging cells that have an apically placed nucleus and a high nuclear/cytoplasmic ratio. Distant metastases from these tumors are more likely to be iodine-refractory with high rates of disease-specific mortality (115). These tumors are reported to be more common in women and have a higher likelihood of transformation to a poorly differentiated carcinoma (113). There have been numerous molecular alterations described in these tumors including *BRAF*, *TERT*, and *TP53* (116–118).

Solid variant of PTC

Commonly seen in children, the solid variant of PTC requires a growth pattern in >50% of the tumor with solid nests of cells separated by collagenous bands (119). The areas of solid growth may be confused with features of insular carcinoma (109). However, the distinguishing factor is that insular tumors do not demonstrate nuclear features of PTC, whereas solid variant does. Initially, this tumor was identified in patients with a prior exposure to nuclear fallout from the Chernobyl accident. Vascular invasion and extrathyroidal extension are commonly seen in these tumors (120). The *RET/PTC* rearrangement frequently has been associated with this variant (121).

Follicular thyroid carcinoma

The second most common thyroid cancer histotype, follicular thyroid carcinomas, are solid, invasive tumors which tend to be solitary and encapsulated. On surgical pathology, these tumors are highly cellular, composed of microfollicles, trabeculae, and solid masses of cells. These tumors are indistinguishable from adenomas on FNA due to the inability to identify capsular or vascular invasion on cytology.

Most FTC tumors harbor either *RAS* mutations or *PAX8/PPARγ* gene rearrangements (11). *RAS* mutations can be seen in all stages of differentiation of thyroid tumors, from follicular adenomas, to well-differentiated tumors such as FTC and FVPTC, as well as poorly differentiated tumors and anaplastic carcinoma (122, 123). This finding across the spectrum of neoplasms points to the possible role of *RAS* mutations as an early event in tumorigenesis. Others have opined that the presence of a *RAS* mutation in a follicular adenoma represents a precursor lesion to the development of FTC (123, 124). There are three main isoforms in the *RAS* family, *H-*, *N-*, and *K-RAS*; all are encoded by different genes. *PAX8/PPARγ* rearrangements may also be seen in both adenomas and carcinomas (125). The mechanisms triggering the oncogenic activity of this rearrangement are poorly delineated.

Follicular carcinomas are divided into three major categories: minimally invasive, moderately invasive, and widely invasive. Those tumors exhibiting only capsular invasion are termed minimally invasive and are associated with a favorable long-term prognosis (126). Tumors with extensive vascular invasion ($\geq$4 foci), those larger than 4 cm, and those with a widely invasive pattern, are associated with worse 10-year disease-free survival and higher likelihood of distant metastases (126). Those tumors with 1–4 foci of vascular invasion are sometimes also termed "minimally invasive." However, their clinical behavior is distinct from those tumors with only capsular invasion. The tumors with angioinvasion are associated with an increased probability of recurrence and metastases compared to those with only capsular involvement (126). The extent of vascular invasion (<4 or $\geq$4 vessels) is predictive of disease-specific survival and disease-free survival (127–129). Some authors have accordingly dubbed those tumors with 1–4 foci of vascular invasion "moderately invasive" (127).

Compared to PTC, FTC metastasizes about half as often to regional lymph nodes, occurring in approximately 20% of cases and is usually seen with the more aggressive tumors that often have distant metastases as well (68). Because it spreads hematogenously, FTC tends to metastasize to lung, bone, CNS, and other soft tissues with greater frequency than does PTC. Distant metastases at the time of diagnosis may be seen in approximately 20% of patients and in up to 46% of those with extensive vascular invasion (>4 foci) on surgical pathology (130). However, distant metastases are rarely seen with primary tumors measuring <2 cm in diameter (68).

FTC tends to occur in older patients than in PTC; peak incidence is between 40–60 years with FTC, compared to 30–50 years for PTC (131). Iodine deficiency has been identified as a possible risk factor for the development of FTC (132). With the introduction of iodine supplementation programs, some studies have demonstrated a reduction in the incidence of follicular thyroid cancer relative to the frequency of PTC (133, 134).

Hürthle cell carcinoma (HCC)

Hürthle cells are large, polygonal cells with a marked eosinophilic, granular cytoplasm that is characterized by abundant mitochondria (135). Also called oncocytic follicular cells, Hürthle cells are present in both benign and malignant thyroid conditions. Oncocytic metaplasia is frequently seen in chronic lymphocytic thyroiditis and multinodular goiters (136). Oncocytic follicular cells may also be seen in the oncocytic variant of papillary thyroid carcinoma; these tumors are distinguished from their follicular counterparts by the presence of classic nuclear features of PTC. Hürthle cell tumors may be either benign (adenomas) or malignant (carcinomas); the distinction is made based on the presence of capsular and/or vascular invasion, similar to the situation with FTC. Similar to FTC, HCC may be classified as minimally invasive or widely invasive. Those tumors with extensive vascular invasion ($\geq$4 foci) and extrathyroidal extension are classified as widely invasive, whereas those tumors that are fully encapsulated and only demonstrate microscopic foci of capsular (see Figure 8.2c) or vascular invasion are termed minimally invasive (137).

HCCs are considered by many to represent a separate entity rather than a subtype of FTC because of their distinct molecular profile (see Table 8.2), clinical behavior, and prognosis (see Table 8.1). The majority of FTCs harbor either a *RAS* mutation or a *PAX8/PPARγ* rearrangement, whereas HCC demonstrates a more heterogeneous molecular profile, including *TP53*, *RAS*, *TERT*, and *PTEN* mutations (135, 136, 138). In a single institution study, compared to patients with FTC, those with HCC were older at presentation, had more advanced disease including distant metastases, and were more likely to have persistent/recurrent disease (139). Further, several studies demonstrate worse survival with HCC compared to FTC (138, 140). A more recent analysis, however, demonstrated that survival for HCC has improved over time (141). Survival was worse from 1974–1979 in those patients with HCC compared to FTC. In contrast, there was no significant difference in survival between the two histologic subtypes for those patients diagnosed from 2000–2004. HCC survival improved over the time span studied, while FTC mortality rates remained stable (141). The authors were unable to explain the improvement in outcomes for HCC cases. Factors associated with a higher risk of recurrence or death are male gender and higher disease stage (see below) (142).

TUMOR STAGING SYSTEMS AND PROGNOSTIC SCORING SYSTEMS

A number of tumor staging systems have been used to predict mortality with DTC; most commonly utilized is the TNM (tumor, node, metastasis) classification of the American Joint Commission on Cancer (AJCC). Recently modified to better personalize risk of mortality, the 8th edition of the AJCC-TNM staging distinguishes the degree of nodal involvement and extent of extrathyroidal extension (143) (see Table 8.3). The greatest utility of staging systems is in epidemiological studies and as tools to stratify patients for prospective therapy trials. However, all staging systems are of limited utility in forecasting outcome in thyroid cancer patients because they do not predict the risk of recurrence. Since most patients with thyroid cancer will have excellent survival rates, the greater concern in most cases is whether the disease will recur. For this reason, a dynamic risk stratification system was developed to better predict individual prognosis, guiding surveillance decisions, and potentially, informing the need for additional therapeutic interventions (144). (See sections on initial risk assessment and response to therapy.)

As a point of clarification, the terms "recurrent" and "persistent" technically have separate meanings. Recurrence is conceptualized as occurring after a seemingly complete eradication of disease and may be detected up to many years after the initial therapy. Persistent disease is the result of incomplete removal of the tumor and is detected shortly after initial treatment. In reality, however, the two entities may be thought of as one in the same, as "recurrent" disease, even when detected far from the initial therapy, arises from disease which was likely present at the time of the original surgery and has, until this point, remained undetected. For this reason, the terms recurrent and persistent are used interchangeably in this chapter.

FACTORS INFLUENCING PROGNOSIS AND AFFECTING OUTCOME

The prognosis of DTC is determined by an interaction of clinical variables including tumor stage, patient age, and response to therapy. With modern methods for detection of residual disease having such a high sensitivity, the likelihood of identifying recurrent disease after a patient has achieved an excellent response to therapy is very low (144). Age is an important factor in the prognosis of patients with thyroid cancer. Multivariate analysis models from the SEER database confirm a trend of worsening cause-specific survival for each successive decade starting at age 60 (hazard ratio = 7.5, 95% confidence interval 1.0–54.1, $p = 0.047$) compared to younger patients (<20 years old) (145). The presence of distant metastases, advanced stage disease at diagnosis, and decreased cause-specific survival were more likely among older patients (145). A recent analysis of patients from 11 different medical centers in 6 countries found that age-associated mortality risk is dependent upon *BRAF* mutational status; age is a strong, independent mortality risk factor in patients with *BRAF V600E* mutations but not in those with wild-type *BRAF* (13).

Differentiated thyroid cancer in the pediatric age group is typically more advanced at the time of diagnosis, with a higher likelihood of local and distant metastases than found in adults (79, 146). Up to 80% of children develop cervical lymph node metastases and 15% to 20% develop pulmonary metastases (147), rates that are almost twofold higher than those seen in adults. Yet the prognosis for survival in children is excellent, with or without a history of irradiation (148). Even in the presence of pulmonary metastases, pediatric patients have favorable outcomes; a complete response to radioactive iodine (RAI) therapy may be seen in nearly

Table 8.3 *AJCC-TNM Cancer Staging Manual,* 8th Edition

	<55 years old	55 years and older
Stage I	Any T, Any N, M0	T1-2, N0, M0
Stage II	Any T, Any N, M1	T3, N0, M0
		T1-3, N1, M0
Stage III		T4a, Any N, M0
Stage IVa		T4b, Any N, M0
Stage IVb		Any T, Any N, M1

50% and disease-specific mortality was 2.8% in one systematic review of the literature (149).

Gender is an important prognostic factor for thyroid cancer; recurrence and mortality rates are higher in men than in women (150). Ten-year cancer-specific mortality rates for PTC among men and women older than 40 years are 13% and 7%, respectively. Compared with women at the time of diagnosis, men have higher rates of extrathyroidal tumor (51% vs. 39%), including more regional metastases (40% vs. 32%), and twice the rate of distant metastases (9% vs. 4%) (3). The reason for this gender disparity is unclear.

TREATMENT OF PAPILLARY AND FOLLICULAR THYROID CARCINOMAS

Preoperative imaging

Surgery is the initial treatment for essentially all thyroid cancers, and preoperative imaging is essential in determining the extent of disease and therefore guiding the most effective surgical approach. A comprehensive neck ultrasound should be performed in all patients prior to surgery, as the presence of cervical lymph nodes suspicious for metastatic disease will likely dictate the need for more extensive surgery (18). Indeed, the preoperative US may change the surgery in nearly 40% of cases (151, 152). Suspicious-appearing nodes usually feature one or more of the following sonographic characteristics:

round shape, irregular borders, calcification, central cystic necrosis, peripheral vascularity, and loss of the hyperechoic central hilum (153) (see Table 8.4 and Figure 8.3). Fine needle aspiration of such lymph nodes is performed preoperatively to confirm malignancy, via both cytologic analysis as well as measurement of thyroglobulin in the aspirate. Thyroglobulin is produced only by thyroid follicular cells, therefore its presence in a lymph node aspirate signals metastatic thyroid cancer. If advanced cervical disease is suspected based on ultrasound findings, a CT or MRI of the neck should be considered in order to evaluate for neck metastases which may not be visible on ultrasound, most commonly posterior cervical disease and in the mediastinum (18).

Surgery

Surgery is the initial treatment for essentially all thyroid cancers, and in low-risk disease, is often curative. Previously, a bilateral procedure, either total or near-total thyroidectomy, was recommended for nearly all tumors (154). This recommendation was based on retrospective studies suggesting decreased recurrence rates in patients treated with total thyroidectomy as compared to lobectomy or hemi-thyroidectomy (155, 156). Newer evidence, however, has emerged, suggesting that when controlled for tumor size and comorbid conditions, outcomes are comparable in patients with small tumor burden or low-risk disease treated with lobectomy vs. total thyroidectomy (157–159). One

Table 8.4 Sonographic characterization of lymph nodes

Suspicious node features (one or more of following)	Indeterminate node features	Benign node features
Calcifications	Absent hilum AND one of following:	Hilar stripe
Cystic	Rounded shape	Fusiform (ovoid) shape
Peripheral Doppler flow	Increased central vascularization	Absent or hilar vascularity
Hyperechoic		No other suspicious features

From Leenhardt et al. (298).
T1-Tumor is <2 cm; T2 tumor is 2–4 cm and confined to the thyroid; T3 tumor is larger than 4 cm but confined to the thyroid (T3a) or it has grown into the strap muscles around the thyroid (T3b); T4 tumor is any size and has grown extensively beyond the thyroid gland into nearby tissues of the neck (T4a) or toward the spine or into nearby large blood vessels (T4b).

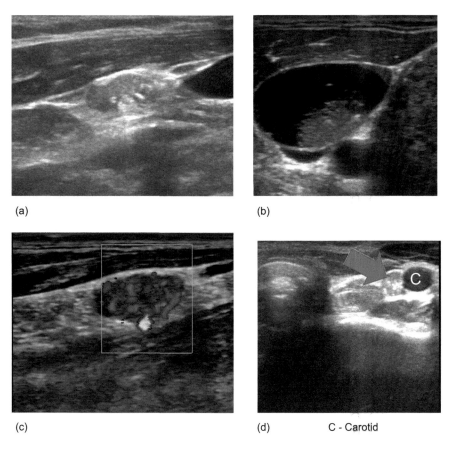

(a)

(b)

(c)

(d)　　　C - Carotid

Figure 8.3 Sonographic images of recurrent or metastatic thyroid cancer. (a) Metastatic cervical lymph node featuring internal microcalcifications and irregular border. (b) Metastatic cervical lymph node featuring cystic necrosis and a solitary microcalcification. (c) Metastatic cervical lymph node featuring intense vascularity. (d) Arrow denotes recurrence of thyroid cancer with microcalcifications within the left thyroid bed, adjacent to the left carotid artery.

study of 23,605 patients with differentiated thyroid cancer found no significant difference in 10-year overall (90.8% vs. 90.4%) or cause-specific (98.6% vs. 96.8%) survival in patients who had undergone lobectomy vs. thyroidectomy (157). This evidence, in combination with an overall movement to utilize less radioiodine therapy, which requires a total thyroidectomy, has obviated the need to remove the entire gland for subsequent treatment and monitoring purposes.

Tumors <1 cm, without evidence of extrathyroidal extension or metastatic lymph nodes, may be safely managed with lobectomy alone (18). In certain cases, total thyroidectomy may be appropriate in patients with a suspicion for intrathyroidal carcinoma in the contralateral lobe, a strong family history of thyroid cancer, or a history of head and neck radiation exposure (18).

Those tumors measuring >1 cm and <4 cm, without evidence of extrathyroidal extension or metastatic lymph nodes, may be considered for lobectomy or total thyroidectomy (18). The decision to pursue a total or near-total thyroidectomy is based on a number of factors, including plan for postoperative radioiodine remnant ablation, older age, more aggressive histological subtype of carcinoma, history of head and neck radiation exposure, and nonspecific findings in the contralateral lobe or the presence of abnormal cervical nodes. Patient preference is also taken into consideration, as some patients fear the certain need for thyroid hormone replacement following a total thyroidectomy, while others feel more comfortable knowing their entire gland has been removed, thus reducing the potential for subsequent surgeries in the future.

Tumors >4 cm, or any size with preoperative evidence of extrathyroidal extension or metastatic lymph nodes, warrant a total thyroidectomy, as postoperative radioiodine therapy is indicated for these patients (18).

LYMPH NODE DISSECTION

Papillary thyroid cancer has a high likelihood of lymph node involvement. Genetic evaluation of lymph nodes in thyroid cancer has determined that up to 90% of patients may have some degree of nodal disease (160). Less stringent criteria, however, still indicate that the majority of thyroid cancer patients have lymph node involvement (151, 161), as evidenced from data from patients undergoing prophylactic central neck nodal dissection (162). Such high rates of nodal involvement have led to ongoing debate over the role of prophylactic neck dissections (71). The ATA Guidelines recently addressed this contentious issue by recommending a "therapeutic" central compartment and/or lateral neck dissection for biopsy-proven or highly clinically suspicious lymph nodes (18). On the other hand, a prophylactic central compartment dissection may be considered in patients with larger intrathyroidal tumors (T3 or T4), or if there are known lateral neck metastases for which a lateral neck dissection will be performed (18).

COMPLETION THYROIDECTOMY

Completion thyroidectomy is performed if pathologic findings from an initial lobectomy create a scenario whereby a total or near total thyroidectomy would have been performed if the diagnosis had been known prior to the initial surgery. This situation occurs most commonly in the setting of a thyroid nodule with indeterminate cytology prior to surgery, which is found to be malignant on final surgical pathology. With the more recent consensus that a lobectomy is sufficient in patients with smaller tumors (18), completion thyroidectomy may be performed less often than in the past. Surgical risks have been reported to be similar in the two-stage thyroidectomy as in a single surgery (163, 164).

SURGICAL COMPLICATIONS

The main complications of thyroidectomy are hypoparathyroidism and recurrent laryngeal nerve damage, which are most common after total thyroidectomy rather than lobectomy. The rates of hypoparathyroidism immediately after surgery are reported to range between 5–52%, depending on the extent of surgery and the experience of the surgeon. However, the rates of persistent hypocalcemia, lasting beyond 6 months, are lower, ranging from 1–16% (165, 166). A retrospective study of 1087 patients who had undergone total thyroidectomy +/− central compartment dissection found significantly higher rates of transient hypoparathyroidism in the patients for whom central compartment dissection was performed (27.7% total thyroidectomy only, 36.1% thyroidectomy plus ipsilateral central compartment dissection, 51.9% thyroidectomy plus bilateral central compartment dissection). When rates of permanent hypoparathyroidism were compared, only the bilateral central compartment group had significantly higher rates (6.3, 7, 16.2%, respectively) (165).

Recurrent laryngeal nerve injury occurs transiently in 2–5% of patients undergoing thyroid surgery, and permanently in 0.5–2% (165, 166). In a review of seven published surgical series, the average rates of permanent recurrent laryngeal nerve injury and hypoparathyroidism, respectively, were 3% and 2.6% after total thyroidectomy and 1.9% and 0.2% after subtotal thyroidectomy (167). A nationwide study of all patients undergoing total thyroidectomy between 2000 and 2009 found that surgeon volume significantly predicts patient outcomes (168). Low volume surgeons (those performing less than 10 cases per year) had postoperative complications in 24% of cases, compared with 14.5% for high-volume surgeons (>100 cases per year). Complication rates were half those of total thyroidectomy when lobectomy was performed for surgeons of all experience levels. This data is of particular importance because over 80% of thyroidectomies in the US are performed by low- or intermediate-volume surgeons (169).

THYROIDECTOMY DURING PREGNANCY

Thyroid carcinoma may occasionally progress rapidly during pregnancy, perhaps due to high maternal serum hCG levels, which have a TSH-like effect. Nonetheless, most DTCs are slow growing and have an excellent prognosis during pregnancy; therefore, surgery can usually be delayed until after delivery (170). If DTC is diagnosed in early pregnancy, the American Thyroid Association recommends that it be re-evaluated via ultrasonography at 24 weeks, and second trimester thyroidectomy be considered only if there is substantial growth or the development of lymph node metastases (171).

Initial risk assessment

RISK STRATIFICATION BASED UPON THE PATIENT'S CLINICAL STATUS AFTER INITIAL THERAPY

The AJCC TNM patient risk stratification and most tumor staging classifications depend heavily upon patient age and tumor stage at the time of diagnosis. While this provides a uniform means of comparing patient mortality, it fails to take into account other important tumor features that predict recurrences in thyroid cancer. For example, the AJCC-TNM system does not account for tumor histology (e.g., tall cell papillary thyroid cancer), tumor molecular features such as *BRAF* mutation, or extent of nodal disease, all of which have an impact on outcomes (see above sections on prognostic features) (143). The ATA thyroid cancer guidelines (18) stratify risk on the basis of these more nuanced factors, as illustrated in Table 8.5. Decision making for subsequent treatment (chiefly, whether radioiodine therapy will be of benefit), and for the appropriate frequency of sonographic and biochemical monitoring for recurrence, are, in large part, dictated by the initial risk assignation. In addition, the target TSH to be achieved with levothyroxine therapy initially is determined by the preliminary risk stratification. It is important to note, however, that the risk estimates outlined in Table 8.5 are based on studies examining the likelihood of recurrence in patients who have had total thyroidectomy, and in many cases, RAI therapy. The risk of recurrent disease in patients who have received less than total thyroidectomy and/or no RAI therapy remains to be determined in many of these categories.

The initial risk for recurrence exists on a spectrum, ranging from 1–55% (18). It is useful to divide the risk into three categories: low, intermediate, and high risk. Tumors considered to be at low

Table 8.5 Risk of structural disease recurrence in those with no evidence of structurally identifiable disease after initial therapy

Tumor features	Risk of recurrence (%)
Unifocal PTMC	1–2
Intrathyroidal, unifocal PTMC, BRAF mutated	1–2
Intrathyroidal, <4 cm, BRAF wild type	1–2
Minimally invasive FTC	2–3
pN1 without ENE, ≤ 3 LN involved	2
Multifocal PTMC	4–6
Intrathyroidal PTC, 2–4 cm	5
pN1, ≤5 LN involved	5
pN1, all LN <0.2 cm	5
pT3 minor ETE	3–8
Intrathyroidal PTC, <4 cm, BRAF mutated	10
pN1, >5 LN involved	20
Clinical N1	20
PTC, vascular invasion	15–30
PTC, ETE, BRAF mutated	10–40
pN1, any LN >3 cm	30
PTC, >1 cm, *TERT* mutated ± BRAF mutated	>40
pN1 with ENE, >3 LN involved	40
pT4a gross ETE	30–40
FTC, extensive vascular invasion	30–55

Extent of surgery and RAI treatment as a component of therapy is variable across the studies in determining these risks of recurrence.
Source: Adapted from Haugen et al. 2015 (18).

risk for recurrence comprise those that are smaller (<4 cm), do not extend beyond the thyroid capsule, and have no or very small lymph node involvement (<0.2 cm foci in <3–5 nodes). Tumors in the high risk for recurrence category exhibit such features as gross extrathyroidal extension, incomplete resection, large nodal burden (>3 cm, extranodal extension), and more aggressive oncogenic mutations (*TERT, BRAF*). Those tumors that fall between these two extremes are considered to be at intermediate risk for recurrence, and it is here where medical decision making is challenging, due to a lack of high quality evidence.

SERUM THYROGLOBULIN IN INITIAL RISK ASSESSMENT

Thyroglobulin (Tg), a thyroid-specific protein, is a product of normal thyroid follicular cells as well as differentiated thyroid cancers. In a postthyroidectomy patient, the presence of serum thyroglobulin is indicative of either residual normal thyroid remnant or persistent carcinoma. Thus, the postoperative serum thyroglobulin (Tg) level is commonly employed as a predictive tool for the achievement of remission (172), and may contribute to subsequent management decisions such as whether to administer radioiodine (173, 174). Serum Tg antibodies, present in up to 25% of patients, particularly in the setting of Hashimoto's disease, must be assessed concomitantly with Tg as their presence almost always invalidates Tg measurement (175). In radioimmunometric Tg assays, anti-Tg antibodies can cause falsely low values for Tg, while Tg levels are falsely elevated in Tg radioimunoassays (176). Recently, thyroglobulin LC-MS/MS assays have been introduced that purport to circumvent the problem of anti-Tg antibody interference (177). However, these assays may still yield falsely low serum Tg levels in patients with known residual disease (178). There is more detailed information about Tg assays in Chapter 1, "The Laboratory and Imaging Approaches to Thyroid Disorders."

Anti-Tg antibodies must be quantitated because they can serve as a (less specific) surrogate marker for Tg, rising when there is a tumor recurrence and falling when the tumor burden declines (175, 179). Postoperative Tg is typically measured 4–6 weeks following surgery in order to facilitate treatment decision making, although it should be noted that serum Tg may continue to decline over years

following surgery without additional intervention (180).

Thyroid-stimulating hormone (TSH) stimulates the production of thyroglobulin from thyroid follicular cells and follicular cell–derived cancers, therefore one expects that thyroglobulin will rise when the TSH is elevated, whether by the administration of recombinant human TSH (rhTSH), or physiologically via thyroid hormone withdrawal (181). By the same mechanism, serum Tg may be low or undetectable when serum TSH is suppressed. It is therefore useful to describe a serum Tg level as *stimulated* or *suppressed*, as the residual tumor may not produce a detectable serum Tg level in the TSH-suppressed state, but the Tg will rise to detection with TSH stimulation. Postoperative Tg was previously routinely measured in the setting of TSH stimulation. However, recent studies suggest that in patients with small disease burden, an unstimulated undetectable serum Tg with a high sensitivity Tg assay is a strong predictor of excellent outcome (173). One study found that stimulated Tg values were not helpful in identifying those with residual disease beyond what was identified with an unstimulated Tg and cervical US in patients with initially low-risk tumors (182). Thus, one may elect to reserve measurement of *stimulated* Tg only in patients with larger tumors or if there is greater suspicion for incomplete tumor removal.

The 2015 ATA guidelines suggest that an unstimulated Tg of <0.2 ng/mL or a stimulated Tg of <1 ng/mL can be considered an excellent response to therapy, while suppressed Tg >1 ng/mL or stimulated Tg >10 ng/mL should prompt an imaging evaluation out of concern for persistent disease. Serum Tg values that fall somewhere in between these levels (i.e., unstimulated Tg >0.2 ng/mL but <1.0 ng/mL and stimulated Tg >1.0 ng/mL but <10 ng/mL), are classified as an indeterminate response to therapy and subsequent management, (e.g., observation vs. pursuit of imaging) is dependent upon the patient's individual risk factors (18). (See the section on Surveillance.)

It is important to recognize that Tg is produced by normal thyroid tissue as well as differentiated thyroid carcinoma. Thus, in patients with a known or suspected normal thyroid remnant, particularly when RAI therapy has not been employed, a detectable Tg does not necessarily reflect persistent thyroid cancer. In patients who have undergone hemithyroidectomy, persistent thyroglobulinemia is to be expected, with serum levels about 50% of normal circulating values. In these cases, there are limited data regarding the role of serial measurement of thyroglobulin and the optimal cutoff value for indicating a disease-free state (183).

IMAGING IN INITIAL RISK ASSESSMENT

Along with serum Tg measurement, neck ultrasonography is a cornerstone of postoperative risk assessment. Utilized as a complement to the biochemical detection of persistent disease with Tg, cervical ultrasound detects persistent anterior neck structural disease. (184, 185).

Postoperative radioiodine diagnostic whole body scanning (DxWBS), using ^{123}I or a low dose of ^{131}I, can provide additional prognostic information as it may reveal iodine avid local and distal thyroid cancer metastases, in addition to thyroid remnant. Given the excellent negative predictive value of serum Tg and neck ultrasound in low risk patients (186), DxWBS is not essential to determine the existence of persistent disease for all patients post thyroid cancer surgery. The DxWBS is a valuable tool, however, when the extent of residual disease cannot be sufficiently determined by surgical pathology, serum Tg or neck ultrasonography, and the information obtained will enhance subsequent treatment decision making. It is frequently utilized prior to RAI therapy to calculate percent uptake and aid in the determination of administered activity (18).

After the administration of RAI, it is critical to perform a post-treatment whole body scan (RxWBS) to identify areas of treated disease. Disease identified prior to therapy on ultrasound or cross-sectional imaging that is not visualized on the RxWBS is highly concerning for the possibility of non-iodine avidity. As such, the RxWBS both provides prognostic information and points to the need for alternative therapies if the disease progresses. The optimal timing of the RxWBS after RAI therapy is unclear, but it is generally performed 5–10 days after therapy, to minimize background uptake in the urinary bladder, nasopharynx, and salivary glands, as discussed below. The addition of SPECT/CT imaging to the RxWBS is being used increasingly as a tool to discriminate between areas of disease and physiologic uptake (see Figure 8.4). The SPECT/CT portion may alter risk stratification and potentially future treatment decisions, particularly when it identifies disease not seen on the planar RxWBS (187, 188).

Thyroid hormone therapy

LEVOTHYROXINE (T4) SUPPRESSION OF TSH

The typical starting dose of levothyroxine following total thyroidectomy is 1.6–2.0 mcg/kg/day, depending on whether the goal is a low-normal or suppressed serum TSH. DTC cells contain TSH receptors that stimulate cell growth and the expression of specific proteins including thyroglobulin and the sodium-iodide symporter. Suppression of TSH with levothyroxine historically has been an important component of the treatment of DTC because of its theoretical inhibition of tumor growth (66). A number of studies support this theory; a meta-analysis of thyroid hormone suppression therapy in thyroid cancer patients showed an association with reduced risk of major adverse clinical events, defined as disease progression and/or recurrence and death (189). Other more recent studies, however, have failed to find a benefit of TSH suppression in patients with low-risk disease (190–192).

TSH suppressive therapy (i.e., serum TSH <0.1 mU/L) must be balanced against the potential for harm. Observational studies have reported increased cardiovascular and all-cause mortality in older patients treated for differentiated thyroid cancer (193). Potential complications of subclinical thyrotoxicosis include an increased risk of atrial fibrillation in older patients (194, 195), a higher 24-hour heart rate, more atrial premature contractions per day, ventricular hypertrophy, diastolic dysfunction, and impaired cardiac reserve (196). Additionally, patients with thyroid carcinoma treated with suppressive doses of levothyroxine have a high rate of bone turnover that decreases acutely after withdrawing treatment (197). A study of patients with low- and intermediate-risk thyroid cancer found that TSH suppression to <0.4 mIU/L was associated with higher rates of osteoporosis, but not decreased cancer recurrence rates (198). Studies of fracture risk in women treated with thyroid hormone indicate an increased risk when suppressive doses are used (195, 199, 200).

Therefore, the target TSH range should be determined on an individual basis, taking into consideration both the initial risk for recurrence as well as

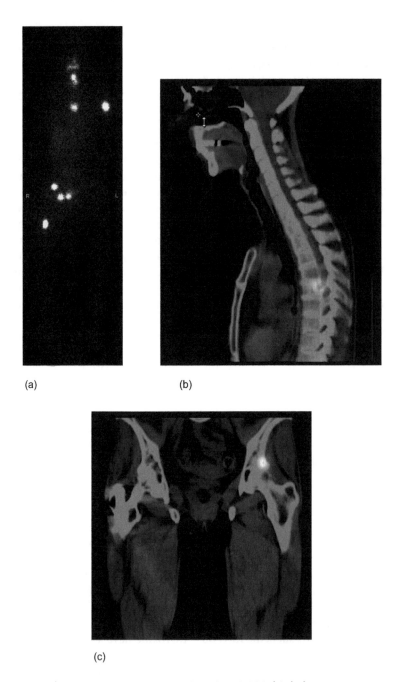

(a)

(b)

(c)

Figure 8.4 Metastatic disease on posttreatment imaging. **(a)** Multiple bony metastases on posttreatment WBS. **(b)** Spinal metastases seen on SPECT/CT. **(c)** Pelvic metastasis seen on SPECT/CT.

response to therapy, while weighing the risk for thyrotoxicosis-related morbidities, namely atrial fibrillation and osteoporosis in older patients (18). The target TSH for an individual may also evolve over time. If, for example, an initially high-risk patient has an excellent response to therapy, their degree of TSH suppression may be lessened over time.

Radioiodine (^{131}I) therapy

GOALS OF THERAPY

Radioiodine therapy is intended to meet one of three similar but distinct goals.

Adjuvant therapy is intended to destroy suspected, but unproven microscopic residual disease.

Radioactive iodine (RAI) therapy is also given to target known persistent or recurrent disease. The patient's individual risk dictates the specific goal of therapy, which then, in combination with patient factors, determines the appropriate administered dose or activity.

Remnant ablation is used when complete surgical removal of the tumor is likely, but the destruction of the small remaining thyroid tissue in the thyroid bed, including normal tissue of thyroglossal duct remnants, is desired. This therapy will augment the ability to detect recurrent or persistent disease via measurement of serum Tg and/or diagnostic iodine scans.

DECISION TO USE ^{131}I THERAPY

In the past, nearly all patients with DTC received RAI therapy following surgery as adjuvant therapy. Strong evidence, albeit not from randomized trials, has emerged showing a minimal impact of RAI therapy on disease-free survival for patients at low risk for recurrence (189, 201–203). Based on these findings, current ATA guidelines do not recommend the routine use of ^{131}I in such patients (18). At the other end of the spectrum, patients with advanced disease, specifically those with gross extrathyroidal extension or distant metastases, clearly do benefit from RAI therapy, with significant improvement in overall and disease specific mortality (189, 204).

RAI is therefore routinely used in this patient population (Table 8.6).

It is the patients who fall between these two ends of the spectrum, classified as either intermediate risk for recurrence, or low risk for recurrence with more aggressive features (e.g., <4 cm tumor with a few nodal micrometastases), for whom data are scant or conflicting, and the best course of action may not be immediately clear. In this setting, it is helpful to place a patient's individual tumor features on the spectrum, outlined in Table 8.5, in order to determine their individual risk for recurrence. In so doing, the potential risk lowering benefit of RAI can be conceptualized. In a patient for whom the risk of recurrence is already less than 5%, for example, the practitioner may feel assured in taking an observational approach following surgery. Individual patient preference and inclusion in decision making also plays an important role in decreasing decisional conflict (205). Subsequent tracking of serum Tg, as discussed later, also contributes to decision making; for example, a persistently elevated serum Tg in a postoperative patient may prompt the decision to administer adjuvant ^{131}I therapy, whereas undetectable Tg levels provide reassurance in continuing to observe without therapy. Indeed, RAI can be administered any time, not just in the immediate postoperative period.

Table 8.6 Indications for radioiodine therapy

ATA staging risk	Features	[131]I recommended?	Dose activity
Low (1–10%)	Papillary microcarcinoma	No	
	1–4 cm confined to thyroid	No	Remnant Ablation, 30–50 mCi
	Tumor size >4 cm, no ETE	Consider	
	Central compartment microscopic nodal metastases (<0.2 cm)	Not routine, may consider	
Intermediate (15–30%)	Aggressive histology Minimal ETE	Consider	Adjuvant therapy, 50–150 mCi
	0.2–3 cm central or lateral nodal metastases, >5 nodes involved	Generally recommended	
High (40–70%)	>3 cm nodal metastases Extranodal extension FTC, extensive vascular invasion Gross ETE Distant Metastases	Yes	RAI therapy, 100–200 mCi empirically, or dosimetry

Modified from Haugen et al. 2015 (18). Decision to administer ^{131}I and dose activity may be further modified by several factors, including patient age and preference, response to initial therapy (postoperative serum Tg/Tg Ab, pre and postoperative sonographic findings), and surgeon experience.

There are no explicit recommendations regarding the use of radioiodine in patients with Hürthle cell carcinoma. It is unclear what percentage of HCC metastases actually are iodine-avid; there are conflicting results in the literature. All of the studies are limited by small sample sizes and retrospective design. A single institution study of 127 patients found that only 38% of HCC metastases are iodine-avid (206). A smaller cohort was found to have uptake in 69% (11 of 16 cases) (207). A more recent analysis of 30 patients found that 53% of the cohort had uptake on iodine scanning in the metastatic areas (208). It appears, however, that the use of RAI in patients with HCC has a beneficial effect on outcomes. Analysis of the National Cancer Data Base found that patients treated with RAI had improved overall survival rates compared to HCC patients who did not. The administration of RAI was associated with a 30% reduction in mortality (209).

PREPARATION FOR ^{131}I THERAPY

Females with childbearing potential must have a negative pregnancy test documented shortly before receiving diagnostic imaging or therapeutic amounts of [131]I. The patient must be queried for recent exposure to iodine: iodinated intravenous CT contrast routinely impairs the uptake of ^{131}I for a month, and iodine-containing drugs should be held for 4-6 weeks prior to treatment (210). Amiodarone-treated patients may take significantly longer (months to years) to achieve a normal urine iodine level (211) If in doubt, a urinary iodine level may be measured, with levels <100 mcg/24 hours being satisfactory for treatment (18). A low-iodine diet should be followed for 1–2 weeks prior to therapy (18), though there are no randomized studies demonstrating this intervention results in improved long-term outcomes. However, retrospective studies have shown an increase in ^{131}I uptake by the remnant tissue in those adhering to a low-iodine diet, compared to those not observing such a diet (212).

The serum TSH levels must be high enough (≥30 mU/L) to stimulate neoplastic and normal thyroid tissues to concentrate an adequate amount of [131]I (181). For decades, the only way to prepare for RAI therapy was via thyroid hormone withdrawal (213), in which levothyroxine is withdrawn, and liothyronine (T3) is given for 4 weeks, then stopped for 2 more weeks, and then ^{131}I is administered. THW causes profound hypothyroidism with TSH levels often well above 100 mU/L. After THW, serum TSH levels must be measured before diagnostic or therapeutic ^{131}I dosing because the TSH response to THW is unpredictable and may fail to rise above 30 mU/L. A TSH level of 30 mI/L or greater is generally regarded as the acceptable threshold for successful ^{131}I therapy; however, the optimal magnitude of TSH elevation is unknown and differs among patients (181). THW can cause severe clinical hypothyroidism, however, and in select populations, the clinical ramifications can be significant. In patients with severe or unstable depression or heart failure, THW may not be tolerated or advisable. Additionally, in patients with central hypothyroidism, an elevation of serum TSH is not feasible (18).

The other method to increase serum TSH levels is by the administration of recombinant human TSH (rhTSH, Thyrogen®) while the patient continues thyroid hormone therapy, and thus avoids symptomatic hypothyroidism (214). The usual protocol is for rhTSH to be administered intramuscularly at a dosage of 0.9 mg for 2 consecutive days, with ^{131}I administration 24 hours after the last injection (215). Mean peak TSH concentrations are reached between 3 and 24 hours after the second injection (median of 10 hours) and the mean half-life is 25 ± 10 hours (216). Measurement of serum TSH levels after rhTSH stimulation is not necessary and there is no optimal value prior to treatment. When given to euthyroid patients taking levothyroxine, rhTSH injection is as effective as thyroid hormone withdrawal in preparing patients for remnant ablation and produces an equally favorable therapeutic response (215, 217, 218). The use of rhTSH reduces total body radiation from ^{131}I by 33% compared with withdrawal-induced hypothyroidism, since hypothyroidism reduces glomerular filtration, thereby delaying the renal excretion of [131]I (215). Despite its cost, the multiple advantages offered by rhTSH make it the more commonly elected method of TSH elevation prior to ^{131}I therapy for patients at a low and intermediate risk for recurrence. A lack of good quality evidence of non-inferiority of this method as compared to THW in patients with high-risk features, however, prevents the universal endorsement for the use of rhTSH in this setting. There are, however, several retrospective studies examining the outcomes in patients with higher risk disease when prepared with rhTSH or withdrawal (219–221). Though limited by the retrospective study design and small sample sizes, each study demonstrated equal or greater efficacy with rhTSH as measured by a nonsignificant difference in the rates of achieving a stimulated Tg <2 after therapy (219); slightly improved rates of freedom from disease (220); and no significant difference in overall survival (221). Until higher quality evidence is available, however, it is recommended that patients with advanced disease receive RAI after THW (18).

DIAGNOSTIC WHOLE-BODY ^{131}I SCAN AND THE STUNNING EFFECT

Prior to ^{131}I therapy, some physicians perform a diagnostic ("pretreatment") whole-body scan (DxWBS) in order to establish the size and iodine avidity of the thyroid remnant, and to search for the presence of cervical nodal, or distant metastatic disease. Pretreatment scans may provide valuable information with regard to disease status, which could inform the decision of whether to treat with radioiodine or not, and/or the activity to be used. Studies of pretreatment scans have shown that they provide potential treatment altering information in 25–53% of patients (222, 223). If a diagnostic scan is ordered, it is usually obtained 24 to 72 hours after giving 2 to 4 mCi of [131]I. Larger amounts of ^{131}I should not be given because ^{131}I doses as small as 3 mCi diminish the subsequent uptake of therapeutic ^{131}I, which is termed the "stunning effect" (224, 225). To avoid stunning, doses of 1 to 3 mCi of ^{131}I have been recommended; however, these doses are slightly less sensitive than larger scanning doses of ^{131}I in identifying thyroid remnants (226). Administration of the therapeutic dose as soon as possible after the diagnostic dose of ^{131}I helps to minimize stunning (226, 227). Alternatively, using the lower energy isotope ^{123}I in doses of ≥1.5 mCi has been reported to yield excellent images without stunning (228).

DETERMINING THE APPROPRIATE ^{131}I ADMINISTERED ACTIVITY

THYROID REMNANT ABLATION

Usually, remnant ablation can be achieved with 30 to 50 mCi of ^{131}I, which is as effective as larger activities in ablating the thyroid remnant (217, 218, 229). A lower dose activity of 30 mCi is also associated with fewer short-term adverse effects when compared to higher activities, typically 100 mCi or greater.

[131]I ADJUVANT THERAPY

Patients with suspected, but unproven microscopic residual disease, most often falling into the intermediate risk category, are candidates for adjuvant RAI therapy. Previously recommended activities in this setting ranged from 100–200 mCi (154). However, recent studies have raised doubt that higher administered activities are associated with improved patient outcomes (230–232). For example, a retrospective review of 181 patients with Nlb disease found no difference in clinical outcomes in younger patients who received a median activity of 102 mCi vs. 150 mci vs. 202 mci (232). As with the data for remnant ablation, there was a trend toward improved outcomes with higher activities in older patients. However, concern for toxicity with activities >150 mCi must be weighed carefully against any potential benefit of therapy. Current guidelines recommend activities of up to 150 mCi for adjuvant ^{131}I therapy (18). One specific patient population in whom to consider higher administered activities are patients over the age of 45 years. A retrospective review showed lower disease specific survival in low and intermediate risk patients >45 years of age who received lower activities (30 mCi as compared to 100 mCi), although overall survival was not significantly different (233).

TREATMENT OF RESIDUAL, RECURRENT, OR METASTATIC CARCINOMA WITH [131]I

Known residual thyroid carcinoma (especially macroscopic disease) should be treated surgically whenever possible. Only 50 to 75% of DTCs and their metastases concentrate [131]I (234–236). Moreover, the larger the tumor mass, the less likely that ^{131}I therapy will successfully ablate the tumor. There are three approaches to radioiodine therapy: empiric fixed doses, upper-bound limits set by blood dosimetry, and quantitative dosimetry (237, 238). Dosimetric methods have not been shown to be more effective on overall survival than empiric dosing (239), and are generally reserved for unusual cases, or where dose limitation is desired from a safety standpoint, such as in renal failure.

Empirical fixed doses

With empirical doses, a fixed amount of ^{131}I is given based on tumor stage; this is the method most commonly employed. While it is established that the efficacy of RAI therapy increases with higher administered activities, the optimal effective and safe activity remains uncertain. In the past, dose activities of 150 mCi routinely were administered for residual carcinoma in cervical nodes or the thyroid bed, and 200 mCi for distant metastases. However, concern has been raised for the potential for doses of 150 mCi or more to exceed the blood exposure limit, particularly in patients 70 years of age or older (240) or in those with reduced renal function (241). Activities which exceed 80 mCi whole body retention at 48 hours increase the risk of pulmonary fibrosis. Consequently, dosimetry-guided ^{131}I therapy may be preferable to fixed-dose ^{131}I treatment in older patients and in patients with ^{131}I-avid diffuse bilateral pulmonary metastases, even when renal function is normal (240, 242).

Upper-bound limits set by blood dosimetry

This approach establishes an upper limit on the amount of ^{131}I in a single dose that can be given safely, which is generally considered to be 200 rad to the whole blood (243). In patients with diffuse pulmonary metastases, the dose is also limited, so that no more than 80 mCi of ^{131}I remains in the whole body after 48 hours to avoid pulmonary fibrosis.

Quantitative tumor dosimetry

This approach calculates the amount of ^{131}I that is required to deliver 30,000 rad to ablate the thyroid remnant or 8,000 to 12,000 rad to treat nodal or discrete soft tissue metastases. For pulmonary metastases, an amount of ^{131}I is administered that will deliver 200 rad to whole blood with no more than 80 mCi of whole blood retention at 48 hours (243). The mass of residual tissue and the effective half time of ^{131}I in that tissue are the two most important factors in determining success (243).

POSTTREATMENT SCANS

A posttreatment scan (RxWBS) is performed 5 to 10 days after ^{131}I therapy, in order to identify iodine-avid tissue. In most patients, an area in the midline corresponding to the thyroid remnant is all that is seen. However, cervical nodal disease may be visualized in the lateral neck or mediastinum in papillary thyroid cancer, and more rarely diffuse lung uptake is seen, especially in children and adolescents. In a study of 60 patients with differentiated thyroid carcinoma, a post-ablation scan provided new information that changed therapeutic approach in 15%, and altered the disease stage

in 8.3% of patients (244). A number of situations can cause false-positive ^{131}I scans, including body secretions, transudates, inflammation, nonspecific mediastinal uptake (e.g., blood pool or the thymus), and neoplasms of nonthyroidal origin, which may uncommonly concentrate ^{131}I (245). This includes physiological secretion of ^{131}I from the nasopharynx, salivary and sweat glands, stomach, and genitourinary tract and from skin and hair contamination with sputum or tears (246).

The use of ^{131}I SPECT/CT is helpful to distinguish iodine-avid disease from physiologic uptake which may be more challenging with traditional planar ^{131}I scanning. In a study of 109 post-ablation patients, the use of ^{131}I SPECT/CT scanning altered the initial risk of recurrence stratification in 6.4% of patients and reduced the need for additional cross-sectional imaging in 20% of patients (187). It may be of most benefit in cases where disease is advanced and/or there are inconclusive findings on the traditional scanning alone.

Complications of ^{131}I

IMMEDIATE COMPLICATIONS

There are few immediate serious risks of ^{131}I therapy except when metastases are in critical locations such as long bones, brain, or the paratracheal area that may not tolerate post-therapeutic swelling. For example, brain or spinal cord metastases can undergo potentially catastrophic edema and hemorrhage 12 hours to 2 weeks after ^{131}I treatment. In patients with disease in critical areas such as the CNS, pretreatment with high doses of glucocorticoids has been recommended (247). Severe radiation thyroiditis may occur within a week of administering a large dose of ^{131}I to a patient who has undergone only lobectomy, causing pain, swelling, and rarely airway compromise that may require glucocorticoid therapy (248). Leukopenia, and a slight drop in the number of platelets, often occurs approximately six weeks after therapy, but ordinarily, these effects are mild and transient unless very large activities of ^{131}I are administered (249). Nasal pain, nasal sores, nasal dryness, and epistaxis have also been described in the acute period after RAI, occurring in up to 10.5% of patients within 11 days of therapy (250). The likelihood of this complication is correlated with the administered activity of radioiodine and is less common in those prepared with rhTSH stimulation versus THW (250).

LONG-TERM COMPLICATIONS

Salivary gland dysfunction occurs commonly after ^{131}I therapy, manifesting as sialadenitis, xerostomia, and altered taste or smell. Duration of symptoms ranges from less than three months to being permanent. The use of sialagogues to stimulate salivary flow is controversial, since increased radiation absorption in the salivary glands following ^{131}I therapy may occur (251). As dental caries are an important complication of xerostomia, patients should be educated about oral hygiene and routine dental care. Complete bilateral nasolacrimal duct obstruction, resulting in epiphora (excessive tearing), has been rarely reported (252). Reported reproductive effects of ^{131}I therapy include transient oligomenorrhea in 10–25% of women (253), delayed time to child bearing (254), and earlier onset of menopause (255). In men, testicular germinal cell function may be transiently impaired, with persistent elevation of follicle stimulating hormone and transient oligospermia with cumulative dose activities of greater than 500 mCi (256), although male infertility related to cumulative radioiodine doses has not been reported (257). As mentioned earlier, pulmonary fibrosis is a potential complication of ^{131}I therapy for diffuse pulmonary metastases when the whole-body retention of ^{131}I is >80 mCi 48 hours after treatment. Neither the cumulative dose nor the number of therapies are predictive of pulmonary fibrosis (258).

LEUKEMIA AND SECOND PRIMARY MALIGNANCY

The development of second primary malignancies, including leukemia, and malignancy of bone, breast, salivary gland, kidney, and colorectum following exposure to ^{131}I has been established in a number of studies (259–261) (262). A meta-analysis of two large studies reported a relative risk of second malignancies of 1.19 (95% CI 1.04–1.36) in long-term thyroid cancer survivors that were treated with RAI compared to those who had not. However, it must be noted that the *absolute* risk of malignancy as compared to the general population remains quite low (263). The risk is dose-related, with one study reporting an excess absolute risk of 14.4 solid cancers and of 0.8 leukemias per GBq (27 mCi) of ^{131}I per 100,000 person-years of follow-up. Cumulative administered activities greater than 500 mCi are associated with a clearly increased risk (262). A SEER database analysis of patients with low

risk disease (T1N0) found increased standardized incident ratio (SIR) of salivary gland malignancies (SIR = 11.13; 95% CI, 1.35–40.2) and leukemia (SIR = 5.68; 95% CI, 2.09–12.37) in patients treated with RAI, and that there was significantly higher risk of leukemia after RAI treatment in younger patients (<45 years) as compared to those over the age of 45 (264).

It is reasonable to give high cumulative doses of ^{131}I to patients with extensive metastatic disease responsive to therapy, as the risk posed by the known thyroid cancer outweighs the risk of a potential second cancer from radiation. However, for patients with low- and intermediate-risk disease, given the potential for development of second primary malignancy, and lack of consensual data strongly supporting the benefit of RAI treatment, it is wise to consider using the minimal effective dose of ^{131}I for each patient, which in some cases may be zero. Strategies to reduce radiation exposure include the use of laxatives and vigorous hydration following RAI administration. Additionally, radiation exposure to the uninvolved tissue and the general public is reduced when rhTSH therapy is used in place of thyroid hormone withdrawal (265). Radiation safety recommendations for reducing exposure to household members and the general public are available in an American Thyroid Association guideline (266).

Therapies for advanced thyroid cancer

EXTERNAL BEAM RADIATION THERAPY (EBRT)

External beam radiation therapy has a limited role in the management of localized DTC after surgical resection and ^{131}I therapy. Typical candidate sites of disease for EBRT include the neck, upper mediastinum, or bone lesions that are symptomatic, or in critical skeletal locations to prevent fracture. In the neck, external beam radiation therapy is mainly reserved for macroscopic, inoperable, non-iodine-avid disease, or in tumors which are iodine-avid but with low iodine uptake insufficient to ablate the tumor. Improvement in locoregional progression has been shown with the use of intensity-modulated radiation therapy in patients with gross residual/unresectable neck metastases (267, 268). The use of adjuvant EBRT following surgery and radioiodine therapy in patients with completely resected disease but with high suspicion for microscopic residual disease, such as T4 disease with extrathyroidal extension, or in aggressive histologic subtypes, is controversial, but there is some evidence of benefit, particularly in patients over the age of 60 (269, 270). Risks of EBRT acutely range from local skin erythema, hyperpigmentation, and esophageal mucositis, to chronic risks for tracheal or esophageal stricture, in some cases requiring a feeding tube, must be taken into consideration. Exposure of neck tissue to EBRT may make subsequent surgeries more challenging, but in some cases, the overall risks of EBRT may be more favorable than those of multiple reoperations.

EBRT may be employed in the palliation of painful bone metastases, or for bony lesions located at weight-bearing sites. Stereotactic radiotherapy, which provides more precise delivery of radiation than EBRT, is the preferred approach for brain metastases (18). Either approach may be appropriate for lung metastases, depending on their size and location.

THERMOABLATION

Thermoablation is a localized, directed therapy of tumor cell destruction by heating (radiofrequency ablation) or cooling (cryoablation). It is a well-established and effective local treatment for lung, liver, and bone metastases from a number of primary carcinomas, and there are some published data on its use specifically for differentiated thyroid cancer metastatic to lung and bone (271). Given the relatively low adverse effects of this procedure when performed by an experienced operator, it may be considered in the treatment of a symptomatic single metastatic lesion in favor of systemic therapy and its inherent systemic toxicities.

Systemic therapies

In progressive disease which is refractory or not amenable to surgery, radioiodine, EBRT, or more localized therapy such as stereotactic radiation or thermoablation, systemic therapies are the next line of treatment. In the past decade, however, the emergence of kinase inhibitors has provided a new means of targeted therapy against persistent disease.

Kinase inhibitors

Kinase inhibitors are agents which target signaling kinases involved in multiple steps in tumor progression, including those related to oncogenic mutations of BRAF, RET and RAS kinases, as well as downstream signaling of the vascular endothelial growth factor receptor (VEGFR). Selection of the appropriate patient to receive these agents is key, as these drugs have multiple side effects which impair quality of life. While several agents have shown promise in the improvement of progression-free survival, an overall survival benefit has yet to be established.

Use of multikinase inhibitors (MKI) is reserved for patients in whom disease is progressive and symptomatic, or likely to cause significant morbidity or mortality in the next six months. If metastases are localized and amenable to targeted therapy such as resection, radiation, or thermoablation, these treatments should be considered prior to administering systemic therapy. When disease is diffuse with a low overall tumor burden, continued observation with TSH suppression as appropriate is recommended for small tumors <1–2 cm with <20% growth per year. Tumors larger than this threshold or with more rapid growth are candidates for kinase inhibitor therapy. The American Thyroid Association recommends that such patients be referred for clinical trials whenever possible (18). When clinical trial participation is not possible or desired, lenvatinib and sorafenib are the two FDA-approved tyrosine kinase inhibitors. In clinical trials, lenvatinib therapy was associated with improved progression free survival by 14.7 months as compared to placebo (272), with a more modest prolongation of progression-free survival of 5 months for sorafenib (273). Other MKIs have shown some benefit for DTC or are currently under investigation, including pazopanib, vandetinib, sunitinib, and the selective inhibitor of the V600E mutant BRAF kinase venmurafenib. In this fast-moving area, the best way to get current information on clinical trials for thyroid cancer is to use the website of the National Cancer Institute (http://www.cancer.gov/clinicaltrials), or that of the ATA (http://www.thyroid.org).

Toxicities of the kinase inhibitors are specific to each agent, but in general, the most common are hypertension, diarrhea, taste alteration, weight loss, bleeding and thrombosis, increased levothyroxine requirement, and hand and foot cutaneous manifestations. The phase III trial of lenvatinib reported a therapy-attributed mortality rate of 2.3% (272). Therefore, a discussion in which both the physician and patient agree that the potential for benefit outweighs the potential for detriment with these agents is of the utmost importance.

Cytotoxic agents

The previously minor role cytotoxic agents played in the treatment of advanced DTC has been further eclipsed by the introduction of tyrosine kinase inhibitors. Doxorubicin may occasionally be used in a patient with refractory, progressive DTC which is not responsive to tyrosine kinase inhibitors, or in a patient for whom these agents are contraindicated. There is some evidence that concurrent doxorubicin administration with EBRT improves outcomes (274). A recent study comparing patients with gross residual thyroid cancer treated with EBRT vs. EBRT with concurrent chemotherapy (the majority of which was doxorubicin) reports improved locoregional progression-free survival 73% vs. 90%, although this difference did not reach statistical significance (267).

"Redifferentiation" therapy

A promising area of active research is the targeted blockade of the MAP kinase pathway to restore iodine avidity in radioiodine-refractory disease. The MEK inhibitor selumetinib and the BRAF inhibitor dabrafenib have both been shown to improve RAI uptake in RAI refractory patients (275, 276). A benefit of this approach is the limited timeframe of taking a systemic agent (typically one month), minimizing the risk and side effect profile of these potent agents. This approach remains experimental, and further studies are needed to determine if it will become an effective therapy.

Long-term follow-up and monitoring

THYROGLOBULIN MONITORING

Serum Tg, along with Tg antibodies are measured at routine intervals in order to detect recurrence of carcinoma. The frequency at which Tg should be measured depends on the patient's initial risk for recurrence and response to therapy (see Table 8.7). In patients who have undergone radioiodine remnant ablation, an unstimulated serum Tg <0.2 ng/mL or stimulated Tg <1.0 ng/mL, is consistent with biochemical disease-free status. Measurement of Tg following stimulation with rhTSH may increase the sensitivity of detecting dormant residual malignancy and is often done in conjunction with administration of rhTSH for radioiodine diagnostic scanning. However, routine use of stimulation in the follow-up of patients with low- or intermediate-risk disease with excellent response to therapy is probably not necessary (277). Other factors to be considered when interpreting thyroglobulin levels are the sensitivity of the assay, which can be quite variable, the presence of thyroglobulin antibodies, and the trend and rate of increase (doubling time) of the Tg level (278). The use of high sensitivity Tg assays with functional sensitivities of 0.1–0.2 ng/ml is recommended.

The interpretation of serum Tg levels in patients who have undergone less than a total thyroidectomy (e.g., lobectomy) or a total thyroidectomy without radioiodine remnant ablation can be challenging, as the optimal cutoff value to designate freedom from disease has not been clearly defined. This problem is amplified by the fact that this patient population is expected to grow with the current trend of more restrained use of ^{131}I and less than total thyroidectomy. There is evidence to support the definition of biochemical excellent response to therapy as an unstimulated Tg <0.2 ng/mL and stimulated <2 ng/mL in patients who have undergone a total thyroidectomy without ablation, or unstimulated Tg <30 ng/mL in a patient who has undergone a lobectomy (183, 279). Following the trend of Tg over time is of particular importance in this patient population.

Poorly differentiated follicular cell derived cancers may not produce thyroglobulin or lose this capacity as they dedifferentiate. For this reason, in addition to biochemical surveillance, imaging is a central component in long-term monitoring for all such patients.

IMAGING

Ultrasound

A postoperative central and lateral neck ultrasound is highly sensitive for the detection of cancer in the thyroid bed and cervical lymph nodes. It is typically performed at 3–6 months postoperatively, and then at regular intervals in the first several years following initial therapy. The recommended frequency varies with the initial risk of recurrence and the biochemical response to therapy. Suspicious sonographic features indicative of malignant lymph nodes were reviewed earlier (see preoperative imaging, Figure 8.3). If the information will change management, aspiration of such nodes, with cytologic analysis and measurement of Tg in the aspirate, is recommended when the smallest diameter is >8 mm for

Table 8.7 Long-term thyroid cancer monitoring

Response category	Tg monitoring	Imaging	TSH goal*
Excellent (*low and intermediate risk for recurrence*)	Every 12–24 months	Ultrasound at 6–12 months following surgery, routine WBS not recommended unless higher risk features are present	0.5–2 mU/L
Excellent (*high risk for recurrence*)	Every 6–12 months, consider stimulation testing	Yearly ultrasound, consider periodic cross-sectional imaging	0.1–0.5 mU/L
Indeterminate	Every 6–12 months, consider stimulation	Ultrasound every 6–12 months, more comprehensive imaging may be appropriate based on individual patient factors	0.5–2.0 mU/L if low risk 0.1–0.5 mU/L if high risk
Biochemical Incomplete	Every 6–12 months, consider stimulation	WBS or PET, other cross sectional imaging to evaluate for source of Tg	0.1–0.5 mU/L
Structural Incomplete	Every 6–12 months, consider stimulation	Individualized per patient factors; if observation selected, short surveillance intervals recommended	<0.1 mU/L

*Appropriate TSH suppression may need to be modified in the setting of increased risk for thyrotoxic complications (e.g., atrial fibrillation, osteoporosis, age >60 years). Length of TSH suppression in the biochemical incomplete group varies depending on the degree of Tg elevation and trend in Tg.
Source: Modified from Haugen et al. 2015 (18).

central neck nodes and >10 mm for lateral neck nodes (18); otherwise they may be serially followed with ultrasound. Sonographic findings may be less specific, for example, a rounded lymph node which lacks a central hilum but without any other suspicious features, or a hypoechoic structure within the thyroid bed which may represent normal thyroid remnant vs. recurrent disease. These findings generally categorize the patient as having an indeterminate structural response to therapy. Continued observation of such findings will typically reveal their true nature, with stability or disappearance suggesting benignity, and growth prompting further investigation (280).

Diagnostic radioiodine WBS

While an initial posttreatment scan is performed in all patients receiving ^{131}I treatment, subsequent routine diagnostic scanning has not shown to be useful in patients with low risk disease, as well as many with intermediate risk disease that had no iodine uptake outside of the thyroid bed on initial post treatment scanning, and who are shown to have had an excellent response to therapy (281). If done, a follow-up scan is best performed at 6–12 months after initial RAI therapy in patients with an initial high risk for recurrence (or intermediate risk with higher risk features), if there is suspicion for recurrent or metastatic disease as evidenced by rising Tg or Tg Ab, or previous iodine uptake outside the thyroid bed. Use of SPECT/CT radioiodine imaging has been shown to improve diagnostic accuracy compared to planar imaging alone (282) (see Figure 8.4).

Whole-body positron emission tomography

Positron emission tomography (PET) scanning is of most value in the setting of high serum Tg levels and negative neck ultrasonography and cross-sectional imaging (CT and MRI). Scanning with ^{18}F-deoxyglucose (FDG-PET) provides two important pieces of information. First, it may identify DTC metastasis that cannot be identified by ^{131}I scintigraphy. Second, ^{18}F-FDG uptake in thyroid cancer is an indicator of poor functional differentiation and poor prognosis (283). A retrospective study of 400 patients with thyroid cancer studied at one institution (81) found an inverse relationship between patient survival and the glycolytic rate (standard uptake value or SUV) of the most active lesion. FDG avidity has been identified as an independent negative predictor of survival (81, 284). The likelihood of observing an FDG-avid lesion increases with the serum Tg level, especially when the serum Tg is >10 ng/mL (285). False-positive [18] F-DG uptake may occur with benign lung disease, inflammatory conditions, and other malignancies (286). A clinical benefit of TSH stimulation prior to PET scanning has not been shown (287).

Response to therapy

While TNM staging is designed to predict the risk of mortality, and the initial ATA risk categorization predicts recurrence, both are static and based only on data that exist at the time of resection. The ATA has developed a third classification system, Response to Therapy, which recognizes that outcomes and risk are dynamic and thus allows for an individualized approach to monitoring intensity and intervals based on real-time outcomes (18, 144) (Table 8.7, also see Figure 8.5).

Markers of response to therapy are twofold: biochemical, with measurement of serum thyroglobulin (Tg), and radiographic (see below). Response to therapy categories consist of:

- Excellent: No biochemical (serum Tg <0.2 ng/mL unstimulated or stimulated <1.0 mg/mL) and no radiographic evidence of disease
- Biochemical incomplete: Rising or elevated serum Tg, or rising Tg Antibodies without an imaging correlate
- Structural incomplete: Known structural persistent tumor or recurrent metastatic disease
- Indeterminate: Nonspecific findings, either biochemical, structural, or both, which could represent recurrent disease, including the presence of anti-Tg antibodies

EXCELLENT RESPONSE TO THERAPY

Those patients who have had an excellent response to therapy, have no biochemical (serum Tg <0.2 ng/mL unstimulated or stimulated <1.0 mg/mL) and no radiographic evidence of disease. Patients in this category with initial low or intermediate risk for recurrence are recommended to have serum Tg monitored every 12–24 months, although it should be noted that the utility and ideal timing of Tg monitoring for these patients is not well established (18).

BIOCHEMICAL INCOMPLETE RESPONSE TO THERAPY—ELEVATED TG AND NEGATIVE IMAGING

When serum Tg is elevated or rising, the clinician should endeavor to identify the source with sonography of the neck and cross-sectional imaging (18). In some cases, however, a structural correlate cannot be identified, and empiric radioiodine administration may be considered. Prior to empiric radioiodine administration, a PET/CT is recommended, as tumors that are FDG-avid are much less likely to concentrate iodine (288), and identification of such disease eliminates radioiodine as an effective option (285). In a patient with a negative PET scan and other cross-sectional imaging, and serum Tg >5–10 ng/mL, or rising Tg antibodies, empiric doses of 100–200 mCi, or otherwise as determined by dosimetry, may be given, with a posttreatment scan obtained in order to identify possible uptake (18). The posttreatment scan is successful in identifying the recurrent or persistent disease in about 50% of patients, and even among patients for whom uptake is not seen, serum Tg decreases following empiric radioiodine in about half of patients (289).

STRUCTURAL INCOMPLETE RESPONSE TO THERAPY—RECURRENT OR METASTATIC DISEASE

Cervical node disease

When persistent or recurrent disease is found in cervical lymph nodes, resection is generally recommended, as this offers the best chance for cure. Risks of revision surgery, however, must be weighed against potential benefit. Smaller suspicious appearing lymph nodes, such as those <8–10 mm, may be elected to be observed closely (18, 290). Larger nodes should be biopsied, with both cytologic analysis and Tg measurement of the aspirate to confirm malignancy. Once confirmed, nodes of this size should be considered for resection, although size is not the sole determinant of observation vs. surgery. The number of suspicious nodes, initial risk of the tumor, presence of distant disease, risk of revision surgery, patient anxiety, and proximity of nodes to vital structures should all be taken into consideration. The extent of surgery will vary by individual patient and surgeon factors, but overall,

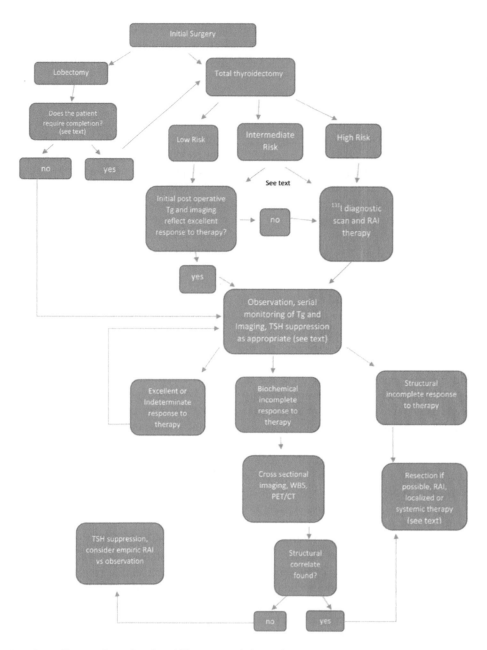

Figure 8.5 Surveillance algorithm for differentiated thyroid cancer.

comprehensive compartmental surgery is supe-rior to "berry-picking," in which only the known macroscopic foci are removed, since macroscopic nodal disease is usually associated with clinically or radiographically unapparent disease with potential to grow over time (291) (see Chapter 11, "Surgical Approach to Thyroid Disorders"). Radioiodine therapy, for iodine-avid lesions, is an additional therapeutic option, whether as an adjuvant treatment following resection or as primary ther-apy for neck recurrence in patients who are poor surgical candidates. The decision to use radioiodine in this setting, and dose activity administered, is highly variable across providers (292). There are a paucity of prospective studies guiding clinicians on the appropriate indications for RAI in patients with persistent disease. Other therapies, including percu-taneous ethanol injection of neck metastases (293),

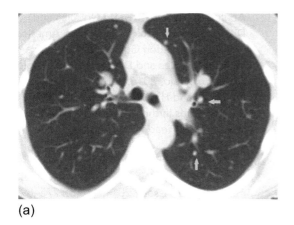

(a)

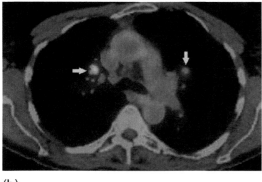

(b)

Figure 8.6 Pulmonary metastases as seen on CT (a) and PET (b) imaging.

radiofrequency ablation (294), and EBRT are second or third-line options in the treatment of neck metastases, but may be considered in patients who are poor surgical candidates or for those who desire to avoid additional surgeries (18).

Pulmonary metastases

Pulmonary metastases, which are often multiple (see Figure 8.6), are not typically resectable, and radioiodine is generally the most effective treatment. Administered activities from 100–200 mCi are commonly given, or dosimetry may be used. Repeat treatment every 6–12 months is recommended, as long as a clinical response and continued concentration of iodine is demonstrated (18). Single empiric doses of >200 mCi, or dosimetrically-calculated administered activities that render >80 mCi whole body retention at 48 hours and 200 cGy to the bone marrow are not recommended (18). Pulmonary fibrosis, a risk of exposure to high radioiodine activities,

may limit continued use of [131]I. Pulmonary function testing, as well as monitoring for bone marrow suppression should be performed in patients for whom high administered activities or repeated treatments are being considered (18).

Bone metastases

Radioiodine avid bone metastases may be treated with ^{131}I therapy (295). Bone-directed therapies, specifically the anti-resorptive agents, bisphosphonates and denosumab, are also utilized, specifically in diffuse, radioiodine refractory bone disease. Both agents have been shown to improve symptoms and time to occurrence of fracture in patients with bone metastases from solid tumors, and zoledronic acid has shown a benefit in bone metastases arising from differentiated thyroid cancer (296). Focal bone lesions causing acute symptoms may be treated with focal therapies such as external radiation, thermoablation, or surgery.

REFERENCES

1. *Cancer Facts and Figures 2018*. 2018 [cited 2018 3.]. Available from: https://www.cancer.org/content/dam/cancer-org/research/cancer-facts-and-statistics/annual-cancer-facts-and-figures/2018/cancer-facts-and-figures-2018.pdf.
2. Edwards, B.K., et al., Annual report to the nation on the status of cancer, 1975–2002, featuring population-based trends in cancer treatment. *J. Natl. Cancer Inst.*, 2005; 97(19): 1407–27.
3. *SEER database*. 2018 [03/20/2018]. Available from: https://seer.cancer.gov/statfacts/html/thyro.html.
4. Aschebrook-Kilfoy, B., et al., The clinical and economic burden of a sustained increase in thyroid cancer incidence. *Cancer Epidemiol. Biomarkers Prev.*, 2013; 22(7): 1252–9.
5. Pazaitou-Panayiotou, K., M. Capezzone, and F. Pacini, Clinical features and therapeutic implication of papillary thyroid microcarcinoma. *Thyroid*, 2007; 17(11): 1085–92.
6. Davies, L. and H.G. Welch, Increasing incidence of thyroid cancer in the United States, 1973–2002. *JAMA*, 2006; 295(18): 2164–7.
7. La Vecchia, C., et al., Thyroid cancer mortality and incidence: A global overview. *Int. J. Cancer*, 2015; 136(9): 2187–95.

8. Lim, H., et al., Trends in Thyroid Cancer Incidence and Mortality in the United States, 1974–2013. *JAMA*, 2017; 317(13): 1338–1348.

9. Frattini, M., et al., Alternative mutations of BRAF, RET and NTRK1 are associated with similar but distinct gene expression patterns in papillary thyroid cancer. *Oncogene*, 2004; 23(44): 7436–40.

10. Puxeddu, E., et al., BRAF(V599E) mutation is the leading genetic event in adult sporadic papillary thyroid carcinomas. *J. Clin. Endocrinol. Metab.*, 2004; 89(5): 2414–20.

11. Penna, G.C., et al., Molecular markers involved in tumorigenesis of thyroid carcinoma: Focus on aggressive histotypes. *Cytogenet. Genome Res.*, 2016; 150(3–4): 194–207.

12. Tufano, R.P., et al., BRAF mutation in papillary thyroid cancer and its value in tailoring initial treatment: A systematic review and meta-analysis. *Medicine (Baltimore)*, 2012; 91(5): 274–86.

13. Shen, X., et al., Patient age-associated mortality risk is differentiated by BRAF V600E status in papillary thyroid cancer. *J. Clin. Oncol.*, 2018; 36(5): 438–445.

14. Elisei, R., et al., The BRAF(V600E) mutation is an independent, poor prognostic factor for the outcome of patients with low-risk intrathyroid papillary thyroid carcinoma: Single-institution results from a large cohort study. *J. Clin. Endocrinol. Metab.*, 2012; 97(12): 4390–8.

15. Gouveia, C., et al., Lack of association of BRAF mutation with negative prognostic indicators in papillary thyroid carcinoma: The University of California, San Francisco, experience. *JAMA Otolaryngol. Head Neck Surg.*, 2013; 139(11): 1164–70.

16. Henke, L.E., et al., BRAF mutation is not predictive of long-term outcome in papillary thyroid carcinoma. *Cancer Med.*, 2015; 4(6): 791–9.

17. Kim, T.H., et al., The association of the BRAF(V600E) mutation with prognostic factors and poor clinical outcome in papillary thyroid cancer: A meta-analysis. *Cancer*, 2012; 118(7): 1764–73.

18. Haugen, B.R., et al., 2015 American Thyroid Association Management Guidelines for Adult Patients with Thyroid Nodules and Differentiated Thyroid Cancer: The American Thyroid Association Guidelines Task Force on Thyroid Nodules and Differentiated Thyroid Cancer. *Thyroid*, 2016; 26(1): 1–133.

19. Davies, L. and H.G. Welch, Current thyroid cancer trends in the United States. *JAMA Otolaryngol. Head Neck Surg.*, 2014; 140(4): 317–22.

20. Chen, C.H. and R.J. Chen, Prevalence of telomerase activity in human cancer. *J. Formos Med. Assoc.*, 2011; 110(5): 275–89.

21. Vinagre, J., et al., Telomerase promoter mutations in cancer: An emerging molecular biomarker? *Virchows Arch.*, 2014; 465(2): 119–33.

22. Moyzis, R.K., et al., A highly conserved repetitive DNA sequence, (TTAGGG)n, present at the telomeres of human chromosomes. *Proc. Natl. Acad. Sci. U S A*, 1988; 85(18): 6622–6.

23. Blasco, M.A., Telomeres and human disease: Ageing, cancer and beyond. *Nat. Rev. Genet.*, 2005; 6(8): 611–22.

24. Pestana, A., et al., TERT biology and function in cancer: Beyond immortalisation. *J. Mol. Endocrinol.*, 2017; 58(2): R129–R146.

25. Xing, M., et al., BRAF V600E and TERT promoter mutations cooperatively identify the most aggressive papillary thyroid cancer with highest recurrence. *J. Clin. Oncol.*, 2014; 32(25): 2718–26.

26. de Biase, D., et al., TERT promoter mutations in papillary thyroid microcarcinomas. *Thyroid*, 2015; 25(9): 1013–9.

27. Jin, L., et al., BRAF and TERT promoter mutations in the aggressiveness of papillary thyroid carcinoma: A study of 653 patients. *Oncotarget*, 2016; 7(14): 18346–55.

28. Nasirden, A., et al., In Japanese patients with papillary thyroid carcinoma, TERT promoter mutation is associated with poor prognosis, in contrast to BRAF (V600E) mutation. *Virchows Arch.*, 2016; 469(6): 687–696.

29. Vuong, H.G., et al., A meta-analysis of prognostic roles of molecular markers in papillary thyroid carcinoma. *Endocr. Connect*, 2017; 6(3): R8–R17.

30. Liu, R., et al., Mortality risk stratification by combining BRAF V600E and TERT promoter mutations in papillary thyroid cancer:

Genetic duet of BRAF and *TERT* promoter mutations in thyroid cancer mortality. *JAMA Oncol.*, 2016; 3(2): 202–208.

31. Xing, M., Clinical utility of RAS mutations in thyroid cancer: A blurred picture now emerging clearer. *BMC Med.*, 2016; 14: 12.

32. Medici, M., et al., The variable phenotype and low-risk nature of RAS-positive thyroid nodules. *BMC Med.*, 2015; 13: 184.

33. Medici, M., et al., Long- versus short-interval follow-up of cytologically benign thyroid nodules: A prospective cohort study. *BMC Med.*, 2016; 14: 11.

34. Nagy, R. and M.D. Ringel, Genetic predisposition for nonmedullary thyroid cancer. *Horm. Cancer*, 2015; 6(1): 13–20.

35. Charkes, N.D., On the prevalence of familial nonmedullary thyroid cancer in multiply affected kindreds. *Thyroid*, 2006; 16(2): 181–6.

36. Ito, Y., et al., Biological behavior and prognosis of familial papillary thyroid carcinoma. *Surgery*, 2009; 145(1): 100–5.

37. Lee, Y.M., et al., Familial history of nonmedullary thyroid cancer is an independent prognostic factor for tumor recurrence in younger patients with conventional papillary thyroid carcinoma. *J. Surg. Oncol.*, 2014; 109(2): 168–73.

38. Park, Y.J., et al., The long-term outcomes of the second generation of familial nonmedullary thyroid carcinoma are more aggressive than sporadic cases. *Thyroid*, 2012; 22(4): 356–62.

39. Sung, T.Y., et al., Surgical management of familial papillary thyroid microcarcinoma: A single institution study of 94 cases. *World J. Surg.*, 2015; 39(8): 1930–5.

40. Schneider, A.B., et al., Dose-response relationships for radiation-induced thyroid cancer and thyroid nodules: Evidence for the prolonged effects of radiation on the thyroid. *J. Clin. Endocrinol. Metab.*, 1993; 77(2): 362–9.

41. Somerville, H.M., et al., Thyroid neoplasia following irradiation in adolescent and young adult survivors of childhood cancer. *Med. J. Aust.*, 2002; 176(12): 584–7.

42. White, M.G., et al., Radiation-induced differentiated thyroid cancer is associated with improved overall survival but not thyroid cancer-specific mortality or disease-free survival. *Thyroid*, 2016; 26(8): 1053–60.

43. Shaha, M.A., et al., Previous external beam radiation treatment exposure does not confer worse outcome for patients with differentiated thyroid cancer. *Thyroid*, 2017; 27(3): 412–417.

44. Jung, C.K., et al., The increase in thyroid cancer incidence during the last four decades is accompanied by a high frequency of BRAF mutations and a sharp increase in RAS mutations. *J. Clin. Endocrinol. Metab.*, 2014; 99(2): E276–85.

45. Kowalska, A., et al., Increase in papillary thyroid cancer incidence is accompanied by changes in the frequency of the BRAF V600E mutation: A single-institution study. *Thyroid*, 2016; 26(4): 543–51.

46. Romei, C., et al., Modifications in the papillary thyroid cancer gene profile over the last 15 years. *J. Clin. Endocrinol. Metab.*, 2012; 97(9): E1758–65.

47. Pappa, T. and M. Alevizaki, Obesity and thyroid cancer: A clinical update. *Thyroid*, 2014; 24(2): 190–9.

48. Kitahara, C.M. and J.A. Sosa, The changing incidence of thyroid cancer. *Nat. Rev. Endocrinol.*, 2016; 12(11): 646–653.

49. Peterson, E., P. De, and R. Nuttall, BMI, diet and female reproductive factors as risks for thyroid cancer: A systematic review. *PLoS One*, 2012; 7(1): e29177.

50. Kwon, H. and J.E. Pessin, Adipokines mediate inflammation and insulin resistance. *Front. Endocrinol. (Lausanne)*, 2013; 4: 71.

51. Proces, S., et al., Minor alterations in thyroid-function tests associated with diabetes mellitus and obesity in outpatients without known thyroid illness. *Acta Clin. Belg.*, 2001; 56(2): 86–90.

52. Fiore, E. and P. Vitti, Serum TSH and risk of papillary thyroid cancer in nodular thyroid disease. *J. Clin. Endocrinol. Metab.*, 2012; 97(4): 1134–45.

53. McLeod, D.S., et al., Prognosis of differentiated thyroid cancer in relation to serum thyrotropin and thyroglobulin antibody status at time of diagnosis. *Thyroid*, 2014; 24(1): 35–42.

54. Malaguarnera, R., et al., Insulin Resistance: Any Role in the Changing Epidemiology of Thyroid Cancer? *Front. Endocrinol. (Lausanne)*, 2017; 8: 314.

55. Zimmermann, M.B. and V. Galetti, Iodine intake as a risk factor for thyroid cancer: A comprehensive review of animal and human studies. *Thyroid Res.*, 2015; 8: 8.

56. Schmidt, J.A., et al., Insulin-like growth factor-i and risk of differentiated thyroid carcinoma in the European prospective investigation into cancer and nutrition. *Cancer Epidemiol. Biomarkers. Prev.*, 2014; 23(6): 976–85.

57. Cho, Y.A. and J. Kim, Thyroid cancer risk and smoking status: A meta-analysis. *Cancer Causes Control*, 2014; 25(9): 1187–95.

58. Ng, M., et al., Smoking prevalence and cigarette consumption in 187 countries, 1980–2012. *JAMA*, 2014; 311(2): 183–92.

59. Hoffman, K., J.A. Sosa, and H.M. Stapleton, Do flame retardant chemicals increase the risk for thyroid dysregulation and cancer? *Curr. Opin. Oncol.*, 2017; 29(1): 7–13.

60. Moreno, A., et al., Encapsulated papillary neoplasm of the thyroid: Retrospective clinicopathological study with long term follow up. *Eur. J. Surg.*, 1996; 162(3): 177–80.

61. Schroder, S., et al., The encapsulated papillary carcinoma of the thyroid. A morphologic subtype of the papillary thyroid carcinoma. *Cancer*, 1984; 54(1): 90–3.

62. Kim, K.J., et al., Prognostic significance of tumor multifocality in papillary thyroid carcinoma and its relationship with primary tumor size: A retrospective study of 2,309 consecutive patients. *Ann. Surg. Oncol.*, 2015; 22(1): 125–31.

63. Shi, X., et al., Differential clinicopathological risk and prognosis of major papillary thyroid cancer variants. *J. Clin. Endocrinol. Metab.*, 2016; 101(1): 264–74.

64. Wang, F., et al., The prognostic value of tumor multifocality in clinical outcomes of papillary thyroid cancer. *J. Clin. Endocrinol. Metab.*, 2017; 102(9): 3241–3250.

65. La Greca, A., et al., Patients with multifocal macroscopic papillary thyroid carcinoma have a low risk of recurrence at early follow-up after total thyroidectomy and radioactive iodine treatment. *Eur. Thyroid J.*, 2017; 6(1): 31–39.

66. Mazzaferri, E.L. and S.M. Jhiang, Long-term impact of initial surgical and medical therapy on papillary and follicular thyroid cancer. *Am. J. Med.*, 1994; 97(5): 418–28.

67. Qubain, S.W., et al., Distribution of lymph node micrometastasis in pN0 well-differentiated thyroid carcinoma. *Surgery*, 2002; 131(3): 249–56.

68. Machens, A., H.J. Holzhausen, and H. Dralle, The prognostic value of primary tumor size in papillary and follicular thyroid carcinoma. *Cancer*, 2005; 103(11): 2269–73.

69. Arch-Ferrer, J., et al., Accuracy of sentinel lymph node in papillary thyroid carcinoma. *Surgery*, 2001; 130(6): 907–13.

70. Mirallie, E., et al., Localization of cervical node metastasis of papillary thyroid carcinoma. *World J. Surg.*, 1999; 23(9): 970–3; discussion 973–4.

71. Randolph, G.W., et al., The prognostic significance of nodal metastases from papillary thyroid carcinoma can be stratified based on the size and number of metastatic lymph nodes, as well as the presence of extranodal extension. *Thyroid*, 2012; 22(11): 1144–52.

72. Leboulleux, S., et al., Prognostic factors for persistent or recurrent disease of papillary thyroid carcinoma with neck lymph node metastases and/or tumor extension beyond the thyroid capsule at initial diagnosis. *J. Clin. Endocrinol. Metab.*, 2005; 90(10): 5723–9.

73. Yamashita, H., et al., Extracapsular invasion of lymph node metastasis is an indicator of distant metastasis and poor prognosis in patients with thyroid papillary carcinoma. *Cancer*, 1997; 80(12): 2268–72.

74. Ito, Y., et al., Prognosis of patients with papillary thyroid carcinoma having clinically apparent metastasis to the lateral compartment. *Endocr. J.*, 2009; 56(6): 759–66.

75. Wada, N., et al., Lymph node metastasis from 259 papillary thyroid microcarcinomas: Frequency, pattern of occurrence and recurrence, and optimal strategy for neck dissection. *Ann. Surg.*, 2003; 237(3): 399–407.

76. Cranshaw, I.M. and B. Carnaille, Micrometastases in thyroid cancer. An important finding? *Surg. Oncol.*, 2008; 17(3): 253–8.

77. Moreno, M.A., et al., Preoperative lateral neck ultrasonography as a long-term outcome predictor in papillary thyroid cancer. *Arch. Otolaryngol. Head Neck Surg.*, 2011; 137(2): 157–62.

78. Yu, X.M., et al., Should all papillary thyroid microcarcinomas be aggressively treated? An analysis of 18,445 cases. *Ann. Surg.*, 2011; 254(4): 653–60.

79. Durante, C., et al., Long-term outcome of 444 patients with distant metastases from papillary and follicular thyroid carcinoma: Benefits and limits of radioiodine therapy. *J. Clin. Endocrinol. Metab.*, 2006; 91(8): 2892–9.

80. Lang, B.H., et al., Evaluating the prognostic factors associated with cancer-specific survival of differentiated thyroid carcinoma presenting with distant metastasis. *Ann. Surg. Oncol.*, 2013; 20(4): 1329–35.

81. Robbins, R.J., et al., Real-time prognosis for metastatic thyroid carcinoma based on 2-[18F]fluoro-2-deoxy-D-glucose-positron emission tomography scanning. *J. Clin. Endocrinol. Metab.*, 2006; 91(2): 498–505.

82. Ronga, G., et al., Lung metastases from differentiated thyroid carcinoma. A 40 years' experience. *Q. J. Nucl. Med. Mol. Imaging*, 2004; 48(1): 12–9.

83. Shoup, M., et al., Prognostic indicators of outcomes in patients with distant metastases from differentiated thyroid carcinoma. *J. Am. Coll. Surg.*, 2003; 197(2): 191–7.

84. Ito, Y., et al., Patient age is significantly related to the progression of papillary microcarcinoma of the thyroid under observation. *Thyroid*, 2014; 24(1): 27–34.

85. Tuttle, R.M., et al., Natural history and tumor volume kinetics of papillary thyroid cancers during active surveillance. *JAMA Otolaryngol. Head Neck Surg.*, 2017; 143(10): 1015–1020.

86. Brito, J.P., et al., A clinical framework to facilitate risk stratification when considering an active surveillance alternative to immediate biopsy and surgery in papillary microcarcinoma. *Thyroid*, 2016; 26(1): 144–9.

87. Chow, S.M., et al., Papillary microcarcinoma of the thyroid-Prognostic significance of lymph node metastasis and multifocality. *Cancer*, 2003; 98(1): 31–40.

88. Gui, C.Y., et al., Clinical and pathologic predictors of central lymph node metastasis in papillary thyroid microcarcinoma: A retrospective cohort study. *J. Endocrinol. Invest.*, 2018; 41(4): 403–409.

89. Zhang, L., et al., Risk factors for neck nodal metastasis in papillary thyroid microcarcinoma: A study of 1066 patients. *J. Clin. Endocrinol. Metab.*, 2012; 97(4): 1250–7.

90. Mazzaferri, E.L., Thyroid cancer in thyroglossal duct remnants: A diagnostic and therapeutic dilemma. *Thyroid*, 2004; 14(5): 335–6.

91. Doshi, S.V., R.M. Cruz, and R.L. Hilsinger, Jr., Thyroglossal duct carcinoma: A large case series. *Ann. Otol. Rhinol. Laryngol.*, 2001; 110(8): 734–8.

92. Patel, S.G., et al., Management of well-differentiated thyroid carcinoma presenting within a thyroglossal duct cyst. *J Surg Oncol*, 2002; 79(3): 134–9; discussion 140–1.

93. Pellegriti, G., et al., Thyroid cancer in thyroglossal duct cysts requires a specific approach due to its unpredictable extension. *J. Clin. Endocrinol. Metab.*, 2013; 98(2): 458–65.

94. Rayess, H.M., et al., Thyroglossal duct cyst carcinoma: A systematic review of clinical features and outcomes. *Otolaryngol. Head Neck Surg.*, 2017; 156(5): 794–802.

95. Burningham, A.R., et al., Papillary and follicular variant of papillary carcinoma of the thyroid: Initial presentation and response to therapy. *Otolaryngol. Head Neck Surg.*, 2005; 132(6): 840–4.

96. Chem, K.T. and J. Rosai, Follicular variant of thyroid papillary carcinoma: A clinicopathologic study of six cases. *Am. J. Surg. Pathol.*, 1977; 1(2): 123–30.

97. Zidan, J., et al., Pure versus follicular variant of papillary thyroid carcinoma: Clinical features, prognostic factors, treatment, and survival. *Cancer*, 2003; 97(5): 1181–5.

98. Passler, C., et al., Follicular variant of papillary thyroid carcinoma: A long-term follow-up. *Arch. Surg.*, 2003; 138(12): 1362–6.

99. Rivera, M., et al., Encapsulated papillary thyroid carcinoma: A clinico-pathologic study of 106 cases with emphasis on its morphologic subtypes (histologic growth pattern). *Thyroid*, 2009; 19(2): 119–27.

100. Nikiforov, Y.E., et al., Nomenclature revision for encapsulated follicular variant of papillary thyroid carcinoma: A paradigm shift to reduce overtreatment of indolent tumors. *JAMA Oncol*, 2016; 2(8): 1023–9.

101. Seethala, R.R., et al., Noninvasive follicular thyroid neoplasm with papillary-like nuclear features: A review for pathologists. *Mod. Pathol.*, 2018; 31(1): 39–55.

102. Haugen, B.R., et al., American thyroid association guidelines on the management of thyroid nodules and differentiated thyroid cancer task force review and recommendation on the proposed renaming of encapsulated follicular variant papillary thyroid carcinoma without invasion to noninvasive follicular thyroid neoplasm with papillary-like nuclear features. *Thyroid*, 2017; 27(4): 481–483.

103. Kazaure, H.S., S.A. Roman, and J.A. Sosa, Aggressive variants of papillary thyroid cancer: Incidence, characteristics and predictors of survival among 43,738 patients. *Ann. Surg. Oncol.*, 2012; 19(6): 1874–80.

104. Silver, C.E., et al., Aggressive variants of papillary thyroid carcinoma. *Head Neck*, 2011; 33(7): 1052–9.

105. Burman, K.D., M.D. Ringel, and L. Wartofsky, Unusual types of thyroid neoplasms. *Endocrinol. Metab. Clin. North Am.*, 1996; 25(1): 49–68.

106. Nikiforova, M.N., et al., BRAF mutations in thyroid tumors are restricted to papillary carcinomas and anaplastic or poorly differentiated carcinomas arising from papillary carcinomas. *J. Clin. Endocrinol. Metab.*, 2003; 88(11): 5399–404.

107. Jalisi, S., T. Ainsworth, and M. Lavalley, Prognostic outcomes of tall cell variant papillary thyroid cancer: A meta-analysis. *J. Thyroid Res.*, 2010; 2010: 325602.

108. Bongiovanni, M., et al., Columnar cell variant of papillary thyroid carcinoma: Cytomorphological characteristics of 11 cases with histological correlation and literature review. *Cancer Cytopathol.*, 2017; 125(6): 389–397.

109. Baloch, Z.W. and V.A. LiVolsi, Special types of thyroid carcinoma. *Histopathology*, 2018; 72(1): 40–52.

110. Chen, J.H., et al., Clinicopathological and molecular characterization of nine cases of columnar cell variant of papillary thyroid carcinoma. *Mod. Pathol.*, 2011; 24(5): 739–49.

111. Vuong, H.G., et al., Prognostic significance of diffuse sclerosing variant papillary thyroid carcinoma: A systematic review and meta-analysis. *Eur. J. Endocrinol.*, 2017; 176(4): 431–439.

112. Nikiforov, Y.E., et al., Distinct pattern of ret oncogene rearrangements in morphological variants of radiation-induced and sporadic thyroid papillary carcinomas in children. *Cancer Res.*, 1997; 57(9): 1690–4.

113. Asioli, S., et al., Papillary thyroid carcinoma with prominent hobnail features: A new aggressive variant of moderately differentiated papillary carcinoma. A clinicopathologic, immunohistochemical, and molecular study of eight cases. *Am. J. Surg. Pathol.*, 2010; 34(1): 44–52.

114. Motosugi, U., et al., Thyroid papillary carcinoma with micropapillary and hobnail growth pattern: A histological variant with intermediate malignancy? *Thyroid*, 2009; 19(5): 535–7.

115. Ambrosi, F., et al., Hobnail variant of papillary thyroid carcinoma: A literature review. *Endocr. Pathol.*, 2017; 28(4): 293–301.

116. Asioli, S., et al., Cytomorphologic and molecular features of hobnail variant of papillary thyroid carcinoma: Case series and literature review. *Diagn. Cytopathol.*, 2014; 42(1): 78–84.

117. Morandi, L., et al., Somatic mutation profiling of hobnail variant of papillary thyroid carcinoma. *Endocr. Relat. Cancer*, 2017; 24(2): 107–117.

118. Teng, L., et al., Hobnail variant of papillary thyroid carcinoma: Molecular profiling and comparison to classical papillary thyroid carcinoma, poorly differentiated thyroid carcinoma and anaplastic thyroid carcinoma. *Oncotarget*, 2017; 8(13): 22023–22033.

119. Nikiforov, Y.E., et al., Solid variant of papillary thyroid carcinoma: Incidence, clinical-pathologic characteristics, molecular analysis, and biologic behavior. *Am. J. Surg. Pathol.*, 2001; 25(12): 1478–84.

120. LiVolsi, V.A., et al., The Chernobyl thyroid cancer experience: Pathology. *Clin. Oncol. (R. Coll. Radiol.)*, 2011; 23(4): 261–7.

121. Romei, C. and R. Elisei, RET/PTC translocations and clinico-pathological features in human papillary thyroid carcinoma. *Front. Endocrinol. (Lausanne)*, 2012; 3: 54.

122. Nikiforov, Y.E., et al., Impact of mutational testing on the diagnosis and management of patients with cytologically indeterminate thyroid nodules: A prospective analysis of 1056 FNA samples. *J. Clin. Endocrinol. Metab.*, 2011; 96(11): 3390–7.

123. Zhu, Z., et al., Molecular profile and clinical-pathologic features of the follicular variant of papillary thyroid carcinoma. An unusually high prevalence of ras mutations. *Am. J. Clin. Pathol.*, 2003; 120(1): 71–7.

124. Burns, J.S., et al., Stepwise transformation of primary thyroid epithelial cells by a mutant Ha-ras oncogene: An in vitro model of tumor progression. *Mol. Carcinog.*, 1992; 6(2): 129–39.

125. Najafian, A., et al., RAS Mutations, and RET/PTC and PAX8/PPAR-gamma chromosomal rearrangements are also prevalent in benign thyroid lesions: Implications thereof and a systematic review. *Thyroid*, 2017; 27(1): 39–48.

126. Ito, Y., et al., Prognostic factors of minimally invasive follicular thyroid carcinoma: Extensive vascular invasion significantly affects patient prognosis. *Endocr. J.*, 2013; 60(5): 637–42.

127. D'Avanzo, A., et al., Follicular thyroid carcinoma: Histology and prognosis. *Cancer*, 2004; 100(6): 1123–9.

128. Lee, Y.M., et al., Risk factors for distant metastasis in patients with minimally invasive follicular thyroid carcinoma. *PLoS One*, 2016; 11(5): e0155489.

129. Mills, S.C., et al., Hürthle cell carcinoma of the thyroid: Retrospective review of 62 patients treated at the Royal Marsden Hospital between 1946 and 2003. *Eur. J. Surg. Oncol.*, 2009; 35(3): 230–4.

130. Kim, H.J., et al., Association of vascular invasion with increased mortality in patients with minimally invasive follicular thyroid carcinoma but not widely invasive follicular thyroid carcinoma. *Head Neck*, 2014; 36(12): 1695–700.

131. Grani, G., et al., Follicular thyroid cancer and Hürthle cell carcinoma: Challenges in diagnosis, treatment, and clinical management. *Lancet Diabetes Endocrinol.*, 2017; 6(6): 500–514.

132. Harach, H.R. and G.A. Ceballos, Thyroid cancer, thyroiditis and dietary iodine: A review based on the Salta, Argentina model. *Endocr. Pathol.*, 2008; 19(4): 209–20.

133. Harach, H.R., et al., Thyroid carcinoma and thyroiditis in an endemic goitre region before and after iodine prophylaxis. *Acta Endocrinol. (Copenh)*, 1985; 108(1): 55–60.

134. Pettersson, B., et al., Trends in thyroid cancer incidence in Sweden, 1958–1981, by histopathologic type. *Int. J. Cancer*, 1991; 48(1): 28–33.

135. Ahmadi, S., et al., Hürthle cell carcinoma: Current perspectives. *Onco Targets Ther.*, 2016; 9: 6873–6884.

136. Montone, K.T., Z.W. Baloch, and V.A. LiVolsi, The thyroid Hürthle (oncocytic) cell and its associated pathologic conditions: A surgical pathology and cytopathology review. *Arch. Pathol. Lab. Med.*, 2008; 132(8): 1241–50.

137. Baloch, Z.W. and V.A. LiVolsi, Follicular-patterned afflictions of the thyroid gland: Reappraisal of the most discussed entity in endocrine pathology. *Endocr. Pathol.*, 2014; 25(1): 12–20.

138. Kushchayeva, Y., et al., Comparison of clinical characteristics at diagnosis and during follow-up in 118 patients with Hürthle cell or follicular thyroid cancer. *Am. J. Surg.*, 2008; 195(4): 457–62.

139. Ernaga Lorea, A., et al., Comparison of clinical characteristics of patients with follicular thyroid carcinoma and Hürthle cell carcinoma. *Endocrinol. Diabetes Nutr.*, 2018; 65(3): 136–142.

140. Kutun, S., et al., The predicting factors for clinical outcomes in patients with Hürthle cell carcinoma: How we do it. *Clin. Otolaryngol.*, 2011; 36(1): 73–7.

141. Nagar, S., et al., Hürthle cell carcinoma: An update on survival over the last 35 years. *Surgery*, 2013; 154(6): 1263–71; discussion 1271.

142. Hundahl, S.A., et al., A National Cancer Data Base report on 53,856 cases of thyroid carcinoma treated in the U.S., 1985–1995 [see commetns]. *Cancer*, 1998; 83(12): 2638–48.

143. *AJCC Cancer Staging Manual (8th edition)*. 8th ed. 2017. Springer International Publishing: American Joint Commission on Cancer.

144. Tuttle, R.M., et al., Estimating risk of recurrence in differentiated thyroid cancer after total thyroidectomy and radioactive iodine remnant ablation: Using response to therapy variables to modify the initial risk estimates predicted by the new American Thyroid Association staging system. *Thyroid*, 2010; 20(12): 1341–9.

145. Shi, R.L., et al., The trend of age-group effect on prognosis in differentiated thyroid cancer. *Sci. Rep.*, 2016; 6: 27086.

146. Bal, C.S., et al., Is chest x-ray or high-resolution computed tomography scan of the chest sufficient investigation to detect pulmonary metastasis in pediatric differentiated thyroid cancer? *Thyroid*, 2004; 14(3): 217–25.

147. Dottorini, M.E., et al., Differentiated thyroid carcinoma in children and adolescents: A 37-year experience in 85 patients. *J. Nucl. Med.*, 1997; 38(5): 669–75.

148. Golpanian, S., et al., Pediatric papillary thyroid carcinoma: Outcomes and survival predictors in 2504 surgical patients. *Pediatr. Surg. Int.*, 2016; 32(3): 201–8.

149. Pawelczak, M., et al., Outcomes of children and adolescents with well-differentiated thyroid carcinoma and pulmonary metastases following (1)(3)(1)I treatment: A systematic review. *Thyroid*, 2010; 20(10): 1095–101.

150. Liu, C., et al., Reevaluating the prognostic significance of male gender for papillary thyroid carcinoma and microcarcinoma: A SEER database analysis. *Sci. Rep.*, 2017; 7(1): 11412.

151. Kouvaraki, M.A., et al., Role of preoperative ultrasonography in the surgical management of patients with thyroid cancer. *Surgery*, 2003; 134(6): 946–54; discussion 954–5.

152. Stulak, J.M., et al., Value of preoperative ultrasonography in the surgical management of initial and reoperative papillary thyroid cancer. *Arch. Surg.*, 2006; 141(5): 489–94; discussion 494–6.

153. Leboulleux, S., et al., Ultrasound criteria of malignancy for cervical lymph nodes in patients followed up for differentiated thyroid cancer. *J. Clin. Endocrinol. Metab.*, 2007; 92(9): 3590–4.

154. American Thyroid Association Guidelines Taskforce on Thyroid, N., et al., Revised American Thyroid Association management guidelines for patients with thyroid nodules and differentiated thyroid cancer. *Thyroid*, 2009; 19(11): 1167–214.

155. Bilimoria, K.Y., et al., Extent of surgery affects survival for papillary thyroid cancer. *Ann. Surg.*, 2007; 246(3): 375–81; discussion 381–4.

156. Handkiewicz-Junak, D., et al., Total thyroidectomy and adjuvant radioiodine treatment independently decrease locoregional recurrence risk in childhood and adolescent differentiated thyroid cancer. *J. Nucl. Med.*, 2007; 48(6): 879–88.

157. Barney, B.M., et al., Overall and cause-specific survival for patients undergoing lobectomy, near-total, or total thyroidectomy for differentiated thyroid cancer. *Head Neck*, 2011; 33(5): 645–9.

158. Mendelsohn, A.H., et al., Surgery for papillary thyroid carcinoma: Is lobectomy enough? *Arch. Otolaryngol. Head Neck Surg.*, 2010; 136(11): 1055–61.

159. Nixon, I.J., et al., Thyroid lobectomy for treatment of well differentiated intrathyroid malignancy. *Surgery*, 2012; 151(4): 571–9.

160. Arturi, F., et al., Early diagnosis by genetic analysis of differentiated thyroid cancer metastases in small lymph nodes. *J. Clin. Endocrinol. Metab.*, 1997; 82(5): 1638–41.

161. Bardet, S., et al., Macroscopic lymph-node involvement and neck dissection predict lymph-node recurrence in papillary thyroid carcinoma. *Eur. J. Endocrinol.*, 2008; 158(4): 551–60.

162. Ito, Y., et al., Preoperative ultrasonographic examination for lymph node metastasis: Usefulness when designing lymph node dissection for papillary microcarcinoma of the thyroid. *World J. Surg.*, 2004; 28(5): 498–501.

163. Erdem, E., et al., Comparison of completion thyroidectomy and primary surgery for differentiated thyroid carcinoma. *Eur. J. Surg. Oncol.*, 2003; 29(9): 747–9.

164. Untch, B.R., et al., Oncologic outcomes after completion thyroidectomy for patients with well-differentiated thyroid carcinoma. *Ann. Surg. Oncol.*, 2014; 21(4): 1374–8.

165. Giordano, D., et al., Complications of central neck dissection in patients with papillary

thyroid carcinoma: Results of a study on 1087 patients and review of the literature. *Thyroid*, 2012; 22(9): 911–7.

166. Rosato, L., et al., Complications of thyroid surgery: Analysis of a multicentric study on 14,934 patients operated on in Italy over 5 years. *World J. Surg.*, 2004; 28(3): 271–6.

167. Pattou, F., et al., Hypocalcemia following thyroid surgery: Incidence and prediction of outcome. *World J. Surg.*, 1998; 22(7): 718–24.

168. Hauch, A., et al., The importance of surgical volume on outcomes in thyroid surgery revisited: Old is in again: Editorial response to "what's old is new again" by Julie Ann Sosa (doi: 10.1245/s10434–014-3850-z). *Ann. Surg. Oncol.*, 2014. 21(12): 3721–2.

169. Kandil, E., et al., The impact of surgical volume on patient outcomes following thyroid surgery. *Surgery*, 2013; 154(6): 1346–52; discussion 1352–3.

170. Moosa, M. and E.L. Mazzaferri, Outcome of differentiated thyroid cancer diagnosed in pregnant women. *J. Clin. Endocrinol. Metab.*, 1997; 82(9): 2862–6.

171. Alexander, E.K., et al., 2017 Guidelines of the American Thyroid Association for the diagnosis and management of thyroid disease during pregnancy and the postpartum. *Thyroid*, 2017; 27(3): 315–389.

172. Polachek, A., et al., Prognostic value of post-thyroidectomy thyroglobulin levels in patients with differentiated thyroid cancer. *J. Endocrinol. Invest.*, 2011; 34(11): 855–60.

173. Ibrahimpasic, T., et al., Undetectable thyroglobulin after total thyroidectomy in patients with low- and intermediate-risk papillary thyroid cancer--is there a need for radioactive iodine therapy? *Surgery*, 2012; 152(6): 1096–105.

174. Rosario, P.W., et al., Postoperative stimulated thyroglobulin of less than 1 ng/ml as a criterion to spare low-risk patients with papillary thyroid cancer from radioactive iodine ablation. *Thyroid*, 2012; 22(11): 1140–3.

175. Spencer, C.A., et al., Serum thyroglobulin autoantibodies: Prevalence, influence on serum thyroglobulin measurement, and prognostic significance in patients with differentiated thyroid carcinoma. *J. Clin. Endocrinol. Metab.*, 1998; 83(4): 1121–7.

176. Netzel, B.C., et al., Thyroglobulin (Tg) testing revisited: Tg assays, TgAb assays, and correlation of results with clinical outcomes. *J. Clin. Endocrinol. Metab.*, 2015; 100(8): E1074–83.

177. Clarke, N.J., Y. Zhang, and R.E. Reitz, A novel mass spectrometry-based assay for the accurate measurement of thyroglobulin from patient samples containing antithyroglobulin autoantibodies. *J. Investig. Med.*, 2012; 60(8): 1157–63.

178. Azmat, U., et al., Thyroglobulin liquid chromatography-tandem mass spectrometry has a low sensitivity for detecting structural disease in patients with antithyroglobulin antibodies. *Thyroid*, 2017; 27(1): 74–80.

179. Spencer, C.A., Recoveries cannot be used to authenticate thyroglobulin (Tg) measurements when sera contain Tg autoantibodies. *Clin. Chem.*, 1996; 42(5): 661–3.

180. Padovani, R.P., et al., Even without additional therapy, serum thyroglobulin concentrations often decline for years after total thyroidectomy and radioactive remnant ablation in patients with differentiated thyroid cancer. *Thyroid*, 2012; 22(8): 778–83.

181. Valle, L.A., et al., In thyroidectomized patients with thyroid cancer, a serum thyrotropin of 30 muU/mL after thyroxine withdrawal is not always adequate for detecting an elevated stimulated serum thyroglobulin. *Thyroid*, 2013; 23(2): 185–93.

182. Dominguez, J.M., et al., Neck sonography and suppressed thyroglobulin have high sensitivity for identifying recurrent/persistent disease in patients with low-risk thyroid cancer treated with total thyroidectomy and radioactive iodine ablation, making stimulated thyroglobulin unnecessary. *J. Ultrasound Med.*, 2017; 36(11): 2299–2307.

183. Momesso, D.P., et al., Dynamic risk stratification in patients with differentiated thyroid cancer treated without radioactive iodine. *J. Clin. Endocrinol. Metab.*, 2016; 101(7): 2692–700.

184. Lee, J.I., et al., Postoperative-stimulated serum thyroglobulin measured at the time of ^{131}I ablation is useful for the prediction of disease status in patients with differentiated thyroid carcinoma. *Surgery*, 2013; 153(6): 828–35.

185. Lepoutre-Lussey, C., et al., Postoperative neck ultrasound and risk stratification in differentiated thyroid cancer patients with initial lymph node involvement. *Eur. J. Endocrinol.*, 2014; 170(6): 837–46.

186. Pacini, F., et al., Recombinant human thyrotropin-stimulated serum thyroglobulin combined with neck ultrasonography has the highest sensitivity in monitoring differentiated thyroid carcinoma. *J. Clin. Endocrinol. Metab.*, 2003; 88(8): 3668–73.

187. Grewal, R.K., et al., The effect of posttherapy ^{131}I SPECT/CT on risk classification and management of patients with differentiated thyroid cancer. *J. Nucl. Med.*, 2010; 51(9): 1361–7.

188. Maruoka, Y., et al., Incremental diagnostic value of SPECT/CT with ^{131}I scintigraphy after radioiodine therapy in patients with well-differentiated thyroid carcinoma. *Radiology*, 2012; 265(3): 902–9.

189. Jonklaas, J., et al., Outcomes of patients with differentiated thyroid carcinoma following initial therapy. *Thyroid*, 2006; 16(12): 1229–42.

190. Carhill, A.A., et al., Long-term outcomes following therapy in differentiated thyroid carcinoma: NTCTCS registry analysis 1987–2012. *J. Clin. Endocrinol. Metab.*, 2015; 100(9): 3270–9.

191. Diessl, S., et al., Impact of moderate vs stringent TSH suppression on survival in advanced differentiated thyroid carcinoma. *Clin. Endocrinol. (Oxf)*, 2012; 76(4): 586–92.

192. Sugitani, I. and Y. Fujimoto, Does postoperative thyrotropin suppression therapy truly decrease recurrence in papillary thyroid carcinoma? A randomized controlled trial. *J. Clin. Endocrinol. Metab.*, 2010; 95(10): 4576–83.

193. Klein Hesselink, E.N., et al., Long-term cardiovascular mortality in patients with differentiated thyroid carcinoma: An observational study. *J. Clin. Oncol.*, 2013; 31(32): 4046–53.

194. Collet, T.H., et al., Subclinical hyperthyroidism and the risk of coronary heart disease and mortality. *Arch. Intern. Med.*, 2012; 172(10): 799–809.

195. Flynn, R.W., et al., Serum thyroid-stimulating hormone concentration and morbidity from cardiovascular disease and fractures in patients on long-term thyroxine therapy. *J. Clin. Endocrinol. Metab.*, 2010; 95(1): 186–93.

196. Sawin, C.T., et al., Low serum thyrotropin concentrations as a risk factor for atrial fibrillation in older persons. *N. Engl. J. Med.*, 1994; 331(19): 1249–52.

197. Biondi, B., et al., Cardiac effects of long term thyrotropin-suppressive therapy with levothyroxine. *J. Clin. Endocrinol. Metab.*, 1993; 77(2): 334–8.

198. Wang, L.Y., et al., Thyrotropin suppression increases the risk of osteoporosis without decreasing recurrence in ATA low- and intermediate-risk patients with differentiated thyroid carcinoma. *Thyroid*, 2015; 25(3): 300–7.

199. Uzzan, B., et al., Effects on bone mass of long term treatment with thyroid hormones: A meta-analysis. *J. Clin. Endocrinol. Metab.*, 1996; 81(12): 4278–89.

200. Blum, M.R., et al., Subclinical thyroid dysfunction and fracture risk: A meta-analysis. *JAMA*, 2015; 313(20): 2055–65.

201. Lamartina, L., et al., Low-risk differentiated thyroid cancer and radioiodine remnant ablation: A systematic review of the literature. *J. Clin. Endocrinol. Metab.*, 2015; 100(5): 1748–61.

202. Sacks, W., et al., The effectiveness of radioactive iodine for treatment of low-risk thyroid cancer: A systematic analysis of the peer-reviewed literature from 1966 to April 2008. *Thyroid*, 2010; 20(11): 1235–45.

203. Schvartz, C., et al., Impact on overall survival of radioactive iodine in low-risk differentiated thyroid cancer patients. *J. Clin. Endocrinol. Metab.*, 2012; 97(5): 1526–35.

204. Podnos, Y.D., et al., Survival in patients with papillary thyroid cancer is not affected by the use of radioactive isotope. *J. Surg. Oncol.*, 2007; 96(1): 3–7.

205. Sawka, A.M., et al., Thyroid cancer patient perceptions of radioactive iodine treatment choice: Follow-up from a decision-aid randomized trial. *Cancer*, 2015; 121(20): 3717–26.

206. Lopez-Penabad, L., et al., Prognostic factors in patients with Hürthle cell neoplasms of the thyroid. *Cancer*, 2003; 97(5): 1186–94.

207. Besic, N., et al., The role of radioactive iodine in the treatment of Hürthle cell carcinoma of the thyroid. *Thyroid*, 2003; 13(6): 577–84.

208. Besic, N., et al., Treatment and outcome of 32 patients with distant metastases of Hürthle cell thyroid carcinoma: A single-institution experience. *BMC Cancer*, 2016; 16: 162.

209. Jillard, C.L., et al., Radioactive iodine treatment is associated with improved survival for patients with hürthle cell carcinoma. *Thyroid*, 2016; 26(7): 959–64.

210. Padovani, R.P., et al., One month is sufficient for urinary iodine to return to its baseline value after the use of water-soluble iodinated contrast agents in post-thyroidectomy patients requiring radioiodine therapy. *Thyroid*, 2012; 22(9): 926–30.

211. Toubert, M.E., et al., Plasma exchanges overcome persistent iodine overload to enable ^{131}I ablation of differentiated thyroid carcinoma. *Thyroid*, 2008; 18(4): 469–72.

212. Sawka, A.M., et al., Dietary iodine restriction in preparation for radioactive iodine treatment or scanning in well-differentiated thyroid cancer: A systematic review. *Thyroid*, 2010; 20(10): 1129–38.

213. Edmonds, C.J., et al., Measurement of serum TSH and thyroid hormones in the management of treatment of thyroid carcinoma with radioiodine. *Br. J. Radiol.*, 1977; 50(599): 799–807.

214. Pilli, T., et al., A comparison of 1850 (50 mCi) and 3700 MBq (100 mCi) 131-iodine administered doses for recombinant thyrotropin-stimulated postoperative thyroid remnant ablation in differentiated thyroid cancer. *J. Clin. Endocrinol. Metab.*, 2007; 92(9): 3542–6.

215. Haugen, B.R., et al., A comparison of recombinant human thyrotropin and thyroid hormone withdrawal for the detection of thyroid remnant or cancer. *J. Clin. Endocrinol. Metab.*, 1999; 84(11): 3877–85.

216. Pacini, F., et al., Radioiodine ablation of thyroid remnants after preparation with recombinant human thyrotropin in differentiated thyroid carcinoma: Results of an international, randomized, controlled study. *J. Clin. Endocrinol. Metab.*, 2006; 91(3): 926–32.

217. Mallick, U., et al., Ablation with low-dose radioiodine and thyrotropin alfa in thyroid cancer. *N. Engl. J. Med.*, 2012; 366(18): 1674–85.

218. Schlumberger, M., et al., Strategies of radioiodine ablation in patients with low-risk thyroid cancer. *N. Engl. J. Med.*, 2012; 366(18): 1663–73.

219. Bartenstein, P., et al., High-risk patients with differentiated thyroid cancer T4 primary tumors achieve remnant ablation equally well using rhTSH or thyroid hormone withdrawal. *Thyroid*, 2014; 24(3): 480–7.

220. Pitoia, F., et al., Radioiodine thyroid remnant ablation after recombinant human thyrotropin or thyroid hormone withdrawal in patients with high-risk differentiated thyroid cancer. *J. Thyroid Res.*, 2012; 2012: 481568.

221. Tala, H., et al., Five-year survival is similar in thyroid cancer patients with distant metastases prepared for radioactive iodine therapy with either thyroid hormone withdrawal or recombinant human TSH. *J. Clin. Endocrinol. Metab.*, 2011; 96(7): 2105–11.

222. Chen, M.K., et al., The utility of I-123 pretherapy scan in I-131 radioiodine therapy for thyroid cancer. *Thyroid*, 2012; 22(3): 304–9.

223. Van Nostrand, D., et al., The utility of radioiodine scans prior to iodine 131 ablation in patients with well-differentiated thyroid cancer. *Thyroid*, 2009; 19(8): 849–55.

224. Maxon, H.R., et al., Relation between effective radiation dose and outcome of radioiodine therapy for thyroid cancer. *N. Engl. J. Med.*, 1983; 309(16): 937–41.

225. Medvedec, M., Thyroid stunning in vivo and in vitro. *Nucl. Med. Commun.*, 2005; 26(8): 731–5.

226. Morris, L.F., A.D. Waxman, and G.D. Braunstein, Thyroid stunning. *Thyroid*, 2003; 13(4): 333–40.

227. Muratet, J.P., et al., Predicting the efficacy of first iodine-131 treatment in differentiated thyroid carcinoma. *J. Nucl. Med.*, 1997; 38(9): 1362–8.

228. Urhan, M., et al., Iodine-123 as a diagnostic imaging agent in differentiated thyroid carcinoma: A comparison with iodine-131 post-treatment scanning and serum thyroglobulin measurement. *Eur. J. Nucl. Med. Mol. Imaging*, 2007; 34(7): 1012–7.

229. Cheng, W., et al., Low- or high-dose radio-iodine remnant ablation for differentiated thyroid carcinoma: A meta-analysis. *J. Clin. Endocrinol. Metab.*, 2013; 98(4): 1353–60.

230. Castagna, M.G., et al., Post-surgical thyroid ablation with low or high radioiodine activities results in similar outcomes in intermediate risk differentiated thyroid cancer patients. *Eur. J. Endocrinol.*, 2013; 169(1): 23–9.

231. Han, J.M., et al., Effects of low-dose and high-dose postoperative radioiodine therapy on the clinical outcome in patients with small differentiated thyroid cancer having microscopic extrathyroidal extension. *Thyroid*, 2014; 24(5): 820–5.

232. Sabra, M.M., et al., Higher administered activities of radioactive iodine are associated with less structural persistent response in older, but not younger, papillary thyroid cancer patients with lateral neck lymph node metastases. *Thyroid*, 2014; 24(7): 1088–95.

233. Verburg, F.A., et al., Long-term survival in differentiated thyroid cancer is worse after low-activity initial post-surgical ^{131}I therapy in both high- and low-risk patients. *J. Clin. Endocrinol. Metab.*, 2014; 99(12): 4487–96.

234. Ruegemer, J.J., et al., Distant metastases in differentiated thyroid carcinoma: A multivariate analysis of prognostic variables. *J. Clin. Endocrinol. Metab.*, 1988; 67(3): 501–8.

235. Samaan, N.A., et al., Pulmonary metastasis of differentiated thyroid carcinoma: Treatment results in 101 patients. *J. Clin. Endocrinol. Metab.*, 1985; 60(2): 376–80.

236. Simpson, W.J., et al., Papillary and follicular thyroid cancer: Impact of treatment in 1578 patients. *Int. J. Radiat. Oncol. Biol. Phys.*, 1988; 14(6): 1063–75.

237. Lassmann, M., C. Reiners, and M. Luster, Dosimetry and thyroid cancer: The individual dosage of radioiodine. *Endocr. Relat. Cancer*, 2010; 17(3): R161–72.

238. Van Nostrand, D., et al., Dosimetrically determined doses of radioiodine for the treatment of metastatic thyroid carcinoma. *Thyroid*, 2002; 12(2): 121–34.

239. Deandreis, D., et al., Comparison of empiric versus whole-body/-blood clearance dosimetry-based approach to radioactive iodine treatment in patients with metastases from differentiated thyroid cancer. *J. Nucl. Med.*, 2017; 58(5): 717–722.

240. Tuttle, R.M., et al., Empiric radioactive iodine dosing regimens frequently exceed maximum tolerated activity levels in elderly patients with thyroid cancer. *J. Nucl. Med.*, 2006; 47(10): 1587–91.

241. Holst, J.P., et al., Radioiodine therapy for thyroid cancer and hyperthyroidism in patients with end-stage renal disease on hemodialysis. *Thyroid*, 2005; 15(12): 1321–31.

242. Kulkarni, K., et al., The relative frequency in which empiric dosages of radioiodine would potentially overtreat or undertreat patients who have metastatic well-differentiated thyroid cancer. *Thyroid*, 2006; 16(10): 1019–23.

243. Maxon, H.R., 3rd and H.S. Smith, Radioiodine-131 in the diagnosis and treatment of metastatic well differentiated thyroid cancer. *Endocrinol. Metab. Clin. North Am.*, 1990; 19(3): 685–718.

244. Souza Rosario, P.W., et al., Ovarian function after radioiodine therapy in patients with thyroid cancer. *Exp. Clin. Endocrinol. Diabetes*, 2005; 113(6): 331–3.

245. Greenler, D.P. and H.A. Klein, The scope of false-positive iodine-131 images for thyroid carcinoma. *Clin. Nucl. Med.*, 1989; 14(2): 111–7.

246. Carlisle, M.R., C. Lu, and I.R. McDougall, The interpretation of ^{131}I scans in the evaluation of thyroid cancer, with an emphasis on false positive findings. *Nucl. Med. Commun.*, 2003; 24(6): 715–35.

247. Luster, M., et al., rhTSH-aided radioiodine ablation and treatment of differentiated thyroid carcinoma: A comprehensive review. *Endocr. Relat. Cancer*, 2005; 12(1): 49–64.

248. DiRusso, G. and K.A. Kern, Comparative analysis of complications from I-131 radioablation for well-differentiated thyroid cancer. *Surgery*, 1994; 116(6): 1024–30.

249. Allweiss, P., et al., Sialadenitis following I-131 therapy for thyroid carcinoma: Concise communication. *J. Nucl. Med.*, 1984; 25(7): 755–8.

250. Jonklaas, J., Nasal symptoms after radioiodine therapy: A rarely described side effect with similar frequency to lacrimal dysfunction. *Thyroid*, 2014; 24(12): 1806–14.

251. Jentzen, W., et al., The influence of saliva flow stimulation on the absorbed radiation dose to the salivary glands during radioiodine therapy of thyroid cancer using 124I PET(/CT) imaging. *Eur. J. Nucl. Med. Mol. Imaging*, 2010; 37(12): 2298–306.

252. Kloos, R.T., et al., Nasolacrimal drainage system obstruction from radioactive iodine therapy for thyroid carcinoma. *J. Clin. Endocrinol. Metab.*, 2002; 87(12): 5817–20.

253. Sawka, A.M., et al., A systematic review examining the effects of therapeutic radioactive iodine on ovarian function and future pregnancy in female thyroid cancer survivors. *Clin. Endocrinol. (Oxf)*, 2008; 69(3): 479–90.

254. Wu, J.X., et al., Reproductive outcomes and nononcologic complications after radioactive iodine ablation for well-differentiated thyroid cancer. *Thyroid*, 2015; 25(1): 133–8.

255. Ceccarelli, C., et al., ^{131}I therapy for differentiated thyroid cancer leads to an earlier onset of menopause: Results of a retrospective study. *J. Clin. Endocrinol. Metab.*, 2001; 86(8): 3512–5.

256. Rosario, P.W., et al., Testicular function after radioiodine therapy in patients with thyroid cancer. *Thyroid*, 2006; 16(7): 667–70.

257. Sawka, A.M., et al., A systematic review of the gonadal effects of therapeutic radioactive iodine in male thyroid cancer survivors. *Clin. Endocrinol. (Oxf)*, 2008; 68(4): 610–7.

258. Jang, E.K., et al., Changes in the pulmonary function test after radioactive iodine treatment in patients with pulmonary metastases of differentiated thyroid cancer. *PLoS One*, 2015; 10(4): e0125114.

259. Brown, A.P., et al., The risk of second primary malignancies up to three decades after the treatment of differentiated thyroid cancer. *J. Clin. Endocrinol. Metab.*, 2008; 93(2): 504–15.

260. Lang, B.H., et al., Risk of second primary malignancy in differentiated thyroid carcinoma treated with radioactive iodine therapy. *Surgery*, 2012; 151(6): 844–50.

261. Sawka, A.M., et al., Second primary malignancy risk after radioactive iodine treatment for thyroid cancer: A systematic review and meta-analysis. *Thyroid*, 2009; 19(5): 451–7.

262. Rubino, C., et al., Second primary malignancies in thyroid cancer patients. *Br. J. Cancer*, 2003; 89(9): 1638–44.

263. Hall, P. and L.E. Holm, Cancer in iodine-131 exposed patients. *J. Endocrinol. Invest.*, 1995; 18(2): 147–9.

264. Iyer, N.G., et al., Rising incidence of second cancers in patients with low-risk (T1N0) thyroid cancer who receive radioactive iodine therapy. *Cancer*, 2011; 117(19): 4439–46.

265. Taieb, D., et al., Iodine biokinetics and radioiodine exposure after recombinant human thyrotropin-assisted remnant ablation in comparison with thyroid hormone withdrawal. *J. Clin. Endocrinol. Metab.*, 2010; 95(7): 3283–90.

266. American Thyroid Association Taskforce On Radioiodine, S., et al., Radiation safety in the treatment of patients with thyroid diseases by radioiodine [131]I: Practice recommendations of the American Thyroid Association. *Thyroid*, 2011; 21(4): 335–46.

267. Romesser, P.B., et al., External beam radiotherapy with or without concurrent chemotherapy in advanced or recurrent non-anaplastic non-medullary thyroid cancer. *J. Surg. Oncol.*, 2014; 110(4): 375–82.

268. Schwartz, D.L., et al., Postoperative external beam radiotherapy for differentiated thyroid cancer: Outcomes and morbidity with conformal treatment. *Int. J. Radiat. Oncol. Biol. Phys.*, 2009; 74(4): 1083–91.

269. Brierley, J., et al., Prognostic factors and the effect of treatment with radioactive iodine and external beam radiation on patients with differentiated thyroid cancer seen at a single institution over 40 years. *Clin. Endocrinol. (Oxf)*, 2005; 63(4): 418–27.

270. Sia, M.A., et al., Differentiated thyroid cancer with extrathyroidal extension: Prognosis and the role of external beam radiotherapy. *J. Thyroid Res.*, 2010; 2010: 183461.

271. Monchik, J.M., et al., Radiofrequency ablation and percutaneous ethanol injection treatment for recurrent local and distant well-differentiated thyroid carcinoma. *Ann. Surg.*, 2006; 244(2): 296–304.

272. Schlumberger, M., et al., A phase II trial of the multitargeted tyrosine kinase inhibitor Lenvatinib (E7080) in advanced medullary thyroid cancer. *Clin. Cancer Res.*, 2016; 22(1): 44–53.

273. Brose, M.S., et al., Sorafenib in radioactive iodine-refractory, locally advanced or

metastatic differentiated thyroid cancer: A randomised, double-blind, phase 3 trial. *Lancet*, 2014; 384(9940): 319–28.

274. Kim, J.H. and R.D. Leeper, Treatment of locally advanced thyroid carcinoma with combination doxorubicin and radiation therapy. *Cancer*, 1987; 60(10): 2372–5.

275. Ho, A.L., et al., Selumetinib-enhanced radio-iodine uptake in advanced thyroid cancer. *N. Engl. J. Med.*, 2013; 368(7): 623–32.

276. Rothenberg, S.M., et al., Redifferentiation of iodine-refractory BRAF V600E-mutant metastatic papillary thyroid cancer with dabrafenib. *Clin. Cancer Res.*, 2015; 21(5): 1028–35.

277. Chindris, A.M., et al., Undetectable sensitive serum thyroglobulin (<0.1 ng/ml) in 163 patients with follicular cell-derived thyroid cancer: Results of rhTSH stimulation and neck ultrasonography and long-term biochemical and clinical follow-up. *J. Clin. Endocrinol. Metab.*, 2012; 97(8): 2714–23.

278. Giovanella, L., Thyroglobulin-guided (131) I ablation in low-risk differentiated thyroid carcinoma: Is the yardstick accurate enough? *Head Neck*, 2011; 33(9): 1379–80; author reply 1380–1.

279. Park, H.J., et al., Early stimulated thyroglobulin for response prediction after recombinant human thyrotropin-aided radioiodine therapy. *Ann. Nucl. Med.*, 2017; 31(8): 616–622.

280. Robenshtok, E., et al., Suspicious cervical lymph nodes detected after thyroidectomy for papillary thyroid cancer usually remain stable over years in properly selected patients. *J. Clin. Endocrinol. Metab.*, 2012; 97(8): 2706–13.

281. Pacini, F., et al., Diagnostic 131-iodine whole-body scan may be avoided in thyroid cancer patients who have undetectable stimulated serum Tg levels after initial treatment. *J. Clin. Endocrinol. Metab.*, 2002; 87(4): 1499–501.

282. Jeong, S.Y., et al., Clinical applications of SPECT/CT after first I-131 ablation in patients with differentiated thyroid cancer. *Clin. Endocrinol. (Oxf)*, 2014; 81(3): 445–51.

283. Feine, U., et al., Fluorine-18-FDG and iodine-131-iodide uptake in thyroid cancer. *J. Nucl. Med.*, 1996; 37(9): 1468–72.

284. Deandreis, D., et al., Do histological, immuno-histochemical, and metabolic (radioiodine and fluorodeoxyglucose uptakes) patterns of metastatic thyroid cancer correlate with patient outcome? *Endocr. Relat. Cancer*, 2011; 18(1): 159–69.

285. Kloos, R.T., Approach to the patient with a positive serum thyroglobulin and a negative radioiodine scan after initial therapy for differentiated thyroid cancer. *J. Clin. Endocrinol. Metab.*, 2008; 93(5): 1519–25.

286. Bakheet, S.M. and J. Powe, Fluorine-18-fluorodeoxyglucose uptake in rheumatoid arthritis-associated lung disease in a patient with thyroid cancer. *J. Nucl. Med.*, 1998; 39(2): 234–6.

287. Leboulleux, S., et al., Assessment of the incremental value of recombinant thyrotropin stimulation before 2-[18F]-Fluoro-2-deoxy-D-glucose positron emission tomography/computed tomography imaging to localize residual differentiated thyroid cancer. *J. Clin. Endocrinol. Metab.*, 2009; 94(4): 1310–6.

288. Wang, W., et al., Resistance of [18f]-fluoro-deoxyglucose-avid metastatic thyroid cancer lesions to treatment with high-dose radioactive iodine. *Thyroid*, 2001; 11(12): 1169–75.

289. Ma, C., J. Xie, and A. Kuang, Is empiric ^{131}I therapy justified for patients with positive thyroglobulin and negative ^{131}I whole-body scanning results? *J. Nucl. Med.*, 2005; 46(7): 1164–70.

290. Tufano, R.P., et al., Management of recurrent/persistent nodal disease in patients with differentiated thyroid cancer: A critical review of the risks and benefits of surgical intervention versus active surveillance. *Thyroid*, 2015; 25(1): 15–27.

291. Eskander, A., et al., Pattern of spread to the lateral neck in metastatic well-differentiated thyroid cancer: A systematic review and meta-analysis. *Thyroid*, 2013; 23(5): 583–92.

292. Haymart, M.R., et al., The role of clinicians in determining radioactive iodine use for low-risk thyroid cancer. *Cancer*, 2013; 119(2): 259–65.

293. Kim, S.Y., et al., Long-term outcomes of ethanol injection therapy for locally recurrent papillary thyroid cancer. *Eur. Arch. Otorhinolaryngol.*, 2017; 274(9): 3497–3501.

294. Jeong, S.Y., et al., Ethanol and thermal ablation for malignant thyroid tumours. *Int. J. Hyperthermia*, 2017; 33(8): 938–945.

295. Bernier, M.O., et al., Survival and therapeutic modalities in patients with bone metastases of differentiated thyroid carcinomas. *J. Clin. Endocrinol. Metab.*, 2001; 86(4): 1568–73.

296. Orita, Y., et al., Zoledronic acid in the treatment of bone metastases from differentiated thyroid carcinoma. *Thyroid*, 2011; 21(1): 31–5.

297. Gilliland, F.D., W.C. Hunt, D.M. Morris, and C.R. Key, Prognostic factors for thyroid carcinoma. A population-based study of 15,698 cases from the Surveillance, Epidemiology and End Results (SEER) program 1973–1991. *Cancer*, 1997; 79(3): 564–73.

298. Leenhardt, L., et al., 2013 European thyroid association guidelines for cervical ultrasound scan and ultrasound-guided techniques in the postoperative management of patients with thyroid cancer. *Eur. Thyroid J.*, 2013; 2(3): 147–59.

299. Kasaian K, Chindris AM, Wiseman SM, et al. MEN1 mutations in Hürthle cell (oncocytic) thyroid carcinoma. *J Clin Endocrinol Metab.* Apr 2015;100(4):E611–615.

300. Ganly I, Ricarte Filho J, Eng S, et al. Genomic dissection of Hürthle cell carcinoma reveals a unique class of thyroid malignancy. *J Clin Endocrinol Metab.* May 2013;98(5):E962–972.

301. Wei S, LiVolsi VA, Montone KT, Morrissette JJ, Baloch ZW. Detection of Molecular Alterations in Medullary Thyroid Carcinoma Using Next-Generation Sequencing: an Institutional Experience. *Endocrine pathology.* Dec 2016;27(4):359–362.

Medullary thyroid carcinoma in medical management of thyroid disease

MIMI I. HU, ELIZABETH G. GRUBBS, AND JULIE ANN SOSA

Introduction	225	Regional site-specific or symptom-specific therapies	231
Germline RET mutation associated with hereditary MTC	226	Systemic therapies for advanced, progressive disease	233
MEN2A and associated features and variants	*226*	*Approved multikinase inhibitors (MKI) for MTC*	*233*
MEN2B and associated features	*227*	*When should an MKI be initiated?*	*234*
2015 ATA risk stratification of RET codon mutations	*228*	*Adverse effects of MKI*	*235*
		Monitoring for response to targeted therapy	*236*
Clinical presentation and diagnostic workup of MTC	228	*Other agents in clinical trials*	*237*
Surgical management as initial treatment	229	Conclusion and future directions	238
Active surveillance of MTC	230	References	238
Prognostic indicators beyond doubling times	*231*		

INTRODUCTION

Medullary thyroid cancer (MTC), a neuroendocrine malignancy of thyroid C cells, accounts for approximately 1–2% of all thyroid malignancies (1). Since it is estimated that 53,990 new cases of thyroid cancer will be diagnosed in 2018 in the United States, we can anticipate that approximately 540–1080 incident cases will be MTC (2). Despite the rarity of MTC, it is one of the most well-characterized solid tumors with respect to its pathologic, biochemical, molecular, and genetic properties and clinical correlations.

MTC was first described histologically in 1959 by Hazard et al. as a distinct pleomorphic neoplasm with amyloid stroma (3). In 1966, Williams showed that MTC originates from the neural crest-derived parafollicular C cells of the thyroid gland (4). These C cells secrete calcitonin (Ctn), the primary biochemical tumor marker used in the evaluation of MTC. Twenty-five years ago, the hereditary form of MTC, which represents 25% of all MTC cases and which is associated with the multiple endocrine neoplasia (MEN) types 2A and 2B syndromes, was causally linked to activating germline point mutations in the *RET* (*RE*arranged during Transfection) proto-oncogene (5–7). Recommendations for prophylactic thyroidectomy in patients with MEN2A and 2B have evolved over time with greater understanding of genotype–phenotype correlations, most recently updated in the 2015 American Thyroid Association (ATA) guidelines (1). Of patients with sporadic MTC (75% of MTC cases), mutually exclusive somatic mutations occur in *RET* or *RAS* along with overexpression of various other receptor tyrosine kinases which mediate cell cycle progression, inhibition of apoptosis, angiogenesis, and cell proliferation and migration (8, 9). Improved understanding of the pathogenesis of MTC has led to a rapid expansion in the number of clinical trials investigating various multikinase inhibitors (MKIs) and ultimately the approval of two agents (cabozantinib and vandetanib) by the United States Food and Drug Administration and the European Medicines Agency for advanced, progressive, or symptomatic MTC.

This chapter provides a comprehensive review of MTC, including its clinical presentation and the different behaviors of hereditary versus sporadic disease, initial surgical management, prognostic indicators, surveillance and treatment strategies for persistent or recurrent disease, and the systemic treatments now available as a standard of care for patients with advanced and progressive MTC.

GERMLINE RET MUTATION ASSOCIATED WITH HEREDITARY MTC

The *RET* proto-oncogene, located on chromosome 10q11.2 and comprised of 21 exons spanning almost 55,000 base pairs, encodes for a single transmembrane receptor with an intracellular domain that contains two tyrosine kinase regions. When the tyrosine kinase regions are auto-phosphorylated, the activated RET receptor drives intracellular signal transduction through the mitogen-activated protein kinase (MAPK) and phosphoinositide 3-kinases/AKT (PI3K/AKT) pathways (5–7). Hereditary MTC and its associated MEN2A and 2B syndromes are caused by an activating point mutation of *RET*, which is transmitted in an autosomal dominant fashion from one affected parent to an offspring. *De novo* mutations of *RET* can occur in 5–9% of MEN2A and 75% of MEN2B patients, predominantly arising from the paternal allele (10, 11). In addition, 1–7% of patients with apparently sporadic MTC (i.e., no personal or family history of other MEN-related endocrine neoplasias) will have a germline *RET* mutation when tested, indicating hereditary disease (12–14). There is a significant correlation of genotype with phenotypic expression regarding the likelihood of developing other endocrine neoplasias, manifesting other MEN2A variants, and predicting the aggressive potential of MTC (see the later sections on MEN2A and 2B) (15). In the end, all patients with MTC should be tested for germline *RET* mutations to allow for proper counseling of other family members if there is a mutation identified and to inform proper recommendations around surveillance of affected individuals.

In contrast to sporadic (non-hereditary) MTC, hereditary MTC is often multifocal (>90% of cases) and bilateral in the thyroid gland, with a background of nodular C cell hyperplasia, the precursor of hereditary MTC. The C cells, which are concentrated in the upper two-thirds of the lateral thyroid lobes, initially undergo hyperplasia in the hereditary syndromes before developing into MTC. These patients may present with MTC across a spectrum of age groups but commonly present at a younger age compared with sporadic MTC patients. Similar to sporadic cases, hereditary MTC tends to metastasize to lymph nodes in the neck and mediastinum, lungs, liver, and bones. In addition to having MTC, these patients may have a personal or family history of other endocrine neoplasias or a distinctive MEN2-related phenotype.

MEN2A and associated features and variants

MEN2A is the most common type of MEN2 syndrome, accounting for approximately 90–95% of MEN2 cases. It is characterized by MTC in >90% of *RET*-mutated carriers, unilateral or, more often, bilateral pheochromocytomas in 50% of carriers, and primary hyperparathyroidism (PHPT) due to single or multigland parathyroid hyperplasia in 10–20% of carriers (16). MTC is most often the first endocrine neoplasia that is clinically manifested; however, pheochromocytoma may be the incident neoplasia in 10% of MEN2A patients. In patients with MEN2A, the *RET* 634 codon mutation is the one most commonly associated with the development of MEN2A syndrome, characterized by MTC, pheochromocytomas, and PHPT. In *RET*-634-mutated patients, the presence of a pheochromocytoma is not associated with the more aggressive, advanced stage of MTC or with worse overall survival (17). Pheochromocytomas in MEN2A are rarely malignant. *RET* mutations of codons 609, 611, 618, and 620 are also associated with pheochromocytomas and PHPT but with lower penetrance of these associated tumors than that seen with the 634 mutation.

There are three additional variants of MEN2A: MEN2A with cutaneous lichen amyloidosis, MEN2A with Hirschsprung disease, and familial

MTC (FMTC). MEN2A with cutaneous lichen amyloidosis, a highly pruritic pigmented patch of skin typically across the upper back between the shoulder blades due to amyloid deposition, has been reported predominantly with the *RET* 634 mutation, and in one case with a V804M mutation (18, 19). MEN2A with Hirschsprung disease develops in childhood in MEN2A patients who have exon 10 mutations (codons 609, 611, 618, or 620) due to the congenital absence of enteric innervation, causing chronic bowel obstruction in infancy; these patients may require colon surgery and can have chronic problems with intestinal motility issues and malabsorption. FMTC consists of the presence of a *RET* germline mutation without the development of pheochromocytomas or hyperparathyroidism in (1) families with MTC or (2) a single individual with MTC and no family history of MTC. FMTC was historically a freestanding hereditary syndrome, but the 2015 ATA guidelines reclassified it as a variant of MEN2A (1). FMTC represents only 5–15% of all hereditary forms of MTC, and it tends to be the least aggressive form of MTC, with an older age of onset, on average.

MEN2B and associated features

MEN2B is associated with a distinctive phenotype, and it is associated with the most aggressive-behaving MTC. Fortunately, it is also the least common of the MEN2 syndromes (5%). It demonstrates 100% penetrance of MTC and 50% penetrance of pheochromocytomas, without PHPT. The prominent and classic phenotype is due to the development of mucosal neuromas and gastrointestinal ganglioneuromas affecting the tongue, lips, eyelids, salivary glands, pancreas, intestine, gallbladder, upper respiratory tract, and urinary bladder (Figure 9.1). Alimentary ganglioneuromas lead to chronic problems with constipation, diarrhea, feeding problems, and megacolon (Figure 9.2). Opioid therapies for pain control should be avoided to prevent intestinal obstruction. MEN2B patients have a marfanoid habitus, with a decreased upper/lower body segment ratio, long limbs, hyperextending joints, scoliosis, narrow and long faces, and anterior chest deformities; however, they do not have the lens subluxation or cardiovascular abnormalities that are characteristic of Marfan syndrome. In addition, these patients are unable to make tears. As 75% of MEN2B cases

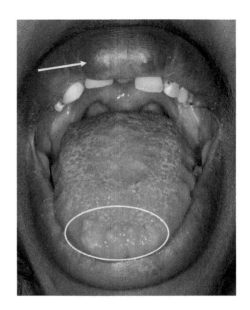

Figure 9.1 Mucosal neuromas of tongue and lips in an MEN2B Patient. Mucosal neuromas on tongue (within yellow circle) and on the lips (yellow arrow) in an MEN2B patient. (Courtesy of Steven G. Waguespack, MD.)

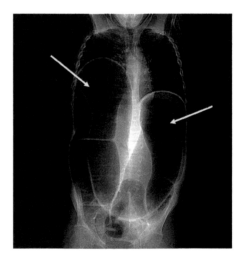

Figure 9.2 Megacolon in an MEN2B Patient. Dilated colon (yellow arrows) elevating bilateral diaphragms.

are due to *de novo RET* mutations, neither parent typically will have the classic phenotype nor a *RET* mutation. The cause of MEN2B in the majority of patients is due to one of two *RET* codon mutations, most commonly M918T (>95%) and rarely A883F (5%). In comparison with MEN2A patients, M918T-mutated MEN2B patients are associated with the following aggressive MTC features: earlier average age of diagnosis in the second decade of life (about 10 years earlier than MEN2A patients), younger onset of lymph node and distant metastases, and higher morbidity and mortality rates, typically due to the advanced stage at presentation rather than it being a more aggressive cancer (20, 21). MTC with an A833F mutation is less aggressive compared with germline M918T-mutated MTC (22).

2015 ATA risk stratification of RET codon mutations

Since 1993, strong correlations observed between RET mutations and their respective clinical expression drove consensus recommendations for evaluation and treatment to prevent morbidity and mortality associated with hereditary MTC. The aggressive potential of MTC associated with a specific RET mutation is estimated by identifying the earliest age of MTC diagnosis and the earliest age at which metastases have been demonstrated (23). Originally designated as levels A through D in the 2009 ATA guidelines, RET mutations are now stratified to a specific risk of aggressive MTC, using the terms "highest risk," "high risk," and "moderate risk" (1, 24). The "highest risk" category is comprised of only the codon M918T mutation seen with MEN2B; it is associated with the earliest age of MTC diagnosis (2 months of age), lymph node metastasis (3 months of age), and distant metastasis (5 years of age) (23). The "high risk" category includes 2 codons, C634 and A883F, associated with MEN2A and MEN2B, respectively. All other codon mutations are considered to be "moderate risk," as the MTC associated with risk level tends to present later in life, have less extensive disease at diagnosis, and a more indolent pace of progression. Based on these risk categories, there are guideline recommendations regarding timing of prophylactic thyroidectomy, which will be described later in this chapter.

CLINICAL PRESENTATION AND DIAGNOSTIC WORKUP OF MTC

Sporadic MTC most often occurs between the fourth and sixth decades of life, with slightly under half of patients presenting with stage III or IV disease (25, 26). There has been no trend toward detection at earlier stages and no improvement

in patient survival. An analysis of the population-based Surveillance, Epidemiology, and End Results Registry from 1973 to 2002 showed the mean overall survival rate for MTC was 8.6 years. Patients with localized or regional disease at the time of diagnosis experienced a superior 10-year survival rate of 95.6% and 75.5%, respectively, compared with patients with distant metastases, who had a 10-year survival rate of 40% (26).

Most cases are identified during the evaluation of a palpable nodule or a nodule identified incidentally on imaging for unrelated reasons (27). Individuals who present with a thyroid nodule harboring suspicious sonographic findings should undergo a fine needle aspiration (FNA). When histological analysis shows features suggestive of, but not diagnostic of, MTC, diagnostic accuracy can be markedly improved by measuring Ctn levels in the FNA washout fluid, as well as by performing immunohistochemical staining to look for the presence of markers including Ctn, chromogranin, and carcinoembryonic antigen (CEA), as well as the absence of thyroglobulin (28). In studies of small numbers of patients, Thyroseq v3 genomic classifier demonstrated accurate detection of medullary thyroid cancer in a training set of 15 samples, all of which were identified correctly, and Veracyte Afirma's MTC classifier (part of its Gene Expression Classifier) demonstrated a sensitivity of 96%, with 26 of 27 specimens appropriately diagnosed (29, 30).

When a diagnosis of MTC has been confirmed or is highly suspicious, serum Ctn and CEA levels (both secretory products of the C cells) should be measured. Ctn can be elevated in non-MTC conditions, such as chronic renal failure, autoimmune thyroiditis, primary hyperparathyroidism, presence of heterophilic antibodies, other malignancies (e.g., lung, prostate, neuroendocrine tumors). Additionally, children under 3 years of age can have markedly elevated Ctn levels, which should be carefully interpreted when considering thyroid surgery in this population. The issue of whether a serum Ctn should be evaluated in patients with thyroid nodules is controversial; there is no consensus recommendation for checking it routinely as a screening test in nodular disease (1). In a study of 10,864 patients with thyroid nodules in whom Ctn was measured, 0.4% of patients were found to have MTC with Ctn screening (31).

With regard to imaging, comprehensive neck ultrasound including nodal mapping of the central and lateral neck compartments is essential in all patients diagnosed with MTC. When there is a clinical or radiographic concern for locally advanced tumor extension into surrounding structures or suspicion for disease extending posteriorly or into the mediastinum, additional cross-sectional imaging, such as computed tomography (CT) of the neck with intravenous contrast or magnetic resonance imaging (MRI), should be considered. Elevated levels of Ctn greater than 500 picograms (pg)/milliliter (ml) suggest a higher likelihood that there is disease outside of the neck and should prompt the performance of CT of the chest and abdomen or MRI of the liver (1). Evidence of distant metastatic disease does not necessarily preclude treatment of the primary tumor. Such findings should prompt the multidisciplinary clinical team to jointly determine the most appropriate course of action, which should balance the removal of the primary tumor to avoid potential morbidity from continued locoregional growth and any urgency to treat distant disease burden with systemic therapy. In addition, the information provided by preoperative biochemical evaluation and imaging allows an informed discussion between clinicians and the patient about whether surgery is intended for cure or palliation.

Patients diagnosed with MTC should be evaluated for symptoms of dysphagia, dyspnea, and hoarseness, which may indicate the presence of locally advanced disease. Symptoms of flushing, diarrhea, or bone pain may be suggestive of distant metastatic disease. The physical exam should include palpation of the thyroid to determine the size of the mass and possible fixation to surrounding structures suggestive of locally advanced disease, as well as evaluation for associated lymphadenopathy in the anterior and lateral neck.

Because 1–7% of patients with presumed sporadic MTC have the hereditary form of the disease, all patients diagnosed with MTC should undergo genetic testing and direct DNA analysis to detect activating mutations in the *RET* proto-oncogene. Initial screening testing should include single- or multi-tiered analysis to detect known pathogenic *RET* mutations in, at least, exons 8, 10, 11, and 13–16. Ideally, testing would be performed prior to surgical intervention, and if no mutations are identified, treatment for MTC may proceed. If a MEN2A-associated *RET* mutation is identified, further biochemical workup for the associated diseases of primary hyperparathyroidism and pheochromocytoma should be performed prior to surgery; for MEN2B, pheochromocytoma should be ruled out. If genetic testing is not available prior to surgery, evaluation for the associated diseases should be performed prior to surgery, specifically albumin-corrected serum calcium and intact parathyroid hormone for primary hyperparathyroidism and urine or plasma metanephrines for pheochromocytoma.

SURGICAL MANAGEMENT AS INITIAL TREATMENT

Initial thyroid surgery in patients with known MTC is total thyroidectomy and central neck dissection. In a patient found to have MTC diagnosed after an initial diagnostic lobectomy, completion thyroidectomy is recommended if the patient harbors a *RET* proto-oncogene mutation, has an elevated Ctn 3–6 months postoperatively, or if there is imaging concerning for residual cancer. With regards to the extent of lymph node dissection, a bilateral central neck Level VI lymph node dissection is appropriate in all cases of operable MTC, regardless of the size of the primary tumor. As with all thyroid surgery, the extent of operation within the central neck must be weighed carefully against the potential risks of hypoparathyroidism and recurrent laryngeal nerve compromise; it must also factor in the therapeutic versus the palliative goal of the operation. While the recommendation in favor of a central neck dissection is well established and endorsed by the 2015 ATA guidelines, the threshold for performance of a lateral neck dissection is more controversial. The ATA guidelines recommend using radiographic and biopsy-proven evidence of disease to determine performance of a therapeutic compartment-oriented lateral neck dissection (Level II–V) (1). However, the guidelines "recommended neither for nor against" lateral compartment dissection in individuals with no radiographically concerning lateral neck disease based on basal Ctn levels. Risks associated with surgery in the lateral neck include injury to the vagus, phrenic, spinal accessory, and hypoglossal nerves and the brachial plexus, as well as bleeding and lymphatic and thoracic duct leaks. If a surgeon is not experienced at performing a central or lateral neck dissection, consideration should be made for referral to a high-volume surgeon; complication rates are decreased when surgeries are performed by high-volume surgeons and in high-volume centers (32).

It is sometimes appropriate to perform a thyroidectomy with/without neck dissection even in the setting of distant metastatic disease. Some patients will experience morbidity from compression or invasion of the aerodigestive tract from uncontrolled locoregional disease before they are affected by indolent distant metastases. The decision for surgery in these cases should be discussed in a multidisciplinary context and informed by measurement of the pace of growth of distant disease.

In the setting of hereditary MTC, patients often are encountered before they demonstrate clinical evidence of the disease. Early fastidious thyroidectomy can prevent the development of MTC altogether or be curative for early stage disease. Debate exists around the optimal timing of surgery for MEN2 patients with mutations in codons other than 918 and 634, especially as rarer and less virulent *RET* mutations are becoming more prevalent in the genetic testing era (23). The primary oncologic goal of early intervention is to render the patient free of MTC and the implied risk of death from metastatic disease. A truly prophylactic thyroidectomy is performed with the goal of preventing malignancy from occurring in the first place, but it may be argued that the most important goal is to remove the thyroid before metastasis occurs. Surgery performed in this setting may be called an early thyroidectomy. The 2015 ATA guidelines suggest performing a total thyroidectomy in the first year of life in asymptomatic carriers with the highest risk *RET* 918 mutation and at or before 5 years of age for those with a high-risk mutation (1). With all other *RET* mutations, the timing of surgery can be determined by the detection of an elevated Ctn level and/or concerning features on ultrasonography; the final decision should be made by the multidisciplinary team in consultation with the child's parents, who may opt for earlier intervention.

ACTIVE SURVEILLANCE OF MTC

Given the propensity for recurrent disease, especially when cervical lymph nodes are already involved at the time of diagnosis, and the indolent disease course observed in most patients with MTC, long-term surveillance with laboratory testing and imaging at appropriate intervals is warranted. Serum Ctn is the primary biomarker used for postoperative surveillance and prediction of persistent, recurrent, and/or progressive disease; generally speaking, it correlates well with tumor burden. CEA, a less specific biomarker for MTC, should be measured concurrently with Ctn to understand tumor differentiation status, as a tumor that expresses relatively high amounts of CEA to Ctn tends to be poorly differentiated and can have a more aggressive course over time. Tumor markers should be assessed 3 months after initial surgery to identify nadir levels, given the long half-lives of each, and repeated every 6 months for the first 2 years after surgery.

Ctn and CEA doubling times generally correlate with the rate of progression, recurrence, and survival (33). Doubling times >1 year are associated with superior disease-specific survival and recurrence-free survival rates; the CEA doubling time appears to have a higher predictive value than Ctn doubling time. Although there are no formal published guidelines on how often to follow MTC patients for progression, it is generally accepted that measurement of doubling times can help guide surveillance intervals. Patients with long doubling times (>1 year) may have clinical evaluations with imaging studies performed every 6–12 months. However, if a patient has a short doubling time of less than 6–9 months, closer follow-up at intervals of 3–6 months are indicated with a variety of imaging studies to identify sites of progressive metastases, as per the practice patterns of the authors.

Radiologic surveillance for metastatic disease includes a variety of studies. Ultrasound of the neck is the most sensitive imaging modality for detecting thyroid bed or nodal recurrences (most frequent sites of recurrences after initial surgery) with minimal risk to the patient; thus, it is routinely performed in MTC patients even if tumor markers remain undetectable or stable. If the postoperative Ctn level is >150 pg/mL and/or CEA levels are persistently elevated or rising without any evidence of progression in the neck on ultrasound, then additional imaging studies are needed (1). Contrast-enhanced computed tomography of the neck can identify metastatic disease in the retropharyngeal region or superior mediastinum, which are areas not visualized well by ultrasound (34). Fine-section contrast-enhanced CT or MRI of the chest and abdomen with a 3-phase liver protocol are valuable studies to detect pulmonary, intrathoracic lymph nodes and hepatic metastases. There is a 19% prevalence of bone metastases in MTC; these are often multifocal (77%), predominantly involving the spine and pelvis, and typically occur in the setting of other distant metastases (89%) (35). A bone scan or MRI of the spine should be done to screen for bone metastases and to follow lesions over time for progression. Fluorodeoxyglucose positron emission tomography/CT (FDG PET/CT) and L-6-[^{18}F]-fluoro-3,4-dihydroxyphenylalanine (F-DOPA) PET/CT are less sensitive for MTC metastases compared with the aforementioned studies; however, they may correlate with progressive disease, compromised survival, or greater disease burden (36, 37). Scintigraphy with radiolabeled octreotide, a somatostatin analog (^{111}In-Octreoscan), has low sensitivity for metastatic MTC and is not recommended for routine surveillance (1). A somatostatin analog-labeled PET/CT with ^{68}Gallium (^{68}Ga) (^{68}Ga-DOTATATE PET/CT) has a predominant affinity for somatostatin-receptor subtype 2, which is frequently found on MTC cell membranes. It was demonstrated to be superior to ^{111}In-Octreoscan in detecting recurrent MTC in one small study (38, 39).

Response Evaluation Criteria In Solid Tumors (RECIST) version 1.1 is a standardized and broadly accepted set of criteria used in oncology and radiology for determining radiologic response or progression of soft tissue metastases in solid tumors, including thyroid cancer (40). Notably, osteoblastic bone lesions are not considered measurable, but osteolytic bone lesions with an identifiable soft tissue component evaluable by CT or MRI can be considered as a measurable lesion. Progressive disease is defined as a $\geq$20% increase in target lesion measurements. A partial response is defined as a $\geq$30% decrease in the sum of all target lesions. Stable disease is any response between $-$29 and $+$19% change in the sum of target lesions. A real-life clinical dilemma is that radiologists often do not report findings based on RECIST criteria outside of a clinical trial, making it necessary for the clinician to personally determine overall stability, response, or progression of MTC.

Prognostic indicators beyond doubling times

With the development of targeted drug therapies, it is unclear if the conventional use of Ctn and CEA is effective in the measurement of response to therapy. This is a general concern that is shared across many different cancer types and has led to the development of a new generation of tumor biomarkers that include circulating cell-free DNA (cfDNA), which contain DNA derived from dying tumors (41, 42). It is now widely accepted for several types of cancer that tumor cfDNA levels provide prognostic information in untreated patients and also may be predictive of response to treatment. Liquid biopsy has been shown to detect *RET* M918T mutations in patient plasma with high specificity but low sensitivity (43). In individuals with known somatic *RET* M918T mutations, the allelic fraction of circulating tumor DNA is prognostic for overall survival and may play a role in monitoring response to treatment.

The presence of a somatic *RET* mutation has been found to be associated with a lower survival rate (44). The role of somatic copy number alteration as a mechanism for MTC tumorigenesis has been recently studied; the loss of somatic cyclin-dependent kinase inhibitor 2C (CDKN2C), an inhibitor of the retinoblastoma pathway necessary for tumor cell cycle activation, is associated with the presence of distant metastasis at presentation as well as decreased overall survival, a relationship enhanced by concomitant *RET* M918T mutation (45).

REGIONAL SITE-SPECIFIC OR SYMPTOM-SPECIFIC THERAPIES

Locoregional persistence and recurrence of MTC is not uncommon, and the decision regarding the appropriateness of remedial surgery should balance the anatomic threat of local invasion into vital structures with the elevated risks of hypoparathyroidism and nerve injury associated with reoperation (Figure 9.3) (46).

Adjunctive external beam radiation therapy (EBRT) to the neck is controversial and poorly studied, largely in a retrospective and non-randomized setting. It is not recommended when further surgery can successfully extirpate residual or recurrent disease. Although it may reduce

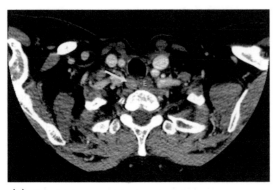

(a)

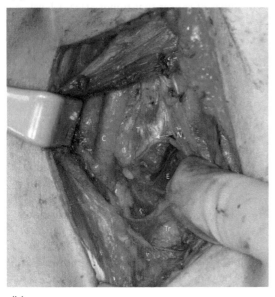

(b)

Figure 9.3 (a) Growing persistent disease (denoted by arrow) requiring reoperation given location adjacent to esophagus and course of right recurrent laryngeal nerve and risk of future invasiveness into the esophagus and/or nerve. (b) Intraoperative findings of tumor posterior to recurrent laryngeal nerve, nerve able to be preserved. E: Esophagus, T: Tumor, N: Recurrent laryngeal nerve, Tr: Trachea.

locoregional recurrences, there is no evidence demonstrating improved overall survival, and it certainly can lead to significant morbidity, such as esophageal stricture (47). With the availability of anti-angiogenic MKIs for progressive MTC, we recommend deferring EBRT in the absence of tracheal or esophageal wall disease, due to the risk for tracheoesophageal or tracheo-tumor fistula development (48).

Brain metastases should be irradiated using EBRT or stereotactic radiosurgery to prevent potentially catastrophic neurologic events. Additionally, if systemic therapy with an MKI is being considered, brain imaging should be performed before initiation and irradiation completed for occult brain metastases, as there is concern for potential increased bleeding risk into these lesions due to the MKI targeting the vascular endothelial growth factor receptor (VEGFR), although some clinical trials indicated that antiangiogenic therapies were not associated with an increased risk of intracranial bleeding in patients with known brain metastases (49).

Distant metastases to the lung and liver that are indolent and asymptomatic can be followed with serial imaging. Progressive pulmonary metastases can cause symptoms of dyspnea, hemoptysis, or cause post-obstructive pneumonia. In selected cases where localized pulmonary metastases compromise pulmonary function, palliative surgical resection or radiotherapy may be considered. For patients with progressive or symptomatic liver metastases, transarterial chemoembolization (TACE) or radioembolization can be considered (50).

Bone metastases in MTC are often clinically silent. In a retrospective study of over 1000 patients with MTC from a single center, 25% of patients with bone metastases were identified within 3 months of MTC diagnosis (35). Skeletal-related events (SREs) (defined as spinal cord compression, pathological fracture, radiation or surgery to bone, and hypercalcemia of malignancy) occurred in 48% of the patients; radiotherapy was most common, followed by a pathologic fracture. Spinal cord compression was extremely rare (1.6%). Overall, patients with SREs did not experience compromised survival compared to patients without SREs. EBRT, stereotactic radiotherapy, vertebroplasty, radiofrequency ablation, cryosurgery, arterial embolization, or surgical resection can be considered to palliate painful bone metastases or to prevent fracture or neurological compromise. Anti-resorptive therapies that inhibit osteoclast activity, such as bisphosphonates or denosumab, are employed in patients with osteolytic bone metastases from several different types of neoplasms (lung, breast, prostate, kidney, and multiple myeloma); anecdotal experience supports their use in MTC, as these treatments can reduce pain associated with bone metastases. There are no prospective controlled trials available studying these agents in metastatic bone disease in thyroid cancer.

Diarrhea, a common (30% of MTC patients) paraneoplastic syndrome seen in MTC, can cause weight loss, dehydration, and poor quality of life. Tumoral co-secretion of peptides (e.g., prostaglandins, 5-hydroxytryptamin, vasoactive intestinal peptide, and calcitonin gene-related peptide) is associated with hypersecretory diarrhea and increased gastrointestinal motility. It is frequently present in patients with advanced, metastatic disease, typically involving the liver. Anti-motility drugs (loperamide, diphenoxylate/atropine or tincture of opium) are effective first-line agents. Somatostatin analogs may provide some benefit based on small, nonrandomized studies (51, 52). Surgical debulking or hepatic TACE is helpful in some patients (50). Diarrhea can decrease with MKI therapy, a clinical indicator of response.

Ectopic Cushing's syndrome is a rare paraneoplastic syndrome that can be associated with MTC (less than 1%); it is caused by tumoral production of adrenocorticotropic hormone or corticotropin-releasing hormone. It is associated with dramatic clinical findings, such as hypertension, hypokalemia, proximal muscle wasting, hyperglycemia, opportunistic infections, and hypercoagulability; it conveys a poor prognosis if not aggressively treated. When associated with a localized tumor, resection or ablation can cause clinical remission of this paraneoplastic syndrome. In the presence of widely metastatic disease, medical therapy (ketoconazole or metyrapone) or bilateral adrenalectomy may be necessary.

SYSTEMIC THERAPIES FOR ADVANCED, PROGRESSIVE DISEASE

Patients with rapidly progressive, widely metastatic, or symptomatic disease that is not amenable to focal or targeted palliative treatments should be considered for systemic chemotherapy. Prior to 2000, studies with chemotherapeutic regimens typically combining dacarbazine with other agents (e.g., cyclophosphamide, vincristine, 5-fluorouracil) demonstrated a reduction in tumor size in approximately 25% of patients (53). However, significant toxicity profiles and lack of complete responses made these treatments unfavorable for use.

Subsequent studies revealed promising antitumoral responses to small molecule tyrosine kinase inhibitors (TKIs), which compete with the ATP-binding site of the catalytic domain of a tyrosine kinase, which in turn inhibit autophosphorylation and activation of the tyrosine kinase domain of various transmembrane receptors (e.g., VEGFR, RET, c-Kit, epidermal growth factor receptor [EGFR], c-Met). These receptors are critical for activating intracellular signaling pathways that drive cell activation, division, migration, and survival. The TKIs target more than one type of tyrosine protein kinase with varying potencies, thus designating them as multikinase inhibitors; however, all target VEGFR-2, the primary mediator of angiogenesis. Although numerous MKIs have been investigated in MTC in various phases of clinical trials, both vandetanib and cabozantinib were studied robustly in phase III placebo-controlled trials, and subsequently were approved for commercial use in the United States in April 2011 and November 2012, respectively, for the treatment of advanced, progressive, or symptomatic MTC. These are notable achievements for a rare cancer that historically had no viable therapeutic options other than surgery.

Approved multikinase inhibitors (MKI) for MTC

Vandetanib targets RET (IC_{50} 100nM), VEGFR-2 (IC_{50} 40nM) and EGFR (IC_{50} 500nM) (54). Given the activity against RET, the drug was first studied in hereditary MTC patients. Two phase II clinical trials evaluated hereditary MTC patients using two different doses: 100-mg and 300 mg daily (55, 56). Encouraging findings from these trials led to the ZETA study, a large, multicenter, randomized controlled phase III trial for patients with advanced MTC (hereditary and non-hereditary), measurable by RECIST and a Ctn of at least 500 pg/mL (n=331) (57). Radiologic progression prior to enrollment was not required, a distinguishing feature of this trial. Patients were randomized in a 2:1 ratio to vandetanib or placebo between 12/2006 and 11/2007 with the ability to crossover to the active drug if placebo-treated patients demonstrated progression while on the study. Vandetanib led to a significantly prolonged progression-free survival of 30.5 months (predicted) compared with placebo (19.3 months) (HR 0.46; 95% CI, 0.31–0.69, P<0.001). The overall response rate observed in the trial was 45% in the vandetanib group compared with 13% in the placebo group. Although it was not designed to evaluate overall survival, there was no difference in overall survival between the treatment groups.

Cabozantinib inhibits RET (IC_{50} 4.5nM), VEGFR-2 (IC_{50} 0.035nM) and c-MET (IC_{50} 1.8) (54). A phase I clinical trial evaluating cabozantinib in patients with solid tumors became enriched for MTC patients once favorable responses were observed (58). Of the 37 MTC patients enrolled, all of whom had progressive disease prior to study entry, 29% had a partial response with a combined benefit (partial response plus stable disease) seen in 68% of patients. The subsequent multicenter, randomized controlled phase III EXAM trial randomized MTC (hereditary and non-hereditary) patients, who had progressive disease within 14 months of study enrollment, to cabozantinib or placebo in a 2:1 allocation (n=330) (59). The median progression-free survival was significantly longer in the cabozantinib-treated patients (11.2 months) compared with the placebo group (4.0 months) (HR 0.28; 95% CI 0.19–0.40, P<0.001), with a partial response of 28% for cabozantinib and 0% in placebo-treated patients. Responses were observed regardless of *RET* mutation status. Overall survival, a secondary endpoint in this study as crossover from placebo to active drug was not permitted, was not different between the treatment groups (HR 0.85; 95% CI, 0.64–1.12; P=0.24) 60.

Due to the differences in enrollment criteria and protocol designs, it is not possible to compare the outcomes from these two trials or to determine whether one agent is more effective than the other (Table 9.1). The patients in the EXAM trial had more aggressive disease, as progression prior to enrollment was required, whereas ZETA included patients with stable disease at baseline. The EXAM trial did not allow crossover to active drug if a placebo-treated patient demonstrated progression, which the ZETA study permitted.

When should an MKI be initiated?

Patients who have rising tumor markers alone, without documented structural disease, or have stable or indolent metastatic disease with prolonged Ctn and CEA doubling times greater than 2 years, do not require systemic therapy; they require routine active surveillance for progression as described in an earlier section (1). The 2015 ATA guidelines recommend that patients with symptomatic or progressive metastatic disease with a high tumor burden are candidates for either vandetanib or cabozantinib as first-line systemic therapy. The following are indications for initiating systemic chemotherapy (61):

1. Radiologically progressive (based on RECIST) and clinically significant disease within 12 to 14 months

Table 9.1 Comparison of the phase III cabozantinib and vandetanib trials

	EXAM trial		ZETA trial	
	Cabozantinib (n=219)	Placebo (n=111)	Vandetanib (n=231)	Placebo (n=100)
Inclusion Criteria	Documented RECIST progression within 14 months of enrollment		Locally advanced or metastatic disease and calcitonin ≥500 pg/mL (no requirement for RECIST progression)	
Crossover at Progression	Not Allowed		Allowed	
Median PFS (months)	11.2	4.0	Not reached; estimated 30.5	19.3
1-year PFS	47%	7%	83%	63%
HR (95% CI)	0.28 (0.19, 0.40)		0.35 (0.24, 0.53)	
ORR	28%	0%	45%	13%

EXAM: **E**fficacy of **X**L184 in **A**dvanced **M**edullary Thyroid Carcinoma; ZETA: **Z**actima **E**fficacy in **T**hyroid Cancer **A**ssessment; RECIST: **R**esponse **E**valuation **C**riteria **I**n **S**olid **T**umors; PFS: progression-free survival; HR: hazard ratio; CI: confidence interval; ORR: objective response rate.

2. Symptomatic metastatic disease not amenable to, or that has failed, local or symptom-specific therapies (e.g., surgery, radiotherapy, embolization, cryoablation, or antidiarrheals)
3. Bulky disease compromising or threatening organ function not manageable with localized therapies.

In selected cases, additional reasons to embark on systemic therapy include (61):

1. Ctn doubling time of less than 6 months and structural evidence of clinically significant disease not treatable with local therapies
2. Severe, intractable MTC-related diarrhea or ectopic Cushing's syndrome and lack of efficacy with other medical treatments and presence of structural and clinically significant disease.

Adverse effects of MKI

Compared with cytotoxic chemotherapeutic agents, the adverse events (AEs) associated with MKIs are generally better tolerated and manageable. Some AEs are serious or can worsen quality of life. While patients with progressive metastatic disease may benefit from an MKI and the potential AEs are considered acceptable risks, potential serious AEs of these drugs outweigh the marginal benefits in patients with indolent or stable disease.

Common toxicities with MKIs include the following: dermatologic (palmar-plantar erythrodysesthesia, photosensitivity), mucocutaneous (stomatitis, taste changes), cardiovascular (hypertension), gastrointestinal (diarrhea, nausea, anorexia), systemic (fatigue), and uncontrolled hypothyroidism (Table 9.2; Figure 9.4). With vandetanib, the most common side effects (≥20%) noted in the phase III trial included (in order of descending frequency): diarrhea, rash, nausea, hypertension, fatigue, headache, diminished appetite, and acne (57). QTc prolongation was observed in 14% of patients treated with vandetanib, although there were no reports of torsades de pointes. There is a black box warning on the package insert for vandetanib specifying the necessity to: (1) monitor electrocardiograms (ECGs) routinely when treating with this agent; (2) avoid medications known

Table 9.2 Adverse events (all grades) with cabozantinib and vandetanib (57, 59)

Adverse event	Cabozantinib (n=214), %	Placebo (n=109), %	Adverse event	Vandetanib (n=231), %	Placebo (n=99), %
Diarrhea	63.1	33.0	Diarrhea	56	26
Palmar-plantar erythrodysesthesia	50.0	1.8	Rash	45	11
Decreased weight	47.7	10.1	Nausea	33	16
Decreased appetite	45.8	15.6	Hypertension	32	5
Nausea	43.0	21.1	Fatigue	24	23
Fatigue	40.7	28.4	Headache	26	9
Dysgeusia	34.1	5.5	Decreased appetite	21	12
Hair color changes	33.6	0.9	Acne	20	5
Hypertension	32.7	4.6	Asthenia	14	11
Stomatitis	29.0	2.8	Vomiting	14	7
Constipation	26.6	5.5	Back pain	9	20
Hemorrhage	25.2	15.6	Dry skin	15	5
Vomiting	24.3	1.8	Insomnia	13	10
Mucosal inflammation	23.4	3.7	Abdominal pain	14	5
Asthesia	21.0	14.7	Dermatitis acneiform	15	2
Dysphonia	20.1	9.2	Cough	10	10

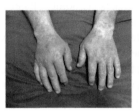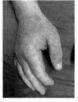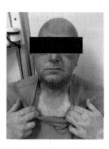

Figure 9.4 Skin adverse effect with vandetanib. Photosensitivity skin adverse event arising 55 days after starting vandetanib therapy. There are erythematous plaques and bullae on the face, scalp, neck, dorsal hands, and palms, sparing the upper back/chest with well-demarcated borders.

to prolong the QT interval; (3) correct electrolyte abnormalities (hypocalcemia, hypokalemia, hypomagnesemia); and (4) correct hypothyroidism. Cabozantinib was associated with the following common side effects in the phase III trial ($\geq$ 20%, in order of descending frequency): diarrhea, palmar-plantar erythrodysesthesia, weight loss, diminished appetite, nausea, fatigue, taste change, hair color changes, hypertension, stomatitis, constipation, hemorrhage, vomiting, mucosal inflammation, asthenia, and dysphonia (59). Cabozantinib is a more potent inhibitor of VEGFR-2, which is likely why it is associated with hemorrhage, venous thrombosis, gastrointestinal (GI) perforation, and fistula formation (Figure 9.5). There is a black box warning on the package insert for cabozantinib for the risks of GI perforation, fistula, and hemorrhage. Given the side effect profiles of each of these drugs and the variable propensity for specific side effects, recommendations regarding starting systemic chemotherapy for a patient must be patient-centered and account for multiple factors, including patient's medical history, physical examination findings, baseline laboratory data, ECG, concomitant medications, radiation history, and extension of tumor into surrounding tissues, especially vascular structures (61). From this evaluation, it is possible to select a drug with the least risk for side effects while providing oncologic benefit.

As neither agent is curative, chronic use is required for control of disease. Patient quality of life, compliance, and optimal response to drug therapy can all be limited without implementation of regular preventative strategies and aggressive management of AEs. The management of AEs associated with MKIs used for metastatic thyroid cancer is well described by Cabanillas et al. (62).

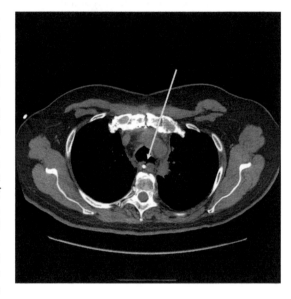

Figure 9.5 Tracheoesophageal fistula with cabozantinib. Patient taking cabozantinib with a tracheoesophageal fistula (yellow arrow identifies the tract between the trachea and the esophagus, which has an hyper-enhancing nasogastric tube within it).

Monitoring for response to targeted therapy

While on systemic treatment, routine monitoring for response with high-resolution imaging studies (CT, MRI) should be performed every 2 to 3 months. The response should be determined based on radiologic findings, not on biomarker changes alone, as Ctn and CEA levels can be discordant and may not correlate with radiologic responses in some cases. The challenge is that some lesions will demonstrate response while other sites may progress in an individual patient, termed a "mixed response."

It is generally accepted that soft tissue metastases respond more effectively to MKIs than bone metastases. These mixed responses may be due to variable tissue distribution of drug or tumor heterogeneity, a problem identified in other solid tumors, papillary thyroid cancer, and MTC (63–66). There is also the possibility of tumor resistance, such as that seen with a gatekeeper mutation like V804 *RET* mutations (67). In patients with mixed responses, targeted treatment of focal areas of progression (e.g., radiation or resection) can be considered. Eventually, most patients will become refractory to treatment, and the clinician should be prepared to recommend the next treatment, either by switching to the other approved agent or referring the patient for consideration for a clinical trial.

Other agents in clinical trials

In MTC, various somatic mutations are potential therapeutic targets (Table 9.3). Although targeting multiple kinases leads to a multi-faceted attack on oncogenic pathways, this can also lead to off-target effects on normal cells, manifesting as AEs, as described earlier. There is growing interest in developing highly specific RET inhibitors, especially since RET fusion proteins are found in more prevalent malignancies such as papillary thyroid cancer and non-small cell lung adenocarcinomas. Highly specific RET inhibitors may demonstrate greater antitumoral efficacy with more tolerable side effect profiles, especially if there is less anti-angiogenic effect (68). Two separate phase I trials studying RET-specific inhibitors (BLU-667 and LOXO-292) in solid tumors, including MTC, are currently actively enrolling (www.clinicaltrials.gov). The results of these two trials are highly anticipated.

In various solid tumors, including MTC, activation of tyrosine kinase receptors leads to downstream upregulation of *RAS* and activation of the MAPK and PI3K/Akt/mTOR pathways. The mammalian target of rapamycin (mTOR) plays a role in cell proliferation and inhibiting apoptosis. Additionally, MTC can be associated with *RAS* mutations (most commonly *HRAS* type), mutually exclusive from *RET* mutations, in approximately 14% of patients (8). In a single-arm, multicenter, phase II trial with everolimus (an mTOR inhibitor), metastatic thyroid cancer patients of all histologies, with evidence of progression by RECIST criteria within the prior 6 months, were enrolled (69). Ten of 33 patients had MTC. Nine had a *RET* mutation, and four had prior treatment with an MKI. One patient had a partial response, while eight others had stable disease, with a median progression-free survival of 13.1 months (range: 1.8–49.2 months). Another phase II trial of everolimus in patients with thyroid cancers of any histology reported that the eight patients with MTC all had stable disease as the best response (70). A Dutch phase II study of everolimus in thyroid cancer included seven MTC patients with progression within 12 months prior to enrollment (71). Five patients had stable disease, and the other two had continued progressive disease. There is an ongoing study of the combination of everolimus with vandetanib, which may have a synergistic effect. Larger studies with everolimus are needed to understand the benefit of this agent for MTC.

Immunotherapy agents targeting cytotoxic T-lymphocyte-associated antigen 4 (CTLA-4; ipilimumab), programmed cell death protein 1 (PD-1; pembrolizumab and nivolumab), or programmed cell death ligand 1 (PD-L1; atezolizumab, avelumab, and durvalumab) have led to remarkable responses in melanoma, non-small cell lung, renal cell, bladder, and head and neck cancers. There are currently ongoing trials using either single agent or combination immunotherapies for thyroid (medullary and non-medullary) cancers.

Table 9.3 Somatic mutations identified in medullary thyroid carcinoma (8)

Gene	Mutated samples	Tested samples	Mutation frequency
RET	1007	2304	44%
HRAS	111	1033	11%
KRAS	36	1039	3%
NRAS	4	824	0.5%
BRAF	31	508	6%
CDKN2C	5	83	6%

CONCLUSION AND FUTURE DIRECTIONS

The era of targeted therapy for thyroid cancer began at the turn of the century with the recognition that neoplastic growth depended on the upregulation of angiogenesis and pathogenic "driver" mutations encoding kinases that activate critical intracellular pathways. With this new understanding, there was an exponential development of targeted systemic therapies studied in successfully completed clinical trials led by an international community of investigators. Since 2011, four drugs were approved for use in advanced, progressive MTC (cabozantinib and vandetanib) and radioiodine-refractory differentiated thyroid cancer (lenvatinib and sorafenib) not amenable to surgery or other treatments. However, the holy grail of a curative treatment has yet to be identified.

These achievements attained over a relatively short time promise a hopeful future for patients with MTC. Further research is much needed in the following areas: evaluating patient-reported outcomes to develop individualized care models, identifying more effective early prognostic indicators of tumoral behavior, establishing other targetable mechanisms of oncogenesis, understanding how intratumoral heterogeneity may influence responses to therapy, clarifying mechanisms of drug resistance, and (most important) finding a treatment regimen that leads to a cure for what has long been considered a chronic cancer.

REFERENCES

1. Wells SA, Jr., Asa SL, Dralle H, Elisei R, Evans DB, Gagel RF, Lee N, et al. Revised American Thyroid Association guidelines for the management of medullary thyroid carcinoma. *Thyroid* 2015; 25(6):567–610.
2. Siegel RL, Miller KD, Jemal A. Cancer statistics, 2018. *CA Cancer J. Clin.* 68(1):7–30.
3. Hazard JB, Hawk WA, Crile G, Jr. Medullary (solid) carcinoma of the thyroid; a clinicopathologic entity. *J. Clin. Endocrinol. Metab.* 1959; 19(1):152–61.
4. Williams ED. Histogenesis of medullary carcinoma of the thyroid. *J. Clin. Pathol.* 1966; 19(2):114–18.
5. Donis-Keller H, Dou S, Chi D, Carlson KM, Toshima K, Lairmore TC, Howe JR, et al. Mutations in the RET proto-oncogene are associated with MEN2A and FMTC. *Hum. Mol. Genet.* 1993; 2(7):851–6.
6. Mulligan LM, Kwok JB, Healey CS, Elsdon MJ, Eng C, Gardner E, Love DR, et al. Germ-line mutations of the RET proto-oncogene in multiple endocrine neoplasia type 2A. *Nature* 1993; 363(6428):458–60.
7. Eng C, Smith DP, Mulligan LM, Nagai MA, Healey CS, Ponder MA, Gardner E, et al. Point mutation within the tyrosine kinase domain of the RET proto-oncogene in multiple endocrine neoplasia type 2B and related sporadic tumors. *Hum. Mol. Genet.* 1994; 3(2):237–41.
8. [cited 01/09/2018]. Available from: https://cancer.sanger.ac.uk/cosmic/browse/tissue?wgs=off&sn=thyroid&ss=all&hn=carcinoma&sh=medullary_carcinoma&in=t&src=tissue&all_data=n.
9. Cabanillas ME, Hu MI, Jimenez C, Grubbs EG, Cote GJ. Treating medullary thyroid cancer in the age of targeted therapy. *Int. J. Endocr. Oncol.* 2014; 1(2):203–16.
10. Carlson KM, Bracamontes J, Jackson CE, Clark R, Lacroix A, Wells SA, Jr., Goodfellow PJ. Parent-of-origin effects in multiple endocrine neoplasia type 2B. *Am. J. Hum. Genet.* 1994; 55(6):1076–82.
11. Schuffenecker I, Ginet N, Goldgar D, Eng C, Chambe B, Boneu A, Houdent C, et al. Prevalence and parental origin of de novo RET mutations in multiple endocrine neoplasia type 2A and familial medullary thyroid carcinoma. Le Groupe d'Etude des Tumeurs a calcitonine. *Am. J. Hum. Genet.* 1997; 60(1):233–7.
12. Wohllk N, Cote GJ, Bugalho MM, Ordonez N, Evans DB, Goepfert H, Khorana S, et al. Relevance of RET proto-oncogene mutations in sporadic medullary thyroid carcinoma. *J. Clin. Endocrinol. Metab.* 1996; 81(10):3740–5.
13. Elisei R, Romei C, Cosci B, Agate L, Bottici V, Molinaro E, Sculli M, et al. RET genetic screening in patients with medullary thyroid cancer and their relatives: Experience with 807 individuals at one center. *J. Clin. Endocrinol. Metab.* 2007; 92(12):4725–9.
14. Eng C, Mulligan LM, Smith DP, Healey CS, Frilling A, Raue F, Neumann HPH, Ponder

MA, Ponder BAJ. Low frequency of germ-line mutations in the *RET* proto-oncogene in patients with apparently sporadic medullary thyroid carcinoma. *Clin. Endocrinol* 1995; 43(1):123–7.

15. Kouvaraki MA, Shapiro SE, Perrier ND, Cote GJ, Gagel RF, Hoff AO, Sherman SI, Lee JE, Evans DB. *RET* proto-oncogene: A review and update of genotype-phenotype correlations in hereditary medullary thyroid cancer and associated endocrine tumors. *Thyroid* 2005; 15(6):531–44.

16. Brandi ML, Gagel RF, Angeli A, Bilezikian JP, Beck-Peccoz P, Bordi C, Conte-Devolx B, et al. Guidelines for diagnosis and therapy of MEN type 1 and type 2. *J. Clin. Endocrinol. Metab.* 2001; 86(12):5658–71.

17. Thosani S, Ayala-Ramirez M, Palmer L, Hu MI, Rich T, Gagel RF, Cote G, et al. The characterization of pheochromocytoma and its impact on overall survival in multiple endocrine neoplasia type 2. *J. Clin. Endocrinol. Metab.* 2013; 98(11):E1813–9.

18. Rothberg AE, Raymond VM, Gruber SB, Sisson J. Familial medullary thyroid carcinoma associated with cutaneous lichen amyloidosis. *Thyroid* 2009;19 (6):651–5.

19. Donovan DT, Levy ML, Furst EJ, Alford BR, Wheeler T, Tschen JA, Gagel RF. Familial cutaneous lichen amyloidosis in association with multiple endocrine neoplasia type 2A: A new variant. *Henry Ford Hosp. Med. J.* 1989; 37(3–4):147–50.

20. Zenaty D, Aigrain Y, Peuchmaur M, Philippe-Chomette P, Baumann C, Cornelis F, Hugot JP, et al. Medullary thyroid carcinoma identified within the first year of life in children with hereditary multiple endocrine neoplasia type 2A (codon 634) and 2B. *Eur. J. Endocrinol.* 2009; 160(5):807–13.

21. Raue F. German medullary thyroid carcinoma/multiple endocrine neoplasia registry. German MTC/MEN study group. Medullary thyroid carcinoma/multiple endocrine neoplasia type 2. *Langenbecks Arch. Surg.* 1998; 383(5):334–6.

22. Jasim S, Ying AK, Waguespack SG, Rich TA, Grubbs EG, Jimenez C, Hu MI, Cote G, Habra MA. Multiple endocrine neoplasia type 2B with a *RET* proto-oncogene A883F mutation displays a more indolent form of medullary thyroid carcinoma compared with a *RET* M918T mutation. *Thyroid* 2011; 21(2):189–92.

23. Waguespack SG, Rich TA, Perrier ND, Jimenez C, Cote GJ. Management of medullary thyroid carcinoma and MEN2 syndromes in childhood. *Nat. Rev. Endocrinol.* 2011; 7(10):596–607.

24. Task F, Kloos RT, Eng C, Evans DB, Francis GL, Gagel RF, et al. Medullary thyroid cancer: Management guidelines of the American Thyroid Association. *Thyroid* 2009; 19(6):565–612.

25. Kebebew E, Greenspan FS, Clark OH, Woeber KA, Grunwell J. Extent of disease and practice patterns for medullary thyroid cancer. *J. Am. Coll. Surg.* 2005; 200(6):890–6.

26. Roman S, Lin R, Sosa JA. Prognosis of medullary thyroid carcinoma: Demographic, clinical, and pathologic predictors of survival in 1252 cases. *Cancer* 2006; 107(9):2134–42.

27. Moley JF, DeBenedetti MK. Patterns of nodal metastases in palpable medullary thyroid carcinoma: Recommendations for extent of node dissection. *Ann. Surg.* 1999; 229(6):880–7.

28. Trimboli P, Cremonini N, Ceriani L, Saggiorato E, Guidobaldi L, Romanelli F, Ventura C, et al. Calcitonin measurement in aspiration needle washout fluids has higher sensitivity than cytology in detecting medullary thyroid cancer: A retrospective multicentre study. *Clin. Endocrinol. (Oxf.)* 2014; 80(1):135–40.

29. Nikiforova MN, Mercurio S, Wald AI, Barbi de Moura M, Callenberg K, Santana-Santos L, Gooding WE, et al. Analytical performance of the ThyroSeq v3 genomic classifier for cancer diagnosis in thyroid nodules. *Cancer* 2018; 124(8):1682–90.

30. Pankratz DG, Hu Z, Kim SY, Monroe RJ, Wong MG, Traweek ST, Kloos RT, Walsh PS, Kennedy GC. Analytical performance of a gene expression classifier for medullary thyroid carcinoma. *Thyroid* 2016; 26(11):1573–80.

31. Elisei R, Bottici V, Luchetti F, Di Coscio G, Romei C, Grasso L, Miccoli P, et al. Impact of routine measurement of serum calcitonin on the diagnosis and outcome of medullary

thyroid cancer: Experience in 10,864 patients with nodular thyroid disorders. *J. Clin. Endocrinol. Metab.* 2004; 89(1):163–8.

32. Sosa JA, Bowman HM, Tielsch JM, Powe NR, Gordon TA, Udelsman R. The importance of surgeon experience for clinical and economic outcomes from thyroidectomy. *Ann. Surg.* 1998; 228(3):320–30.

33. Meijer JA, le Cessie S, van den Hout WB, Kievit J, Schoones JW, Romijn JA, Smit JW. Calcitonin and carcinoembryonic antigen doubling times as prognostic factors in medullary thyroid carcinoma: A structured meta-analysis. *Clin. Endocrinol. (Oxf.)* 2010; 72(4):534–42.

34. Ahn JE, Lee JH, Yi JS, Shong YK, Hong SJ, Lee DH, Choi CG, Kim SJ. Diagnostic accuracy of CT and ultrasonography for evaluating metastatic cervical lymph nodes in patients with thyroid cancer. *World J. Surg.* 2008; 32(7):1552–8.

35. Xu JY, Murphy WA, Jr., Milton DR, Jimenez C, Rao SN, Habra MA, Waguespack SG, et al. Bone metastases and skeletal-related events in medullary thyroid carcinoma. *J. Clin. Endocrinol. Metab.* 2016; 101(12):4871–7.

36. Treglia G, Castaldi P, Villani MF, Perotti G, de Waure C, Filice A, Ambrosini V, et al. Comparison of 18F-DOPA, 18F-FDG and 68Ga-somatostatin analog PET/CT in patients with recurrent medullary thyroid carcinoma. *Eur. J. Nucl. Med. Mol. Imaging* 2012; 39(4):569–80.

37. Verbeek HH, Plukker JT, Koopmans KP, de Groot JW, Hofstra RM, Muller Kobold AC, van der Horst-Schrivers AN, Brouwers AH, Links TP. Clinical relevance of 18F-FDG PET and 18F-DOPA PET in recurrent medullary thyroid carcinoma. *J. Nucl. Med.* 2012; 53(12):1863–71.

38. Yamaga LYI, Cunha ML, Campos Neto GC, Garcia MRT, Yang JH, Camacho CP, Wagner J, Funari MBG. Ga-DOTATATE PET/CT in recurrent medullary thyroid carcinoma: A lesion-by-lesion comparison with ^{111}In-octreotide SPECT/CT and conventional imaging. *Eur. J. Nucl. Med. Mol. Imaging* 2017; 44(10):1695–701.

39. Tran K, Khan S, Taghizadehasl M, Palazzo F, Frilling A, Todd JF, Al-Nahhas A. Gallium-68 Dotatate PET/CT is superior to other imaging modalities in the detection of medullary carcinoma of the thyroid in the presence of high serum calcitonin. *Hell. J. Nucl. Med.* 2015; 18(1):19–24.

40. [Available from: http://recist.eortc.org/wp-content/uploads/2015/03/RECISTGuidelines.pdf.

41. Schwarzenbach H, Hoon DS, Pantel K. Cell-free nucleic acids as biomarkers in cancer patients. *Nat. Rev. Cancer* 2011; 11(6):426–37.

42. Jung K, Fleischhacker M, Rabien A. Cell-free DNA in the blood as a solid tumor biomarker – A critical appraisal of the literature. *Clin. Chim. Acta* 2010; 411(21–22):1611–24.

43. Cote GJ, Evers C, Hu MI, Grubbs EG, Williams MD, Hai T, Duose DY, et al. Prognostic significance of circulating *RET* M918T mutated tumor DNA in patients with advanced medullary thyroid carcinoma. *J. Clin. Endocrinol. Metab.* 2017; 102(9):3591–9.

44. Elisei R, Cosci B, Romei C, Bottici V, Renzini G, Molinaro E, Agate L, et al. Prognostic significance of somatic *RET* oncogene mutations in sporadic medullary thyroid cancer: A 10-year follow-up study. *J. Clin. Endocrinol. Metab.* 2008; 93(3):682–7.

45. Grubbs EG, Williams MD, Scheet P, Vattathil S, Perrier ND, Lee JE, Gagel RF, et al. Role of CDKN2C copy-number in sporadic medullary thyroid carcinoma. *Thyroid* 2016; 26(11):1553–62.

46. Hughes DT, Laird AM, Miller BS, Gauger PG, Doherty GM. Reoperative lymph node dissection for recurrent papillary thyroid cancer and effect on serum thyroglobulin. *Ann. Surg. Oncol.* 2012; 19(9):2951–7.

47. Schwartz DL, Rana V, Shaw S, Yazbeck C, Ang KK, Morrison WH, Rosenthal DI, et al. Postoperative radiotherapy for advanced medullary thyroid cancer – Local disease control in the modern era. *Head Neck* 2008;30(7):883–8.

48. Blevins DP, Dadu R, Hu M, Baik C, Balachandran D, Ross W, Gunn B, Cabanillas ME. Aerodigestive fistula formation as a rare side effect of antiangiogenic tyrosine kinase inhibitor therapy for thyroid cancer. *Thyroid* 2014; 24(5):918–22.

49. Askoxylakis V, Arvanitis CD, Wong CSF, Ferraro GB, Jain RK. Emerging strategies for delivering antiangiogenic therapies to primary and metastatic brain tumors. *Adv. Drug Deliv. Rev.* 2017; 119:159–74.

50. Fromigue J, De Baere T, Baudin E, Dromain C, Leboulleux S, Schlumberger M. Chemoembolization for liver metastases from medullary thyroid carcinoma. *J. Clin. Endocrinol. Metab.* 2006; 91(7):2496–9.

51. Mahler C, Verhelst J, de Longueville M, Harris A. Long-term treatment of metastatic medullary thyroid carcinoma with the somatostatin analog octreotide. *Clin. Endocrinol. (Oxf.)* 1990; 33(2):261–9.

52. Vainas I, Koussis Ch, Pazaitou-Panayiotou K, Drimonitis A, Chrisoulidou A, Iakovou I, Boudina M, Kaprara A, Maladaki A. Somatostatin receptor expression in vivo and response to somatostatin analog therapy with or without other antineoplastic treatments in advanced medullary thyroid carcinoma. *J. Exp. Clin. Cancer Res.* 2004; 23(4):549–59.

53. Vitale G, Caraglia M, Ciccarelli A, Lupoli G, Abbruzzese A, Tagliaferri P, Lupoli G. Current approaches and perspectives in the therapy of medullary thyroid carcinoma. *Cancer* 2001; 91(9):1797–808.

54. Sherman SI. Advances in chemotherapy of differentiated epithelial and medullary thyroid cancers. *J. Clin. Endocrinol. Metab.* 2009; 94(5):1493–9.

55. Robinson BG, Paz-Ares L, Krebs A, Vasselli J, Haddad R. Vandetanib (100 mg) in patients with locally advanced or metastatic hereditary medullary thyroid cancer. *J. Clin. Endocrinol. Metab.* 2010; 95(6):2664–71.

56. Wells SA, Jr., Gosnell JE, Gagel RF, Moley J, Pfister D, Sosa JA, Skinner M, et al. Vandetanib for the treatment of patients with locally advanced or metastatic hereditary medullary thyroid cancer. *J. Clin. Oncol.* 2010;28(5):767–72.

57. Wells SA, Jr., Robinson BG, Gagel RF, Dralle H, Fagin JA, Santoro M, Baudin E, et al. Vandetanib in patients with locally advanced or metastatic medullary thyroid cancer: A randomized, double-blind phase III trial. *J. Clin. Oncol.* 2012; 30(2):134–41.

58. Kurzrock R, Sherman SI, Ball DW, Forastiere AA, Cohen RB, Mehra R, Pfister DG, et al. Activity of XL184 (cabozantinib), an oral tyrosine kinase inhibitor, in patients with medullary thyroid cancer. *J. Clin. Oncol.* 2011; 29(19):2660–6.

59. Elisei R, Schlumberger MJ, Muller SP, Schoffski P, Brose MS, Shah MH, Licitra L, et al. Cabozantinib in progressive medullary thyroid cancer. *J. Clin. Oncol.* 2013; 31(29):3639–46.

60. Schlumberger M, Elisei R, Muller S, Schoffski P, Brose M, Shah M, Licitra L, et al. Overall survival analysis of EXAM, a phase III trial of cabozantinib in patients with radiographically progressive medullary thyroid carcinoma. *Ann. Oncol.* 2017; 28(11):2813–9.

61. Cabanillas ME, Hu MI, Jimenez C. Medullary thyroid cancer in the era of tyrosine kinase inhibitors: To treat or not to treat – And with which drug – Those are the questions. *J. Clin. Endocrinol. Metab.* 2014; 99(12):4390–6.

62. Cabanillas ME, Hu MI, Durand JB, Busaidy NL. Challenges associated with tyrosine kinase inhibitor therapy for metastatic thyroid cancer. *J. Thyroid Res.* 2011; 2011:985780.

63. Le Pennec S, Konopka T, Gacquer D, Fimereli D, Tarabichi M, Tomas G, Savagner F, et al. Intratumor heterogeneity and clonal evolution in an aggressive papillary thyroid cancer and matched metastases. *Endocr. Relat. Cancer* 2015; 22(2):205–16.

64. Walts AE, Pao A, Sacks W, Bose S. BRAF genetic heterogeneity in papillary thyroid carcinoma and its metastasis. *Hum. Pathol.* 2014; 45(5):935–41.

65. McGranahan N, Swanton C. Clonal heterogeneity and tumor evolution: Past, present, and the future. *Cell* 2017; 168(4):613–28.

66. Romei C, Ciampi R, Casella F, Tacito A, Torregrossa L, Ugolini C, Basolo F, et al. *RET* mutation heterogeneity in primary advanced medullary thyroid cancers and their metastases. *Oncotarget* 2018; 9(11):9875–84.

67. Carlomagno F, Guida T, Anaganti S, Vecchio G, Fusco A, Ryan AJ, Billaud M, Santoro M. Disease associated mutations at valine 804

in the RET receptor tyrosine kinase confer resistance to selective kinase inhibitors. *Oncogene* 2004; 23(36):6056–63.

68. Roskoski R, Jr., Sadeghi-Nejad A. Role of *RET* protein-tyrosine kinase inhibitors in the treatment *RET*-driven thyroid and lung cancers. *Pharmacol. Res.* 2018; 128:1–17.

69. Hanna GJ, Busaidy NL, Chau NG, Wirth LJ, Barletta JA, Calles A, Haddad RI, et al. Genomic correlates of response to everolimus in aggressive radioiodine-refractory thyroid cancer: A phase II study. *Clin. Cancer Res.* 2018; 24(7):1546–53.

70. Lim SM, Chang H, Yoon MJ, Hong YK, Kim H, Chung WY, Park CS, et al. A multi-center, phase II trial of everolimus in locally advanced or metastatic thyroid cancer of all histologic subtypes. *Ann. Oncol.* 2013; 24(12):3089–94.

71. Schneider TC, de Wit D, Links TP, van Erp NP, van der Hoeven JJ, Gelderblom H, van Wezel T, et al. Beneficial effects of the mTOR inhibitor everolimus in patients with advanced medullary thyroid carcinoma: Subgroup results of a Phase II trial. *Int. J. Endocrinol.* 2015; 2015:348124.

Anaplastic thyroid carcinoma and thyroid lymphoma

ASHISH V. CHINTAKUNTLAWAR AND KEITH C. BIBLE

Case example	244	Hashimoto's/chronic lymphocytic thyroiditis	
Diagnostic approach to a rapidly enlarging		and PTL	251
thyroid mass	244	Pathology	251
Anaplastic thyroid carcinoma	244	Lymphoma cell types and histologic features	251
Incidence and demographics	244	Clinical features	251
Natural history and mortality rates	244	Symptoms and signs	251
Prognostic factors	245	Thyroid dysfunction	252
Diagnosis	245	Diagnosis	252
Fine needle aspiration	245	Serum chemistries and immunoglobulins	252
Radionuclide studies	246	Imaging studies	252
Thyroid ultrasonography	246	Timing of studies	252
Other radiologic studies	246	Ultrasonography	252
Fiberoptic examination of airway and/or		Computed tomography	252
esophagus	246	Magnetic resonance imaging	252
Pathology	246	Radionuclide scanning	253
Gross features	246	Staging	253
Histology	246	Initial disease stage	253
Genetics	247	Therapy	253
Airway management	248	Surgery	253
Concurrent chemoradiotherapy	248	Airway protection	253
Primary thyroid lymphoma	250	Radiotherapy	253
Case example	250	Chemotherapy	253
Incidence	251	Failure patterns	254
Age and sex distribution	251	References	254

Thyroid cancer incidence is increasing worldwide, likely due to more frequent incidentally detected papillary microcarcinoma (1). Within this "epidemic" a small apparent increase in differentiated thyroid cancer (DTC) incidence is possible (2). Fortunately, the incidence of aggressive thyroid malignancies (anaplastic thyroid cancer [ATC] and thyroid lymphomas) has remained low, comprising <2% of all thyroid cancers. However, mortality from aggressive thyroid carcinomas, especially ATC, continues to be high (3). In this chapter, we discuss our approach to the diagnosis and management of ATCs and primary thyroid lymphomas (PTL). Aggressive tumors such as ATC and PTL tend to present similarly, most often with a symptomatic rapidly growing neck mass requiring expeditious evaluation, diagnosis, and therapy.

CASE EXAMPLE

A 59-year-old gentleman presented with a rapidly enlarging neck mass associated with hoarseness, reddening of the overlying skin, and neck swelling, without prior history of thyroid disorders. Examination showed a large right anterior neck mass (Figure 10.1); the right vocal cord was paralyzed.

DIAGNOSTIC APPROACH TO A RAPIDLY ENLARGING THYROID MASS

Almost all patients with aggressive thyroid malignancies present with a rapidly growing neck mass; incidental detection is uncommon. Other symptoms can include hoarseness, ear pain, erythema, dyspnea and/or swallowing difficulties, and neck pain. Emergent multidisciplinary evaluation and care are most often needed.

In addition to vocal cord assessment, imaging of the brain, neck, chest, and abdomen is required to rule out disseminated disease (4). Pathologic confirmation of the diagnosis has to be obtained concurrently and expeditiously, accomplished by directed biopsy of the neck mass—or biopsy of distant disease if present. A core biopsy reviewed by an expert thyroid pathologist is best to distinguish between aggressive thyroid carcinoma, sarcoma, lymphoma, or metastasis to the thyroid from another site. The following sections discuss

evaluation and management of ATC and thyroid lymphomas, separately and in detail.

ANAPLASTIC THYROID CARCINOMA

Incidence and demographics

The frequency of ATC relative to other thyroid cancers was higher in the past, but more recently it has been 1–2% in the United States (5). Part of this apparent reduction in incidence may be due to improvements in discrimination of this tumor from other poorly differentiated tumors of the thyroid and because of earlier diagnosis of smaller DTCs. The median age at ATC diagnosis from a Surveillance, Epidemiology, and End Results (SEER) program was 62 years (6). However, anaplastic thyroid cancers can also present in people in their mid-forties and, extremely rarely, in their thirties. There might be a slight female preponderance (7).

ATC incidence appears influenced by dietary iodine. In one study (8), the frequency of ATC was three times higher in an iodine-deficient area compared with an iodine-rich area; however, a more recent study demonstrated no such differences (9).

Natural history and mortality rates

ATC has a dismal prognosis. In a population-based study from British Columbia, almost all patients not referred for treatment died within 1 month; the 1-year overall survival rate was 19% (10). In 1961, Woolner et al. reported from the Mayo Clinic that 61% were dead within 6 months and 77% within

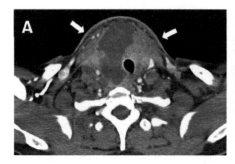
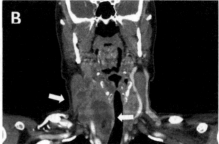

Figure 10.1 Computed tomographic (CT) scan with axial (A) and coronal (B) views demonstrating anaplastic thyroid cancer characterized by a large invasive mass (white arrows) associated with central necrosis (darker) and leftward tracheal deviation.

1 year from diagnosis (11). Almost 50 years later, a study from MD Anderson reported a mean survival of 7 months (12). Only 8% (20 of 240 patients) from both series survived longer than 1 year. The median survival in a later Mayo Clinic studies was only 3 months (13). The overall cause-specific mortality of 516 patients from the SEER database was 69.3% at 6 months and 80.7% at 12 months (7). Although improvements have been shown in specific publications (14, 15), population-based studies continue to show poor prognosis even today. In a National Cancer Database (NCDB) study from 2017, 1-year survival was still dismal at 11% (5).

If left untreated, death occurs most commonly from the effects of local tumor invasion, particularly asphyxiation, with over half of patients dying from suffocation from invasive neck tumor (16, 17). However, in most recent studies wherein patients were treated with chemoradiation therapy with or without surgery, patients instead died from distant metastases, suggesting progress in affecting locoregional tumor control (14, 15, 18).

Prognostic factors

In single institutional studies, the presence of DTC component (11), younger patient age (19), and earlier tumor stage at the time of diagnosis (14) have been associated with better prognosis. In a study of 516 patients from the SEER database, multivariate analysis showed that only: age <60, lesser disease extent, and combined modality therapy with surgical resection and external beam radiotherapy were independent prognostic factors (7). In the recent NCDB study, age, presence of distant metastasis, administration of chemotherapy, surgical resection, and radiation dose were similarly shown to be independently associated with survival per multivariable analysis (5). In summary, younger age, limited stage disease (AJCC stage IVA and IVB), and multimodality treatment seem to be associated with better survival.

DIAGNOSIS

History

Patients most often present with a rapidly enlarging neck mass; symptoms of tracheal compression or invasion are most common. A study from the Mayo Clinic also found that about two-thirds had a rapidly enlarging neck mass, either with (37%) or without (32%) pre-existing goiter; about half had dyspnea at the time of diagnosis (20), with symptoms present <3 months in almost half. Rapid tumor enlargement often causes neck and/or ear pain, erythema, and local tissue edema, probably due to venous congestion and/or jugular venous thrombosis, tumor necrosis, and invasion of neck tissues. Hoarseness due to vocal cord paralysis, stridor due to laryngeal edema, or airway compromise are also often present. Some patients undergo initial surgical resection of a presumed DTC, later to experience rapidly recurrent neck tumor later confirmed to be ATC. Any patient with rapidly growing thyroid mass should be considered operationally to have ATC or thyroid lymphoma until proven otherwise.

Physical examination

ATC primary tumors are typically hard, poorly circumscribed, and fixed to surrounding structures. In the Mayo Clinic series, 60% presented as a multinodular goiter and 38% presented as an apparently unifocal thyroid mass; only 2% caused diffuse thyroid enlargement (20). ATCs are characteristically quite large and may be associated with palpable cervical lymph nodes. In the Mayo Clinic series, approximately 80% of ATCs were >5 cm; half had palpably enlarged cervical lymph nodes; one-third had vocal cord paralysis upon initial presentation (20). Stridor portends serious airway compromise and raises the question of elective tracheostomy to protect the airway (4).

Only about one-third of ATC patients have evident distant metastases at diagnosis, mostly to the lung, but about half eventually developed them (12, 20). In an MD Anderson cohort, nearly 8% of ATC patients demonstrated brain metastases, almost uniformly symptomatic at detection (21). The diagnosis of malignancy is usually obvious because of ominous symptoms, physical findings, and aggressive behavior. The main diagnostic challenge is in differentiating ATC from less aggressive—but still poorly differentiated—thyroid cancers and from extremely rare primary thyroid lymphoma, squamous cell carcinoma, sarcoma, or sometimes aggressive thyroid metastasis.

Fine needle aspiration

Fine needle aspiration (FNA) can be helpful in identifying ATC, but when ATC is suspected, a core (or occasionally open) biopsy with immuno-histochemical staining (IHC, including TTF-1, thyroglobulin, p53, PAX8) is required to confirm the diagnosis (22). ATC may sometimes be difficult to distinguish from thyroid lymphoma, medullary thyroid carcinoma (MTC), and other forms of poorly differentiated thyroid carcinoma or cancers metastatic to the thyroid. Giant- and spindle-cell patterns of ATC predominate, sometimes with multinucleated giant cells, suggesting the correct diagnosis. MTC can be distinguished by calcitonin IHC staining and elevated serum calcitonin. Non-Hodgkin's thyroid lymphoma can be identified by FNA, but a core biopsy and IHC are often necessary to differentiate it from ATC, especially for large cell lymphoma. Critically, ATC is expected to show no or minimal immunohistochemical staining for thyroglobulin and TTF-1, positive staining for PAX8 and cytokeratin, and to be histologically indistinguishable from poorly differentiated carcinoma of any site of origin.

RADIONUCLIDE STUDIES

Diagnostic scanning with radioiodine is not indicated in ATC and can delay diagnosis, but it is sometimes helpful later in the disease course in the event of recurrent coexistent DTC. Positron emission tomography (PET) with 18F-fluorodeoxyglucose (18F-FDG) has emerged as the most overall useful modality to stage and follow ATC (23, 24).

THYROID ULTRASONOGRAPHY

Ultrasound plays a lesser role in ATC evaluation than do CT and FDG-PET imaging. The majority of differentiated carcinomas and ATCs present as hypoechoic masses by ultrasonography. Invasive or infiltrating tumors strongly suggest a malignant process and should prompt biopsy.

OTHER RADIOLOGIC STUDIES

CT may be needed preoperatively for surgical planning, especially when the tumor extends into the thorax, is invasive, involves adjacent lymph nodes, or is associated with vocal cord paralysis. ATC generally appears as a large low attenuation mass, accompanied by dense calcification in over half the patients, most also showing central tumor necrosis (48). Neck MRI can alternatively be used but is not routinely needed. However, brain MRI is recommended proactively, especially if symptoms are suggestive of intracranial metastasis (4, 21).

Fiberoptic examination of airway and/or esophagus

Assessment of vocal cord function should always be performed upon ATC diagnosis (4). Esophagoscopy is helpful in defining the extent of esophageal invasion, while fiberoptic visualization of trachea permits the detection of the extent of tracheal invasion—especially important if surgery is of consideration.

Pathology

GROSS FEATURES

ATCs often involve both thyroid lobes and are typically invasive and poorly delineated. Extensive local invasion into the soft tissues, trachea, and esophagus is common. On gross examination, the tumors are gray-white, fibrous, calcified, or even ossified, and they frequently show areas of necrosis.

HISTOLOGY

About half of ATCs arise from pre-existing DTCs, while some appear to arise *de novo*. ATCs are composed wholly or in part of undifferentiated cells and tend to behave according to their most aggressive tumor element. The three major types of ATC are spindle cells, giant cells, and squamoid—but other histologic variants such as paucicellular, lymphoepithelioma-like, and carcinosarcoma exist. Subdivision, however, carries no prognostic value. ATCs are pleomorphic and may resemble fibrosarcoma or rhabdomyosarcoma, or may contain multinucleated giant cells resembling osteoclasts. Cytoplasm can be varied and nuclei are usually large, with frequent mitoses. Necrosis within a biopsy or necrotic material in a cytopathology specimen is quite common, favoring imaging-guided core biopsy.

The IHC proof of the follicular origin of ATC is its staining with epithelial markers, the most useful of which is low-molecular-weight keratin (cytokeratin), expressed in up to 80% of ATC cases (25, 26). TTF-1 and thyroglobulin IHC is expected negative, more often staining for p53 and/or paired box gene 8 (PAX8). ATC is also heavily infiltrated with inflammatory cells, including macrophages, and demonstrates high expression of programmed death-ligand 1 (PD-L1) (Figure 10.2) (27). It is critical to differentiate ATC from lymphoma and MTC due to differential therapy and prognosis.

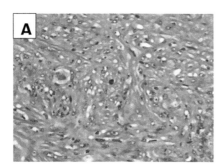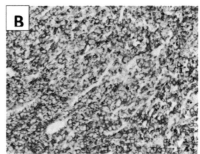

Figure 10.2 Hematoxylin and eosin stained section of ATC (**A**) with IHC demonstrating high expression of programmed death-ligand 1 (PD-L1) on ATC cells (**B**). (Photomicrograph courtesy of Dr. Michael Rivera, Mayo Clinic.)

GENETICS

Poorly differentiated thyroid cancers and ATCs harbor characteristic somatic mutations, including p53 and telomerase reverse transcriptase (*TERT*), present in 70–80%, which lead to dedifferentiation, tumorigenesis, and rapid growth. *BRAF* mutations are also seen in 40–50%, thought to arise from preexisting papillary thyroid carcinoma (PTC). *RAS* mutations are seen exclusive of *BRAF* mutations; other mutations, including neurofibromatosis type 1 (*NF1*), Phosphatase and tensin homolog (*PTEN*), Eukaryotic translation initiation factor 1A, X-chromosomal (*EIF1AX*), DNA mismatch repair pathway genes (*MSH2, MSH6, MLH1*), and translocations involving anaplastic lymphoma kinase (*ALK*) genes are also sometimes seen (28–30). There is preliminary evidence that these mutations could also be assessed by circulating tumor-free DNA, especially in the case of *BRAF* (30).

Treatment

ATCs are therapy-resistant, rarely cured, and remain almost universally fatal. Surgery, chemotherapy, or radiotherapy used separately have generally not been effective; however, early multimodal therapy combining surgery when feasible, external beam irradiation (usually intensity-modulated radiation therapy [IMRT]), and cytotoxic chemotherapy are associated with improved outcomes; see Scheme 10.1 for our suggested initial approach. Mutation-specified salvage therapy for metastatic disease is emerging as promising, but limited.

Surgical therapy

Thyroid surgery
In principle, we feel that near-total thyroidectomy, with resection of the involved adjacent neck tissues and cervical lymph nodes, should be done if possible; however, *radical surgery (laryngectomy, tracheal resection or reconstruction) is inadvisable in ATC.* There is emerging evidence that chemoradiation therapy is effective in controlling locoregional disease and that rapid initiation after surgery is important. More extensive surgery may delay initiation of chemoradiation. Moreover, we generally do not recommend surgery in metastatic ATCs.

In an earlier Mayo Clinic series, 41% of the patients underwent surgical resection—mostly partial or total thyroidectomy (11); in a later Mayo series, 62% underwent surgical resection (13). In one MD Anderson series, approximately 59% of patients underwent surgery (12). In population-based studies, however, surgical resection has been reported less frequently. For example, a Canadian study reported surgery in only 22% (10), and a SEER study reported primary surgery in only 10%, suggesting differential care at community versus academic centers (7).

The role of surgical resection in ATC is poorly defined because of inherent biases in published studies; moreover, with increasing evidence of the efficacy of chemoradiation, the role of surgery may be evolving. Previous single institution studies did not show benefit for surgery (11, 12). Similar results were also demonstrated in population-based studies (7). However, newer studies suggest that surgery may provide benefit when part of multimodality treatment (5, 31). We are unlikely to have a definitive answer without a randomized study; it is reasonable to plan total thyroidectomy and selective neck dissection with an intention of removal of gross disease and rapid initiation of adjuvant chemoradiotherapy thereafter. When a more radical surgery or complications are expected, or in the

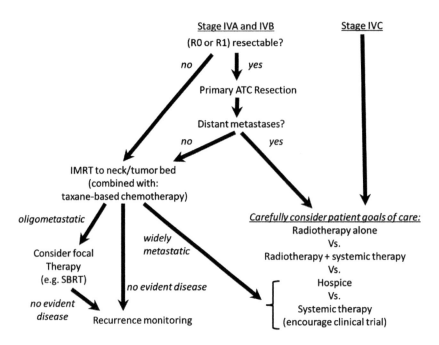

Scheme 10.1 Suggested initial approach to ATC management.

setting of metastatic ATC, chemoradiation may be the best initial approach, foregoing surgery.

AIRWAY MANAGEMENT

Per the American Thyroid Association (ATA) guidelines, prophylactic tracheostomy is not indicated when airway compromise is not an immediate issue (4). The tumor may, however, compromise the airway by compression, displacement, infiltration, and, less often, via bilateral vocal cord paralysis. Management involves thyroid gland resection with decompression of the airway. The minority of patients require a tracheostomy.

Radiotherapy may cause tumor edema that acutely exacerbates airway obstruction; palliative corticosteroids can be tried in such instances. More than half of ATC patients in the Mayo Clinic series required tracheostomy during the course of their disease (20). In patients who are not surgical candidates or who do not wish to have invasive procedures, tracheal stenting may be an alternative to provide symptomatic relief while maintaining quality of life (32).

Chemoradiation therapy

Radiotherapy
Radiotherapy, in particular IMRT, has become a cornerstone of treatment in ATC. Effective local control can be achieved by combined modality treatment partnering radiation and chemotherapy with or without surgery. Based on the population- and single-institutional-based studies, about 20% of patients with ATC survive 2 years or beyond after multimodality therapy (5, 14, 15, 33–35). Alternative fractionation of radiotherapy has also been investigated, but toxicity is high, with benefits uncertain (15, 19, 36–38). With IMRT now widely available in the United States and Europe, it is feasible to include combination chemotherapy with radiation therapy as demonstrated by Mayo Clinic protocol (3, 14, 39). The utility of IMRT perhaps points to the fact that total dose, rather than fractionation approach, may be of greater importance; total radiation dosage >40–60 Gy has been associated with improved survival (5, 19, 35, 37). At the Mayo Clinic, stage IVA and IVB patients are routinely given a radiation dose of >60 Gy (14). Similar dosage is also reasonable in selected IVC patients, to attain locoregional control, but it does not seem to improve survival (14, 15, 35).

CONCURRENT CHEMORADIOTHERAPY

There is no consensus regarding the selection of chemotherapeutic(s) to be given concurrently with radiotherapy. The selection of drugs is often based upon side effects, the fitness of the patients, and institutional preferences. Doxorubicin, platins, and taxanes remain the most commonly used agents, administered either alone or in combination. Our practice, in general, is to offer docetaxel and doxorubicin (20 mg/m² each, weekly) or paclitaxel and carboplatin (50 mg/m² and AUC 2 respectively, weekly) concurrently with radiotherapy.

Studies from multiple institutions describe apparent benefit from multimodality therapy in ATC, but most are retrospective and subject to potential biases. In 1983, a regimen consisting of combining weekly doxorubicin (10 mg/m²) and hyperfractionated radiation (160 cGy twice daily 3 days/week) was reported for ATC (40, 41), delivering 5760 cGy over 40 days. The protocol was well tolerated with little morbidity. Median survival was 1 year, but most patients ultimately developed distant metastases and died.

Multiple studies by Swedish groups (38, 42, 43) have used hyperfractionated radiotherapy, chemotherapy (Bleomycin, cyclophosphamide and 5-fluorouracil [BCF]), or, most recently, with 20 mg/week doxorubicin, and debulking surgery. Radiotherapy was administered preoperatively to 30 Gy in 3 weeks, and postoperatively with an additional 16 Gy, else the same cumulative radiation dose preoperatively. Death was attributed to local failure in eight patients (24%), but the median survival was only 2–3 months.

In 1991, a French group (18) reported results in 20 ATC patients treated; depending on the patient's age, two types of chemotherapy were used every 4 weeks: those <65 years received doxorubicin (60 mg/m²) and cisplatin (90 mg/m²); those >65 received mitoxantrone (14 mg/m²) alone. Radiotherapy (17.5 Gy) was given in seven fractions to the neck and superior mediastinum intercurrently. Three patients (15%) survived longer than 20 months. All developed pharyngoesophagitis and tracheitis after the first or second cycle of radiotherapy. The same group published another prospective study in 2004 involving 30 ATC patients. Two cycles of doxorubicin (60 mg/m²) and cisplatin (120 mg/m²) were delivered before radiotherapy, four cycles following radiotherapy. Radiotherapy consisted of two daily fractions of 1.25 Gy, 5 days per week to a total dose of 40 Gy. Surgical resection was possible in 24 (80%). Median survival with this protocol was 10 months and only 5% succumbed to locoregional disease (15).

In the newer studies from the Mayo Clinic, chemoradiotherapy (doxorubicin and docetaxel at 20 mg/m²/week each or at 60 mg/m² every 3 weeks each, and combined with IMRT to 60–66 Gy) has been combined with surgery as feasible. A pilot study published in 2011 demonstrated promise (39), prompting an expanded cohort of 48 patients confirming these results; median overall survival was 21 months in the patients with multimodal therapy compared to 4 months in patients treated with palliative therapy or best supportive care. Locoregional relapse was seen in only 2 of 27 evaluable patients treated with multimodal therapy (14). Similar results were seen from a Memorial Sloan Kettering study, where patients (n=7) treated with doxorubicin (20 mg/m²/week) and radiotherapy of >60 Gy had a median survival of 17 months (19).

Palliative systemic therapies

Cytotoxics have had low efficacy in metastatic ATC, with no FDA-approved systemic agents other than doxorubicin. Doxorubicin, however, has low efficacy and a response rate of 16% in a phase 2 trial (44). In the same study, the combination of cisplatin and doxorubicin demonstrated the numerically higher response rate of 26%. Paclitaxel has been shown to have a 50% response rate in ATC (45); however, in another multi-institution study, paclitaxel demonstrated a lower response rate of 21% and median overall survival of 6.7 months (46). Based on these studies, taxanes and anthracyclines could be considered for palliative ATC treatment, but modest benefit is anticipated.

Personalized therapies are emerging in metastatic ATC. Recently, targeted therapy was investigated in BRAF-mutated ATC, showing a 69% response rate with the combination of the MEK inhibitor trametinib and the BRAF inhibitor dabrafenib in a basket study (47). This combination needs confirmation in a dedicated study for ATC. There are also reports of BRAF inhibitors used as single agent in ATC, but most responses are brief (48–50). Multikinase inhibitors (MKIs) also have emerged as effective in DTC (51–53), but MKI treatment of ATC has been disappointing (48, 54–57).

Future ATC treatment strategies

With better understanding of the outcomes achieved from initial chemoradiation (15, 39), the ATC genetic landscape (28), the pathogenesis and molecular drivers of ATC (58), and the outcomes from molecularly targeted personalized therapies (47), further innovative treatment strategies are being planned and studied (59, 60). The first fully accrued randomized study involving ATC patients, RTOG 0912, examining the potential benefit from adding the MKI pazopanib (or not) to initial chemoradiation therapy in ATC, completed accrual in 2016, with results awaited. Another trial involving upfront treatment of ATC with chemoradiation plus immunotherapy (the anti-PD-1 agent pembrolizumab) is now accruing, in the hopes that heightened antigen presentation from surgery and/or radiotherapy will prime for more effective immunotherapy and thereby further improve survival (NCT03211117). Another study is building on the phase 1 study examining PPAR-gamma agonist efatutazone combined with paclitaxel as salvage therapy in ATC (NCT02152137). Lessons learned from these and other studies have fostered new interest in systemic therapies in ATC for the first time in several decades, hopefully leading to an emerging renaissance in ATC therapeutic innovation.

PRIMARY THYROID LYMPHOMA

Primary thyroid lymphoma (PTL)—along with ATC—should be considered prominently in the differential diagnosis of any rapidly expanding thyroid mass. PTL is a rare, but potentially life-threatening, malignancy that often poses diagnostic challenges based on paucicellular FNA samples alone, making a core biopsy critical (68). PTL typically arises in the setting of chronic thyroiditis, sometimes in patients with long-standing hypothyroidism (61). Treatments and prognoses differ vastly between ATC and PTL, but expeditious diagnosis and therapy of PTL are generally associated with an excellent prognosis, unlike ATC (62–64), making it imperative that PTL is considered and correctly identified.

Case example

An 81-year-old woman noted a rapidly expanding neck mass, first detected upon showering; imaging including CT and FDG-PET demonstrated a thyroid mass with involvement of L4 (Figure 10.3) but no bone marrow involvement. Suspicion was raised over anaplastic thyroid cancer versus lymphoma; FNA was initially nondiagnostic, but a biopsy later

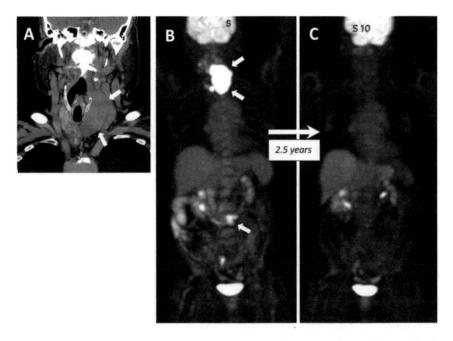

Figure 10.3 Thyroid (diffuse large B-cell non-Hodgkin's) lymphoma; **(A)** CT at diagnosis, showing large left thyroid mass (white arrows) and right thyroid multinodular goiter; **(B)** FDG-PET at diagnosis, showing primary PTL and involved lumbar vertebra (white arrows), absent upon reimaging; **(C)** 2.5 years after diagnosis in response to R-CHOP.

showed clear evidence of diffuse large B-cell lymphoma. The patient was since treated with R-CHOP, attaining a complete response after two cycles; four more cycles were administered with complete response ongoing over 2.5 years later.

Incidence

The annual incidence of PTL in the United States is less than one in two million, accounting for only 1–2% of all extranodal lymphomas (62). The thyroid gland is sometimes secondarily involved by widespread lymphoma; in such cases, origin is difficult to determine. Therefore, we limit discussion to stage IE and IIE, and not IIIE or IVE, PTL. Although many PTLs were incorrectly diagnosed in the past as anaplastic small-cell thyroid carcinoma, adequate pathological materials and appropriate IHC interrogation allow differentiation. Pathologists have also become more adept at distinguishing lymphoma from advanced Hashimoto's thyroiditis, which is absolutely critical since PTL typically develops in the setting of coexisting lymphocytic thyroiditis.

Age and sex distribution

Contrary to other lymphomas, females predominate in PTL (62), probably because it originates from active lymphoid cells in chronic lymphocytic thyroiditis, which occurs more often in women. The median age is 60–70, but a wide age range has been reported (62, 63).

Hashimoto's/chronic lymphocytic thyroiditis and PTL

In one study, the relative risk of PTL among people in Sweden with Hashimoto's thyroiditis was 67-fold greater than expected (mean follow-up 8.5 years) (61). Another study from Japan found an 80-fold increased frequency of PTL among 5592 women aged 25 years or older with chronic thyroiditis (65). The average interval between the diagnosis of chronic thyroiditis and PTL was 9.2 years.

Pathology

LYMPHOMA CELL TYPES AND HISTOLOGIC FEATURES

Virtually all PTLs are B-cell non-Hodgkin's lymphomas, which can be identified and characterized using monoclonal antibodies (63, 66). Most PTLs are diffuse large B-cell lymphomas (DLBCL), with MALT lymphoma less common—pointing to the embryonal origin of the thyroid from the endodermal epithelium in the primitive pharynx. Rarely, DLBCL and MALT lymphoma coexist, likely resulting from transformation; this is associated with a poor prognosis (63, 67). Less common PTLs include indolent B-cell lymphomas and others such as T-cell and Hodgkin's lymphomas.

The histologic features of Hashimoto's disease and PTL are often difficult to differentiate. PTL demonstrates normal thyroid tissue that is extensively infiltrated with abnormal and invasive lymphoid cells that often penetrate the thyroid capsule, extending into adjacent soft tissues. PTL is usually composed of monotonous small cells, distinct from autoimmune thyroiditis.

The interface between lymphocytic thyroiditis and PTL may be sharply defined, or there may be a transitional zone in which elements of both are intermixed. Lymphoma cells tend to displace, distort, and replace the thyroid epithelium. Classification can be performed using IHC for CD5, CD10, CD20, CD23, CD43, CD30, BCL-2, c-myc, and cyclin-D1 (68).

Clinical features

SYMPTOMS AND SIGNS

Much like ATC, most PTLs present with compressive symptoms caused by a rapidly expanding goiter over the course of days or a few weeks (67). Common symptoms include dysphagia, dyspnea, stridor, neck pressure, and neck pain—potential indicators of extrathyroidal tumor extension that should alert clinicians to possible malignant goiter. Stridor and hoarseness often occur together, and when they do, laryngeal nerve paralysis is of concern. The disease may present focally, with only one thyroid lobe or a discrete nodule involved, or there may be diffuse thyromegaly. By palpation, the gland is nearly always firm or hard, usually nontender, and often fixed—a sign of local invasion. Other signs of extrathyroidal spread include ill-defined thyroid borders with extension laterally or retrosternally on imaging. Nodal involvement is often present but B-symptoms are uncommon (66). Almost all patients with PTL have clinical or histologic evidence of lymphocytic thyroiditis at the time of diagnosis (62).

Thyroid dysfunction

Although laboratory evidence of autoimmune thyroiditis is common, most are euthyroid or only mildly hypothyroid, showing minimal elevation in serum thyroid-stimulating hormone (TSH) and otherwise normal thyroid function tests (62, 64). Thyrotoxicosis is extremely uncommon, but can occur in PTL (63).

DIAGNOSIS

Differential diagnosis

The diagnostic possibilities of a rapidly enlarging thyroid mass are PTL, ATC, MTC, multinodular goiter, or colloid nodule with acute hemorrhage, and also inflammatory disorders including acute, subacute, and Hashimoto's thyroiditis.

SERUM CHEMISTRIES AND IMMUNOGLOBULINS

Routine serum chemistries and hematologic studies are usually normal. Lactate dehydrogenase may be elevated. Thyroid function testing may disclose subclinical or overt hypothyroidism, and serum antimicrosomal and antithyroglobulin antibodies are often positive.

FNA/core biopsy

In general, when ATC or PTL are of consideration, it is best to obtain a core biopsy rather than FNA (69). Immunophenotyping with IHC markers is crucial in classifying lymphoma for accurate diagnosis and treatment. Occasionaly an open (surgical) biopsy is necessary to obtain sufficient architectural detail to allow for accurate histologic subtype (70).

Imaging studies

TIMING OF STUDIES

Once PTL is diagnosed, imaging is required to define disease extent. CT scan, MRI, and ultrasonography could be used, but (18)F-fluorodeoxyglucose (FDG) positron emission tomography/computed tomography (PET/CT) is best used to determine disease extent (71). Radioactive iodine diagnostic thyroid imaging is typically not appropriate or helpful.

ULTRASONOGRAPHY

PTL may appear as a markedly hypoechoic solid mass with significant posterior acoustic enhancement intermingled with coexisting Hashimoto's

thyroiditis in the remainder of the gland. Most PTLs are discrete solid nodules/masses occurring in a diffuse goiter. The findings of PTL are similar to those seen with Hashimoto's thyroiditis but to a much more dramatic extent—typically, the gland is markedly hypoechoic, with dense fibrotic bands, and prominent adenopathy (72). Ultrasonography may disclose contiguous tumor spread into both thyroid lobes, is sensitive in detecting abnormal cervical lymph nodes, and represents an important adjunct to physical examination.

COMPUTED TOMOGRAPHY

PTL is usually manifest as one or more areas of low thyroid density, either as areas of iso- or low-attenuation on contrast-enhanced CT scan of the neck (Figure 10.4) (73). CT scan appearances are of three types: solitary nodules, multiple nodules, and diffuse goiter. Both lobes are usually involved with advanced disease and often have extrathyroidal extension. The tumors have a strong tendency to compress or infiltrate surrounding structures and infrequently show calcification.

MAGNETIC RESONANCE IMAGING

Lymphomas appear as homogeneous iso- or high-intensity areas on T1-weighted images compared with uninvolved thyroid tissue, which appears homogeneously high-intensity on T2-weighted images. The distinction between tumor and uninvolved thyroid gland is sometimes more apparent

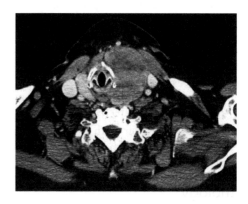

Figure 10.4 Contrast CT, axial section, of patient with primary thyroid lymphoma (PTL). Note that: PTL mass is hypodense relative to normal thyroid and moreover contains heterogeneous areas of even lower CT density.

by MRI than CT scan, but the two are comparable in identifying extrathyroidal extension, cervical lymphadenopathy, and in staging of lymphoma (73). Hashimoto's thyroiditis often shows homogeneous signal intensities on MRI that are indistinguishable from those of lymphoma.

RADIONUCLIDE SCANNING

FDG-PET is perhaps the most useful approach to staging in both ATC and PTL and in assessing treatment response (23, 24, 71, 74). Various radionuclides, including compounds labeled with radioactive iodine, ^{201}Tl, ^{67}Ga, ^{111}In-octreotide, FDG-PET, MIBG, and ^{99m}Tc, may be used to study patients with PTL, but none is specific for the diagnosis. Lymphoma appears as a hypofunctional lesion with ^{123}I or ^{99m}Tc-pertechnetate thyroid scanning. Like ^{99m}Tc-labeled compounds, ^{201}Tl may demonstrate uptake in PTL.

Staging

INITIAL DISEASE STAGE

Staging for PTL is according to the Ann Arbor classification system (Table 10.1) (75, 76). PTL is macroscopically confined to the thyroid gland (stage IE) in almost 60%, with spread to regional lymph nodes (stage IIE) in the other 40% (63).

THERAPY

Large, randomized, multicenter trials for PTL have not yet been done; thus, therapy in PTL is generally based upon that performed for similar histological lymphoma types otherwise occurring at other locations. As in other lymphomas, chemotherapy—and sometimes external beam radiation therapy—have emerged as preferred therapies, especially for high-grade PTLs (63). Overall survival for stage I disease approaches 90%, for stage II 60–80%, depending on the lymphoma subtype and the therapeutic modality (66, 77).

SURGERY

Surgery is now less commonly undertaken in PTL due to improved efficacies of systemic therapies. Earlier reports (78), however, suggested that patients undergoing total macroscopic tumor removal fared considerably better than those with persistent tumor after surgery; 5-year survival rates in the two groups, respectively, were approximately 65% and 22%. Similar results were reported from the Mayo

Clinic (79), where 5-year survival rates were lower (49% vs. 75%) when patients had obvious residual disease postoperatively. Perhaps the least controversial reasons for surgery are for diagnosis and tumor staging and to relieve airway obstruction. In the largest population-based analysis, 68% underwent resection with statistically better disease-specific survival reported (66). However, surgery as monotherapy is of consideration only in stage I disease.

AIRWAY PROTECTION

Patients commonly present with a rapidly enlarging thyroid mass. Occasionally, tracheal compression with respiratory distress may necessitate emergency surgery or tracheostomy. Almost 25% of the patients in a large series from the Mayo Clinic required an elective tracheostomy (80).

RADIOTHERAPY

Radiation therapy is employed in the setting of lymphoma subtypes with a lesser risk of systemic dissemination, especially for patients with stage IE or IIE PTL. Control of disease in the neck is related both to radiation dosage and selection of radiation fields and may also be dependent upon the degree of surgical debulking (if performed) prior to radiotherapy. The thyroid, bilateral neck, and mediastinum are treated with at least 40 Gy (4000 rad) given in divided doses over 4 to 5 weeks in earlier studies. An earlier Mayo Clinic study achieved a 59% disease-free survival with about 40 (24–60) Gy in 38 patients, most of whom had intermediate-grade histology and stage IE or IIE disease (79). None experienced substantial side effects. Results are best for patients with stage IE and IIE disease. Another study reported 5-year survival rates of 91% in patients with stage IE disease who were treated with 40 Gy (81).

CHEMOTHERAPY

Historically, based upon recent reviews (63, 82) chemotherapy was administered to almost half of the patients with PTL. The most commonly used regimens were CHOP or R-CHOP (rituximab, cyclophosphamide, doxorubicin, vincristine, and prednisone). These regimens are well tolerated even in elderly patients with PTL and can be curative even in disseminated PTL (64). A review of the published literature suggested that the addition of chemotherapy to radiation therapy significantly lowered distant and overall recurrence (83). More recent studies indicate

Table 10.1 Ann Arbor classification system for non-Hodgkin's lymphoma

Ann Arbor non-Hodgkin's lymphoma stage	Features
I	Single nodal or visceral site of lymphoma only (thyroid)
II	Two or more nodal sites of disease, both on same side of the diaphragm
III	Nodal involvement on both sides of the diaphragm
IV	Involvement of additional distant visceral sites (beyond E)

A = no symptoms, B = fever, drenching sweats and/or >10% loss of body weight in 6 months; E = a single, extranodal site (thyroid in this instance) contiguous or proximal to known nodal site.

5-year overall survival rates of 74–87% (63, 64, 77). Older age, advanced stage, aggressive histologic subtype, and lack of combined modality treatment were associated with worse survival (66).

FAILURE PATTERNS

Recurrence rates vary dramatically; most recurrences (75%) are detected within the first 2 years following therapy, and recurrences were detected by both physical exam and imaging studies (79, 84, 85). However, routine use of PET-CT for surveillance is being increasingly discouraged, especially in low-grade lymphomas (86).

Local disease failure usually occurs in 25 to 35% of patients after 40 Gy of external radiation (78, 81, 83). The rate of local failure appears related to the amount of residual disease after initial thyroidectomy, to the tailoring of radiation fields, and to the use of chemotherapy. A Mayo Clinic study reported no failures within the treatment fields in patients without residual disease when radiation therapy was started, but otherwise, there were twice as many failures following radiotherapy to the neck alone compared with radiotherapy to both the neck and mediastinum (60% vs. 36%) (79).

Distant recurrences can occur in the lungs, gastrointestinal tract, liver, central nervous system, and kidneys. One study (84) of 245 patients found that the gastrointestinal tract was infrequently involved. An autopsy study, however (87), found the most common sites of involvement to be the gastrointestinal tract (100%), lung and kidney (each 63%), and liver and pancreas (each 50%).

REFERENCES

1. Vaccarella, S., S. Franceschi, F. Bray, C.P. Wild, M. Plummer, and L. Dal Maso, Worldwide thyroid-cancer epidemic? The increasing impact of overdiagnosis. N. Engl. J. Med., 2016; 375(7): 614–17.
2. Lim, H., S.S. Devesa, J.A. Sosa, D. Check, and C.M. Kitahara, Trends in thyroid cancer incidence and mortality in the United States, 1974–2013. JAMA, 2017; 317(13): 1338–48.
3. Bible, K.C., R.L. Foote, and R.C. Smallridge, Toward improved outcomes in patients with anaplastic thyroid cancer. Oncology, 2012; 26(4): 398, 401, 406.
4. Smallridge, R.C., K.B. Ain, S.L. Asa, K.C. Bible, J.D. Brierley, K.D. Burman, E. Kebebew, et al., American Thyroid Association guidelines for management of patients with anaplastic thyroid cancer. Thyroid, 2012; 22(11): 1104–39.
5. Pezzi, T.A., A.S.R. Mohamed, T. Sheu, P. Blanchard, V.C. Sandulache, S.Y. Lai, M.E. Cabanillas, et al., Radiation therapy dose is associated with improved survival for unresected anaplastic thyroid carcinoma: Outcomes from the National Cancer Data Base. Cancer, 2017; 123(9): 1653–61.
6. Arora, S., P. Christos, A. Pham, P. Desai, A.G. Wernicke, D. Nori, K.S. Chao, and B. Parashar, Comparing outcomes in poorly-differentiated versus anaplastic thyroid cancers treated with radiation: A surveillance, epidemiology, and end results analysis. J. Cancer Res. Ther., 2014; 10(3): 526–30.
7. Kebebew, E., F.S. Greenspan, O.H. Clark, K.A. Woeber, and A. McMillan, Anaplastic thyroid carcinoma. Treatment outcome and prognostic factors. Cancer, 2005; 103(7): 1330–5.
8. Belfiore, A., G.L. La Rosa, G. Padova, L. Sava, O. Ippolito, and R. Vigneri, The frequency of cold thyroid nodules and thyroid malignancies in patients from an iodine-deficient area. Cancer, 1987; 60(12): 3096–102.

9. Tavarelli, M., P. Malandrino, P. Vigneri, P. Richiusa, A. Maniglia, M.A. Violi, G. Sapuppo, et al., Anaplastic thyroid cancer in Sicily: The role of environmental characteristics. *Front. Endocrinol. (Lausanne)*, 2017; 8: 277.

10. Goutsouliak, V. and J.H. Hay, Anaplastic thyroid cancer in British Columbia 1985–1999: A population-based study. *Clin. Oncol.*, 2005; 17(2): 75–8.

11. Woolner, L.B., O.H. Beahrs, B.M. Black, W.M. McConahey, and F.R. Keating, Classification and prognosis of thyroid carcinoma. A study of 885 cases observed in a thirty year period. *Am. J. Surg.*, 1961; 102: 354–87.

12. Venkatesh, Y.S., N.G. Ordonez, P.N. Schultz, R.C. Hickey, H. Goepfert, and N.A. Samaan, Anaplastic carcinoma of the thyroid. A clinicopathologic study of 121 cases. *Cancer*, 1990; 66(2): 321–30.

13. McIver, B., I.D. Hay, D.F. Giuffrida, C.E. Dvorak, C.S. Grant, G.B. Thompson, J.A. van Heerden, and J.R. Goellner, Anaplastic thyroid carcinoma: A 50-year experience at a single institution. *Surgery*, 2001; 130(6): 1028–34.

14. Prasongsook, N., A. Kumar, A.V. Chintakuntlawar, R.L. Foote, J. Kasperbauer, J. Molina, Y. Garces, et al., Survival in response to multimodal therapy in anaplastic thyroid cancer. *J. Clin. Endocrinol. Metab.*, 2017; 102(12): 4506–14.

15. De Crevoisier, R., E. Baudin, A. Bachelot, S. Leboulleux, J.P. Travagli, B. Caillou, and M. Schlumberger, Combined treatment of anaplastic thyroid carcinoma with surgery, chemotherapy, and hyperfractionated accelerated external radiotherapy. *Int. J. Radiat. Oncol. Biol. Phys.*, 2004; 60(4): 1137–43.

16. Silverberg, S.G., R.V. Hutter, and F.W. Foote, Jr., Fatal carcinoma of the thyroid: Histology, metastases, and causes of death. *Cancer*, 1970; 25(4): 792–802.

17. Tallroth, E., G. Wallin, G. Lundell, T. Löwhagen, and J. Einhorn, Multimodality treatment in anaplastic giant cell thyroid carcinoma. *Cancer*, 1987; 60(7): 1428–31.

18. Schlumberger, M., C. Parmentier, M.J. Delisle, J.E. Couette, J.P. Droz, and D. Sarrazin, Combination therapy for anaplastic giant cell thyroid carcinoma. *Cancer*, 1991; 67(3): 564–6.

19. Sherman, E.J., S.H. Lim, A.L. Ho, R.A. Ghossein, M.G. Fury, A.R. Shaha, M. Rivera, et al., Concurrent doxorubicin and radiotherapy for anaplastic thyroid cancer: A critical re-evaluation including uniform pathologic review. *Radiother. Oncol. J. Eur. Soc. Ther. Rad. Oncol.*, 2011; 101(3): 425–30.

20. Nel, C.J., J.A. van Heerden, J.R. Goellner, H. Gharib, W.M. McConahey, W.F. Taylor, and C.S. Grant, Anaplastic carcinoma of the thyroid: A clinicopathologic study of 82 cases. *Mayo Clin. Proc.*, 1985; 60(1): 51–8.

21. Chiu, A.C., E.S. Delpassand, and S.I. Sherman, Prognosis and treatment of brain metastases in thyroid carcinoma. *J. Clin. Endocrinol. Metab.*, 1997; 82(11): 3637–42.

22. Saglietti, C., A.M. Onenerk, W.C. Faquin, G.P. Sykiotis, S. Ziadi, and M. Bongiovanni, FNA diagnosis of poorly differentiated thyroid carcinoma. A review of the recent literature. *Cytopathology*, 2017; 28(6): 467–74.

23. Poisson, T., D. Deandreis, S. Leboulleux, F. Bidault, G. Bonniaud, S. Baillot, A. Aupérin, et al., 18F-fluorodeoxyglucose positron emission tomography and computed tomography in anaplastic thyroid cancer. *Eur. J. Nucl. Med. Mol. Imaging*, 2010; 37(12): 2277–85.

24. Bogsrud, T.V., D. Karantanis, M.A. Nathan, B.P. Mullan, G.A. Wiseman, J.L. Kasperbauer, C.C. Reading, I.D. Hay, and V.J. Lowe, 18F-FDG PET in the management of patients with anaplastic thyroid carcinoma. *Thyroid*, 2008; 18(7): 713–19.

25. Ragazzi, M., A. Ciarrocchi, V. Sancisi, G. Gandolfi, A. Bisagni, and S. Piana, Update on anaplastic thyroid carcinoma: Morphological, molecular, and genetic features of the most aggressive thyroid cancer. *Int. J. Endocrinol.*, 2014 : 790834.

26. Bishop, J.A., R. Sharma, and W.H. Westra, PAX8 immunostaining of anaplastic thyroid carcinoma: A reliable means of discerning thyroid origin for undifferentiated tumors of the head and neck. *Hum. Pathol.*, 2011; 42(12): 1873–7.

27. Chintakuntlawar, A.V., K.M. Rumilla, C.Y. Smith, S.M. Jenkins, R.L. Foote, J.L. Kasperbauer, J.C. Morris, et al., Expression

of PD-1 and PD-L1 in anaplastic thyroid cancer patients treated with multimodal therapy: Results From a retrospective study. *J. Clin. Endocrinol. Metab.*, 2017; 102(6): 1943–50.

28. Landa, I., T. Ibrahimpasic, L. Boucai, R. Sinha, J.A. Knauf, R.H. Shah, S. Dogan, et al., Genomic and transcriptomic hallmarks of poorly differentiated and anaplastic thyroid cancers. *J. Clin. Invest.*, 2016; 126(3): 1052–66.

29. Jeon, M.J., S.M. Chun, D. Kim, H. Kwon, E.K. Jang, T.Y. Kim, W.B. Kim, et al., Genomic alterations of anaplastic thyroid carcinoma detected by targeted massive parallel sequencing in a BRAF mutation-prevalent area. *Thyroid Off. J. Am. Thyroid Assoc.*, 2016; 26(5): 683–90.

30. Sandulache, V.C., M.D. Williams, S.Y. Lai, C. Lu, W.N. William, N.L. Busaidy, G.J. Cote, et al., Real-time genomic characterization utilizing circulating cell-free DNA in patients with anaplastic thyroid carcinoma. *Thyroid*, 2017; 27 (1): 81–7.

31. Hu, S., S.N. Helman, E. Hanly, and I. Likhterov, The role of surgery in anaplastic thyroid cancer: A systematic review. *Am. J. Otolaryngol.*, 2017; 38(3): 337–50.

32. Ribechini, A., V. Bottici, A. Chella, R. Elisei, P. Vitti, A. Pinchera, N. Ambrosino, Interventional bronchoscopy in the treatment of tracheal obstruction secondary to advanced thyroid cancer. *J. Endocrinol. Invest.*, 2006; 29(2): 131–5.

33. Rao, S.N., M. Zafereo, R. Dadu, N.L. Busaidy, K. Hess, G.J. Cote, M.D. Williams, et al., Patterns of treatment failure in anaplastic thyroid carcinoma. *Thyroid*, 2017; 27(5): 672–81.

34. Mohebati, A., M. Dilorenzo, F. Palmer, S.G. Patel, D. Pfister, N. Lee, R.M. Tuttle, et al., Anaplastic thyroid carcinoma: A 25-year single-institution experience. *Ann. Surg. Oncol.*, 2014; 21(5): 1665–70.

35. Wendler, J., M. Kroiss, K. Gast, M.C. Kreissl, S. Allelein, U. Lichtenauer, R. Blaser, et al., Clinical presentation, treatment and outcome of anaplastic thyroid carcinoma: Results of a multicenter study in Germany. *Eur. J. Endocrinol.*, 2016; 175(6): 521–9.

36. Dandekar, P., C. Harmer, Y. Barbachano, P. Rhys-Evans, K. Harrington, C. Nutting, and K. Newbold, Hyperfractionated Accelerated Radiotherapy (HART) for anaplastic thyroid carcinoma: Toxicity and survival analysis. *Int. J. Radiat. Oncol. Biol. Phys.*, 2009; 74(2): 518–21.

37. Bhatia, A., A. Rao, K.K. Ang, A.S. Garden, W.H. Morrison, D.I. Rosenthal, D.B. Evans, et al., Anaplastic thyroid cancer: Clinical outcomes with conformal radiotherapy. *Head Neck*, 2010; 32(7): 829–36.

38. Tennvall, J., E. Tallroth, A. el Hassan, G. Lundell, M. Akerman, A. Biörklund, H. Blomgren, et al., Anaplastic thyroid carcinoma. Doxorubicin, hyperfractionated radiotherapy and surgery. *Acta oncol.*, 1990; 29(8): 1025–8.

39. Foote, R.L., J.R. Molina, J.L. Kasperbauer, R.V. Lloyd, B. McIver, J.C. Morris, C.S. Grant, et al., Enhanced survival in locoregionally confined anaplastic thyroid carcinoma: A single-institution experience using aggressive multimodal therapy. *Thyroid*, 2011; 21(1): 25–30.

40. Kim, J.H., and R.D. Leeper, Treatment of locally advanced thyroid carcinoma with combination doxorubicin and radiation therapy. *Cancer*, 1987; 60(10): 2372–5.

41. Kim, J.H., and R.D. Leeper, Treatment of anaplastic giant and spindle cell carcinoma of the thyroid gland with combination Adriamycin and radiation therapy. A new approach. *Cancer*, 1983; 52(6): 954–7.

42. Tennvall, J., G. Lundell, A. Hallquist, P. Wahlberg, G. Wallin, and S. Tibblin, Combined doxorubicin, hyperfractionated radiotherapy, and surgery in anaplastic thyroid carcinoma. Report on two protocols. The Swedish Anaplastic Thyroid Cancer Group *Cancer*, 1994. 74(4): 1348–54.

43. Tennvall, J., G. Lundell, P. Wahlberg, A. Bergenfelz, L. Grimelius, M. Akerman, A.L. Hjelm Skog, and G. Wallin, Anaplastic thyroid carcinoma: Three protocols combining doxorubicin, hyperfractionated radiotherapy and surgery. *Br. J. Cancer*, 2002; 86(12): 1848–53.

44. Shimaoka, K., D.A. Schoenfeld, W.D. DeWys, R.H. Creech, and R. DeConti, A randomized trial of doxorubicin *versus*

doxorubicin plus cisplatin in patients with advanced thyroid carcinoma. *Cancer*, 1985; 56(9): 2155–60.

45. Ain, K.B., M.J. Egorin, and P.A. DeSimone, Treatment of anaplastic thyroid carcinoma with paclitaxel: Phase 2 trial using ninety-six-hour infusion. Collaborative Anaplastic thyroid Cancer Health Intervention Trials (CATCHIT) Group. *Thyroid*, 2000; 10(7): 587–94.

46. Onoda, N., K. Sugino, T. Higashiyama, M. Kammori, K. Toda, K. Ito, A. Yoshida, et al., The safety and efficacy of weekly paclitaxel administration for anaplastic thyroid cancer patients: A nationwide prospective study. *Thyroid*, 2016; 26(9): 1293–9.

47. Subbiah, V., R.J. Kreitman, Z.A. Wainberg, J.Y. Cho, J.H.M. Schellens, J.C. Soria, P.Y. Wen, et al., Dabrafenib and trametinib treatment in patients with locally advanced or metastatic BRAF V600-mutant anaplastic thyroid cancer. *J. Clin. Oncol.*, 2018; 36(1): 7–13.

48. Iyer, P.C., R. Dadu, R. Ferrarotto, N.L. Busaidy, M.A. Habra, M. Zafereo, N. Gross, et al., Real world experience with targeted therapy for the treatment of anaplastic thyroid carcinoma. *Thyroid*, 2018; 28(1): 79–87.

49. Agarwal, R., J. Wang, K. Wilson, W. Barrett, and J.C. Morris, Response to targeted therapy in BRAF mutant anaplastic thyroid cancer. *J. Natl. Compr. Canc. Netw.*, 2016; 14(10): 1203–7.

50. Falchook, G.S., M. Millward, D. Hong, A. Naing, S. Piha-Paul, S.G. Waguespack, M.E. Cabanillas, et al., BRAF inhibitor dabrafenib in patients with metastatic BRAF-mutant thyroid cancer. *Thyroid*, 2015; 25(1): 71–7.

51. Brose, M.S., C.M. Nutting, B. Jarzab, R. Elisei, S. Siena, L. Bastholt, C. de la Fouchardiere, et al., Sorafenib in radioactive iodine-refractory, locally advanced, or metastatic differentiated thyroid cancer: A randomized, double-blind, phase 3 trial. *Lancet*, 2014. 384(9940): 319–28.

52. Schlumberger, M., M. Tahara, L.J. Wirth, B. Robinson, M.S. Brose, R. Elisei, M.A. Habra, et al., Lenvatinib *versus* placebo in radioiodine-refractory thyroid cancer. *N. Engl. J. Med.*, 2015; 372(7): 621–30.

53. Bible, K.C., V.J. Suman, J.R. Molina, R.C. Smallridge, W.J. Maples, M.E. Menefee, J. Rubin, et al., Efficacy of pazopanib in progressive, radioiodine-refractory, metastatic differentiated thyroid cancers: Results of a phase 2 consortium study. *Lancet. Oncol.*, 2010; 11(10): 962–72.

54. Bible, K.C., V.J. Suman, M.E. Menefee, R.C. Smallridge, J.R. Molina, W.J. Maples, N.J. Karlin, et al., A multi-institutional phase 2 trial of pazopanib monotherapy in advanced anaplastic thyroid cancer. *J. Clin. Endocrinol. Metab.*, 2012; 97(9): 3179–84.

55. Iniguez-Ariza, N.M., M.M. Ryder, C.R. Hilger, and K.C. Bible, Salvage lenvatinib therapy in metastatic anaplastic thyroid cancer. *Thyroid*, 2017; 27(7): 923–7.

56. Tahara, M., N. Kiyota, T. Yamazaki, N. Chayahara, K. Nakano, L. Inagaki, K. Toda, et al., Lenvatinib for anaplastic thyroid cancer. *Front. Oncol.*, 2017; 7: 25.

57. Takahashi, S., K.N., Yamazaki, T., Chayahara, N., Nakano, K., INAGAKI, L., Toda, et al., Phase II study of lenvatinib in patients with differentiated, medullary, and anaplastic thyroid cancer: Final analysis results. *J. Clin. Oncol.* In *2016 ASCO Annual Meeting*; Chicago, IL.

58. Isham, C.R., A.R. Bossou, V. Negron, K.E. Fisher, R. Kumar, L. Marlow, W.L. Lingle, et al., Pazopanib enhances paclitaxel-induced mitotic catastrophe in anaplastic thyroid cancer. *Sci. Transl. Med.*, 2013; 5(166): 166ra3.

59. Bible, K.C., A.V. Chintakuntlawar, and M. Ryder, Promises and perils of molecularly targeted therapeutics in anaplastic thyroid cancer. *J. Oncol. Practice*, 2016; 12(6): 521–2.

60. Bible, K.C., and M. Ryder, Evolving molecularly targeted therapies for advanced-stage thyroid cancers. *Nat. Rev. Clin. Oncol.*, 2016; 13(7): 403–16.

61. Holm, L.E., H. Blomgren, and T. Lowhagen, Cancer risks in patients with chronic lymphocytic thyroiditis. *N. Engl. J. Med.*, 1985; 312(10): 601–4.

62. Watanabe, N., J.Y. Noh, H. Narimatsu, K. Takeuchi, T. Yamaguchi, K. Kameyama, K. Kobayashi, et al., Clinicopathological features of 171 cases of primary thyroid

lymphoma: A long-term study involving 24,553 patients with Hashimoto's disease. *Br. J. Haematol.*, 2011; 153(2): 236–43.

63. Onal, C., Y.X. Li, R.C. Miller, P. Poortmans, N. Constantinou, D.C. Weber, B.M. Atasoy, et al., Treatment results and prognostic factors in primary thyroid lymphoma patients: A rare cancer network study. *Ann. Oncol.*, 2011; 22(1): 156–64.

64. Watanabe, N., H. Narimatsu, J.Y. Noh, Y. Kunii, K. Mukasa, M. Matsumoto, M. Suzuki, et al., Rituximab-including combined modality treatment for primary thyroid lymphoma: An effective regimen for elderly patients. *Thyroid*, 2014; 24(6): 994–9.

65. Kato, I., K. Tajima, T. Suchi, K. Aozasa, F. Matsuzuka, K. Kuma, and S. Tominaga, Chronic thyroiditis as a risk factor of B-cell lymphoma in the thyroid gland. *Jpn. J. Cancer Res.*, 1985; 76(11): 1085–90.

66. Graff-Baker, A., S.A. Roman, D.C. Thomas, R. Udelsman, and J.A. Sosa, Prognosis of primary thyroid lymphoma: Demographic, clinical, and pathologic predictors of survival in 1,408 cases. *Surgery*, 2009. 146(6): 1105–15.

67. Derringer, G.A., L.D. Thompson, R.A. Frommelt, K.E. Bijwaard, C.S. Heffess, and S.L. Abbondanzo, Malignant lymphoma of the thyroid gland: A clinicopathologic study of 108 cases. *Am. J. Surg. Pathol.*, 2000; 24(5): 623–39.

68. Green, L.D., L. Mack, and J.L. Pasieka, Anaplastic thyroid cancer and primary thyroid lymphoma: A review of these rare thyroid malignancies. *J. Surg. Oncol.*, 2006; 94(8): 725–36.

69. Sharma, A., S. Jasim, C.C. Reading, K.M. Ristow, J.C. Villasboas Bisneto, T.M. Habermann, V. Fatourechi, and M. Stan, Clinical presentation and diagnostic challenges of thyroid lymphoma: A cohort study. *Thyroid*, 2016; 26(8): 1061–7.

70. Pavlidis, E.T., and T.E. Pavlidis, A review of primary thyroid lymphoma: Molecular factors, diagnosis and management. *J. Invest. Surg.*, 2017: 1–6.

71. Naswa, N., P. Sharma, A.H. Nazar, T.K. Mohapatra, C. Bal, and R. Kumar, ^{18}F-FDG PET/CT for initial assessment and response monitoring in a case of high grade primary lymphoma of the thyroid gland: A case report and review of literature. *Indian J. Nucl. Med.*, 2014; 29(2): 94–6.

72. Ma, B., Y. Jia, Q. Wang, and X. Li, Ultrasound of primary thyroid non-Hodgkin's lymphoma. *Clin. Imaging*, 2014; 38(5): 621–6.

73. Takashima, S., N. Nomura, Y. Noguchi, F. Matsuzuka, and T. Inoue, Primary thyroid lymphoma: Evaluation with US, CT, and MRI. *J. Comput. Assist. Tomogr.*, 1995; 19(2): 282–8.

74. Levy, A., S. Leboulleux, C. Lepoutre-Lussey, E. Baudin, A.A. Ghuzlan, D. Hartl, E. Deutsch, et al., (18)F-fluorodeoxyglucose positron emission tomography to assess response after radiation therapy in anaplastic thyroid cancer. *Oral Oncol.*, 2015; 51(4): 370–5.

75. Carbone, P.P., H.S. Kaplan, K. Musshoff, D.W. Smithers, and M. Tubiana, Report of the committee on Hodgkin's disease staging classification. *Cancer Res.*, 1971; 31(11): 1860–1.

76. Armitage, J.O., Staging non-Hodgkin lymphoma. *CA Cancer J. Clin.*, 2005; 55(6): 368–76.

77. Sun, T.Q., X.L. Zhu, Z.Y. Wang, C.F. Wang, X.Y. Zhou, Q.H. Ji, and Y. Wu, Characteristics and prognosis of primary thyroid non-Hodgkin's lymphoma in Chinese patients. *J. Surg. Oncol.*, 2010; 101(7): 545–50.

78. Tupchong, L., F. Hughes, and C.L. Harmer, Primary lymphoma of the thyroid: Clinical features, prognostic factors, and results of treatment. *Int. J. Radiat. Oncol. Biol. Phys.*, 1986; 12(10): 1813–21.

79. Blair, T.J., R.G. Evans, S.J. Buskirk, P.M. Banks, and J.D. Earle, Radiotherapeutic management of primary thyroid lymphoma. *Int. J. Radiat. Oncol. Biol. Phys.*, 1985; 11(2): 365–70.

80. Devine, R.M., A.J. Edis, and P.M. Banks, Primary lymphoma of the thyroid: A review of the Mayo Clinic experience through 1978. *World J. Surg.*, 1981; 5(1): 33–8.

81. Vigliotti, A., J.S. Kong, L.M. Fuller, and W.S. Velasquez, Thyroid lymphomas stages IE and IIE: Comparative results for radiotherapy only, combination chemotherapy only,

and multimodality treatment. *Int. J. Radiat. Oncol. Biol. Phys.*, 1986; 12(10): 1807–12.

82. Alzouebi, M., J.R. Goepel, J.M. Horsman, and B.W. Hancock, Primary thyroid lymphoma: The 40 year experience of a UK lymphoma treatment centre. *Int. J. Oncol.*, 2012; 40(6): 2075–80.

83. Doria, R., J.F. Jekel, and D.L. Cooper, Thyroid lymphoma. The case for combined modality therapy. *Cancer*, 1994; 73(1): 200–6.

84. Compagno, J., and J.E. Oertel, Malignant lymphoma and other lymphoproliferative disorders of the thyroid gland. A clinico-pathologic study of 245 cases. *Am. J. Clin. Pathol.*, 1980; 74(1): 1–11.

85. Thompson, C.A., H. Ghesquieres, M.J. Maurer, J.R. Cerhan, P. Biron, S.M. Ansell, C. Chassagne-Clément, et al., Utility of routine post-therapy surveillance imaging in diffuse large B-cell lymphoma. *J. Clin. Oncol.*, 2014; 32(31): 3506–12.

86. Thanarajasingam, G., N. Bennani-Baiti, and C.A. Thompson, PET-CT in staging, response evaluation, and surveillance of lymphoma. *Curr. Treat. Options Oncol.*, 2016; 17(5): 24.

87. Souhami, L., W.J. Simpson, and J.S. Carruthers, Malignant lymphoma of the thyroid gland. *Int. J. Radiat. Oncol. Biol. Phys.*, 1980; 6(9): 1143–7.

11

Surgical approach to thyroid disorders

VANINDER K. DHILLON AND RALPH P. TUFANO

Introduction	261	Approach to well-differentiated thyroid	
Surgical technique	261	carcinomas	265
Identifying the superior and recurrent		*Medullary thyroid carcinoma*	266
laryngeal nerves and parathyroid glands	262	*Neck dissection*	266
Closure of the wound	262	*Approach to thyroid carcinomas with*	
Preoperative considerations for		*aerodigestive invasion*	267
thyroid surgery	262	*Approach to anaplastic thyroid carcinoma*	
Postoperative considerations for thyroid		*(ATC)*	269
surgery	262	*Reoperative thyroid surgery in patients with*	
Postoperative levothyroxine therapy	263	*DTC*	269
Approach to hyperthyroidism	263	*Thyroid surgery in pediatric patients*	269
Approach to thyroid nodules	263	*Advances in thyroid surgery—Scarless*	
Approach to multinodular goiter (substernal		*thyroid surgery*	269
component)	264	References	270

INTRODUCTION

Surgery for the thyroid gland began pre-Renaissance and was advanced with modern techniques by renowned surgeons, including Kocher, Billroth, and Halstead (1). Indeed, the 1909 Nobel Prize in Medicine was awarded to Theodor Kocher for his work on thyroid physiology and surgery. The role of surgery as a definitive treatment for certain thyroid diseases is well documented. Thyroid surgery is technically challenging, but a systematic approach to the anatomy enables accurate resection with low morbidity. The surgical indications and approaches to different diseases of the thyroid will be discussed in this chapter. The pre- and postoperative considerations, risks, and complications will be reviewed. Lastly, new advancements in the surgical approach to thyroid diseases, including transoral surgery, will be highlighted.

SURGICAL TECHNIQUE

Surgical technique may vary to some extent, although the goals are the same—to remove the thyroid, and all diseased lymph node tissue in the case of thyroid carcinoma, without compromising the structure and function of adjacent structures (2). In thyroid cancer surgery, it is important to begin on the side of the presumed malignancy to ensure resection of the pathology in question in the event of damage to the recurrent laryngeal nerve (RLN). In the case of RLN damage, the surgery may need to be modified to a hemithyroidectomy, with resection of the remaining thyroid only after RLN function has fully recovered. Failure to take this approach risks injury to bilateral RLNs and increases the likelihood of requiring a tracheostomy.

Identifying the superior and recurrent laryngeal nerves and parathyroid glands

During dissection of the superior pole of the thyroid, it is important to identify and stimulate the superior laryngeal nerve. As an adjunct during thyroid surgery, intraoperative nerve monitoring (IONM) may be used to track and identify the neurophysiologic integrity of the superior and recurrent laryngeal nerves. Although the impact of nerve monitoring on reducing permanent recurrent laryngeal nerve palsy rates is highly debated, its use can identify impending nerve injury as it transpires, allowing for surgical maneuvers to avoid further damage (3, 4). An additional technique to identify the RLN is to locate the inferior thyroid artery, which courses perpendicular to the nerve; blunt dissection deep to the artery will lead to the RLN. Identification of the parathyroid glands also allows mapping of the RLN, as the superior parathyroid lies deep to the nerve, and the inferior parathyroid superficial to it. During dissection, it is critical to identify intracapsular parathyroid glands that may be adherent to the thyroid capsule and/or whose vascular supply arises from the thyroid gland itself, as these glands will require intracapsular dissection off of the thyroid capsule. The parathyroid gland will need to be placed in normal saline on ice for later auto-transplantation into adjacent neck musculature at the end of the surgery. Intracapsular parathyroid glands ultimately share the same vascular supply as the thyroid and without which the parathyroid gland is not viable. The tissue, if diced and minced, can be reimplanted into the rich vascular supply of the adjacent neck musculature. Typically, the secretory function of the gland is preserved and parathyroid hormone function is maintained.

Closure of the wound

The strap muscles are reapproximated with a running 3–0 vicryl stitch, making sure to re-oppose the fascia over the musculature appropriately and leave a space inferiorly. It is then important to verify the absence of any further bleeding within the subplatysmal space before closing the skin with 3–0 vicryl subdermal sutures. Surgeon preference guides the decision for stitches or glue alone in skin closure. Stitches can be placed in a subcuticular fashion underneath the skin for closure of the wound and/or tissue adhesive glue may be placed over the skin after meticulously everting the edges for final wound closure. The goal is to have a watertight seal with an aesthetically pleasing closure.

Preoperative considerations for thyroid surgery

Successful postoperative management of patients undergoing thyroid surgery relies on an informed consent and an outline of expectations during the preoperative period. The main risks of thyroid surgery include hypoparathyroidism and recurrent laryngeal nerve injury, which are low in experienced high-volume surgical hands (5). The likelihood of hypoparathyroidism is highly variable in the literature, with a range from 1.5% to 15% (6). However, the majority of these cases will have a resolution of symptoms within a few months. Permanent hypoparathyroidism is typically reported as occurring in less than 2% of cases but is highly operator-dependent (6). Recurrent laryngeal nerve injury is described in relation to the incidence of postoperative vocal fold weakness, with a reported range between 3 and 5% for temporary injury and <1% permanent damage (3). Other risks associated with thyroid surgery include a scar, pain, bleeding, hematoma formation, and infection, with rates of less than 1% for each (2).

Prior to performing thyroidectomy, it is important to obtain a serum TSH. If low, a free T4 and total T3 will further clarify the degree of underlying thyroid dysfunction and determine whether medical therapy is indicated prior to the surgery. Treatment of overt hypothyroidism is optimally executed prior to an operation, except in urgent situations. Concomitant parathyroid disease is seen in 3–5% of patients with nodular thyroid disease (6, 7); due to costs and morbidity associated with reoperation in the central compartment, many experts recommend preoperative measurement of serum calcium. If hyperparathyroidism is identified, the surgical management can be altered accordingly.

Postoperative considerations for thyroid surgery

Restrictions on strenuous activity and diet as well as bathing instructions are important for good wound healing in the first few weeks after surgery. It is generally recommended that the patient not participate in contact sports or weightlifting, with avoidance of extreme bending or twisting in order to prevent increased pressure within the neck, which can increase the risk for the development of a hematoma. The use of dermal glue on the incision allows for normal bathing with water and soap in direct contact with the incision. The role of certain ointments and creams for scar care is debated, but a non-oil-based moisturizer may help to keep the scar hydrated and sunscreen may prevent hyperpigmentation of the scar. A recent systematic review of six prospective studies evaluating the role of vitamin E has found that there is not yet sufficient evidence that monotherapy with topical vitamin E has a significant beneficial effect on scar cosmesis to justify its widespread use (8). All postoperative details should be discussed with the patient before and after surgery in order to ensure patient expectations and compliance.

Postoperative levothyroxine therapy

The need for postoperative levothyroxine therapy is dependent upon the underlying thyroid abnormality requiring surgery and the extent of surgery. For patients undergoing total thyroidectomy, levothyroxine therapy is necessary at a daily replacement dose of approximately 1.6 mcg/kg (0.8 mcg/lb) body weight. When a diagnosis of cancer is certain and radioiodine therapy is desired, some providers may delay the initiation of thyroid hormone replacement until after the adjunctive therapy is administered. However, this approach is becoming far less common with the introduction of recombinant human TSH to stimulate uptake of iodine in follicular cells, obviating the need for thyroid hormone withdrawal (9) (see Chapter 8, "Differentiated Thyroid Carcinoma"). After hemithyroidectomy, the need for levothyroxine therapy is uncertain and immediate institution of LT4 is not necessary. It is estimated that 15% of patients ultimately will become hypothyroid; those with a higher preoperative TSH (>2.6 mU/L) and underlying Hashimoto's thyroiditis are more likely to require supplementation (10). It is important, therefore, to measure the TSH preoperatively and six weeks after surgery to ascertain the need for hormone therapy.

APPROACH TO HYPERTHYROIDISM

Indications for surgical management of hyperthyroidism may include: (a) pregnant patients requiring high doses of an antithyroid drug or who are intolerant to antithyroid drugs, (b) patients with a concomitant thyroid nodule that is malignant or suspicious for malignancy, (c) failure of radioiodine therapy, (d) massive thyroid enlargement with compressive symptoms, (e) severe ophthalmopathy, (f) large toxic multinodular goiter, and (g) patient preference (1). The risks, benefits, and alternatives for total thyroidectomy should be discussed frankly with patients considering surgery for Graves' disease. Surgery may be slightly more difficult in Graves' as the gland may be inflamed and highly vascular (11–13). With some studies suggesting a higher risk profile in Graves' patients undergoing surgery (13), it is crucial that patients are evaluated by an experienced, high-volume thyroid surgeon (>100 cases per year) who can discuss the risk–benefit profile in detail (12).

In the preoperative evaluation of patients with Graves', it is important to acknowledge the potential for thyroid storm. Thyroid storm is a life-threatening condition which leads to an excess release of thyroid hormone, often occurring in a suboptimally controlled hyperthyroid patient. Characterized by severe clinical manifestations of hyperthyroidism, symptoms include fever, gastrointestinal disturbances, tachyarrhythmias, congestive heart failure, agitation, and altered mental status (11; see Thyrotoxicosis chapter). The risk of thyroid storm is reduced by adequate preoperative preparation, initially with antithyroid medications followed by potassium iodide treatment for up to 10 days prior to surgery. An acute iodine load after pretreatment with thionamides reduces the thyroid vascularity and intraoperative blood loss (13). It is known that patients who are thyrotoxic prior to surgery have a higher mortality, but there is no compelling evidence to delay surgery for the sole purpose of adding iodine to decrease vascularity in patients otherwise adequately treated for their thyrotoxicosis (12, 13).

Approach to thyroid nodules

The majority of patients with thyroid nodules are managed conservatively with serial sonographic examinations. However, some patients may seek surgical removal, even in the setting of a benign lesion. Enlarging nodules that are benign after repeat fine needle aspiration (FNA) may prompt removal, particularly for those that are large (>4 cm) or causing compressive symptoms (9). On the other hand, patients with asymptomatic benign nodules that demonstrate growth may safely opt for surveillance (14). Patients with nodules harboring atypical or indeterminate cytology (Bethesda III or IV) (see Table 11.1) (15), may opt for surgical intervention to obtain a definitive histologic diagnosis. In the absence of suspicious lymphadenopathy in the neck, it is reasonable to proceed with a diagnostic lobectomy (9). In the presence of bilateral nodules, a total thyroidectomy may be considered (9). Alternatively, molecular testing can provide patients with guidance on the need for or the extent of surgery (16–20) (see Chapter 7, "Thyroid Nodules and Multinodular Goiter"). The determination of the extent of surgery should begin with a careful discussion with the patient, including the operative complications as well as the postoperative surveillance and management associated with each type of procedure. Final pathological findings after a diagnostic lobectomy may indicate a need for completion thyroidectomy, usually after discussion between the surgeon, patient, and endocrinologist.

Approach to multinodular goiter (substernal component)

Benign multinodular goiter affects 5–7% of the world's population and may be seen in up to 4% of the US population (21). Surgical management generally is recommended for goiters causing compressive symptoms (22). Symptoms of dyspnea, orthopnea, and dysphagia may be associated with thyromegaly. In a substernal goiter, tracheal compression or impingement on thoracic vasculature causing superior vena cava syndrome are also indications for surgery (22). This may be detected at the bedside by directing the patient to hold their arms above their head. With this maneuver, the goiter extends further into the substernal compartment, causing compression and obstruction of venous outflow at the level of the thoracic inlet. When present, the venous outflow obstruction will manifest with facial plethora, a finding known as Pemberton's sign (23) (Figure 11.1).

The approach to a goiter should include a preoperative assessment of breathing, swallowing, and phonation. Preoperative voice assessment, which should include both the patient's and the physician's assessment of voice, should be performed in all patients undergoing thyroidectomy. Laryngoscopy may be indicated in certain high-risk patients, including those with preoperative voice changes, a history of prior cervical surgery, or known thyroid cancer with potential posterior extrathyroidal extension or extensive nodal metastases (24). A bronchoscopy can be performed by the surgeon in the clinic using topical anesthesia in order to assess for any narrowing of the sub-cricoid airway (24). Bronchoscopy is a critical portion of the preoperative or intraoperative evaluation for patients with concern for airway complaints, or extrathyroidal extension with the potential for aerodigestive or laryngotracheal involvement in cases of malignancy (25). This procedure will also help the surgeon inform the anesthesia team of a potentially difficult airway. A preoperative modified barium swallow and esophogram are useful to determine the etiology of swallowing complaints. A substernal component of multinodular goiter often is not detectable on physical examination or

Table 11.1 Bethesda classification system for thyroid nodule cytology

Bethesda classification	Description	Risk of malignancy (%)
I	Nondiagnostic	
II	Benign	1–3
III	Atypia of undetermined significance Follicular lesion of undetermined significance	5–10
IV	Follicular neoplasm Suspicious for follicular neoplasm	20–30
V	Suspicious for malignancy	50–75
VI	Malignant	98–100

Adapted from Baloch et al. (15).

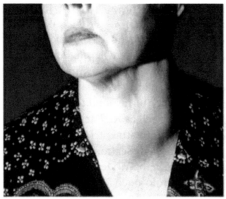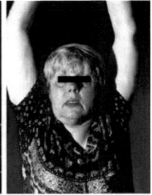

Figure 11.1 Pemberton's sign. (From Pemberton, H.S. (23). Used with permission.)

ultrasound. White et al. reported that 20–30% of substernal goiters were not palpable in the neck or were barely palpable, especially if the extension was posterior (26). For this reason, a preoperative CT of the neck and chest with contrast is beneficial to quantify the caudal extent, reveal the 3D shape, define tracheal compression, and pinpoint the mediastinal compartment(s) that are occupied by the goiter, all of which can aid in surgical planning (22, 26–28). It is important to note that the use of iodinated contrast can induce thyrotoxicosis in patients with untreated Graves' disease or autonomous nodules (29, 30); in patients at risk for cardiovascular complications, careful consideration should be given to whether contrast is essential for the preoperative evaluation.

The majority of goiters, including those with substernal extension, can be removed through a cervical incision. Indications for a sternotomy or cases in which a thoracic surgeon may be consulted are listed in Table 11.2 (22). It is reasonable to counsel patients about performing lobectomy

Table 11.2 Indications for sternotomy

Potential fibrosis of scarring from prior radiation or surgery involving neck or chest
Suspected malignancy with extrathyroidal extension or invasion
Inferior extension below the arotic arch abutting the carina
Involvement of the posterior mediastinum
Ectopic mediastinal goiter not connected to the cervical component

Adapted from Chen et al. (22).

for a bilaterally enlarged gland if there is concern for the integrity of the recurrent laryngeal nerve intraoperatively (22). Patients with asymmetrically enlarged goiters with compressive symptoms biased toward the larger side may opt for a lobectomy in order to preserve an otherwise functional contralateral lobe, to reduce the risk for hypoparathyroidism and hypothyroidism postoperatively.

Approach to well-differentiated thyroid carcinomas

The incidence of differentiated thyroid cancer (DTC) is increasing faster than any other malignancy; however, overall survival remains stable (31). This pattern of change has thus been attributed to over-diagnosis due to increased use of imaging modalities worldwide (32). Indeed, there is a large reservoir of undiagnosed thyroid cancers when autopsy series examine the incidence of thyroid cancer (33). Therefore, the overall focus of new thyroid cancer treatment guidelines is to "minimize potential harm from overtreatment in a majority of patients at low risk for disease-specific mortality and morbidity, while appropriately treating and monitoring those patients at higher risk" (9). This recommendation for a de-escalation in treatment reflects incremental retrospective data indicating similar clinical outcomes following lobectomy versus total thyroidectomy in properly selected patients (34–37). Consequently, it is now considered to be reasonable offer patients either a total thyroidectomy or a hemithyroidectomy for most differentiated thyroid cancers measuring 1–4 cm in the absence of metastatic involvement (9).

Furthermore, less aggressive use of radioactive iodine has allowed for consideration of more conservative surgical management, that is, lobectomy. This trend toward less invasive management of thyroid cancer is further illustrated by the role of active surveillance for certain lesions such as papillary thyroid microcarcinoma (PTMC). A clinical trial in the United States, as well as two large case series in Japan, have been examining the long-term outcomes for patients with tumors measuring less than 1–1.5cm who choose not to undergo surgery (38–41). Initial results are promising, with only a minority of tumors demonstrating evidence of clinically significant progression (38–41).

During the discussion with a patient regarding the risks, benefits, and alternatives of a more conservative approach to thyroid surgery for well-differentiated thyroid cancer, it is important to take into account other clinically relevant factors. For example, patients with a multinodular goiter, hyperthyroidism, and/or Hashimoto's with a concomitant fine needle aspiration of a unifocal lesion for papillary thyroid carcinoma may benefit from a total thyroidectomy. Patients with a first-degree relative with DTC and a unifocal lesion may consider total thyroidectomy, given the risk for multifocality and the potentially increased risk due to the family history (9). In a patient who has a history of head and neck irradiation and multiple thyroid nodules, consideration may be given to proceed with total thyroidectomy (9).

The optimal initial surgical management of Hürthle cell neoplasms on cytology is not clear. Based upon retrospective studies with small numbers of patients, the risk for cancer with an FNA diagnosis of Hürthle cell neoplasm is 20–30% (15, 42). The use of molecular testing to better stratify the malignancy risk of indeterminate nodules with a Hürthle cell cytology remains controversial (43). With a low risk of malignancy, many prefer a less aggressive initial surgery, that is, a hemithyroidectomy. However, this approach carries a risk of requiring a second surgery for completion thyroidectomy if the neoplasm is ultimately malignant. The risk profile associated with a two-step procedure should not be different from an initial total thyroidectomy in an experienced surgeon's hands (44). However, with a malignancy rate of only 30%, committing all patients with a Hürthle cell neoplasm on cytology to a total thyroidectomy would result in a significant rate of over-treatment.

Medullary thyroid carcinoma

The diagnosis of medullary thyroid carcinoma (MTC) can be challenging on FNA as cytology is often indeterminate (45). When the diagnosis is made preoperatively, all patients should have a neck ultrasound to identify suspicious adenopathy as well as *RET* testing prior to surgery; the definitive treatment is total thyroidectomy and central neck dissection (46). In those family members who have been identified as having inherited the *RET* proto-oncogene, there is a role for prophylactic thyroidectomy (46). It is important that patients with medullary thyroid carcinoma or concern for its inheritance be evaluated by a multidisciplinary group of specialists with expertise on medullary thyroid carcinoma. Please see Chapter 9, "Medullary Thyroid Carcinoma in Medical Management of Thyroid Disease" for more details.

Neck dissection

A compartmentalized neck dissection is indicated when there is clinical and/or radiological evidence of lymph node disease in patients with DTC. In spite of the high rates of nodal involvement in patients with papillary thyroid cancer, there is no strong evidence supporting the routine use of prophylactic neck dissection in the operative approach (9).

For patients with FNA-proven medullary thyroid carcinoma, there is a role for prophylactic bilateral central neck dissections with total thyroidectomy, given the high likelihood of central neck disease at the time of initial presentation (46). In contrast, the role of prophylactic lateral neck dissection in MTC is controversial for patients with sonographically normal-appearing lymph nodes or those without biopsy-proven lymph node metastases (46). Instead, a lateral neck dissection should be reserved for cases of biopsy-proven disease. In those circumstances where the likelihood of metastatic disease in the lateral neck is high enough to outweigh the risks of surgery, prophylactic lateral neck dissection may considered (46).

Central and lateral neck dissections are categorized by anatomical level (Figure 11.1) (2, 5). Preoperative or intraoperative identification of locoregional disease justifies a comprehensive neck dissection of the involved compartment. There is no role for attempting to remove only the involved nodes, also referred to as "berry picking"; this approach leads to increased rates of recurrence (9). Any suspicious lymph nodes identified pre-operatively should undergo FNA with thyroglobulin (or calcitonin in cases of suspected MTC) measurement in the needle washout. In selected cases with proven nodal involvement or a high suspicion of nodal involvement, cross-sectional imaging in the form of a neck CT with contrast should be obtained preoperatively (47–49). This enables visualization of any retropharyngeal or upper mediastinal nodes not visualized with ultrasound. It is important that all disease be removed at the time of the initial thyroidectomy since a comprehensive dissection of the involved compartments decreases the risk for recurrence (2, 47). Surgeon experience in performing the neck dissection is also related to improved recurrence-free survival (9, 47, 48).

A comprehensive central neck dissection should be performed when central neck (level VI) lymph nodes are involved on preoperative physical exam or imaging (9). An intraoperative finding of pathologic central lymph nodes is also an indication for central neck dissection. The main risks of central neck dissection are similar to thyroidectomy, although with a higher risk for vocal cord weakness secondary to an intimate dissection of the recurrent laryngeal nerve from the cricothyroid joint down to the sternum, and a higher likelihood of hypoparathyroidism due to the variable location of the inferior parathyroid glands (3, 9, 50, 51).

Lateral neck levels IIA through VB should be resected during a compartmental neck dissection if disease is discovered in those levels (5). Evidence of level IIB disease requires resection of levels IIA/B; resection of level VA is included only if there is biopsy-proven disease in that level (5) (see Figure 11.2).

The main risks of lateral neck dissection include shoulder weakness or palsy secondary to accessory nerve injury or stretching, facial droop, weakness of tongue movement, thoracic duct injury and subsequent chyle leak, Horner's syndrome from sympathetic chain injury along the carotid sheath, seroma, hematoma, and infection (2). The risk of these complications is typically less than 5% (52); however, one prospective study described the rate of chyle leak to be 13.5% (53). A postoperative referral to a physical therapist for range of motion exercises, with continued outpatient therapy for most patients, also may be beneficial. Placement of patients on a regular diet within the first

postoperative day is very helpful to rule out a chyle leak. Chyle leaks are diagnosed based upon the caliber and volume of output in neck drains placed at the time of surgery. Chylous output may be serous or milky with variability in output. To confirm the presence of chylous material, the fluid can be sent from drains in sterile containers and tested for amylase and lipase. If chylous output does not decrease with conservative management in the form of diet changes and octreotide, then surgical intervention may be necessary to ligate the thoracic duct or tributaries in order to prevent a chylothorax or infection (53, 54). A suction drain may be placed in each dissected lateral neck compartment to ameliorate the leak; they are typically removed within 5–7 days depending on output.

Approach to thyroid carcinomas with aerodigestive invasion

The incidence of well-differentiated thyroid carcinomas with invasion of the neck viscera and/or the upper aerodigestive tract is approximately 5–15% (55, 56). Tumors with extrathyroidal extension invading the neck and aerodigestive tract are known to have high rates of recurrence, with low responsiveness to radioactive iodine (9, 55). Furthermore, the surgical morbidity associated with its management is associated with a decreased quality of life.

Suspicion for aerodigestive tract invasion should prompt an evaluation of symptoms, physical examination, and imaging. Patients with evidence of visceral invasion of the trachea, larynx, or esophagus may variably report symptoms of

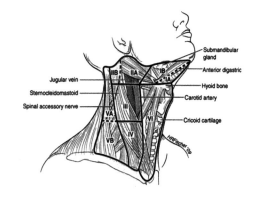

Figure 11.2 Anatomic compartments of the neck. (From Haugen et al. (9). Used with permission.)

voice, swallowing, or breathing complaints, as well as pain (57). A thorough physical examination is important, with attention to palpation of deep cervical structures. While laryngoscopy is indicated when there are associated voice complaints, an in-office tracheobronchoscopy using topical anesthesia for airway assessment is a useful adjunct if there is a concern for tracheal invasion. The goal is to visualize structures distal to the vocal cords in order to identify any submucosal and/or transmural involvement. Shin et al. developed a staging system for papillary thyroid carcinoma based upon the extent of tracheal invasion, where increased stage is correlated to greater extent of transmural invasion (58) (Figure 11.3). A CT with contrast of the neck and chest is important for visualization of the neck viscera as well as the anatomy and proximity of major vessels in the neck and chest (55, 56). Lastly, a swallowing study is important to evaluate esophageal function. Furthermore, every patient with aerodigestive involvement should undergo direct laryngoscopy, bronchoscopy, and esophagoscopy at the onset of surgery in order to assess the degree of visceral involvement prior to beginning resection. Patients should be advised during the consenting process that the surgical plan may change depending on intraoperative findings.

The aim of surgery for locally advanced DTC is to achieve an optimal oncological outcome, minimize surgical morbidity, and maximize quality of life. It is widely accepted that incomplete resection of gross disease compromises oncological outcome; however, the prognostic significance of residual microscopic disease is not well defined (56). If there is distant metastatic disease present at the time of surgical resection, the patient should be counseled preoperatively that the locoregional control is not curative, but surgical management is necessary in order to prevent future airway or esophageal compromise.

A recommendation for surgical resection of the larynx and/or upper airway depends on the extent of aerodigestive tract involvement by the tumor (58). It is important that a multidisciplinary team be involved in the management of these complex patients (9). Indications for total laryngectomy include: bilateral vocal cord paralysis, submucosal involvement of the cricoid (with 180-degree involvement [especially posteriorly]), and involvement of the inferior surface of the vocal cords (55, 56). Tracheal resection is indicated when there is transmural involvement of one or more tracheal rings, or if the integrity or margins of the inner perichondrium of the trachea is questionable after a shave resection (56). Transmural involvement of the esophagus or pharynx also requires pharyngectomy and/or esophagectomy with reconstruction. When there is possible need of visceral resection because of extensive tumor involvement, a multi-surgical team approach is optimal, with preoperative consultation

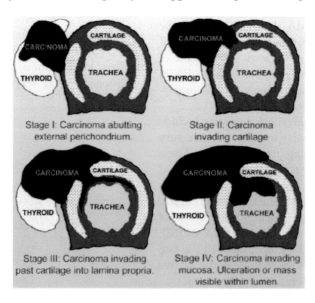

Stage I: Carcinoma abutting external perichondrium.

Stage II: Carcinoma invading cartilage

Stage III: Carcinoma invading past cartilage into lamina propria.

Stage IV: Carcinoma invading mucosa. Ulceration or mass visible within lumen.

Figure 11.3 Shin classification for aerodigestive invasion of thyroid carcinoma. (From Shin et al. (58). Used with permission.)

and intraoperative availability of reconstructive, head and neck, thoracic, and endocrine surgery. The role of such extensive surgery may be changing in the modern era of systemic multikinase inhibitor therapy, however (59, 60).

Approach to anaplastic thyroid carcinoma (ATC)

Surgical management of anaplastic thyroid carcinoma is contingent on the stage of the primary disease and the assessment of the airway. Once the diagnosis is established, patients should be staged rapidly and the airway quickly assessed by fiberoptic laryngoscopy (61). The surgeon needs to balance the possibility of local control with the likelihood of advanced distant metastatic disease. If the primary tumor is thought to be resectable, then this should take precedence, with combined postoperative radiotherapy and chemotherapy. If the primary tumor is unresectable, dependent on rapid growth, extension, and involvement of the tumor with other structures, it is important to stabilize the airway with a tracheostomy prior to beginning systemic treatment (61). As with many aggressive malignancies, patients and family members need to understand the poor prognosis, and advanced directives and wishes of the patient should be discussed thoroughly (61).

Reoperative thyroid surgery in patients with DTC

Development of metastatic disease in the cervical lymph nodes represents the most common location for recurrent/persistent DTC (62). The rate of locoregional metastasis at time of presentation for DTC may be as high as 30% and the rate of recurrence within cervical lymph nodes can be 5–15% (9, 62, 63). The thyroid bed and previously dissected neck compartments are the most likely sites of recurrence (62, 64). Consequently, the American Thyroid Association (ATA) and the National Cancer Comprehensive Network (NCCN) have stressed the importance of a comprehensive compartmentalized neck dissection (9, 65). The decision for reoperative surgery must take into account the clinical significance of the local disease progression and distant metastatic disease, when present, and the morbidity of reoperative surgery. The ATA Surgical Affairs Committee recommends that the surgeon only dissect compartments with identifiable disease

in a reoperative setting and that the entirety of that compartment be resected if possible (62). Exposure and identification of the recurrent laryngeal nerve in a central neck reoperation, as well as preservation of the superior parathyroid glands to prevent hypoparathyroidism, are critically important (64). Furthermore, each surgeon is responsible for formulating a risk–benefit analysis when considering observation versus reoperation. With a reoperation, the rate of hypoparathyroidism is 0–9.5%, the average rate of transient vocal cord paralysis is 3.6% and the rate of permanent vocal cord paralysis is 1.2% (62). The risk of disease progression with observation is typically low: only 9% demonstrated a median growth of 3mm with a mean follow up of 5 years at one high-volume center (66, 67). The provider should have a careful discussion with the patient, outlining these risks and benefits to determine the optimal management strategy.

Thyroid surgery in pediatric patients

The ATA has developed guidelines specific to the management of pediatric patients with thyroid disease (68). A good understanding of the age-specific differences in thyroid cancer is critical, as children and adolescents with this malignancy are more likely to present with disseminated disease, especially to the lung (68–70). In spite of this seemingly more aggressive initial presentation, long-term survival, even in the presence of distant metastatic involvement, is excellent (71). Optimal initial surgical management of the thyroid bed and thorough dissection of all involved neck compartments is crucial for both high survival rates and successful postoperative radioactive iodine therapy. The ATA guidelines highlight the importance of a multidisciplinary team for the workup of a pediatric thyroid cancer patient, the need for a high-volume surgeon to minimize complications, and the centralization of care for pediatric thyroid disease within a center of excellence (68, 72). With the appropriate team and surgical expertise, pediatric thyroid surgery has the same outcomes as adults, with low morbidity and excellent survival.

Advances in thyroid surgery—Scarless thyroid surgery

Remote access and minimally invasive thyroid surgery are a recent phenomenon, challenging and reinventing the traditional cervical incision for thyroid surgery. The advantage of any minimally invasive or remote-access approach is the diminution or absence of a cutaneous incision in the anterior neck. Minimally invasive incisions are typically smaller (66), and remote access approaches will use more distant incisions (axillary, breast, retroauricular, oral, or any combination of these) to place the final scar in a less conspicuous location. The ATA has published a statement on remote-access thyroid surgery (73). The risks of remote-access surgery are specific to each approach and should be discussed thoroughly with the patient. Additionally, surgeon experience with each approach, or the lack thereof, should be clearly defined. The experience with a transoral endoscopic approach for thyroid and parathyroid surgery was recently published in a case series, with the results showing excellent outcomes and minimal complications (74). The risks associated with this specific procedure include injury to lips or teeth. There is also a risk for mental nerve injury resulting in regional hypoesthesia, which has been temporary in all cases to date (74). There should always be a discussion of the possible need for conversion to open surgery if difficulties arise intraoperatively. The value of experience and the presence of a learning curve are clear, and the informed consent process should detail the risks of any new procedure, including the potential for novel or unanticipated risks (75). The functional outcome must be at least as good as one could achieve with a traditional transcervical approach.

REFERENCES

1. Sarkar, S., S. Banerjee, R. Sarkar, and B. Sikder, A review on the history of "thyroid surgery." *Indian J. Surg.*, 2016; 78(1): 32–6.

2. American Thyroid Association, American Association of Endocrine Surgeons, American Academy of Otolaryngology–Head and Neck Surgery, American Head and Neck Society, S.E. Carty, D.S. Cooper, G.M. Doherty, et al., Consensus statement on the terminology and classification of central neck dissection for thyroid cancer. *Thyroid*, 2009; 19(11): 1153–8.

3. Dralle, H., C. Sekulla, J. Haerting, W. Timmermann, H.J. Neumann, E. Kruse, S. Grond, et al., Risk factors of paralysis and functional outcome after recurrent laryngeal nerve monitoring in thyroid surgery. *Surgery*, 2004; 136(6): 1310–22.

4. Mirallie, É C. Caillard, F. Pattou, L. Brunaud, A. Hamy, M. Dahan, M. Prades, et al., Does intraoperative neuromonitoring of recurrent nerves have an impact on the postoperative palsy rate? Results of a prospective multicenter study. *Surgery*, 2018; 163(1): 124–9.

5. Stack, B.C., Jr., R.L. Ferris, D. Goldenberg, M. Haymart, A. Shaha, S. Sheth, J.A. Sosa, R.P. Tufano, and American Thyroid Association Surgical Affairs Committee, American Thyroid Association consensus review and statement regarding the anatomy, terminology, and rationale for lateral neck dissection in differentiated thyroid cancer. *Thyroid*, 2012; 22(5): 501–8.

6. Stack, B.C., Jr., D.N. Bimston, D.L. Bodenner, E.M. Brett, H. Dralle, L.A. Orloff, J. Pallota, et al., American Association of Clinical Endocrinologists and American College of Endocrinology disease state clinical review: Postoperative hypoparathyroidism—Definitions and management. *Endocr. Pract.*, 2015; 21(6): 674–85.

7. Murray, S.E., R.S. Sippel, and H. Chen, Incidence of concomitant hyperparathyroidism in patients with thyroid disease requiring surgery. *J. Surg. Res.*, 2012; 178(1): 264–7.

8. Tanaydin, V., J. Conings, M. Malyar, R. van der Hulst, and B. van der Lei, The role of topical vitamin E in scar management: A systematic review. *Aesthet. Surg. J.*, 2016; 36(8): 959–65.

9. Haugen, B.R., E.K. Alexander, K.C. Bible, G.M. Doherty, S.J. Mandel, Y.E. Nikiforov, F. Pacini, et al., 2015 American Thyroid Association management guidelines for adult patients with thyroid nodules and differentiated thyroid cancer: The American Thyroid Association guidelines task force on thyroid nodules and differentiated thyroid cancer. *Thyroid*, 2016; 26(1): 1–133.

10. Stoll, S.J., Thyroid hormone replacement after thyroid lobectomy. *Surgery*, 2009; 146(4): 554–8; discussion 558. discussion: 558–60.

11. Akamizu, T., T. Satoh, O. Isozaki, A. Suzuki, S. Wakino, T. Iburi, K. Tsuboi, et al.,

Diagnostic criteria, clinical features, and incidence of thyroid storm based on nation-wide surveys. *Thyroid*, 2012; 22(7): 661–79.

12. Langley, R.W., and H.B. Burch, Perioperative management of the thyrotoxic patient. *Endocrinol. Metab. Clin. North Am.*, 2003; 32(2): 519–34.

13. Marigold, J.H., A.K. Morgan, D.J. Earle, A.E. Young, and D.N. Croft, Lugol's iodine: Its effect on thyroid blood flow in patients with thyrotoxicosis. *Br. J. Surg.*, 1985; 72(1): 45–7.

14. Durante, C., G. Costante, G. Lucisano, R. Bruno, D. Meringolo, A. Paciaroni, E. Puxeddu, et al., The natural history of benign thyroid nodules. *JAMA*, 2015; 313(9): 926–35.

15. Baloch, Z.W., V.A. LiVolsi, S.L. Asa, J. Rosai, M.J. Merino, G. Randolph, P. Vielh, et al., Diagnostic terminology and morphologic criteria for cytologic diagnosis of thyroid lesions: A synopsis of the National Cancer Institute thyroid fine needle aspiration state of the science conference. *Diagn. Cytopathol.*, 2008; 36(6): 425–37.

16. Alexander, E.K., G.C. Kennedy, Z.W. Baloch, E.S. Cibas, D. Chudova, J. Diggans, L. Friedman, et al., Preoperative diagnosis of benign thyroid nodules with indeterminate cytology. *N. Engl. J. Med.*, 2012; 367(8): 705–15.

17. Jung, C.K., M.P. Little, J.H. Lubin, A.V. Brenner, S.A. Wells, A.J. Sigurdson, and Y.E. Nikiforov, The increase in thyroid cancer incidence during the last four decades is accompanied by a high frequency of BRAF mutations and a sharp increase in RAS mutations. *J. Clin. Endocrinol. Metab.*, 2014; 99(2): E276–85.

18. Nikiforov, Y.E., S.E. Carty, S.I. Chiosea, C. Coyne, U. Duvvuri, R.L. Ferris, W.E. Gooding, et al., Impact of the multi-gene ThyroSeq next-generation sequencing assay on cancer diagnosis in thyroid nodules with atypia of undetermined significance/follicular lesion of undetermined significance cytology. *Thyroid*, 2015; 25(11): 1217–23.

19. Steward, D.L., and R.T. Kloos, Clinical diagnostic gene expression thyroid testing. *Otolaryngol. Clin. North Am.*, 2014; 47(4): 573–93.

20. Valderrabano, P., L. Khazai, M.E. Leon, Z.J. Thompson, Z. Ma, C.H. Chung, J.E. Hallanger-Johnson, et al., Evaluation of ThyroSeq v2 performance in thyroid nodules with indeterminate cytology. *Endocr. Relat. Cancer*, 2017; 24(3): 127–36.

21. Vanderpump, M.P., The epidemiology of thyroid disease. *Br. Med. Bull.*, 2011; 99: 39–51.

22. Chen, A.Y., V.J. Bernet, S.E. Carty, T.F. Davies, I. Ganly, W.B. Inabnet, A.R. Shaha, and Surgical Affairs Committee of the American Thyroid Association, American Thyroid Association statement on optimal surgical management of goiter. *Thyroid*, 2014; 24(2): 181–9.

23. Pemberton, H.S., Sign of submerged goiter. *Lancet*, 1946; 248(6423): 509.

24. Randolph, G.W., and D. Kamani, The importance of preoperative laryngoscopy in patients undergoing thyroidectomy: Voice, vocal cord function, and the preoperative detection of invasive thyroid malignancy. *Surgery*, 2006; 139(3): 357–62.

25. Avenia, N., J. Vannucci, M. Monacelli, R. Lucchini, A. Polistena, S. Santoprete, R. Potenza, M. Andolfi, and F. Puma, Thyroid cancer invading the airway: Diagnosis and management. *Int. J. Surg.*, 2016; 28.Suppl 1: S75–8.

26. White, M.L., G.M. Doherty, and P.G. Gauger, Evidence-based surgical management of substernal goiter. *World J. Surg.* 2008; 32(7): 1285–300.

27. Cooper, J.C., R. Nakielny, and C.H. Talbot, The use of computed tomography in the evaluation of large multinodular goiters. *Ann. R. Coll. Surg. Engl.*, 1991; 73(1): 32–5.

28. Stang, M.T., M.J. Armstrong, J.B. Ogilvie, L. Yip, K.L. McCoy, C.N. Faber, and S.E. Carty, Positional dyspnea and tracheal compression as indications for goiter resection. *Arch. Surg.*, 2012; 147(7): 621–6.

29. Adler, J., and D.J. Colegrove, Contrast induced thyrotoxicosis in a patient with new onset atrial fibrillation: A case report and review. *J. ATR Fibrillation*, 2013; 6(1): 379.

30. van der Molen, A.J., H.S. Thomsen, S.K. Morcos, and Contrast Media Safety Committee, European Society of Urogenital

Radiology (ESUR), Effect of iodinated contrast media on thyroid function in adults. *Eur. Radiol.*, 2004; 14(5): 902–7.

31. Lim, H., S.S. Devesa, J.A. Sosa, D. Check, and C.M. Kitahara, Trends in thyroid cancer incidence and mortality in the United States, 1974–2013. *JAMA*, 2017; 317(13): 1338–48.

32. Davies, L., and H.G. Welch, Current thyroid cancer trends in the United States. *JAMA Otolaryngol. Head Neck Surg.*, 2014; 140(4): 317–22.

33. Pazaitou-Panayiotou, K., M. Capezzone, and F. Pacini, Clinical features and therapeutic implication of papillary thyroid microcarcinoma. *Thyroid*, 2007; 17(11): 1085–92.

34. Kovatch, K.J., C.W. Hoban, and A.G. Shuman, Thyroid cancer surgery guidelines in an era of de-escalation. *Eur. J. Surg. Oncol.*, 2018; 44(3): 297–306.

35. Adam, M.A., J. Pura, L. Gu, M.A. Dinan, D.S. Tyler, S.D. Reed, R. Scheri, S.A. Roman, and J.A. Sosa., Extent of surgery for papillary thyroid cancer is not associated with survival: An analysis of 61,775 patients. *Ann. Surg.*, 2014; 260(4): 601–5. discussion: 605–7.

36. Matsuzu, K., K. Sugino, K. Masudo, M. Nagahama, W. Kitagawa, H. Shibuya, K. Ohkuwa, et al., Thyroid lobectomy for papillary thyroid cancer: Long-term follow-up study of 1,088 cases. *World J. Surg.*, 2014; 38(1): 68–79.

37. Nixon, I.J., I. Ganly, S.G. Patel, F.L. Palmer, M.M. Whitcher, R.M. Tuttle, A. Shaha, and J.P. Shah, Thyroid lobectomy for treatment of well-differentiated intrathyroid malignancy. *Surgery*, 2012; 151(4): 571–9.

38. Ito, Y., A. Miyauchi, M. Kihara, T. Higashiyama, K. Kobayashi, and A. Miya, Patient age is significantly related to the progression of papillary microcarcinoma of the thyroid under observation. *Thyroid*, 2014; 24(1): 27–34.

39. Ito, Y., T. Uruno, K. Nakano, Y. Takamura, A. Miya, K. Kobayashi, T. Yokozawa, et al., An observation trial without surgical treatment in patients with papillary microcarcinoma of the thyroid. *Thyroid*, 2003; 13(4): 381–7.

40. Miyauchi, A., T. Kudo, Y. Ito, H. Oda, H. Sasai, T. Higashiyama, M. Fukushima, et al., Estimation of the lifetime probability of disease progression of papillary microcarcinoma of the thyroid during active surveillance. *Surgery*, 2018; 163(1): 48–52.

41. Shaha, A.R., and R.M. Tuttle. Editorial: Risk of disease progression during active surveillance of papillary thyroid cancer. *Surgery*, 2018; 163(1): 53–4.

42. Wang, C.C., L. Friedman, G.C. Kennedy, H. Wang, E. Kebebew, D.L. Steward, M.A. Zeiger, et al., A large multicenter correlation study of thyroid nodule cytopathology and histopathology. *Thyroid*, 2011; 21(3): 243–51.

43. Ferris, R.L., and S.E. Carty, Response to letter to the editor on COI for American Thyroid Association statement on surgical application of molecular profiling for thyroid nodules. *Thyroid*, 2015; 25(11): 1266.

44. Sosa, J.A., H.M. Bowman, J.M. Tielsch, N.R. Powe, T.A. Gordon, and R. Udelsman, The importance of surgeon experience for clinical and economic outcomes from thyroidectomy. *Ann. Surg.*, 1998; 228(3): 320–30.

45. Trimboli, P., G. Treglia, L. Guidobaldi, F. Romanelli, G. Nigri, S. Valabrega, R. Sadeghi, et al., Detection rate of FNA cytology in medullary thyroid carcinoma: A meta-analysis. *Clin. Endocrinol. (Oxf.)*, 2015; 82(2): 280–5.

46. Wells, S.A., Jr., S.L. Asa, H. Dralle, R. Elisei, D.B. Evans, R.F. Gagel, N. Lee, et al., Revised American Thyroid Association guidelines for the management of medullary thyroid carcinoma. *Thyroid*, 2015; 25(6): 567–610.

47. Clayman, G.L., G. Agarwal, B.S. Edeiken, S.G. Waguespack, D.B. Roberts, and S.I. Sherman, Long-term outcome of comprehensive central compartment dissection in patients with recurrent/persistent papillary thyroid carcinoma. *Thyroid*, 2011; 21(12): 1309–16.

48. Segal, K., T. Shpitzer, A. Hazan, G. Bachar, G. Marshak, and A. Popovtzer, Invasive well-differentiated thyroid carcinoma: Effect of treatment modalities on outcome. *Otolaryngol. Head Neck Surg.*, 2006; 134(5): 819–22.

49. Wu, G., S. Fraser, S.I. Pai, T.Y. Farrag, P.W. Ladenson, and R.P. Tufano, Determining the

extent of lateral neck dissection necessary to establish regional disease control and avoid reoperation after previous total thyroidectomy and radioactive iodine for papillary thyroid cancer. *Head Neck*, 2012; 34(10): 1418–21.

50. Falk, S.A., and T.V. McCaffrey, Management of the recurrent laryngeal nerve in suspected and proven thyroid cancer. *Otolaryngol. Head Neck Surg.*, 1995; 113(1): 42–8.

51. Pai, S.I., and R.P. Tufano, Central compartment neck dissection for thyroid cancer. Technical considerations. *ORL J. Otorhinolaryngol. Relat. Spec.*, 2008; 70(5): 292–7.

52. Madenci, A.L., D. Caragacianu, J.O. Boeckmann, B.C. Stack, and J.J. Shin, Lateral neck dissection for well-differentiated thyroid carcinoma: A systematic review. *Laryngoscope*, 2014; 124(7): 1724–34.

53. Roh, J.L., D.H. Kim, and C.I. Park, Prospective identification of chyle leakage in patients undergoing lateral neck dissection for metastatic thyroid cancer. *Ann. Surg. Oncol.*, 2008; 15(2): 424–9.

54. Smoke, A., and M.H. Delegge, Chyle leaks: Consensus on management? *Nutr. Clin. Pract.*, 2008; 23(5): 529–32.

55. Nixon, I.J., R. Simo, K. Newbold, A. Rinaldo, C. Suarez, L.P. Kowalski, C. Silver, J.P. Shah, and A. Ferlito, Management of invasive differentiated thyroid cancer. *Thyroid*, 2016; 26(9): 1156–66.

56. Czaja, J.M., and T.V. McCaffrey, The surgical management of laryngotracheal invasion by well-differentiated papillary thyroid carcinoma. *Arch. Otolaryngol. Head Neck Surg.*, 1997; 123(5): 484–90.

57. Gaissert, H.A., J. Honings, H.C. Grillo, D.M. Donahue, J.C. Wain, C.D. Wright, and D.J. Mathisen, Segmental laryngotracheal and tracheal resection for invasive thyroid carcinoma. *Ann. Thorac. Surg.*, 2007; 83(6): 1952–9.

58. Shin, D.H., E.J. Mark, H.C. Suen, and H.C. Grillo, Pathologic staging of papillary carcinoma of the thyroid with airway invasion based on the anatomic manner of extension to the trachea: A clinicopathologic study based on 22 patients who underwent thyroidectomy and airway resection. *Hum. Pathol.*, 1993; 24(8): 866–70.

59. Cabanillas, M.E., M.I. Hu, C. Jimenez, E.G. Grubbs, and G.J. Cote, Treating medullary thyroid cancer in the age of targeted therapy. *Int. J. Endocr. Oncol.*, 2014; 1(2): 203–16.

60. Lirov, R., F.P. Worden, and M.S. Cohen, The treatment of advanced thyroid cancer in the age of novel targeted therapies. *Drugs*, 2017; 77(7): 733–45.

61. Smallridge, R.C., K.B. Ain, S.L. Asa, K.C. Bible, J.D. Brierley, K.D. Burman, E. Kebebew, et al., American Thyroid Association guidelines for management of patients with anaplastic thyroid cancer. *Thyroid*, 2012; 22(11): 1104–39.

62. Tufano, R.P., G. Clayman, K.S. Heller, W.B. Inabnet, E. Kebebew, A. Shaha, D.L. Steward, R.M. Tuttle, and American Thyroid Association Surgical Affairs Committee Writing Task Force, Management of recurrent/persistent nodal disease in patients with differentiated thyroid cancer: A critical review of the risks and benefits of surgical intervention versus active surveillance. *Thyroid*, 2015; 25(1): 15–27.

63. Lamartina, L., I. Borget, H. Mirghani, A. Al Ghuzlan, A. Berdelou, F. Bidault, D. Deandreis, et al., Surgery for neck recurrence of differentiated thyroid cancer: Outcomes and risk factors. *J. Clin. Endocrinol. Metab.*, 2017; 102(3): 1020–31.

64. Tufano, R.P., J. Bishop, and G. Wu, Reoperative central compartment dissection for patients with recurrent/persistent papillary thyroid cancer: Efficacy, safety, and the association of the BRAF mutation. *Laryngoscope*, 2012; 122(7): 1634–40.

65. Tuttle, R.M., et al., Thyroid carcinoma, version 2.2014. *J. Natl. Compr. Canc. Netw.*, 2014; 12(12): 1671–80; quiz 1680. quiz: 1680.

66. Robenshtok, E., S. Fish, A. Bach, J.M. Domínguez, A. Shaha, R.M. Tuttle, Suspicious cervical lymph nodes detected after thyroidectomy for papillary thyroid cancer usually remain stable over years in properly selected patients. *J. Clin. Endocrinol. Metab.*, 2012; 97(8): 2706–13.

67. Rondeau, G., S. Fish, L.E. Hann, J.A. Fagin, and R.M. Tuttle, Ultrasonographically detected small thyroid bed nodules identified after total thyroidectomy for differentiated thyroid cancer seldom show clinically significant structural progression. *Thyroid*, 2011; 21(8): 845–53.

68. Francis, G.L., S.G. Waguespack, A.J. Bauer, P. Angelos, S. Benvenga, J.M. Cerutti, C.A. Dinauer, et al., Management guidelines for children with thyroid nodules and differentiated thyroid cancer. *Thyroid*, 2015; 25(7): 716–59.

69. Al-Qurayshi, Z., A national perspective of the risk presentation, and outcomes of pediatric thyroid cancer. *JAMA Otolaryngol. Head Neck Surg.*, 2016; 142(5): 472–8.

70. Feinmesser, R., E. Lubin, K. Segal, and A. Noyek, Carcinoma of the thyroid in children:—A review. *J. Pediatr. Endocrinol. Metab.*, 1997; 10(6): 561–8.

71. Golpanian, S., E.A. Perez, J. Tashiro, J.I. Lew, J.E. Sola, and A.R. Hogan, Pediatric papillary thyroid carcinoma: Outcomes and survival predictors in 2504 surgical patients. *Pediatr. Surg. Int.*, 2016; 32(3): 201–8.

72. Hogan, A.R., Y. Zhuge, E.A. Perez, L.G. Koniaris, J.I. Lew, and J.E. Sola, Pediatric thyroid carcinoma: Incidence and outcomes in 1753 patients. *J. Surg. Res.*, 2009; 156(1): 167–72.

73. Berber, E., V. Bernet, T.J. Fahey, E. Kebebew, A. Shaha, B.C. Stack, M. Stang, et al., American Thyroid Association statement on remote-access thyroid surgery. *Thyroid*, 2016; 26(3): 331–7.

74. Russell, J.O., J. Clark, S.I. Noureldine, A. Anuwong, M.G. Al Khadem, H. Yub Kim, V.K. Dhillon, et al., Transoral thyroidectomy and parathyroidectomy—A North American series of robotic and endoscopic transoral approaches to the central neck. *Oral Oncol.*, 2017; 71: 75–80.

75. Tufano, R.P., S.I. Noureldine, and P. Angelos, Incidental thyroid nodules and thyroid cancer: Considerations before determining management. *JAMA Otolaryngol. Head Neck Surg.*, 2015; 141(6): 566–72.

12

Thyroid disease and pregnancy

ALISHA N. WADE AND SUSAN J. MANDEL

Thyroid hormone physiology during gestation 275
Thyroid autoimmunity and euthyroidism 277
Hypothyroidism 277
Diagnosis 277
Pregnancy outcome 278
Treatment 280
Hyperthyroidism 281
HCG-associated thyrotoxicosis and
    hyperemesis gravidarum 281
Graves' disease 282
Diagnosis 282
Pregnancy outcome 283
Treatment 283
Lactation 287
Fetal/neonatal hyperthyroidism 287
Thyroid nodules and thyroid cancer 289
References 289

When pregnancy is associated with alterations in maternal thyroid function, the fetus can be affected in two ways: either directly by transplacental passage of maternal thyroid hormone, antithyroid antibodies, or medications, or indirectly by adverse influences on maternal physiology. It is important to recognize the expected alterations in thyroid hormone levels during gestation. The clinician must be able to differentiate normal physiological changes from true thyroid disease; however, hyperthyroidism and hypothyroidism may first be detected during pregnancy. Pregnant patients with pre-existing thyroid dysfunction require close monitoring and frequently need adjustment of therapy.

THYROID HORMONE PHYSIOLOGY DURING GESTATION

During normal gestation, there are changes in thyroid hormone physiology that are reversible after delivery. Serum thyroxine-binding globulin (TBG) levels begin to increase within the first weeks after conception, usually more than doubling

in concentration, with peak levels reached at the middle of gestation (1). Levels remain elevated until delivery and then normalize in the postpartum period. The rise in serum TBG concentration results from an estrogen-induced increase in the sialylation of the protein, which subsequently decreases its hepatic clearance and prolongs its serum half-life (2).

Associated with the rise in TBG are increases in both serum total T4 and T3 levels, which also plateau at the mid-trimester or slightly earlier (1, 3). Because of these TBG changes, normal serum T4 and T3 levels throughout pregnancy are predictably about 1.5 times the normal nonpregnant reference range (Figure 12.1) (4, 5). Interestingly, it has been observed that the serum T4 and T3 concentrations do not increase as much during pregnancy as would be expected given the rise in TBG, and this may be due to decreased TBG saturation (6). The increase in maternal T4 production that occurs in normal gestation is most evident from observations of levothyroxine-replaced hypothyroid women who require a 25–45% dosage increase to maintain normal serum TSH levels during pregnancy (7, 8). Furthermore, the findings of relative hypothyroxinemia and slightly increased serum TSH levels during pregnancy in women from areas of borderline iodine sufficiency (<100mcg/day) support the view that pregnancy constitutes a stress for the maternal thyroid by stimulating thyroidal production (9). There are several possible explanations for this increased T4 requirement. Early in pregnancy, the rise in serum TBG results in the expansion of the extrathyroidal T4 pool. In addition, transplacental passage of T4 and placental T4 degradation may contribute to the increased demand on maternal thyroidal production to maintain euthyroid status. Lastly, the renal clearance of iodide increases because of the higher glomerular filtration rate in pregnancy (10).

Determination of free T4 (FT4) levels may reflect both methodological differences as well as alterations due to gravid physiology. With their sensitivity to binding proteins, however, automated assays appear to show a decrease in serum FT4 levels as pregnancy progresses compared to their own nonpregnant reference range. By the third trimester, serum FT4 levels are often lower than the normal nonpregnant reference range (Figure 12.1) (5, 11, 12).

Serum thyroid stimulating hormone (TSH) levels also fluctuate during pregnancy. The human chorionic gonadotropin (hCG)-mediated increased thyroid hormone synthesis coinciding with the first trimester peak in hCG is reflected by a reciprocal fall in serum TSH levels. It has been hypothesized that hCG has thyrotropic activity because of its structural similarity to TSH, and that the high serum hCG levels stimulate the TSH receptor via a hormone specificity "spillover" syndrome (13). In fact, a positive correlation between individual free T4 and hCG levels in early gestation has been reported, consistent with the TSH-like activity of hCG (6).

Both the upper and lower reference limits of TSH decrease in pregnancy, with the upper limit being approximately 4.0 mIU/l at the end of the 1st trimester (14). TSH reference ranges in pregnancy likely differ by ethnicity (15), and the use of ethnic-specific reference ranges, where available, is preferred to prevent the misclassification of thyroid status.

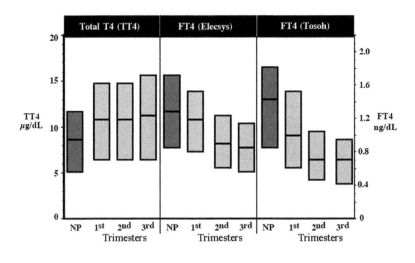

Figure 12.1 Serum thyroxine (TT4) and free thyroxine (FT4) levels by trimester. Interquartile ranges are shown by the shaded boxes, with the median value indicated by the line. Serum TT4 levels rise to approximately 1.5 times the normal nonpregnant reference range. Although serum FT4 ranges were method-dependent, as shown by the differences in measurement by the Elecsys (Roche, Basel, Switzerland) and Tosoh (Fisher Scientific International, Hampton, NH) methods, both methods show a consistent decrease in FT4 as pregnancy progresses. NP = nonpregnant (n = 62), 1st = first trimester (n = 105), 2nd = second trimester (n = 39), 3rd = third trimester (n = 64). (With permission from Chan GW, Mandel SJ. Therapy insight: Management of Graves' disease during pregnancy. *Nat. Clin. Pract. Endocrinol. Metab.* 2007;3(6):470–8.)

Renal iodine clearance increases as a result of an increase in the glomerular filtration rate and there is transplacental passage of iodine and iodothyronines as the fetal-placental unit grows (10). In areas of borderline iodine sufficiency, such as in many European countries, this loss of iodine, combined with the increase in thyroid hormone pools from the marked increase in serum TBG levels, may result in goiter formation. In areas where iodine intake is more than sufficient, such as the United States, a palpable goiter should not occur during normal gestation and, if present, this should direct the clinician to investigate possible thyroid hormone abnormalities (16).

THYROID AUTOIMMUNITY AND EUTHYROIDISM

The prevalence of thyroid autoantibodies in pregnant women ranges between 5 and 17% (17–21). These asymptomatic euthyroid women with thyroid autoimmunity have been reported to be at risk for four complications during or after pregnancy: increased rates of spontaneous miscarriage and very preterm delivery (<32 weeks gestation), possible development of subclinical hypothyroidism during gestation, and development of postpartum thyroiditis (see Chapter 3, "Thyroiditis").

Several meta-analyses have reported a two- to threefold increase in the spontaneous miscarriage rate early in pregnancy among those euthyroid women who have serum antithyroid antibodies (either antithyroid peroxidase or anti-thyroglobulin) detected in the first trimester (22–24) and approximately double the risk of preterm delivery (23, 25). Risk of miscarriage is also increased in euthyroid women with thyroid autoantibodies who undergo assisted reproduction (26). The mechanism linking thyroid autoimmunity and miscarriage is not known. The presence of antithyroid antibodies either prior to pregnancy or in the first trimester is not correlated with anticardiolipin antibody positivity, which is also known to be associated with pregnancy loss (27, 28). Thyroid autoimmunity may be a marker either for a more generalized activation of the immune system or for subtle changes in maternal/fetal thyroid metabolism. In a small randomized controlled trial, levothyroxine therapy decreased miscarriage rates in euthyroid women with positive serum antithyroid peroxidase antibodies, but the benefit appears to be limited to those women with a serum TSH level in the upper normal reference range (>2.5 mIU/L to < the upper limit of normal) (20, 29).

Euthyroid women with detectable antithyroid antibodies may have slightly higher first trimester serum TSH values, still remaining within the normal range, compared to normal pregnant controls. Despite the decrease in antithyroid antibody titers with pregnancy progression in these antibody positive women, thyroid function parameters have been reported to show a progressive deterioration toward hypothyroidism (18). At term, up to 16% of previously euthyroid women developed mild subclinical hypothyroidism as indicated by an elevated serum TSH level >4mIU/L (30). However, this study was conducted in an area of borderline iodine sufficiency, which may have further compromised maternal thyroid gland reserve. There are no data on the possible development of subclinical hypothyroidism in an iodine-replete antibody positive pregnant population.

HYPOTHYROIDISM

Overt hypothyroidism (elevated TSH and low FT4) is reported to occur in between 0.06% and 0.3% of pregnancies (31, 32). However, the prevalence of subclinical hypothyroidism (elevated TSH and normal FT4) is reported to be significantly higher, affecting 2.2–2.4% of American women screened at 16–18 weeks gestation (32, 33).

Hypothyroxinemia and increased serum TSH levels may occur if true hypothyroidism is present, or if the mother has been overtreated with antithyroid drugs for hyperthyroidism. The obstetric complications that have been associated with hypothyroidism are linked to the decreased maternal thyroid hormone levels that provide a less than optimal environment for both fetal and maternal health. The majority of cases of hypothyroidism are caused by Hashimoto's thyroiditis and prior radioiodine or surgical treatment of Graves' disease. Transient hypothyroidism may occur as part of autoimmune or postpartum thyroiditis, especially if a woman has had a recent miscarriage.

Diagnosis

It is important to diagnose hypothyroidism because of its potential adverse impact on pregnancy (see below Pregnancy Outcome), and yet most patients are relatively asymptomatic. Only 20–30% of women with overt biochemical hypothyroidism have symptoms (34), and complaints of fatigue and weight gain are often attributed to the pregnancy itself. The majority of patients with subclinical hypothyroidism are asymptomatic as well. The diagnosis of hypothyroidism is confirmed by finding an elevated serum TSH concentration, except in the rare instance when hypothyroidism is secondary to pituitary or hypothalamic disease.

There is considerable debate about the merits of universal screening in pregnancy for hypothyroidism. In one prospective randomized trial, women were assigned to either a universal screening group or a case finding group with immediate thyroid function testing being performed in the universal screening group and those in the case finding group thought to be high-risk. Levothyroxine was initiated in those with TSH >2.5 mIU/l who had antithyroid peroxidase antibodies. There was no reduction in primary adverse fetal or obstetric outcomes in those in the universal screening group (19). In a second study, women at less than 16 weeks gestation were randomized to either screening with immediate thyroid tests or postpartum analysis of stored blood for thyroid function. Women with elevated TSH, low T4, or both were treated with levothyroxine. There was no difference in cognitive function of offspring at 3 years (35).

The recently published American Thyroid Association guidelines for the management of thyroid disorders during pregnancy acknowledged that universal screening based upon the current published evidence could not be justified but did recommend targeted case finding in asymptomatic women at high-risk for thyroid disease (36). These include those with symptoms of hypothyroidism, evidence of thyroid autoimmunity because of either a past history of postpartum thyroiditis, prior detection of antithyroid antibodies, or previous treatment for hyperthyroidism, even if they are euthyroid without levothyroxine therapy. In such women, autoimmune damage may not affect basal thyroid hormone output in the nonpregnant state but may impair the thyroid's ability to compensate for the increased production needed during pregnancy. In addition, case finding is also recommended in women over 30 years of age and those with the following: a goiter, potentially decreased thyroid gland synthetic function because of a prior lobectomy or head and neck irradiation, multiple

prior pregnancies, body mass index >40 kg/m², use of drugs affecting the thyroid such as amiodarone or lithium, and recent iodinated contrast exposure as well as those living in areas of iodine insufficiency. Fifteen percent of women with type 1 diabetes may develop clinical hypothyroidism during pregnancy (37) and should therefore also have thyroid function testing. Testing is also recommended for women with other autoimmune disorders, a family history of thyroid or autoimmune disease, prior miscarriage, preterm delivery, or infertility (see the section, Thyroid Autoimmunity and Euthyroidism). In addition, all levothyroxine-replaced hypothyroid women must be monitored during pregnancy (see the section, Treatment) (38). Unfortunately, such targeted case-finding will still miss up to 30% of women with hypothyroidism in the first trimester (39, 40).

Pregnancy outcome

Overt hypothyroidism can be associated with anovulatory cycles and subsequent infertility. However, hypothyroid women may become pregnant and several retrospective case series have investigated maternal gestational outcomes in these women (Table 12.1). The likelihood of complications is correlated with the severity of the hypothyroidism (overt versus subclinical) and the adequacy of maternal treatment (21, 34, 41–47). The majority of women reported in these studies had less than optimal prenatal care as the average initial antenatal visit occurred between 16–20 weeks gestation. In women with subclinical hypothyroidism, the presence of antithyroid antibodies may also influence pregnancy outcomes, with a reported fivefold increase in miscarriage in women with both of these conditions when compared to euthyroid women and a nearly tenfold increase in women at the higher end of the TSH spectrum ($5.22 \leq TSH<10$), when compared to euthyroid women (48).

Thyroid hormone is also necessary for normal fetal neurologic development and the fetal thyroid does not begin to function until 12 weeks of life. It is now evident that maternal T4 crosses the placenta (49). As early as seven weeks gestation, T3 is present in the fetal neurologic tissues, which originates from the transplacental passage of maternal T4 that undergoes intracellular deiodination in the fetal brain (50). The relative contribution of

Table 12.1 Pregnancy complications reported in hypothyroid women

	Subclinical hypothyroidism	Overt hypothyroidism
Spontaneous abortion (21, 46)	10–70%	60%
Pregnancy-induced hypertension/ preeclampsia (34, 42, 44, 45)	0–17%	0–44%
Abruption (21, 42–45)	0%	0–19%
Stillbirth (34, 42–44)	0–3%	0–12%
Anemia (43, 44)	0–2%	0–31%
Postpartum hemorrhage (43–45)	0–17%	0–19%
Preterm birth (low birth weight) (21, 41, 43, 44) majority from premature delivery due to preeclampsia	0–9%	20–31%

maternal thyroid hormone versus fetal thyroid hormone to fetal neurologic development is unknown. In areas of iodine deficiency where both maternal and fetal thyroid status are compromised, neurologic cretinism occurs. In contrast, infants born with congenital hypothyroidism in areas of iodine adequacy have normal neurologic function at birth and postnatal levothyroxine therapy is required to continue normal neuronal maturation. Therefore, it is presumed that the transplacental passage of maternal T4 is sufficient to maintain normal fetal neurologic development in utero.

The contribution of maternal thyroid hormone to the brain maturation of a fetus with intact thyroid function is inadequately understood. Cognitive function is impaired and brain DNA and protein content are decreased in rats born to thyroidectomized mothers and thereby deprived of maternal thyroid hormone (51). These deficits are not as severe if maternal hypothyroidism occurs only during the second half of gestation, when the rat fetal thyroid gland activity is adequate (52). Data in humans are less direct. Although early studies of children born to women who were hypothyroxinemic during pregnancy reported impaired mental development (53), they have been criticized for their lack of accurate biochemical assessment of hypothyroidism. Haddow and colleagues performed neuropsychological testing of 62 children (average age of 8 years) born to women who had elevated serum TSH levels at 17 weeks gestation and compared these to results for 124 control children matched for maternal educational level and age. Children born to hypothyroid women (partially treated or untreated) scored on average four points lower than control children ($p = 0.06$) on the full-scale IQ score of the Wechsler Intelligence Scale for Children. This difference was even more marked, a decrease of seven IQ points ($p = 0.005$), when the subset of 48 children born to untreated hypothyroid mothers was compared to control children (54). Furthermore, the decrease in the IQ score was inversely proportional to the degree of maternal serum TSH elevation (55). Although differences in the post-natal environment cannot be excluded as etiologic factors, these studies strongly suggest that untreated or inadequately treated maternal hypothyroidism during pregnancy adversely affects fetal brain development.

It is less clear whether subclinical hypothyroidism has a significant effect on the fetal brain. In a recent multicenter prospective study, there was no difference in IQ score at 5 years in children whose mothers received levothyroxine therapy for subclinical hypothyroidism and those who did not (56). It should be noted however that therapy began at a median gestation of 16–17 weeks, after the critical window for brain development, which may have contributed to the lack of effect.

Lastly, a very small percentage of women with atrophic Hashimoto's thyroiditis may have antibodies that block thyroidal stimulation by TSH. These antibodies may be detected by assays for TSH receptor-binding inhibitory immunoglobulins (TBII), which assess the ability of maternal immunoglobulin to block TSH binding to the TSH receptor in vitro. Transient congenital hypothyroidism may be caused by the transplacental passage of these antibodies that then block TSH stimulation of the neonatal thyroid, analogous to but opposite of the situation of neonatal Graves' disease. The estimated prevalence of this disorder is 1 in 180,000 births, or 2% of infants with congenital hypothyroidism (57). The antibodies can be measured in both the mother and the neonate, and if present, may indicate that lifelong levothyroxine therapy may not be necessary for the infant.

Treatment

Several studies have documented that levothyroxine requirements increase in many hypothyroid women during pregnancy (7, 21). There are various possible explanations for this increased requirement and each may have relative importance at different times in gestation. In early pregnancy, the concentration of TBG rapidly increases and more thyroid hormone may be needed to saturate binding sites. Glomerular filtration rate increases, resulting in increased iodide clearance. Later, with placental growth, there is increased metabolism of T4 to its inactive metabolite reverse T3 by the high levels of placental Type III deiodinase (10). In addition, there is transplacental passage of T4 (49). Lastly, there may be alterations in the volume of distribution of thyroid hormone because of both gravid physiology and the fetal/placental unit.

For patients initially diagnosed with overt hypothyroidism during pregnancy, a daily dose of 2mcg/kg per day should be started, which is higher than the full replacement dose in the nonpregnant patient and accounts for the higher requirement in pregnancy (31). If the serum TSH is first found to be only minimally elevated (<10mU/L) in pregnancy, a levothyroxine dose of 0.1 mg per day may be adequate. In those with known hypothyroidism taking levothyroxine replacement, the need for dosage adjustment may depend upon the etiology of hypothyroidism, with an increase needed in 76% of women who have undergone prior radioiodine ablation or surgery, but only in 47% who have Hashimoto's thyroiditis (58). Levothyroxine requirements generally increase in the first trimester and persist through gestation. A recent prospective study documented the median time for levothyroxine dosage increase was 8 weeks gestation. However, this was using the upper limit of a nonpregnant TSH reference range (5.0mIU/L) for dosage adjustment (7). If a trimester-specific reference TSH range was used, then it is possible

that the increased requirement would be manifested earlier. In addition, levothyroxine dosage requirements may increase in women who have undergone pharmacologic ovulation stimulation to facilitate pregnancy, likely due to the more precipitous increase in TBG (7). It is also important to remember that 25% of those with initial normal serum TSH levels in the first trimester and 37% of those with initial normal serum TSH concentrations in the second trimester will later require dosage increases (58). The increased dosage requirement appears to plateau after 20 weeks gestation (7). Women with subclinical hypothyroidism who are taking less than the replacement dosages of levothyroxine may not require a dosage increase during gestation because the residual thyroid gland is able to increase synthesis of thyroid hormone. These women may be at increased risk for postpartum thyroiditis, however, see Chapter 3, "Thyroiditis."

Levothyroxine replaced hypothyroid women should have thyroid function monitored as soon as they become pregnant and again every 4–6 weeks in the first half of pregnancy (Table 12.2) (38, 59). There are two schools of recommendations for the adjustment of levothyroxine dosage requirements during pregnancy. The first is to increase the dose only once the serum TSH is abnormal compared to trimester-specific values; pragmatically, the upper limit of 2.5mIU/L may be used during gestation. Kaplan has proposed that the increment in levothyroxine dosage can be based upon the initial degree of TSH elevation. For those with serum TSH levels <10mU/L, the average increase was ~50mcg/day; for those with serum TSH values between 10–20mU/L, ~75mcg/day; and for those with serum TSH values >20mU/L, ~100mcg/day (58). The second is to recommend that women with hypothyroidism be instructed to increase their usual levothyroxine intake by two additional doses each week immediately on confirmation of pregnancy and to contact their health care provider so that a program of TSH-guided dose adjustments can be instituted (7). Patients should be instructed to separate levothyroxine ingestion from that of prenatal vitamins containing iron and especially iron supplements, calcium supplements, and soy products which may interfere with levothyroxine absorption (59, 60). Thyroid function should be rechecked 4–6 weeks after any dose change. The dose may be lowered to pre-pregnancy levels at

Table 12.2 Guidelines for clinical management of maternal hypothyroidism during pregnancy (36, 38, 59)

1.	Optimize levothyroxine dosage prior to pregnancy (TSH 0.5–2.5 mIU/L)
2.	Check serum TSH level as soon as pregnancy is confirmed OR ask patient to increase dose by two tablets a week (assuming once daily dosing) on confirmation of pregnancy
3.	Adjust levothyroxine dosage to maintain a serum TSH level < 2.5mIU/L. Increment in dosage may depend upon etiology of hypothyroidism
	Athyreosis (Graves' after I-131 therapy, thyroid cancer) ~45% increment
	Hashimoto's thyroiditis ~25% increment
	Subclinical hypothyroidism may not require increment
4.	TSH should be monitored every 4–6 weeks in the first half of pregnancy; subsequently, it can be checked every 8 weeks, unless a dose adjustment is made
5.	Patients should be instructed to separate levothyroxine ingestion and prenatal vitamins containing iron, iron or calcium supplements, or soy products by at least 4 hours
6.	After delivery, the levothyroxine dose should be reduced to the pre-pregnancy dosage and the serum TSH level should be rechecked at 6 weeks postpartum

delivery and thyroid function should be measured at the 6-week postpartum visit.

HYPERTHYROIDISM

HCG-associated thyrotoxicosis and hyperemesis gravidarum

A spectrum of hCG-induced hyperthyroidism occurs during pregnancy and this entity has been referred to as "gestational thyrotoxicosis" (61, 62). As previously noted, it is postulated that hCG activates the TSH receptor by a spill-over mechanism because of the molecular similarity between these two glycoproteins (13). Findings range from an isolated subnormal serum TSH concentration (up to 18% of pregnancies) to elevations of free thyroid hormone levels in the clinical setting of hyperemesis gravidarum. In women without symptoms of thyrotoxicosis, the serum TSH level may be subnormal but detectable in approximately 9% and undetectable (<0.05 mU/L) in an additional 9% (63). Systematic screening of 1900 consecutive pregnant women at their initial antenatal visit demonstrated low serum TSH and elevated free T4 levels in 2.4%, half of whom had weight loss, lack of weight gain, or unexplained tachycardia (62). In all these women, normalization of the free T4 paralleled the decrease in hCG.

It has been observed that hyperemesis gravidarum, defined as severe nausea and vomiting in pregnancy resulting in weight loss and fluid and electrolyte disturbances, has been associated with abnormal thyroid function tests. Suppressed serum TSH levels may occur in 60% of these patients, with elevated FT4 levels in almost 50% (64). Serum hCG concentrations correlate positively with the serum FT4 levels and inversely with serum TSH determinations. The magnitude of the deviation from normal values increases with the severity of nausea and vomiting (65). Furthermore, thyroid-stimulating activity, as measured by adenylate cyclase activity per IU of hCG, is reported to be greatest in women with hyperemesis gravidarum when compared to those with occasional or no vomiting (61). The vomiting may be related to the elevated hCG-mediated estradiol production since estradiol levels are higher in hyperemesis subjects than controls, rather than to the thyroid stimulation itself (66).

Similar thyroid hormone changes and emetic symptoms may be present with multiple gestations, which are associated with higher peak and more sustained hCG levels (7, 61). In addition, case reports of mutations in the extracellular domain of the TSH receptor, which result in a two- to threefold increase in activation when exposed to hCG, lead to recurrent or severe gestational thyrotoxicosis and further support the concept of hCG-induced thyrotoxicosis (67, 68).

Gestational thyrotoxicosis is transient and usually resolves within ten weeks of the diagnosis (64). In one study of 44 women with hyperemesis gravidarum, serum FT4 levels normalized by 15 weeks gestation while serum TSH remained suppressed until 19 weeks gestation (69). Clinically, this disorder differs from Graves' disease in several ways: (1) nonautoimmune origin, with negative antithyroid and anti-TSH receptor antibodies (2) absence of goiter and (3) resolution in almost all patients after 20 weeks gestation (70). Hyperthyroid symptoms such as weight loss or lack of normal pregnancy weight gain and tachycardia are present in 50% of women with gestational thyrotoxicosis (62). However, ophthalmopathy, which is autoimmune in origin, is not seen with this disorder. Treatment with antithyroid drugs is not recommended unless coincident Graves' disease is present (38). Patients with hyperemesis who remain symptomatic after 20 weeks gestation with elevated thyroid hormone concentrations and suppressed TSH levels may be considered for antithyroid drug therapy. More than likely, such patients probably have mild Graves' disease.

Graves' disease

Hyperthyroidism is reported to affect 0.17–1% of pregnancies, with Graves' disease accounting for the vast majority of cases (85%), with less common causes being toxic nodular disease in 10% and thyroiditis in 1–2% (71, 72). Autoimmune thyroiditis should also be considered as a possible cause, especially if a woman has had a recent miscarriage, which has been reported to trigger "postpartum" thyroiditis (see Chapter 3, "Thyroiditis") (73).

The activity of Graves' disease fluctuates through pregnancy with TSH receptor antibody (TRAb) patterns generally reflecting the clinical course of the disease (74). TRAb may be elevated in the first trimester, but values often decrease over the second and third trimesters and may become undetectable before increasing again postpartum (75, 76). Clinically, patients may experience relapse or exacerbation of Graves' disease by 10–15 weeks of gestation. However, Graves' disease may remit in the late second and third trimesters, a time of known immune tolerance (77). This disease pattern is thought to be due to decreases in TRAb, as described above, rather than increases in inhibitory anti-TSH receptor antibodies (75). Often, antithyroid drug dosage can be reduced or even discontinued late in gestation, only to be followed by a worsening of the disease in the postpartum period (77).

Graves' disease may affect a pregnancy in three scenarios. First, women may have active Graves' disease (either treated or untreated) that can be exacerbated in the first trimester. Second, women in remission may experience a relapse during pregnancy. Third, Graves' disease may occur for the first time during gestation (5). In women who have been euthyroid throughout pregnancy, but have been treated with antithyroid drugs for Graves' disease previously, hyperthyroidism may recur in the postpartum period. However, this may represent either the thyrotoxic phase of postpartum thyroiditis in up to 25% or relapse of Graves' disease. Even in those with postpartum thyroiditis, Graves' disease may recur after the resolution of postpartum thyroiditis (78).

DIAGNOSIS

The clinical diagnosis of hyperthyroidism may be difficult because pregnancy is itself a hypermetabolic state with symptoms of palpitations and heat intolerance. In addition, patients will usually have increased irritability, decreased exercise tolerance, and fatigue. Patients may describe an inability to control their emotions, with otherwise small irritants culminating in what may be perceived as exaggerated emotional responses. They are aware of increasing shortness of breath climbing stairs. The astute clinician must be cognizant of this constellation of symptoms so that the patient can be appropriately screened for hyperthyroidism. The exam usually reveals the presence of a diffuse goiter, sometimes with a bruit or thrill. Other clinical signs may be present, as described in Chapter 2, "The Diagnostic Evaluation and Management of Hyperthyroidism..."

Laboratory studies reveal a serum TSH level below the trimester-specific 95% lower confidence limit, usually with elevated serum thyroid hormone concentrations above the trimester-specific reference range. However, it must be remembered that up to 50% of women with hyperemesis gravidarum may have a suppressed serum TSH level and/or elevated FT4 (66). An elevated free T3 index or free T3 level may be the most clinically useful test to distinguish hyperthyroid patients from those with hyperemesis gravidarum as less than 15% of hyperemetic women have elevations in these measures (66). TRAb are usually detectable and may also be of diagnostic utility (79). Radioactive iodine uptake scans are contraindicated in pregnancy.

PREGNANCY OUTCOME

Throughout the discussion of the risks and treatment of Graves' disease during pregnancy, it is important to remember that in reality, there are two patients, the mother and the fetus, both of whom are at risk for increased morbidity. Prior to the development of antithyroid drugs (ATD), it was reported that only about 50% of hyperthyroid women were even able to conceive. Of those who conceived, spontaneous miscarriage and premature delivery occurred in half (80). Other maternal complications include increased risk of pregnancy-induced hypertension, preterm labor, congestive heart failure, placental abruption and thyroid storm (81), and other fetal complications including low birth weight, intrauterine growth restriction, stillbirth, fetal/neonatal hyperthyroidism, and central congenital hypothyroidism (82).

The frequency of poor outcomes for both mother and fetus is correlated with the degree and duration of hyperthyroidism, with the highest rates in those women with uncontrolled disease and a decreased risk in those appropriately treated with ATD (Table 12.3) (72, 82, 83). These results highlight the importance of control of maternal hyperthyroidism to ensure optimal pregnancy outcome. Significantly, subclinical hyperthyroidism, defined as a serum TSH level below the 2.5th percentile for gestational age and a normal serum FT4 level, has not been found to be associated with adverse pregnancy outcomes (84).

TREATMENT

Antithyroid Drugs. Antithyroid drugs are the main treatment for Graves' disease during pregnancy. Propylthiouracil (PTU) and methimazole (or carbimazole, available in countries outside the United States) (MMI, Tapazole [Pfizer]/or CMZ) have both been used during gestation. They inhibit thyroid hormone synthesis via a reduction in iodine organification and iodotyrosine coupling (see Chapter 2, "The Diagnostic Evaluation and Management of Hyperthyroidism..."). Pregnancy itself does not appear to alter the maternal pharmacokinetics of MMI, although serum PTU levels may be lower in the latter part of gestation compared to the first and second trimesters (85). PTU is more extensively bound to albumin at physiologic pH, whereas MMI is less bound, which hypothetically might result in increased transplacental passage

of MMI relative to PTU. Historically, PTU was preferred over MMI, partly due to early experimental data suggesting that PTU, which is more highly protein bound than MMI, had more limited transplacental passage than MMI (86). Since then, however, other studies have found that both drugs readily cross the placenta (87, 88). No such data evaluating simultaneous maternal and cord levels are available for MMI.

The goals of treatment of Graves' disease during pregnancy are to control maternal hyperthyroidism with vigilant monitoring of maternal thyroid function and to optimize fetal outcome with careful surveillance of fetal development. Throughout gestation, it is critical that the endocrinologist and obstetrician communicate frequently so that biochemical and clinical parameters may be correlated. Signs of clinical improvement include maternal weight gain and decrease in pulse rate, as well as appropriate fetal growth. For example, if there is a concern because of the lack of maternal weight gain in conjunction with mild elevations in thyroid hormone levels, the initiation of a low dose of ATD should be discussed.

Antithyroid Drugs: Effect on the Fetus. The clinician must assume that both PTU and MMI cross the placenta and may decrease fetal thyroid hormone production. For women with Graves' disease, fetal thyroid status reflects the influence of two maternal factors, both of which cross the placenta: maternal ATD dosage and maternal TRAb activity. Different assays for maternal TRAb exist. The more commonly used radioreceptor assay is the TSH-binding inhibitory immunoglobulin (TBII). This assay does not distinguish between those antibodies that bind to and block the TSH receptor versus those that stimulate the receptor, resulting in increased thyroid hormone production (89). However, in the majority of women with Graves' disease, TBII levels are reported to represent stimulating antibodies and correlate with maternal disease activity (90). The currently available bioassay is the thyroid stimulating immunoglobulin (TSI), which measures the generation of cyclic adenosine monophosphate by cells that express TSH receptor when incubated with the patient's serum (90).

The transplacental passage of maternal TRAb can result in excessive fetal thyroid stimulation. Clinically, this becomes relevant at 24–26 weeks, and maternal levels reflect the degree of fetal exposure (91). There is a strong correlation between

Table 12.3 Pregnancy complications reported in hyperthyroid women

	Controlled hyperthyroidism on ATD therapy	Untreated hyperthyroidism
Miscarriage (133, 134)	8–10%	21%
Preterm delivery (72, 81, 83)	3–14%	21–88%
Preeclampsia (72)	2%	11%
Heart failure (81)	3%	63%
Stillbirth (81, 133)	0%	7–50%
Small for gestational age (83, 118, 134)	less	more
Thyroid storm	less	more

ATD: Antithyroid drug.

maternal and cord TRAb levels at term with the development of neonatal hyperthyroidism (see the section below Fetal/Neonatal Hyperthyroidism). In contrast, the continued use of maternal ATD therapy at term, in conjunction with low maternal TRAb levels may result in elevated serum TSH levels in ~50–60% of infants (90). In this scenario, fetal thyroid function may reflect the relative importance of maternal ATD dosage when maternal immune thyroid stimulation is low. It is possible that in pregnant women with toxic nodules, a dose relationship may be more likely to be seen since there is no contribution of fetal thyroid stimulation by the maternal immune system.

Based on the literature, current maternal thyroid status, rather than ATD dose, is the most reliable marker for titration of ATD therapy to avoid fetal hypothyroidism (92, 93). An analysis of fetal cord FT4 and TSH levels at birth in relation to maternal serum FT4 levels in 249 women with Graves' disease who continued ATD through delivery reported that low fetal cord blood FT4 levels were avoided only when the maternal serum FT4 concentration was > 1.9 ng/dL, although one infant whose mother's serum FT4 level was 2.1 ng/dL developed central congenital hypothyroidism (94). The normal nonpregnant reference range for FT4 in this study was 0.8–1.9 ng/dL (10.3–24.5 pmol/L). However, if the maternal serum free T4 is in the lower two-thirds of the nonpregnant normal reference range, 36% of neonates have a decreased FT4, and a decreased FT4 is found in all neonates if the maternal FT4 is below normal (92).

In addition, overdosage with ATD alone may result in fetal or neonatal goiter, which may cause respiratory distress at birth if markedly enlarged.

Goiter is more frequently described in older reports where concomitant iodide therapy was used. Because of either transplacental ATD or iodide-induced inhibition of fetal thyroid hormone production, fetal serum TSH levels increase, resulting in the stimulation of thyroid growth. A fetal ultrasound should be obtained for all women who are still receiving ATD therapy at 24–26 weeks (74). If a fetal goiter is detected on a late pregnancy ultrasound, the clinician must consider whether this represents fetal hyperthyroidism (see below) or fetal "hypothyroidism" because of transplacental passage of maternal ATD therapy. Intra-uterine growth retardation may occur with either condition, but fetal tachycardia (>160–180 beats per minute) and advanced fetal bone age are highly suggestive of hyperthyroidism (74, 95–97). In cases where neonatal goiter has occurred because of maternal ATD use, resolution usually occurs within the first two weeks of life with the dissipation of the drug (98). Therefore, one approach is to stop maternal ATD therapy and monitor the fetal goiter by ultrasound.

There are several case reports of intra-amniotic levothyroxine injections for treatment of the fetal goiter due to maternal ATD exposure. However, in two reports (99, 100), the injections occurred while the maternal PTU dose was lowered. Therefore, it is difficult to distinguish the relative importance of each factor on the resolution of the fetal goiter. A third case report demonstrated that cessation of maternal ATD therapy alone resulted in a decrease in the fetal goiter documented ultrasonographically (101). In cases of fetal goiter where hypothyroidism is suspected because of transplacental ATD, it may be prudent to discontinue or substantially decrease maternal ATD and follow the goiter with sequential ultrasounds. If reduction in size does not occur within 2–3 weeks, periumbilical blood sampling should be performed to determine fetal thyroid function. If still low, intra-amniotic levothyroxine therapy should be given.

Antithyroid Drugs: Risk of Congenital Malformations. Congenital malformations have been described in the offspring of mothers treated with antithyroid drugs. In a Danish nation-wide cohort study, the odds of birth defects were 66% higher in those exposed to MMI and 41% higher in those exposed to PTU. Aplasia cutis and methimazole embryopathy, characterized by choanal atresia, trachea-esophageal fistula, omphalocele, hypo/athelia, and distinctive facial features were 21 times more common in those exposed to MMI (102). Therefore, despite the potential fulminant maternal hepatotoxicity that can occur with PTU, the FDA in 2010 recommended using it in preference to MMI in the first trimester when ATD therapy is necessary (103). If there is a continued need for ATD therapy beyond the first trimester, MMI may be used at a conversion ratio of 1:20 (MMI:PTU dose) (36).

Antithyroid Drugs: Treatment Guidelines. (Table 12.4) Antithyroid drug dosage should be titrated to maintain maternal serum FT4 levels at or just above the normal limit of the trimester-specific reference range reported by that laboratory, and if not available, the nonpregnant reference range should be used. Alternatively, maternal total T4 can be maintained at the upper limit of the pregnancy-appropriate reference range (1.5 times the nonpregnant reference range) (36, 38). Maternal serum T3 levels may not be as helpful because there is no correlation with fetal thyroid function (92). If the serum TSH does become detectable, it should be kept at or just below the 95% confidence interval trimester-specific lower limit. (38). Therefore, the therapeutic treatment goal for Graves' disease during pregnancy is actually subclinical hyperthyroidism compared to normal pregnant physiology. There are, as mentioned before, no reported gestational adverse effects of maternal subclinical hyperthyroidism (84, 104) and this slight degree of undertreatment of the mother optimizes fetal outcome.

ATD therapy may be stopped preconception or during early pregnancy in women with active Graves' disease who are euthyroid while taking low doses of antithyroid drugs. The decision to stop should take into consideration the duration of disease, goiter size, duration of ATD treatment,

Table 12.4 Guidelines for clinical management of maternal hyperthyroidism during pregnancy (36, 38)

Treatment goal: Subclinical hyperthyroidism	
Free T4:	Use trimester-specific reference range if available, if not use nonpregnant reference range
	Titrate to or just above upper normal limit
Total T4:	Use pregnant reference range (1.5 times nonpregnant reference range)
	Titrate to upper normal limit
TSH:	May consider measuring TSH after 2–3 months
	Titrate at or just below lower trimester-specific limit
1.	Use the lowest dose of ATD to maintain maternal thyroid hormone levels at above targets. PTU is preferred in the 1st trimester because of the MMI-associated embryopathy, with consideration to change back to MMI after 14–16 weeks gestation (1:20 dose ratio MMI:PTU)
2.	Check maternal function tests monthly
3.	ATD dose can usually be lowered or discontinued (30%) by 32–36 weeks gestation
4.	If either high-maintenance ATD doses are required (PTU > 450 mg/day, MMI > 40 mg/day or if a patient is nonadherent or allergic to ATD therapy, surgery (subtotal thyroidectomy) should be considered
5.	Low doses of iodides may be used transiently, especially preoperatively
6.	Frequent communication between the endocrinologist and obstetrician is essential so that ATD dose titration is done with monitoring of fetal growth
7.	TRAb measurement and fetal ultrasound should be considered as discussed in Table 12.6

ATD: Antithyroid drug; PTU: propylthiouracil; MMI: methimazole; TRAb: TSH receptor antibodies.

Table 12.5 Scenarios associated with the likelihood of Graves' recurrence after ATD cessation

Factor	Lower likelihood of recurrence	Higher likelihood of recurrence
Duration of maternal ATD therapy prior to conception	More than 6 months	Less than 6 months
MMI dose	<5–10 mg/day	>10 mg/day
Serum TSH on MMI	Normal	Low
TRAb	Normal or slightly elevated	High levels

TRAb: TSH receptor antibody; ATD: antithyroid drug; MMI: methimazole.

recent TFTs, and TRAb measurement as these factors all predict the likelihood of recurrence (Table 12.5). If ATDs are stopped, TFTs must be frequently assessed every week for the first trimester and every two weeks in the second and third trimesters (36).

The initial ATD dosage may vary depending upon the degree of hyperthyroidism. The median time to normalization of the maternal free T4 index is 7–8 weeks for both PTU and MMI (105), although improvement in parameters may be seen earlier at 3–4 weeks. One should reassess maternal free T4 or total T4 3–4 weeks later and adjust ATD dosage based upon the decrement in thyroid hormone levels. As in nonpregnant women with Graves' disease, maternal serum TSH levels may remain suppressed for several weeks after normalization of thyroid hormone levels, and it is not helpful to monitor the serum TSH early in treatment. Graves' disease may improve in the third trimester and with progressive decreases in ATD dosage throughout pregnancy, therapy may be stopped by 32–34 weeks gestation in 30% of women (106). Of course, the same spectrum of adverse effects related to ATD therapy in the nonpregnant state applies to use during gestation (see Chapter 2, "The Diagnostic Evaluation and Management of Hyperthyroidism...").

Beta-Adrenergic Blockers. Beta-adrenergic blocking agents may be used transiently to control adrenergic symptoms until ATD therapy decreases thyroid hormone levels. There is a report of a higher rate of spontaneous first trimester miscarriages in women who were treated with combined ATD and propranolol therapy compared to ATD alone, although both groups had similar levels of thyroid hormone (107). However, this was a small series and propranolol was prescribed for 6–12 weeks, which may be longer than would be typically necessary for most patients.

Iodides. Chronic use of iodides during pregnancy has been associated with hypothyroidism and goiter in neonates, sometimes resulting in asphyxiation because of tracheal obstruction (85). However, in a recent report, women with Graves' disease were switched from MMI to low dose potassium iodide (10–30 mg/day) during the first trimester of pregnancy at a median gestation of six weeks with maintenance of maternal FT4 levels in the upper half of the nonpregnant reference range and substitution or addition of ATD in the second trimester when necessary. In this study, the offspring showed significantly fewer anomalies when compared to those who remained on MMI and had no thyroid dysfunction or goiter (108). Since the experience with iodides is more limited, iodides should not be used as a first line therapy for women with Graves' disease but could be used transiently if needed in preparation for thyroidectomy.

Surgery. Subtotal thyroidectomy is usually only considered during pregnancy as a therapy for maternal Graves' disease if consistently high levels of ATD (PTU > 450 mg/day, MMI > 40 mg/day) are required to control maternal hyperthyroidism, if a patient is nonadherent or allergic to ATD therapy, or if compressive symptoms exist because of goiter size. Thyroid surgery during pregnancy, regardless of indication, appears to be associated with poorer clinical outcomes than in nonpregnant women (109). If a woman has experienced severe ATD-related side-effects such as agranulocytosis, she should receive transient therapy with supersaturated potassium iodide solution (50–100 mg per day) for 10–14 days prior to surgery. The timing of surgery is usually in the latter half of the second trimester. The rationale for not performing surgery in the first trimester is that this is the time of the highest spontaneous abortion rate and surgery could possibly further increase the risk. However, there are no definitive data supporting an increased miscarriage rate related to the surgical procedure and anesthesia if performed in the first trimester (110), and subtotal thyroidectomy may be done if clinically indicated.

I-131 Therapy. Because of its adverse effects on the fetus, the use of I-131 therapy is completely contraindicated in pregnancy, especially after 12-weeks gestation when the fetal thyroid begins to concentrate radioiodine with an even greater avidity than the maternal thyroid. In addition, other fetal tissues are generally more radiosensitive (111). A pregnancy test should be performed in all women prior to radioiodine therapy. However, inadvertent administration of I-131 in early pregnancy may occur and a survey was sent to endocrinologists regarding their experience with this situation. Of 237 cases, therapeutic abortion was advised and performed for 55 patients. In the remaining 182 pregnancies, the risk of stillbirths, spontaneous abortions, and fetal abnormalities was not higher than the general population (112), perhaps because the fetal whole-body irradiation from a therapeutic I-131 dose for Graves' disease at this stage is below the threshold associated with increased congenital defects (111). However, six infants were hypothyroid at birth, four of whom had intellectual disabilities. I-131 therapy had been given after 12 weeks in three of the mothers of the hypothyroid infants, at a time when the fetal thyroid had already begun to concentrate iodine (112). Therefore, fetal hypothyroidism is more likely to occur if I-131 treatment is given after 12 weeks and congenital defects would be the major concern after I-131 therapy in the early first trimester. Dosimetry studies could quantitate the actual fetal exposure, but experts have suggested that the "relatively low fetal whole-body irradiation is probably not sufficient to justify termination of pregnancy." (111). If inadvertent I-131 therapy has been administered to a pregnant woman, PTU therapy may be initiated within 7 days of I-131, which may reduce I-131 recycling by the fetal thyroid, thereby lowering radiation exposure (111). All infants exposed to maternal I-131 therapy need to be evaluated immediately at birth with the institution of levothyroxine therapy if congenital hypothyroidism is documented. The therapeutic administration of I-131 to a nursing mother is contraindicated and lactation should be stopped immediately if this occurs.

LACTATION

Traditionally, many texts have advised against breast feeding in women treated with ATDs because of the presumption that the ATD was present in breast milk in concentrations sufficient to affect the infant's thyroid. However, over the last two decades, several studies have prospectively monitored thyroid function in infants nursed by mothers taking ATD therapy. PTU is more tightly protein bound than MMI; consequently, the ratio of milk to serum levels is lower for PTU (0.67) (113) than for MMI (1.0) (114). In addition, the amount of ingested drug secreted in breast milk is approximately six times higher for MMI than for PTU (0.14% versus 0.025% of the ingested dose) (113).

Several studies reported no alteration in thyroid function in a total of 56 newborns breast fed by mothers treated with daily doses of PTU (50–300 mg), MMI (5–20 mg), or carbimazole (5–15 mg) for periods ranging from 3 weeks to 8 months. Even in women who were overtreated and developed elevated serum TSH levels, the babies' thyroid function tests remained normal (115). Therefore, ATD therapy may be considered during lactation, although the number of reported infants is small. The drug should be taken by the mother after a feeding. In addition, the theoretic possibility of the infant developing ATD side-effects via ATD ingestion through lactation has not been reported (116).

FETAL/NEONATAL HYPERTHYROIDISM

In women either with active Graves' disease or those with radioiodine-ablated or surgically treated Graves' disease, fetal or neonatal hyperthyroidism is reported to occur in 2% of pregnancies (117). However, there are no data evaluating whether the incidence rate is higher in those with active versus "thyroidectomized" Graves' disease. This disorder is caused by the transplacental passage of maternal TRAb that stimulate fetal thyroid hormone production and may cause goiter. Maternal to fetal IgG transport becomes clinically significant at the end of the second trimester, which is when fetal hyperthyroidism usually becomes apparent. Measurement of maternal TRAb at mid gestation provides prognostic information about the development of fetal Graves' disease (74, 118). However, the measurement of these antibody levels is not standardized and may depend upon the individual laboratory's reference range. Therefore, the magnitude of the TRAb elevation compared to that assay's normal range may be more practical for prediction of fetal/neonatal hyperthyroidism, with values >3 times the upper limit of normal strongly predictive of neonatal hyperthyroidism (119).

Fetal thyroid ultrasound at 32 weeks in screening for clinically relevant fetal thyroid dysfunction has a reported sensitivity of 92% and a specificity of 100% (74). However, if a fetal goiter is detected, fetal hyper- and hypothyroidism must be differentiated. Signs suggestive of fetal hyperthyroidism include intrauterine growth retardation, arrhythmias, congestive heart failure, advanced bone age, craniosynostosis, and hydrops (95, 96). Another suspicious feature is a diffuse Doppler ultrasound signal throughout the thyroid gland (74). Tachycardia (>160 beats per minute) may indicate, but is not always present in, fetal thyrotoxicosis (74). If necessary, periumbilical blood sampling will confirm the diagnosis. Although there are no established normal ranges for fetal thyroid hormone levels, the serum TSH is greater than 20mU/L in the published cases of fetal hypothyroidism (99) or the serum T4 level is markedly elevated in those of fetal hyperthyroidism (120, 121). Periumbilical blood sampling has risks of fetal bleeding, bradycardia, infection, and death (99) and is usually not indicated as the diagnosis can often be made clinically. A rational approach for the detection of fetal and neonatal hyperthyroidism using TRAb measurement and fetal ultrasound is presented in Table 12.6.

Treatment of fetal hyperthyroidism is accomplished by giving the mother ATD therapy, which then crosses the placenta and inhibits fetal thyroid hormone synthesis. The dose can then be titrated to maintain a normal fetal heart rate. In a woman who has received prior radioablation or surgery for Graves' disease, levothyroxine therapy may have to be initiated or increased if maternal hypothyroxinemia occurs. Since TRAb levels usually decline toward term, ATD dosage can be decreased as fetal heart rate and growth are monitored.

If antibody levels remain elevated at term, the risk of neonatal hyperthyroidism is increased. A recent study measured cord TRAb level in infants born to mothers on ATD therapy at term as a predictor of neonatal Graves' disease. If the cord TRAb level was negative, none of the infants developed neonatal Graves'. However, if the cord TRAb level was elevated at twofold the upper normal limit, neonatal Graves' occurred in 28% of infants at a mean age of 5 days (122) because the manifestations of hyperthyroidism may be masked until the dissipation of maternal ATD.

ATD therapy is necessary for treatment of neonatal Graves' disease. As maternal antibody levels decrease over the first 3 months of life, therapy can usually be discontinued (123).

Table 12.6 TRAb measurement and fetal ultrasound to predict fetal thyroid dysfunction (74, 135)

	Graves' disease on ATD therapy	Graves' disease after I-131 therapy or thyroidectomy	Graves' disease in remission on no therapy
Maternal TRAb measurement	YES	YES	NO
Timing of TRAb measurement	• Early in pregnancy for disease activity • Mid trimester for prediction of fetal thyrotoxicosis • 30–34 weeks (if positive mid trimester) for prediction of neonatal thyrotoxicosis	End of 1st trimester If negative: no repeat If positive: repeat at mid trimester	

If mother is TRAb + or taking ATD ⟶ Fetal ultrasound in 2nd half of pregnancy to check for fetal goiter, tachycardia, and bone age.

TRAb: TSH receptor antibody; ATD: Antithyroid drug.

THYROID NODULES AND THYROID CANCER

Although goiter may occur during pregnancy in areas of borderline iodine deficiency (124), thyroid size does not increase in iodine replete areas (125). The prevalence of nodules has been reported to be higher in middle-aged women with a history of three or more prior pregnancies (126), but solitary thyroid nodules or thyroid cancer do not arise *de novo* more frequently during pregnancy. The detection of thyroid nodules in pregnant women usually reflects the careful examination by an obstetrician of a healthy pregnant woman who had not regularly seen a physician prior to her conception.

As in the nonpregnant patient (see Chapter 7, "Thyroid Nodules and Multinodular Goiter"), diagnostic thyroid ultrasound for nodule characterization and fine-needle aspiration (FNA) as indicated should be performed for diagnosis in nodules identified during pregnancy (127); the spectrum of cytological results is the same as in the nonpregnant patient (128). Radioactive iodine scanning is contraindicated at this time, but ultrasound can be performed either for characterization and monitoring of the nodule or for guidance of the FNA. Nodules with a benign cytology may be observed, and those with cytological diagnoses of atypia of undetermined significance/follicular lesion of undetermined significance (AUS/FLUS) or follicular neoplasm may require further evaluation and probable surgery after delivery.

If the FNA cytology shows evidence of a thyroid cancer, surgery is recommended. However, the timing of surgery, either during or after pregnancy, is debatable, with some recommending surgery during the mid-trimester (128) and others advocating waiting until after delivery (129). One study has reported no significant difference in recurrence or survival rates between women with malignant nodules who had surgery either during or after pregnancy (130). Furthermore, thyroid cancer discovered during pregnancy is not more aggressive than that found in a similarly aged group of nonpregnant women (129). For women with previously treated thyroid cancer, most reports confirm that subsequent pregnancy does not increase recurrence rates (131). However, if a woman has locoregional residual/recurrent disease in the cervical lymph nodes, there is a small likelihood of progression (132).

For a nodule with malignant cytology suggestive of differentiated thyroid cancer, the recently published American Thyroid Association guidelines recommend that "if discovered early in pregnancy, [it] should be monitored sonographically and if it grows substantially by 24–26 weeks gestation, or if cytologically malignant cervical lymph nodes are present, surgery should be considered during pregnancy. However, if the disease remains stable by midgestation or if it is diagnosed in the second half of pregnancy, surgery may be deferred until after delivery" (36). Immediate surgery should be considered for medullary and anaplastic thyroid cancer.

In women with differentiated thyroid cancer who do not undergo immediate surgery, levothyroxine therapy may be considered to maintain the serum TSH level in the lower half of the normal range (0.3–2.0mIU/L), which would theoretically slow TSH-responsive tumor growth and should not be associated with pregnancy complications. Radioactive iodine therapy, if needed, must be delayed until the postpartum period.

REFERENCES

1. Moleti M, Trimarchi F, Vermiglio F. Thyroid physiology in pregnancy. *Endocr. Pract.* 2014;20(6):589–96.
2. Ain KB, Mori Y, Refetoff S. Reduced clearance rate of thyroxine-binding globulin (TBG) with increased sialylation: A mechanism for estrogen-induced elevation of serum TBG concentration. *J. Clin. Endocrinol. Metab.* 1987;65(4):689–96.
3. Korevaar TIM, Medici M, Visser TJ, et al. Thyroid disease in pregnancy: New insights in diagnosis and clinical management. *Nat. Rev. Endocrinol.* 2017;13(10):610–22.
4. Demers LM, Spencer CA. Laboratory medicine practice guidelines: Laboratory support for the diagnosis and monitoring of thyroid disease. *Clin. Endocrinol. (Oxf).* 2003;58(2):138–40.
5. Chan GW, Mandel SJ. Therapy insight: Management of Graves' disease during pregnancy. *Nat. Clin. Pract. Endocrinol. Metab.* 2007;3(6):470–8.

6. Glinoer D, de Nayer P, Bourdoux P, et al. Regulation of maternal thyroid during pregnancy. *J. Clin. Endocrinol. Metab.* 1990;71(2):276–87.

7. Alexander EK, Marqusee E, Lawrence J, et al. Timing and magnitude of increases in levothyroxine requirements during pregnancy in women with hypothyroidism. *N. Engl. J. Med.* 2004;351(3):241–9.

8. Loh JA, Wartofsky L, Jonklaas J, et al. The magnitude of increased levothyroxine requirements in hypothyroid pregnant women depends upon the etiology of the hypothyroidism. *Thyroid* 2009;19(3):269–75.

9. Glinoer D, Delange F, Laboureur I, et al. Maternal and neonatal thyroid function at birth in an area of marginally low iodine intake. *J. Clin. Endocrinol. Metab.* 1992;75(3):800–5.

10. Burrow GN, Fisher DA, Larsen PR. Maternal and fetal thyroid function. *N. Engl. J. Med.* 1994;331(16):1072–8.

11. Mandel SJ, Spencer CA, Hollowell JG. Are detection and treatment of thyroid insufficiency in pregnancy feasible? *Thyroid* 2005;15(1):44–53.

12. Lambert-Messerlian G, McClain M, Haddow JE, et al. First- and second-trimester thyroid hormone reference data in pregnant women: A FaSTER (First- and Second-Trimester Evaluation of Risk for aneuploidy) Research Consortium study. *Am. J. Obstet. Gynecol.* 2008;199(1):62 e1–6.

13. Yoshimura M, Hershman JM. Thyrotropic action of human chorionic gonadotropin. *Thyroid* 1995;5(5):425–34.

14. Medici M, Korevaar TI, Visser WE, et al. Thyroid function in pregnancy: What is normal? *Clin. Chem.* 2015;61(5):704–13.

15. Korevaar TI, Medici M, de Rijke YB, et al. Ethnic differences in maternal thyroid parameters during pregnancy: The Generation R study. *J. Clin. Endocrinol. Metab.* 2013;98(9):3678–86.

16. Nelson M, Wickus GG, Caplan RH, et al. Thyroid gland size in pregnancy. An ultrasound and clinical study. *J. Reprod. Med.* 1987;32 (12):888–90.

17. Ashoor G, Maiz N, Rotas M, et al. Maternal thyroid function at 11 to 13 weeks of gestation and subsequent fetal death. *Thyroid* 2010;20(9):989–93.

18. Negro R, Formoso G, Mangieri T, et al. Levothyroxine treatment in euthyroid pregnant women with autoimmune thyroid disease: Effects on obstetrical complications. *J. Clin. Endocrinol. Metab.* 2006;91(7):2587–91.

19. Negro R, Schwartz A, Gismondi R, et al. Universal screening versus case finding for detection and treatment of thyroid hormonal dysfunction during pregnancy. *J. Clin. Endocrinol. Metab.* 2010;95(4):1699–707.

20. Nazarpour S, Ramezani Tehrani F, Simbar M, et al. Effects of levothyroxine treatment on pregnancy outcomes in pregnant women with autoimmune thyroid disease. *Eur. J. Endocrinol.* 2017;176(2):253–65.

21. Abalovich M, Gutierrez S, Alcaraz G, et al. Overt and subclinical hypothyroidism complicating pregnancy. *Thyroid* 2002;12(1):63–8.

22. Chen L, Hu R. Thyroid autoimmunity and miscarriage: A meta-analysis. *Clin. Endocrinol. (Oxf).* 2011;74(4):513–9.

23. Thangaratinam S, Tan A, Knox E, et al. Association between thyroid autoantibodies and miscarriage and preterm birth: Meta-analysis of evidence. *BMJ* 2011;342:d2616.

24. Prummel MF, Wiersinga WM. Thyroid autoimmunity and miscarriage. *Eur. J. Endocrinol.* 2004;150(6):751–5.

25. He X, Wang P, Wang Z, et al. Thyroid antibodies and risk of preterm delivery: A meta-analysis of prospective cohort studies. *Eur. J. Endocrinol.* 2012;167(4):455–64.

26. Toulis KA, Goulis DG, Venetis CA, et al. Risk of spontaneous miscarriage in euthyroid women with thyroid autoimmunity undergoing IVF: A meta-analysis. *Eur. J. Endocrinol.* 2010;162(4):643–52.

27. Stagnaro-Green A, Roman SH, Cobin RH, et al. Detection of at-risk pregnancy by means of highly sensitive assays for thyroid autoantibodies. *JAMA* 1990;264(11):1422–5.

28. Pratt D, Novotny M, Kaberlein G, et al. Antithyroid antibodies and the association with non-organ-specific antibodies in recurrent pregnancy loss. *Am. J. Obstet. Gynecol.* 1993;168(3 Pt 1):837–41.

29. Negro R, Schwartz A, Stagnaro-Green A. Impact of levothyroxine in miscarriage and preterm delivery rates in first trimester thyroid antibody-positive women with TSH less than 2.5 mIU/L. *J. Clin. Endocrinol. Metab.* 2016;101(10):3685–90.

30. Glinoer D, Riahi M, Grun JP, et al. Risk of subclinical hypothyroidism in pregnant women with asymptomatic autoimmune thyroid disorders. *J. Clin. Endocrinol. Metab.* 1994;79(1):197–204.

31. Montoro MN. Management of hypothyroidism during pregnancy. *Clin. Obstet. Gynecol.* 1997;40(1):65–80.

32. Cleary-Goldman J, Malone FD, Lambert-Messerlian G, et al. Maternal thyroid hypofunction and pregnancy outcome. *Obstet. Gynecol.* 2008;112(1):85–92.

33. Klein RZ, Haddow JE, Faix JD, et al. Prevalence of thyroid deficiency in pregnant women. *Clin. Endocrinol. (Oxf).* 1991;35(1):41–6.

34. Montoro M, Collea JV, Frasier SD, et al. Successful outcome of pregnancy in women with hypothyroidism. *Ann. Intern. Med.* 1981;94(1):31–4.

35. Lazarus JH, Bestwick JP, Channon S, et al. Antenatal thyroid screening and childhood cognitive function. *N. Engl. J. Med.* 2012;366(6):493–501.

36. Alexander EK, Pearce EN, Brent GA, et al. 2017 Guidelines of the American Thyroid Association for the diagnosis and management of thyroid disease during pregnancy and the postpartum. *Thyroid* 2017;27(3):315–89.

37. Jovanovic-Peterson L, Peterson CM. De novo clinical hypothyroidism in pregnancies complicated by type I diabetes, subclinical hypothyroidism, and proteinuria: A new syndrome. *Am. J. Obstet. Gynecol.* 1988;159(2):442–6.

38. Abalovich M, Amino N, Barbour LA, et al. Management of thyroid dysfunction during pregnancy and postpartum: An Endocrine Society Clinical Practice Guideline. *J. Clin. Endocrinol. Metab.* 2007;92(8 Suppl):S1–47.

39. Vaidya B, Anthony S, Bilous M, et al. Detection of thyroid dysfunction in early pregnancy: Universal screening or targeted high-risk case finding? *J. Clin. Endocrinol. Metab.* 2007;92(1):203–7.

40. Nazarpour S, Tehrani FR, Simbar M, et al. Comparison of universal screening with targeted high-risk case finding for diagnosis of thyroid disorders. *Eur. J. Endocrinol.* 2016;174(1):77–83.

41. Stagnaro-Green A, Chen X, Bogden JD, et al. The thyroid and pregnancy: A novel risk factor for very preterm delivery. *Thyroid* 2005;15(4):351–7.

42. Allan WC, Haddow JE, Palomaki GE, et al. Maternal thyroid deficiency and pregnancy complications: Implications for population screening. *J. Med. Screen.* 2000;7(3):127–30.

43. Leung AS, Millar LK, Koonings PP, et al. Perinatal outcome in hypothyroid pregnancies. *Obstet. Gynecol.* 1993;81(3):349–53.

44. Davis LE, Leveno KJ, Cunningham FG. Hypothyroidism complicating pregnancy. *Obstet. Gynecol.* 1988;72(1):108–12.

45. Wasserstrum N, Anania CA. Perinatal consequences of maternal hypothyroidism in early pregnancy and inadequate replacement. *Clin. Endocrinol. (Oxf)* 1995;42(4):353–8.

46. Glinoer D. The regulation of thyroid function in pregnancy: Pathways of endocrine adaptation from physiology to pathology. *Endocr. Rev.* 1997;18(3):404–33.

47. Chan S, Boelaert K. Optimal management of hypothyroidism, hypothyroxinaemia and euthyroid TPO antibody positivity preconception and in pregnancy. *Clin. Endocrinol. (Oxf).* 2015;82(3):313–26.

48. Liu H, Shan Z, Li C, et al. Maternal subclinical hypothyroidism, thyroid autoimmunity, and the risk of miscarriage: A prospective cohort study. *Thyroid* 2014;24(11):1642–9.

49. Vulsma T, Gons MH, de Vijlder JJ. Maternal-fetal transfer of thyroxine in congenital hypothyroidism due to a total organification defect or thyroid agenesis. *N. Engl. J. Med.* 1989;321(1):13–6.

50. Calvo RM, Jauniaux E, Gulbis B, et al. Fetal tissues are exposed to biologically relevant free thyroxine concentrations during early phases of development. *J. Clin. Endocrinol. Metab.* 2002;87(4):1768–77.

51. Porterfield SP, Hendrich CE. The role of thyroid hormones in prenatal and neonatal neurological development—Current perspectives. *Endocr. Rev.* 1993;14(1):94–106.

52. Bonet B, Herrera E. Different response to maternal hypothyroidism during the first and second half of gestation in the rat. *Endocrinology* 1988;122(2):450–5.

53. Man EB, Brown JF, Serunian SA. Maternal hypothyroxinemia: Psychoneurological deficits of progeny. *Ann. Clin. Lab. Sci.* 1991;21(4):227–39.

54. Haddow JE, Palomaki GE, Allan WC, et al. Maternal thyroid deficiency during pregnancy and subsequent neuropsychological development of the child. *N. Engl. J. Med.* 1999;341(8):549–55.

55. Klein RZ, Sargent JD, Larsen PR, et al. Relation of severity of maternal hypothyroidism to cognitive development of offspring. *J. Med. Screen.* 2001;8(1):18–20.

56. Casey BM, Thom EA, Peaceman AM, et al. Treatment of subclinical hypothyroidism or hypothyroxinemia in pregnancy. *N. Engl. J. Med.* 2017;376(9):815–25.

57. Brown RS, Bellisario RL, Botero D, et al. Incidence of transient congenital hypothyroidism due to maternal thyrotropin receptor-blocking antibodies in over one million babies. *J. Clin. Endocrinol. Metab.* 1996;81(3):1147–51.

58. Kaplan MM. Assessment of thyroid function during pregnancy. *Thyroid* 1992;2(1):57–61.

59. Mandel SJ. Hypothyroidism and chronic autoimmune thyroiditis in the pregnant state: Maternal aspects. *Best Pract. Res. Clin. Endocrinol. Metab.* 2004;18(2):213–24.

60. Campbell NR, Hasinoff BB, Stalts H, et al. Ferrous sulfate reduces thyroxine efficacy in patients with hypothyroidism. *Ann. Intern. Med.* 1992;117(12):1010–3.

61. Kimura M, Amino N, Tamaki H, et al. Gestational thyrotoxicosis and hyperemesis gravidarum: Possible role of hCG with higher stimulating activity. *Clin. Endocrinol. (Oxf).* 1993;38(4):345–50.

62. Glinoer D. Thyroid hyperfunction during pregnancy. *Thyroid* 1998;8(9):859–64.

63. Glinoer D, De Nayer P, Robyn C, et al. Serum levels of intact human chorionic gonadotropin (HCG) and its free alpha and beta subunits, in relation to maternal thyroid stimulation during normal pregnancy. *J. Endocrinol. Invest.* 1993;16(11):881–8.

64. Goodwin TM, Montoro M, Mestman JH. Transient hyperthyroidism and hyperemesis gravidarum: Clinical aspects. *Am. J. Obstet. Gynecol.* 1992;167(3):648–52.

65. Mori M, Amino N, Tamaki H, et al. Morning sickness and thyroid function in normal pregnancy. *Obstet. Gynecol.* 1988;72(3 Pt 1):355–9.

66. Goodwin TM, Montoro M, Mestman JH, et al. The role of chorionic gonadotropin in transient hyperthyroidism of hyperemesis gravidarum. *J. Clin. Endocrinol. Metab.* 1992;75(5):1333–7.

67. Rodien P, Bremont C, Sanson ML, et al. Familial gestational hyperthyroidism caused by a mutant thyrotropin receptor hypersensitive to human chorionic gonadotropin. *N. Engl. J. Med.* 1998;339(25):1823–6.

68. Coulon AL, Savagner F, Briet C, et al. Prolonged and severe gestational thyrotoxicosis due to enhanced hCG sensitivity of a mutant thyrotropin receptor. *J. Clin. Endocrinol. Metab.* 2016;101(1):10–1.

69. Tan JY, Loh KC, Yeo GS, et al. Transient hyperthyroidism of hyperemesis gravidarum. *BJOG* 2002;109(6):683–8.

70. Goodwin TM, Hershman JM. Hyperthyroidism due to inappropriate production of human chorionic gonadotropin. *Clin. Obstet. Gynecol.* 1997;40(1):32–44.

71. Stagnaro-Green A. Overt hyperthyroidism and hypothyroidism during pregnancy. *Clin. Obstet. Gynecol.* 2011;54(3):478–87.

72. Millar LK, Wing DA, Leung AS, et al. Low birth weight and preeclampsia in pregnancies complicated by hyperthyroidism. *Obstet. Gynecol.* 1994;84(6):946–9.

73. Marqusee E, Hill JA, Mandel SJ. Thyroiditis after pregnancy loss. *J. Clin. Endocrinol. Metab.* 1997;82(8):2455–7.

74. Luton D, Le Gac I, Vuillard E, et al. Management of Graves' disease during pregnancy: The key role of fetal thyroid gland monitoring. *J. Clin. Endocrinol. Metab.* 2005;90(11):6093–8.

75. Amino N, Izumi Y, Hidaka Y, et al. No increase of blocking type anti-thyrotropin receptor antibodies during pregnancy in patients with Graves' disease. *J. Clin. Endocrinol. Metab.* 2003;88(12):5871–4.

76. Zakarija M, McKenzie JM. Pregnancy-associated changes in the thyroid-stimulating antibody of Graves' disease and the relationship to neonatal hyperthyroidism. *J. Clin. Endocrinol. Metab.* 1983;57(5):1036–40.

77. Amino N, Tanizawa O, Mori H, et al. Aggravation of thyrotoxicosis in early pregnancy and after delivery in Graves' disease. *J. Clin. Endocrinol. Metab.* 1982;55(1):108–12.

78. Momotani N, Noh J, Ishikawa N, et al. Relationship between silent thyroiditis and recurrent Graves' disease in the postpartum period. *J. Clin. Endocrinol. Metab.* 1994;79(1):285–9.

79. Bucci I, Giuliani C, Napolitano G. Thyroid-stimulating hormone receptor antibodies in pregnancy: Clinical relevance. *Front. Endocrinol. (Lausanne).* 2017;8:137.

80. Gardiner-Hill H. Pregnancy complicating simple goiter and Graves' disease. *Lancet* 1929;1:120–4.

81. Davis LE, Lucas MJ, Hankins GD, et al. Thyrotoxicosis complicating pregnancy. *Am. J. Obstet. Gynecol.* 1989;160(1):63–70.

82. Kempers MJ, van Tijn DA, van Trotsenburg AS, et al. Central congenital hypothyroidism due to gestational hyperthyroidism: Detection where prevention failed. *J. Clin. Endocrinol. Metab.* 2003;88(12):5851–7.

83. Aggarawal N, Suri V, Singla R, et al. Pregnancy outcome in hyperthyroidism: A case control study. *Gynecol. Obstet. Invest.* 2014;77(2):94–9.

84. Casey BM, Dashe JS, Wells CE, et al. Subclinical hyperthyroidism and pregnancy outcomes. *Obstet. Gynecol.* 2006;107(2 Pt 1):337–41.

85. Mandel SJ, Brent GA, Larsen PR. Review of antithyroid drug use during pregnancy and report of a case of aplasia cutis. *Thyroid* 1994;4(1):129–33.

86. Marchant B, Brownlie BE, Hart DM, et al. The placental transfer of propylthiouracil, methimazole and carbimazole. *J. Clin. Endocrinol. Metab.* 1977;45(6):1187–93.

87. Gardner DF, Cruikshank DP, Hays PM, et al. Pharmacology of propylthiouracil (PTU) in pregnant hyperthyroid women: Correlation of maternal PTU concentrations with cord serum thyroid function tests. *J. Clin. Endocrinol. Metab.* 1986;62(1):217–20.

88. Mortimer RH, Cannell GR, Addison RS, et al. Methimazole and propylthiouracil equally cross the perfused human term placental lobule. *J. Clin. Endocrinol. Metab.* 1997;82(9):3099–102.

89. Davies TF, Roti E, Braverman LE, et al. Thyroid controversy—Stimulating antibodies. *J. Clin. Endocrinol. Metab.* 1998;83(11):3777–85.

90. Mortimer RH, Tyack SA, Galligan JP, et al. Graves' disease in pregnancy: TSH receptor binding inhibiting immunoglobulins and maternal and neonatal thyroid function. *Clin. Endocrinol. (Oxf).* 1990;32(2):141–52.

91. Fisher DA. Fetal thyroid function: Diagnosis and management of fetal thyroid disorders. *Clin. Obstet. Gynecol.* 1997;40(1):16–31.

92. Momotani N, Noh J, Oyanagi H, et al. Antithyroid drug therapy for Graves' disease during pregnancy. Optimal regimen for fetal thyroid status. *N. Engl. J. Med.* 1986;315(1):24–8.

93. Bliddal S, Rasmussen AK, Sundberg K, et al. Antithyroid drug-induced fetal goitrous hypothyroidism. *Nat. Rev. Endocrinol.* 2011;7(7):396–406.

94. Momotani N, Iwama S, Noh J, et al., editors. Anti-thyroid drug therapy for Graves' disease during pregnancy: Mildest thyrotoxic maternal free thyroxine concentrations to avoid fetal hypothyroidism. 77th Annual Meeting of the American Thyroid Association; 2006 October 11–15; Phoenix, AZ.

95. Chopra IJ. Fetal and neonatal hyperthyroidism. *Thyroid* 1992;2(2):161–3.

96. Nachum Z, Rakover Y, Weiner E, et al. Graves' disease in pregnancy: Prospective evaluation of a selective invasive treatment protocol. *Am. J. Obstet. Gynecol.* 2003;189(1):159–65.

97. Huel C, Guibourdenche J, Vuillard E, et al. Use of ultrasound to distinguish between fetal hyperthyroidism and hypothyroidism on discovery of a goiter. *Ultrasound Obstet. Gynecol.* 2009;33(4):412–20.

98. Cheron RG, Kaplan MM, Larsen PR, et al. Neonatal thyroid function after propylthiouracil therapy for maternal Graves' disease. *N. Engl. J. Med.* 1981;304(9):525–8.

99. Davidson KM, Richards DS, Schatz DA, et al. Successful in utero treatment of fetal goiter and hypothyroidism. *N. Engl. J. Med.* 1991;324(8):543–6.

100. Van Loon AJ, Derksen JT, Bos AF, et al. In utero diagnosis and treatment of fetal goitrous hypothyroidism, caused by maternal use of propylthiouracil. *Prenat. Diagn.* 1995;15(7):599–604.

101. Ochoa-Maya MR, Frates MC, Lee-Parritz A, et al. Resolution of fetal goiter after discontinuation of propylthiouracil in a pregnant woman with Graves' hyperthyroidism. *Thyroid* 1999;9(11):1111–4.

102. Andersen SL, Olsen J, Wu CS, et al. Birth defects after early pregnancy use of antithyroid drugs: A Danish nationwide study. *J. Clin. Endocrinol. Metab.* 2013;98(11):4373–81.

103. FDA Drug Safety Communication: New Boxed Warning on severe liver injury with propylthiouracil 2010 [cited 2017 December 14, 2017]. Available from: https://www.fda.gov/Drugs/DrugSafety/PostmarketDrugSafetyInformationforPatientsandProviders/ucm209023.htm.

104. Casey BM. Subclinical hypothyroidism and pregnancy. *Obstet. Gynecol. Surv.* 2006;61(6):415–20.

105. Wing DA, Millar LK, Koonings PP, et al. A comparison of propylthiouracil versus methimazole in the treatment of hyperthyroidism in pregnancy. *Am. J. Obstet. Gynecol.* 1994; 170 (1 Pt 1): 90–5.

106. Mestman JH. Hyperthyroidism in pregnancy. *Clin. Obstet. Gynecol.* 1997;40(1):45–64.

107. Sherif IH, Oyan WT, Bosairi S, et al. Treatment of hyperthyroidism in pregnancy. *Acta Obstet. Gynecol. Scand.* 1991;70(6):461–3.

108. Yoshihara A, Noh JY, Watanabe N, et al. Substituting potassium iodide for methimazole as the treatment for Graves' disease during the first trimester may reduce the incidence of congenital anomalies: A retrospective study at a single medical institution in Japan. *Thyroid* 2015;25(10):1155–61.

109. Kuy S, Roman SA, Desai R, et al. Outcomes following thyroid and parathyroid surgery in pregnant women. *Arch. Surg.* 2009;144(5):399–406.

110. Brodsky JB, Cohen EN, Brown BW, Jr., et al. Surgery during pregnancy and fetal outcome. *Am. J. Obstet. Gynecol.* 1980;138(8):1165–7.

111. Masiukiewicz US, Burrow GN. Hyperthyroidism in pregnancy: Diagnosis and treatment. *Thyroid* 1999;9(7):647–52.

112. Stoffer SS, Hamburger JI. Inadvertent 131I therapy for hyperthyroidism in the first trimester of pregnancy. *J. Nucl. Med.* 1976;17(02):146–9.

113. Kampmann JP, Johansen K, Hansen JM, et al. Propylthiouracil in human milk. Revision of a dogma. *Lancet* 1980;1(8171):736–7.

114. Johansen K, Andersen AN, Kampmann JP, et al. Excretion of methimazole in human milk. *Eur. J. Clin. Pharmacol.* 1982;23(4):339–41.

115. Azizi F, Khoshniat M, Bahrainian M, et al. Thyroid function and intellectual development of infants nursed by mothers taking methimazole. *J. Clin. Endocrinol. Metab.* 2000;85(9):3233–8.

116. Mandel SJ, Cooper DS. The use of antithyroid drugs in pregnancy and lactation. *J. Clin. Endocrinol. Metab.* 2001;86(6):2354–9.

117. Leger J. Management of fetal and neonatal Graves' disease. *Horm. Res. Paediatr.* 2017;87(1):1–6.

118. Mitsuda N, Tamaki H, Amino N, et al. Risk factors for developmental disorders in infants born to women with Graves disease. *Obstet. Gynecol.* 1992;80(3 Pt 1): 359–64.

119. Abeillon-du Payrat J, Chikh K, Bossard N, et al. Predictive value of maternal second-generation thyroid-binding inhibitory immunoglobulin assay for neonatal autoimmune hyperthyroidism. *Eur. J. Endocrinol.* 2014;171(4):451–60.

120. Porreco RP, Bloch CA. Fetal blood sampling in the management of intrauterine thyrotoxicosis. *Obstet. Gynecol.* 1990;76(3 Pt 2):509–12.

121. Wenstrom KD, Weiner CP, Williamson RA, et al. Prenatal diagnosis of fetal hyperthyroidism using funipuncture. *Obstet. Gynecol.* 1990;76(3 Pt 2):513–7.

122. Besancon A, Beltrand J, Le Gac I, et al. Management of neonates born to women with Graves' disease: A cohort study. *Eur. J. Endocrinol.* 2014;170(6):855–62.

123. Skuza KA, Sills IN, Stene M, et al. Prediction of neonatal hyperthyroidism in infants born to mothers with Graves disease. *J. Pediatr.* 1996;128(2):264–8.

124. Rasmussen NG, Hornnes PJ, Hegedus L. Ultrasonographically determined thyroid size in pregnancy and post partum: The goitrogenic effect of pregnancy. *Am. J. Obstet. Gynecol.* 1989;160(5 Pt 1):1216–20.

125. Berghout A, Endert E, Ross A, et al. Thyroid function and thyroid size in normal pregnant women living in an iodine replete area. *Clin. Endocrinol. (Oxf).* 1994;41(3):375–9.

126. Struve CW, Haupt S, Ohlen S. Influence of frequency of previous pregnancies on the prevalence of thyroid nodules in women without clinical evidence of thyroid disease. *Thyroid* 1993;3(1):7–9.

127. Cooper DS, Doherty GM, Haugen BR, et al. Management guidelines for patients with thyroid nodules and differentiated thyroid cancer. *Thyroid* 2006;16(2):109–42.

128. Tan GH, Gharib H, Goellner JR, et al. Management of thyroid nodules in pregnancy. *Arch. Intern. Med.* 1996;156(20):2317–20.

129. Herzon FS, Morris DM, Segal MN, et al. Coexistent thyroid cancer and pregnancy. *Arch. Otolaryngol. Head Neck Surg.* 1994;120(11):1191–3.

130. Moosa M, Mazzaferri EL. Outcome of differentiated thyroid cancer diagnosed in pregnant women. *J. Clin. Endocrinol. Metab.* 1997;82(9):2862–6.

131. Rosen IB, Korman M, Walfish PG. Thyroid nodular disease in pregnancy: Current diagnosis and management. *Clin. Obstet. Gynecol.* 1997;40(1):81–9.

132. Rakhlin L, Fish S, Tuttle RM. Response to therapy status is an excellent predictor of pregnancy-associated structural disease progression in patients previously treated for differentiated thyroid cancer. *Thyroid* 2017;27(3):396–401.

133. Mestman JH, Manning PR, Hodgman J. Hyperthyroidism and pregnancy. *Arch. Intern. Med.* 1974;134(3):434–9.

134. Sugrue D, Drury MI. Hyperthyroidism complicating pregnancy: Results of treatment by antithyroid drugs in 77 pregnancies. *Br. J. Obstet. Gynaecol.* 1980;87(11):970–5.

135. Laurberg P, Nygaard B, Glinoer D, et al. Guidelines for TSH-receptor antibody measurements in pregnancy: Results of an evidence-based symposium organized by the European Thyroid Association. *Eur. J. Endocrinol.* 1998;139(6):584–6.

Index

AACE, *see* American Association of Clinical Endocrinologists

ACR, *see* American College of Radiology

Acute infectious thyroiditis, 88

Addison's disease, 45

Advanced thyroid cancer, therapies for
external beam radiation therapy, 203–204
imaging
diagnostic radioiodine WBS, 206–207
ultrasound, 205–206
whole-body positron emission tomography, 206–207
long-term follow-up and monitoring, 206
indications for radioiodine therapy, 199
thyrogloublin monitoring, 205
response to therapy, 206
biochemical incomplete response to therapy, 207
excellent, 207
structural incomplete response to therapy, 207–209
thermoablation, 204
kinase inhibitors, 203–204
systemic therapies, 204

Afirma GEC (gene expression classifier), 173

Agranulocytosis, 49, 55

AJCC, *see* American Joint Commission on Cancer

Alemtuzumab, 115, 133

Aluminum hydroxide, 118

American Academy of Family Practice, 143

American Association of Clinical Endocrinologists, 16, 137, 138, 143, 147, 159

American College of Endocrinology, 159

American College of Physicians, 16, 143

American College of Radiology, 159, 167

American Joint Commission on Cancer, 191
TNM (tumor, node, metastasis) classification of, 191

American Thyroid Association, 16, 137, 138, 188
adverse events in patients taking DTE, 147
classification systems, 164
clinical management of nodular thyroid disease, 159
compartmentalized neck dissection, 269
criteria for assessment of the risk of malignancy, 21
on diagnosis of TSH-secreting pituitary adenoma, 97
guidelines for methimazole administration, 102
LT4 as initial treatment, 143
radiation safety recommendations, 203
recommendations
for prophylactic thyroidectomy, 225
for prophylactic tracheostomy, 248

RET codon mutations, 228

risk stratification of thyroid nodules, 22, 21

universal screening, 287

US for nodules, 174, 194

on using radioiodine therapy, 54

on Wilson's syndrome, 150

Amiodarone, 8, 9, 62, 111, 112, 278
to reduce T4 to T3 conversion, 116, 117, 145

Amiodarone-induced hypothyroidism, 112, 131

Amiodarone-induced thyrotoxicosis, 8–9, 21, 83, 87, 112
Type 1 AIT, 112, 113
Type 2 AIT, 112, 113

Anaplastic lymphoma kinase genes, 247

Anaplastic thyroid cancer, 21, 243
computerized tomographic scan, 244
diagnosis
CT scan, 246
fiberoptic examination, 246
fine needle aspiration, 245–246
history, 245
neck MRI, 246
physical examination, 245
radionuclide studies, 246
thyroid ultrasonography, 246
future ATC treatment strategies, 249–250
immediate surgery for, 289
incidence and demographics, 244
malignant pseudothyroiditis, 87

natural history and mortality
    rates, 244–245
palliative systemic therapies, 249
pathology
    genetics, 247
    gross features, 246
    histology, 246, 247
    prognostic factors, 245
    surgical approach, 269
    treatment, 247
        airway management, 248
        chemoradiation therapy, 248
        concurrent chemoradiation
            therapy, 248–249
        initial approach to ATC
            management, 248
        thyroid surgery, 247–248
Androgens, 3, 42, 117
Anticytoplasmic neutrophil
    antibodies, 49, 50
Anti-thyroglobulin (TG-Ab)
    antibodies, 81, 82, 107,
    137, 277
Anti-thyroid antibodies (Tabs),
    81, 150
Antithyroid arthritis syndrome, 50
Antithyroid drugs, 45, 55, 103, 283
    carbimazole, 283
    clinical pharmacology of, 45
    in clinical practice, 46
    effect on fetus, 283–285
    for primary therapy of Graves'
        disease, 46–48
    family planning, 46
    methimazole dosing, 47
    thyroid-stimulating
        immunoglobulin titer, 46
    methimazole (Tapazole), 45, 283
    propylthiouracil, 45, 283
    risk of congenital
        malformations, 285
    side effects, 48–51
        agranulocytosis, 49
        antithyroid arthritis
            syndrome, 50
        drugs used to treat thyroid
            storm, 61
        liver toxicity, 50–51
        points scale for diagnosis of
            thyroid storm, 60
    treatment guidelines, 285–286

Anti-thyroid peroxidase
    antibodies, 81
Anti-TSH receptor antibodies, 15,
    38, 46, 85, 282
    measurements, 44
    testing, 47
Atrial arrhythmias, 38
Atrial diastolic dysfunction, 39
Atrial fibrillation, 42, 51, 53, 58, 59,
    119, 145, 197, 198
Aspergillus, 86
Associazione Medici
    Endocrinologi, 159
ATA, see American Thyroid
    Association
Atezolizumab, 237
Atherogenic lipoprotein, 135, 143
Atypical thyroiditis, 82; see
    also Silent thyroiditis
    (nonpostpartum)
Autoimmune thyroiditis, 12, 14, 15,
    82, 115, 228, 251, 252, 282
    pre-existing asymptomatic, 84
    pre-existing euthyroid, 16
Avelumab, 237
Axitinib, 110, 114

Bacteroides, 86
Benign multinodular goiter,
        surgical approach, 264
    Pemberton's sign, 264, 265
Beta-adrenergic antagonist drugs/
        blockers, 51, 53, 55, 88,
        90, 119
Beta-adrenergic blockers, 84, 86,
        103, 111, 114, 286
Bexarotene, 12, 108, 116, 118, 133
Biotin (vitamin B7), 118, 136–137
    ingestion, 45, 58
    -related assay interference, 8,
        118, 138
    supplement, 8, 137
Bisphosphonates, 209, 232
Bleomycin, 249
"Block-replacement" regimen, 47
Blood dosimetry, 199
Bone metastases, 204, 209, 231, 232,
        233, 237
BRAF mutations, 101, 173, 183, 184,
        189, 191, 195
    in ATCs, 247, 249

kinase inhibitors, 204
    risk of structural disease
        recurrence, 195
BRAF V600E, 161, 170, 183, 191
BRAF V600E-like tumors, 172,
        172–173
Brain metastases, 204, 232, 245
Bromocriptine, 99

Cabozantinib, 226, 233, 234,
        236, 238
    adverse events (all grades)
        with, 235
Calcitonin, 14, 161, 162, 170, 225,
        233, 246, 267
Calcium, 141, 229, 262
    abnormalities, 148
    impact on thyroid hormones, 39
Calcium carbonate, 118
Calcium channel blockers, 51
Calcium supplements, 280, 281
Cancer treatment-related
        drugs, 114
Candida albicans, 86
Carbamazepine, 117, 118
Carney complex, 161
Cat-scratch disease, 87
Ccell hyperplasia, 226
C cells, thyroid, 161, 225, 226, 228
Cediranib, 110, 114
Celiac disease, 45, 148
Cell-free DNA, 231
Central hypothyroidism, 10, 12, 16,
        116, 133, 135, 198
    central adrenal insufficiency, 149
    diagnosis, 137–138
    transient central
        hypothyroidism, 52
    untreated, 139
Cervical lymphadenopathy, 17, 61,
        86, 253
Cervical lymph node
        metastases, 191
Cervical node disease, 207–209
    EBRT, 209
    percutaneous ethanol
        injection, 208
    radiofrequency ablation, 209
    radioiodine therapy, 208
Chemotherapy, 245, 247, 249,
        253–254, 269

combination chemotherapy, 248
concurrent chemotherapy, 205
cytotoxic chemotherapy, 247
    for GTN, 102
    prophylactic chemotherapy, 101
    systemic chemotherapy, 233,
        234, 236
Chernobyl nuclear accident,
    161, 189
Cholestyramine, 55, 61, 118, 119
Choriocarcinoma, 101, 102
Chromium, 118
Chronic lymphocytic thyroiditis,
    81–82, 112, 115, 131,
    147–148, 149, 189, 190, 251
    treatment, 82
Cigarette smoking, 7, 13, 38, 46, 54,
    84, 185
    Graves' ophthalmopathy, 56, 82
Coccidioides immitis, 86
Color flow Doppler sonography, 17,
    18, 19, 112, 163
    in all women with postpartum
        Graves' disease, 85
    in differentiating Graves'
        disease, 63, 83
Columnar cell variant, 189
Congenital hypothyroidism, 139,
    279–280, 283, 284
    levothyroxine therapy, 287
    nongoitrous, 12
Congestive heart failure, 58, 144
    and beta-adrenergic blocking
        drug, 51
    hyperthyroidism and, 283, 288
    LT4 therapy, 143
    mild hypothyroidism and,
        139, 140
    myxedema coma, 151
    older patients with
        thyrotoxicosis, 38
    thyroid storm and, 263
Consumptive hypothyroidism, 114,
    133, 138
Coronary heart disease, 139, 144
    mild hypothyroidism and,
        140, 141
Corticosteroids, 3, 58, 117, 248
    and hypothyroidism, 88
    in mild or moderate
        ophthalmopathy, 54

in severe thyrotoxicosis, 84, 90
Cowden syndrome, 161
Coxsackievirus, 87
Creeping thyroiditis, 87–88
Cushing's syndrome, 233, 235
Cyclin-dependent kinase inhibitor
    2C, 231
Cyclophosphamide, 50, 233,
    249, 253
Cystic nodules, 163, 170–171,
    174–175
Cytotoxic chemotherapy, 247
Cytotoxic T-lymphocyte-associated
    antigen 4, 82, 133, 237

Dasatinib, 110, 114
Decompensated hypothyroidism,
    see Myxedema coma
Denosumab, 207, 232
Diarrhea, 227, 229
    MTC related, 233, 235, 236
    thyroid storm, 59
    as toxicities of kinase
        inhibitors, 205
Differentiated thyroid carcinoma,
    182, 243
    complications of [131]I
        immediate
            complications, 202
        leukemia, 203
        long-term complications, 203
        second primary malignancy,
            203–204
    epidemiology, 182–183
        oncogenesis, 183–185
    factors influencing prognosis
        and affecting outcome,
        191–192
        gender, 192
        radioactive iodine therapy,
            191
    initial risk assessment
        imaging in, 197
        patients' clinical status after
            initial therapy, 195–196
        risk of structural disease
            recurrence, 195
        serum thyroglobulin in,
            196–197
    prognostic scoring systems, 191
    radioiodine (^{131}I) therapy

adjuvant therapy, 198, 201
decision to use, 199–200
determining appropriate [131]I
    administered activity, 201
diagnostic whole-body [131]I
    scan, 201
metastatic carcinoma
    with ^{131}I, 201
posttreatment scans, 202
preparation for, 200–201
radioactive iodine therapy,
    199
remnant ablation, 199,
    200–201
reoperative thyroid surgery in
    patients with, 269
surveillance algorithm for, 208
thyroid hormone therapy
    levothyroxine (T4)
        suppression of TSH, 197
    metastatic disease on
        posttreatment imaging, 198
    tumor staging systems, 191
Diffuse sclerosing variant, 189
Diltiazem, 51
Diphenylhydantoin, 9
Diplopia, 39, 56, 57
Distant metastases, 186, 189, 190,
    191, 232, 245
    RAI therapy, 199
Dobutamine, 116
Dopamine, 3, 10, 58, 116
Dopamine agonists, 98
Down syndrome, 129
Doxorubicin, 205, 249, 253
Drug-induced thyroid
    dysfunction, 107
    assay interference, 118
    cancer treatment-related
        drugs, 114
    drug-related changes in thyroid
        function testing, 108–109
    drugs impacting
        thyroxine-binding
            globulin, 117
        TSH synthesis or release, 116
    drugs used for cancer-related
        treatments, 110
    enhanced metabolic clearance
        of thyroid hormone,
        117–118

enterohepatic circulation, 118
immune system modulating-
    related drugs, 115–116
inhibition
    of T4 to T3 conversion,
        116–117
    of thyroid hormone
        absorption, 118
    iodine-containing products, 107,
        111–113
    lithium, 113–114
    thyroid hormonogenesis, 107
    thyrotoxicosis, 118–119
Durvalumab, 237

EBRT, see External beam radiation
    therapy
eFVPTC, see Encapsulated
    follicular variant
    papillary cancers
Encapsulated follicular variant
    papillary cancers, 188
Endocrine Society, 16, 143, 147
Enterohepatic circulation, 61,
    118, 119
Escherichia coli, 86
Estrogens, 7, 42, 117
Eukaryotic translation
    initiation factor 1A,
    X-chromosome, 247
European Medicines Agency, 226
European Thyroid Association,
    147, 159
Euthyroid hyperthyroxinemia, 6, 7
Euthyroid hypothyroxinemia, 9
Euthyroidism, 46, 55, 59, 60, 62, 63, 65
    and pregnancy, 277
Euthyroid sick syndrome, 58,
    116, 149; see also Non-
    thyroidal illness
External beam radiation therapy,
    90, 99, 203, 231, 253

Familial adenomatous
    polyposis, 161
Familial dysalbuminemic
    hyperthyroxinemia, 6, 7
Familial nonmedullary thyroid
    cancer, 185
FDH, see Familial dysalbuminemic
    hyperthyroxinemia

Ferrous sulfate, 118
Fetal hyperthyroidism, 284,
    287, 288
Fetal hypothyroidism, 284,
    287, 288
Fetal microchimerism, 82
Fetal thyroid function, 284, 285
Fibroblasts, 38, 39, 41, 56, 57
Fine needle aspiration, 13, 83, 186,
    228, 264, 266, 289
    for ATC identification, 245
    US as guide, 17
Fine needle biopsy, 21, 27, 61–62,
    170–171
^{18}Fluorodeoxyglucose (^{18}FDG), 27,
    115, 246
    positron emission tomography/
        CT, 231, 252
5-Fluorouracil, 117, 233
    bleomycin, cyclophosphamide
        and 5-fluorouracil, 249
FNA, see Fine-needle aspiration
FNB, see Fine needle biopsy
FNMTC, see Familial
    nonmedullary thyroid
    cancer
Follicular thyroid carcinoma, 163,
    184, 189–190
    categories, 190
    treatment
        completion
            thyroidectomy, 194
        lymph node dissection, 194
        preoperative imaging,
            192, 193
        surgery, 192–194
        surgical complications, 194
        thyroidectomy during
            pregnancy, 194–195
Follicular variant of papillary
    thyroid carcinoma, 184,
    188, 189
FTC, see Follicular thyroid
    carcinoma
Furosemide, 8, 9, 109, 117
FVPTC, see Follicular variant
    of papillary thyroid
    carcinoma

Gallbladder dyes, 116
^{68}Gallium (^{68}Ga), 231

Gastrointestinal stromal
    tumors, 114
Gene Sequencing Classifier, 173
Germ cell tumors, 102
Germline RET mutation associated
    with MTC, 226
    MEN2A and associated features
        and variants, 226–227
Gestational thyrotoxicosis, 281–282
Glucagon-like peptide-1
    agonists, 161
Glucocorticoids, 9, 50, 54, 55, 57,
    116, 150
    for central adrenal insufficiency
        and hypothyroidism, 115
    for diseases with CNS, 202
    prednisone, 113
    rituximab, 57
    for severe thyrotoxicosis, 114
    to suppress TRH or TSH
        production, 133
GO, see Graves' ophthalmopathy
Goiter, 159; see also Thyroid
    nodules
    computed tomography, 169
        of goiter with mediastinal
            extension, 170
    cytology, 170–173
        Bethesda classification
            system, 171–173
        molecular testing, 172
    fine needle biopsy, 170–171
    history and examination, 161–162
    imaging
        ultrasonography, 162–167
    laboratory testing, 162
    magnetic resonance
        imaging, 169
    pathogenesis, 160–161
    prevalence, 159–160
    thyroid scan, 167–169
        CT imaging, 168
        nuclear thyroid scintigraphy,
            167, 168
Granulocyte-colony stimulating
    factor, 49
Graves' disease, 18, 38
    choice of therapy, 55–56
    diagnosis
        clinical effects of
            hyperthyroidism, 41

signs and symptoms, 38–42
epidemiology, 38
laboratory diagnosis
   pitfalls, 44–45
   thyroid hormone and TSH
      levels, 42–43
   TSH receptor antibody
      measurements, 44
   24-hour radioiodine uptake,
      43–44
pathophysiology, 38
treatment, 45
   antithyroid drug therapy,
      45–51
   beta-adrenergic antagonist
      drugs, 51
   Graves' ophthalmopathy
      and pretibial myxedema,
      56–58
   potassium iodide therapy, 51
   radioiodine (^{131}I) therapy
      for, 51–55 (see also
      Radioiodine (^{131}I)
      therapy)
   thyroidectomy, 55
Graves' disease and pregnancy,
   282–289
   antithyroid drugs, 283
      effect on fetus, 283–285
      risk of congenital
         malformations, 285
      treatment guidelines,
         285–286
   beta-adrenergic blockers, 286
   diagnosis, 282
   fetal/neonatal hyperthyroidism,
      287–288
   I-131 therapy, 287
   iodides, 286
   lactation, 287
   likelihood of recurrence, 286
   pregnancy outcome, 283
   surgery, 286
Graves' ophthalmopathy, 38
   and pretibial myxedema,
      56–58
      "elephantine" pretibial
         myxedema, 58
      intralesional steroids, 58
      "NOSPECS" classification, 56
      orbital radiotherapy, 57

rituximab, 57
radioiodine and, 53–54
GSC, see Gene Sequencing
   Classifier

Hashimoto's encephalopathy,
   see Steroid responsive
   encephalopathy
   associated with
   autoimmune thyroid
   disease
Hashimoto's thyroiditis, 18, 26, 83,
   100, 130, 139, 162, 251
   autoimmune disorders, 148
   chronic lymphocytic
      thyroiditis, 131
   etiology of, 82
   and hypothyroidism, 277
   selenoproteins, 82
   TPO antibodies, 111
Hashitoxicosis, see Hashimoto's
   thyroiditis
HCC, see Hürthle cell carcinoma
Health related quality of life, 135
Hereditary MTC, 226
   MEN2A and associated features
      and variants, 226–227
   MEN2B and associated features,
      227–228
Heroin, 117
HM, see Hydatidiform moles
Hook effect, 13
Hormone-binding protein
   concentrations, 5
Hormone specificity "spillover"
   syndrome, 276
Human chorionic gonadotropin,
   11, 101, 102, 276
   -associated thyrotoxicosis, 281
Hürthle cell carcinoma, 190–191
Hydatidiform moles, 101
   pelvic ultrasound, 102
Hyperdefecation, 38, 39
Hyperparathyroidism, 55, 161,
   227, 274
   primary, 226, 228, 229
Hyperthyroidism
   and pregnancy
      complications, 284
      Graves' disease, 282–288
      (see also Graves' disease)

      guidelines for clinical
         management of, 285
   hCG-associated
      thyrotoxicosis, 281–282
   hyperemesis gravidarum,
      281–282
   surgical approach, 263
Hyperthyrotropinemia, 12–13
Hyperthyroxinemia, 7, 9
Hypokalemia, 233, 236
Hypokalemic periodic paralysis, 39
Hypothalamic-pituitary-thyroid
   axis, 13, 107, 117
   biosynthesis and transport, 2
   physiology of, 2–3
Hypothyroidism, 129–130
   adrenal coverage, 149
   classification and etiology,
      130–133, 132
      central hypothyroidism, 133
      peripheral
         hypothyroidism, 133
      primary hypothyroidism,
         130–131, 133
   clinical manifestations,
      133–135, 134
      acute severe
         hypothyroidism, 135
   combination LT4/LT3 therapy,
      145–147
   conditions that are not
      hypothyroidism
      myxedema coma, 151–153
      non-thyroidal illness, 149
      reverse T3 syndrome,
         150–151
      SREAAT, 149–150
      Wilson's low T3
         syndrome, 150
   diagnosis, 135–138
      diagnostic evaluation of, 137
   facial changes with therapy of, 133
   factors contributing to increased
      LT4 requirements,
      144–145
   management/treatment,
      140–143
      levothyroxine
         monotherapy, 140
      thyroid hormone
         preparations, 141

US Pharmacopoeia
standards, 142
NPO patients, 149
outcomes of untreated
hypothyroidism, 139–140
persistent symptoms in patients
on levothyroxine
replacement therapy,
147–149
autoimmune diseases, 148
possible causes of, 148
and pregnancy, 277
diagnosis, 277–278
guidelines for clinical
management of, 281
pregnancy
complications, 279
pregnancy outcome, 278–280
treatment, 280
recommendations, 144
screening and case finding, 138
recommendations for, 138
severity based classification
mild hypothyroidism, 133
myxedema coma, 133
overt hypothyroidism, 133
treatment outcomes, 143–144
Hypothyrotropinemia, 12
Hypothyroxinemia, 9, 10, 276,
277, 288
Hypotriiodothyroninemia, 9

Iatrogenic thyrotoxicosis, 6, 13, 25,
117, 118
^{123}I imaging,27
^{131}I-iobenguane, 112
Imatinib, 110, 114
Immune system modulating-related
drugs, 115–116
alemtuzumab, 115
ipilimumab, 115
lenalidomide, 116
pembrolizumab, 115
thalidomide, 116
tremelimumab, 115
Immunoassay methods, 5
Immunoglobulins, 11, 15, 252
Immunometric methods, 10
IMRT, see Intensity-modulated
radiation therapy
Infiltrative diseases, 87

Infectious/post-infectious thyroiditis
acute infectious thyroiditis,
86–87
subacute thyroiditis, 87–89
Inflammatory thyroiditis, 6
Inhibition
of apoptosis, 183, 225
fetal thyroid hormone, 284
hormone binding, 9, 61
of T4 to T3 conversion, 51,
116–117
of thyroid hormone
absorption, 118
Insular carcinoma, 101, 189
Insulin-like growth factor-1, 56,
58, 161
Intensity-modulated radiation
therapy, 247, 249
treatment in ATC, 248
Interferon-alpha (α), 12, 38, 115, 131
Interleukin-6 (IL-6), 9
Iodide-induced hyperthyroidism, 6
Iodides, 286
induced hypothyroidism, 6
potassium iodide (KI), 51
sodium-iodide symporter (NIS),
23, 197
Iodinated radiocontrast dyes, 8–9
Iodine and iodine containing
products, 111–113
amiodarone, 112–113
hyperthyroidism, 111
hypothyroidism, 111
recommended daily
allowance, 111
thyrotoxicosis, 113
Iodine excess, 26, 111, 131, 160
Iodine-induced hyperthyroidism, 62,
100, 102, 111, 112, 113
Iodine supplementation, 111, 190
Iodothyronine concentration, total
serum, 9–10
Iopanoic acid, 116, 117, 119
Ipodate,8, 116, 117, 119
Ipilimumab, 110, 115, 116, 133, 237
Ischemic optic neuropathy, 56
^{131}I therapy; see also Radioiodine
(^{131}I) therapy
^{131}I-tositumomab, 112

Jod-Basedow phenomenon, 111

Kocher, Theodor (Nobel Prize in
Medicine), 261

Laboratory evaluation of thyroid
disease, see Thyroid
function, laboratory
evaluation of
Lanreotide, 98
Lanthanum carbonate, 118
L-asparaginase, 117
Latin American Thyroid
Society, 138
Lenalidomide, 116
Lenvatinib, 103, 204, 238
Leptin, 185
Leukopenia, 49, 202
Levothyroxine (LT4), 6, 55, 102,
135, 280
and amiodarone, 117
and LT3 combination
therapy, 147
monotherapy, 140
persistent symptoms in patients
on levothyroxine
replacement therapy,
147–149
during pregnancy, 280
suppression of TSH, 197–198
Lithium, 113–115
L-thyroxine therapy, 114
risk of hypothyroidism, 115
thyrotoxicosis, 114
Liver function tests, 39, 49, 50, 51
Lobectomy, 63, 64, 131, 174,
188, 192
abnormal, 165
to counsel patients, 265
regional, 162
vs. thyroidectomy, 193, 264, 265
L-thyroxine therapy, 114
Lugol solution, 112
Lung metastases, 101, 203
Lymphadenopathy, 229
cervical, 17, 61, 86, 253
generalized, 40
Lymph node metastases, 183, 186,
187, 191, 195, 266
Lymphocytic thyroiditis, see
Silent thyroiditis
(non-postpartum)
Lymphoma, see Thyroid lymphomas

MacroTSH, 11–12
Malignant pseudothyroiditis, 87
Mammalian target of
    rapamycin, 237
Means-Lerman "scratch"
    murmur, 38
Medullary thyroid cancer, 161, 225
    active surveillance of, 230–231
        contrast-enhanced computed
            tomography, 230
        fluorodeoxyglucose positron
            emission tomography/
            CT, 231
        L-6-[¹⁸F]-fluoro-3,
            4-dihydrox-
            yphenylalanine PET/
            CT, 231
        prognostic indicators beyond
            doubling times, 231
        radiologic surveillance, 230
        regional site-specific or
            symptom-specific
            therapies, 231–232
        Response Evaluation Criteria
            In Solid Tumors, 231
        scintigraphy with
            radiolabeled
            octreotide, 231
    adverse effects of MKI, 235–236
    approved multikinase
        inhibitors for
        cabozantinib, 234
        comparison of cabozantinib
            and vandetanib trials, 234
        vandetanib, 233–234
    carcinoembryonic antigen, 228
    chromogranin, 228
    clinical presentation and
        diagnostic workup of,
        228–229
    Ctn, 228, 229
    hereditary MTC, 226
        MEN2A and associated
            features and variants,
            226–227
        MEN2B and associated
            features, 227–228
    monitoring for response to
        targeted therapy, 236–237
    other agents in clinical trials,
        237–238

RET codon mutations, 228
    somatic mutations identified
        in, 237
    surgical approach, 266
    surgical management as initial
        treatment, 229–230
    systemic therapies for advanced,
        progressive disease, 233
    time of MKI initiation, 234–235
MEN2A gene, 161
    and associated features, 226–227
MEN2B gene, 225
    and associated features, 227–228
Metaiodobenzyguanidine, 112, 253
Metastatic carcinoma with ¹³¹I,
        treatment, 201–202
    empirical fixed doses, 201–202
    quantitative tumor
        dosimetry, 202
    upper-bound limits set by blood
        dosimetry, 202
Metastatic disease
    bone metastases, 209
    cervical node disease, 207–209
    pulmonary metastases, 209
    surveillance algorithm for
        DTC, 208
Metastatic thyroid cancer, 23,
        102–103, 236, 237
    differentiated thyroid cancer
        metastases, 102
    sonographic images of, 193
Metformin, 12, 116, 133
Methadone, 117
Methimazole, 45, 48, 49, 60, 102,
        111, 112, 115
    advantages over PTU, 46, 47
    dosing in hyperthyroidism, 47
    interference with radioiodine
        therapy, 52
    and ophthalmopathy, 53, 54
Metoprolol, 51
Mild hypothyroidism, 133, 135
    outcomes of untreated
        hypothyroidism, 139
    progression, 140
    recommendations regarding
        treatment for, 144
    optimal TSH level on
        replacement therapy, 144
    treatment of, 142

Mitral valve prolapse, 38
MKIs, see Multikinase inhibitors
Molar pregnancy, see Hydatidiform
    moles
Molecular testing, 159, 172,
        264, 266
    performance characteristics
        of commercially
        available, 173
Monocarboxylate transporter 8, 130
Motesanib, 110, 114
MTC, see Medullary thyroid cancer
Multikinase inhibitors
    adverse effects of, 235–236
    approved for MTC
        cabozantinib, 234, 236
        comparison of cabozantinib
            and vandetanib trials, 234
        vandetanib, 226,
            233–234, 236
    time of initiation, 234–235
Multinodular goiter, see Thyroid
    nodules; Toxic
    multinodular goiter
Multiple endocrine neoplasia
    syndromes, 225, 226
    type 2 (MEN type 2), 161
Mycobacterium tuberculosis, 86
Myxedema coma, 133, 151–153
    clinical feature scoring system
        1, 151
    clinical feature scoring system
        2, 152
    treatment, 152

Nadolol, 51, 117
National Cancer Comprehensive
    Network, 269
National Cancer Database, 245
National Cancer Institute's
    Surveillance,
    Epidemiology and End
    Results
    analysis, 183, 203
    database, 101, 186, 191
    program, 182, 244
    study, 245, 247
NCCN, see National Cancer
    Comprehensive Network
NCDB, see National Cancer
    Database

Neck dissection, 266–267
    comprehensive, 267
    risks of, 267
Neonatal hyperthyroidism, 15, 44,
        283, 287–288
Neonatal hypothyroidism, 16
Nephrotic syndrome, 9, 42
Neurofibromatosis type 1, 247
Niacin, 117
NIFTP, *see* Noninvasive follicular
        neoplasm with papillary-
        like nuclear features
Nilotinib, 110, 114
Nivolumab, 133, 237
Nocardia spp., 86
Nodular thyroid disease, 17, 48, 54,
        159, 262
Non-Hodgkin's lymphomas, 246,
        250, 251
    Ann Arbor classification system
        for, 254
Noninvasive follicular neoplasm
        with papillary-like
        nuclear features, 172, 188
Nonseminomatous tumors, 102
Nonsteroidal anti-inflammatory
        drugs, 88, 117
Non-thyroidal illness, 149
Nontoxic goiter, 159
NOSPECS classification, 56
Nothing by mouth patients, 149
NSAIDs, *see* Nonsteroidal anti-
        inflammatory drugs
NTI, *see* Non-thyroidal illness
NTRK1 mutation, 172, 189
Nuclear medicine studies
    diffuse thyroid disease, 26
    ectopic thyroid tissue, 27
    indications, 24–25
    normal thyroid appearance,
        25–26
    technique, 23–24
    thyroid cancer, 27–28
    thyroid nodules, 27

Occult subacute thyroiditis,
        see Silent thyroiditis
        (non-postpartum)
Octreotide, 98, 99, 116, 231, 267
Oncogenesis, thyroid
        carcinoma, 183

BRAF, 183–184
    common oncogenic
        mutations, 184
    MAPK (mitogen-activated protein
        kinase) pathway, 183
    RAS oncogenes, 184–185
    telomerase reverse transcriptase
        promoter mutations, 184
Orbital radiotherapy, 57
Organic anion transporter
        P1C1, 130
"Orphan Annie eye" nuclei, 186
Ovarian teratoma, 100
Overt hypothyroidism, 129, 133, 134
    outcomes of untreated
        hypothyroidism, 139
    treatment of, 141

p53 oncogene, 189, 246, 247
Painless thyroiditis, *see*
        Silent thyroiditis
        (non-postpartum)
Paired box gene 8 (PAX8), 246
Papillary cancer within
        thyroglossal duct,
        187–188
Papillary micro-carcinoma, 243
Papillary thyroid cancers/
        carcinoma, 163, 192, 186
    follicular variant papillary
        carcinoma, 188
    metastatic nodal disease, 186
    mutations, 171
    noninvasive follicular neoplasm
        with papillary-like
        nuclear features, 188
    "orphan Annie eye" nuclei, 186
    papillary cancer within
        thyroglossal duct,
        187–188
    papillary thyroid
        microcarcinoma, 186–187
    prognosis, 186
    thyroid scan, 168
    treatment
        completion
            thyroidectomy, 194
        lymph node dissection, 194
        preoperative imaging,
            192, 193
        surgery, 192–194

surgical complications, 194
    thyroidectomy during
        pregnancy, 194–195
variant of PTC
    columnar cell variant of, 189
    diffuse sclerosing variant
        of, 189
    hobnail variant of, 189
    solid variant of, 189
    tall cell variant of, 188–189
Papillary thyroid microcarcinoma,
        186–187
Parathyroid hyperplasia, 226
Pasteurella, 86
Pazopanib, 110, 202, 250
PBDEs, *see* Polybromylated
        diphenyl ethers
PDGFR receptor, *see* Platelet-
        derived growth factor
        receptor
Pediatric patients, 191
    thyroid surgery in, 269
Pembrolizumab, 115, 237, 250
Percutaneous ethanol injection, 64,
        174, 208
Peripheral hypothyroidism,
        133, 138
Phenobarbital, 108, 117, 118
Phenytoin, 108, 117, 118
Pheochromocytomas, 161, 226,
        227, 229
Phosphatase and tensin homolog,
        247
Pituitary or hypothalamic disease,
        12, 278
Pituitary surgery, 98, 99
Platelet-derived growth factor
        receptor, 114
Platins, 249
    cisplatin, 102, 249
Pneumocystis carinii, 86
Polybromylated diphenyl ethers,
        185
Positron emission tomography
        scanning, 27, 168, 206,
        246
    ^{18}F-deoxyglucose, 168, 182, 206,
        246, 253
    PET-CT, 89, 207, 231, 252, 254
Postpartum thyroiditis, 84
    diagnosis, 85

epidemiology, 84
natural history
    of postpartum thyroiditis, 85
    of subacute thyroiditis, 85
pathophysiology, 84
treatment, 86
    selenium, 86
Potassium iodide therapy, 51
Potassium perchlorate, 112
Prednisone, 54
Pregnancy
    hyperthyroidism and, 284
    Graves' disease and, 282–283
    hypothyroidism and,
        278–280, 279
Pretibial myxedema, 56–58
    "elephantine" pretibial
        myxedema, 58
    intralesional steroids, 58
    "NOSPECS" classification, 56
    orbital radiotherapy, 57
    rituximab, 57
Primary hypothyroidism, 11,
        130–131, 133, 149
    classification and etiology
        of, 134
    diagnostic evaluation of, 137
    hormone changes during, 135
Primary thyroid lymphoma, with
        ATC, 243, 250–251
    age and sex distribution, 251
    Ann Arbor classification system,
        253, 254
    B-cell lymphoma, 251
    diagnosis
        differential diagnosis, 252
        FNA/core biopsy, 252
        serum chemistries and
            immunoglobulins, 252
    failure patterns, 254
    Hashimoto's/chronic
        lymphocytic thyroiditis
        and, 251
    imaging studies
        computed tomography, 252
        magnetic resonance imaging,
            252–253
        radionuclide scanning, 253
        timing of studies, 252
        ultrasonography, 252
    incidence, 251

lymphoma cell types
    and histologic
    features, 251
symptoms and signs, 251
therapy, 253
    airway protection, 253
    chemotherapy, 253–254
    radiotherapy, 253
    surgery, 253
    thyroid dysfunction, 252
PRKAR1A (gene), 161
Programmed cell death ligand 1,
        237, 246
Programmed cell death protein 1,
        133, 237
Progressive pulmonary
    metastases, 232
Propranolol, 10, 39, 51, 60, 108, 117,
        119, 286
Propylthiouracil, 10, 45, 60, 108,
        117, 283
Proton pump inhibitors, 118, 145
Psammoma bodies, 168, 186, 188
PTC, see Papillary thyroid cancers/
        carcinoma
PTMC, see Papillary thyroid
        microcarcinoma
Pulmonary metastases, 27, 191, 202,
        203, 209, 232
Pulmonary hypertension, 38

Quantitative tumor dosimetry, 202

Radiation thyroiditis, 89–90
    diagnosis, 90
    epidemiology, 90
    pathophysiology, 90
    treatment, 90
Radioactive iodine therapy, 174,
        191, 195
Radioiodine (131I) therapy
    adjuvant therapy, 198, 201
    decision to use, 199
    determining appropriate 131I
        administered activity, 201
    diagnostic whole-body 131I
        scan, 201
    for Graves' disease, 51–53
        and cancer, 54–55
        and Graves' ophthalmopathy,
            53–54

metastatic carcinoma with
        131I, 201
    posttreatment scans, 202
    preparation for, 200–201
    radioactive iodine therapy, 199
    remnant ablation, 199, 201
Radionuclide scanning, 253
Radiotherapy, 98, 99, 248, 249, 253
Raloxifene, 108, 118
Rapidly enlarging thyroid mass,
        244, 252, 253
RAS-like tumors, 172
RAS mutations, 184–185, 189,
        237, 247
Raynaud's phenomenon, 51
Recombinant human TSH, 15, 27,
        65, 90, 115, 174, 196, 263
Recurrent laryngeal nerve, 55, 64,
        194, 229, 232, 261
    identifying, 262, 265, 267, 269
Renal iodine clearance, 277
Resin-binders, 109, 119
Resistance to thyroid hormone,
        12, 97; see also Thyroid
        hormone resistance
RET codon mutations, 2015
    ATA risk stratification
        of, 228
RET/PTC-positive tumors, 161
Retinoid X receptor, 130
    ligand bexarotene, 116
Reverse T3 dominance syndrome,
        see Reverse T3 syndrome
Reverse T3 syndrome, 150–151
Riedel's thyroiditis
    diagnosis, 89
    etiology, 89
    pathophysiology, 89
    treatment, 89
Rifampin, 108, 118
RTH, see Resistance to thyroid
        hormone

Salicylates, 7, 88, 109
Salmonella, 86
Salvage therapy, 247, 250
Saturated solution of potassium
        iodide, 50, 55, 63, 66, 112
Scarless thyroid surgery, 269–270
Secondary hypothyroidism, see
        Central hypothyroidism

SEER, *see* National Cancer
  Institute's Surveillance,
  Epidemiology and End
  Results
Selenium, 57, 82, 86, 131
Sertraline, 7, 9, 108, 118
Sevelamer, 118
Silent thyroiditis
    (non-postpartum), 82
  diagnosis, 83
  epidemiology, 83
  pathophysiology, 83
  treatment, 84
Skeletal-related events, 232
Sodium-iodine symporter activity,
    2, 111
Solitary autonomous thyroid
    nodules, 61
Solitary toxic nodules, 61
  clinical considerations, 62
  diagnosis, 62–63
  pathogenesis, 62
  pathology, 61–62
  treatment, 63–64
    laser therapy, 63
    percutaneous ethanol
      injection, 63
    radiofrequency ablation, 63
Somatostatin analogs, 58, 98, 99,
    116, 233
Sorafenib, 114, 204, 238
Splenomegaly, 41
SREAAT, *see* Steroid responsive
    encephalopathy associated
    with autoimmune thyroid
    disease
Staphylococcus, 86
Steroid responsive encephalopathy
    associated with
    autoimmune thyroid
    disease, 149–150
Streptococcus, 86
Stroke risk, 140
Struma ovarii, 100–101
  benign struma ovarii, 101
  papillary cancer, 101
Stunning effect, 201
Subacute granulomatous
    thyroiditis, 18
Subacute thyroiditis, 87
  diagnosis, 87–88

epidemiology, 87
pathophysiology, 87
treatment, 88–89
Subclinical hyperthyroidism, 58
  euthyroid sick syndrome, 58
  diagnosis, 58
  treatment, 58
Sucralfate, 109, 145
Sunitinib, 110, 114, 204

Tachycardia, 38, 55, 59, 90, 100, 281,
    282, 284, 288
Tall cell variant, 188–189
Tamoxifen, 7, 89, 108, 117
Taxanes, 249
TBG, *see* Thyroxine-binding
    globulin
TBPA, *see* Thyroid-binding
    prealbumin
Technetium (99mTc) scanning, 23,
    62, 63, 111, 168
Telomerase reverse transcriptase,
    184
  in ATCs, 247
Thalidomide, 110, 116, 132
THBR, *see* Thyroid hormone-
    binding ratio
Thermoablation, 204
  cytotoxic agents, 205
  kinase inhibitors, 204–205
    multikinase inhibitors, 204
  redifferentiation therapy, 205
  systemic therapies, 204
Thrombocytopenia, 51
Thymic enlargement, 41
Thyroglobulin, 13–14, 83, 119, 192,
    196
  thyroid-stimulating hormone,
    196
Thyroid autoantibodies, 14–15
Thyroid autoimmunity, 277
  and pregnancy, 277
Thyroid-binding prealbumin, 2, 3,
    117, 130
Thyroid cancer/carcinoma,
    169, 182; *see also*
    Differentiated thyroid
    carcinoma
  with aerodigestive invasion,
    surgical approach,
    267–269

anatomic compartments of
    neck, 267
  Shin classification, 268
incidence and survival rates
    of, 182
oncogenesis, 183
and pregnancy, 289
risk factors for, 185
  environmental etiologic
    factors, 185
  inheritance, 185
  point mutation, 185
  radiation exposure, 185
tumor histology, 186
  papillary thyroid
    carcinoma, 186
Thyroid disease
  imaging approach to
    nuclear medicine studies,
      23–28
    ultrasonography 17–23
  laboratory evaluation for,
      15–16
    screening and case finding,
      16–17
Thyroid disorders, surgical
    approach, 261
  anaplastic thyroid
    carcinoma, 269
  benign multinodular goiter, 264
    Pemberton's sign, 264, 265
  hyperthyroidism, 263
  medullary thyroid
    carcinoma, 266
  neck dissection, 266–267
  reoperative thyroid
    surgery in patients with
    DT, 269
  scarless thyroid surgery,
    269–270
  surgical technique, 261
    closure of wound, 262
    identifying parathyroid
      glands, 262
    identifying superior and
      recurrent laryngeal
      nerves, 262
    postoperative considerations,
      262–263
    postoperative levothyroxine
      therapy, 263

preoperative considerations, 262
thyroid carcinomas with aerodigestive invasion, 267–269
anatomic compartments of neck, 267
Shin classification, 268
thyroid nodules, 263–264
Bethesda classification system for thyroid nodules, 264
thyroid surgery in pediatric patients, 269
well-differentiated thyroid carcinomas, 265–266
Thyroidectomy, 55, 100, 187
completion thyroidectomy, 194
for Grave's disease, 55
during pregnancy, 194–195
total thyroidectomy, 192, 193
Thyroid function, laboratory evaluation of
specialized studies of thyroglobulin, 13–14
thyroid autoantibodies, 14–15
tissue responses to thyroid hormone action, 15–16
thyroid function test, 116, 287
thyroid hormones, assays of
causes of decreased T_4 and T_3 concentrations, 9–10
causes of increased T_4 and T_3 concentrations, 6–9
free T_4 and T_3 concentrations, 4–6
total serum iodothyronine concentrations, 3–4
thyroid-stimulating hormone, assays of, 10–12
causes of hyperthyrotropinemia, 12–13
causes of hypothyrotropinemia, 12
Thyroid hormone
cost-effective screening, 2
early research, 1
physiology during gestation, 275
renal iodine clearance, 277

thyroid stimulating hormone, 276
thyroxine (TT4) and free thyroxine (FT4) levels, 276
thyroxine-binding globulin, 275
Thyroid hormone-binding ratio, 5, 6, 7, 9, 10
Thyroid Hormone Replacement for Untreated Older Adults with Subclinical Hypothyroidism Study, 143
Thyroid hormone replacement therapy, 16, 111, 112, 116, 117, 118
causes of rising serum TSH levels on, 144
optimal TSH level on, 144
Thyroid hormone resistance, 99–100
impaired sensitivity to thyroid hormone, 99
regulation of thyroid hormone, 99
thyroid function tests, 100
Thyroid hormone therapy, 111, 114, 118, 135
levothyroxine (T4) suppression of TSH, 197–198
treatment outcome, 143, 149
Thyroid hormonogenesis, 107
Thyroid Imaging Reporting and Data Systems, 21, 166
American College of Radiology, 159, 167
thyroid nodule classification system, 166
ultrasound sonographic patterns and risk stratification system, 166
Thyroiditis, 81
chronic lymphocytic thyroiditis, 81–82
infectious/post-infectious thyroiditis, 86–87
postpartum thyroiditis, 84–86
radiation thyroiditis, 89–90
Riedel's thyroiditis, 89

silent thyroiditis (non-postpartum), 82–84
subacute thyroiditis, 87–89
trauma-induced thyroiditis, 90
types of, 82
Thyroid lymphomas, 163, 243, 244
Thyroid nodules, 21, 161
ACR-TIRADS classification system, 166
management and follow-up, 173–175
molecular testing for, 173
and pregnancy, 289
risk stratification systems for, 21–23, 165
surgical approach, 263–264
Bethesda classification system for thyroid nodules, 264
thyroid scan, 169
TSH suppression therapy, 174
US characteristics of, 163, 164
Thyroid peroxidase, 2, 11, 14, 45
antibodies (TPO-Ab), 81, 85, 107, 277, 278
Thyroid sonography, 137
Thyroid stimulating hormone, 3, 107, 129–130
assays of, 10–12
analytical sensitivity, 10
functional sensitivity, 10
immunometric methods, 10, 11
macroTSH, 11–12
optimal reference range, 11
causes of elevated serum TSH, 138
frequency distribution by age, 136
level during pregnancy, 276
levothyroxine (T4) suppression of, 197
macro-TSH, 137
TSH receptors, 130
Thyroid storm, 40, 45, 46, 59–61, 263
drugs used to treat, 61
point scale for the diagnosis of, 60
treatment, 60–61
Thyroid Symptom Score, 143

Thyroid system
  free T4 and T3, 130
  physiology of, 129–130
  production of thyroid
    hormones, 130
  protein-bound T4 and T3, 130
Thyroid transcription factor, 246
ThyroSeq, 173, 228
Thyrotoxicosis related to exogenous
    sources of thyroid
    hormone, 118–119
Thyrotropin-induced
    hyperthyroidism, 97–98
  TSH-secreting pituitary
    adenomas vs. TRH, 98
Thyrotoxicosis factitial, 119
Thyrotropin, see Thyroid
    stimulating hormone
Thyrotropin-binding inhibitory
    immunoglobulin, 44, 279
  assay, 44, 283
Thyrotropin releasing hormone, 3,
    97, 107, 129
  TRH receptors, 129
  TSH-secreting pituitary
    adenomas vs., 98
Thyroxine (T_4), 2, 130, 140
  causes
    of decreased concentrations,
      7, 9–10
    of increased concentrations,
      6–9
  determination of 4–6
  toxicosis, 43
Thyroxine-binding globulin, 2, 117,
    130
  level during pregnancy, 275
  X-linked inherited excess, 7
Thyroxine-binding prealbumin,
    2, 4, 130
TIRADS, see Thyroid Imaging
    Reporting and Data
    Systems
Tiredness Score, 143
Tirosint (Institute
    Biochimique), 133
Tissue responses, to thyroid
    hormone action, 15–16
Total or near-total
    thyroidectomy, 192, 193

Toxic multinodular goiter, 64
  diagnosis, 63
  pathogenesis, 64, 63
  treatment, 63–64
    antithyroidagent therapy, 64
    antithyroid drug
      pretreatment, 63
    near total thyroidectomy, 64
Transient hypothyroidism, 85, 88,
    131, 277
Transient painless thyroiditis, 82;
    see also Silent thyroiditis
    (non-postpartum)
Transient thyrotoxicosis with
    lymphocytic thyroiditis,
    see Silent thyroiditis
    (non-postpartum)
Transthyretin, 2, 6, 7, 9, 117, 130; see
    also Thyroxine-binding
    prealbumin
Trauma-induced thyroiditis, 90
Tremelimumab, 110, 115, 116
Treponema pallidum, 86
TRH, see Thyrotropin-releasing
    hormone
Triiodothyronine (T_3), 2, 130
  causes
    of decreased concentrations,
      7, 9–10
    of increased concentrations,
      6–9
  determination of, 4–6
  free T_3 index, 6, 282
  free T_3/T_4 measurements, 145
  reverse T_3 (rT_3), 2
Trophoblastic tumors, 101–102
TSH, see Thyroid stimulating
    hormone
Turner syndrome, 129
24-Hour radioiodine uptake test,
    43–44
"Two-step" assay method, 5, 8, 9,
    10, 266
Tyrosine-kinase inhibitors, 103,
    110, 114, 119, 233

Ultrasonography, 162–167
  calcification, 163
  diffuse thyroid disease, 17–21
  estimated malignancy risk, 166

  high-resolution US, 163
  indications, 17
  lymph nodes, 23, 24
  normal thyroid appearance, 17, 18
  technique, 17
  thyroid nodules, 21–23
Ultrasound-guided FNB biopsy, 170
UK Royal College of Physicians, 138
United States Food and Drug
    Administration, 226
United States Preventive Services
    Task Force, 138
Unithroid (Jerome Stevens), 141
Uridine diphosphate-
    glucuronosyltransferase
    enzymes, 118

Vandetanib, 110, 226, 233–234, 238
  adverse effects, 235, 236
Variants of MEN2A, 226
  cutaneous lichen
    amyloidosis, 226
  familial MTC, 226–227
  Hirschsprung disease, 226
Variants of PTC
  columnar cell variant of, 189
  diffuse sclerosing variant of, 189
  hobnail variant of, 189
  solid variant of, 189
  tall cell variant of, 188–189
Vascular endothelial growth factor
    receptor, 114, 231
VEGF receptor/VEGFR, see
    Vascular endothelial
    growth factor receptor
Vitiligo, 39, 41, 42

Wechlser Intelligence Scale for
    Children, 279
Well-differentiated thyroid
    carcinomas, surgical
    approach, 265–266
Werner syndrome, 161
Wilson's low T3 syndrome, 150
Wolff-Chaikoff effect, 111,
    112, 131

X-linked complete TBG
    deficiency, 9
X-linked inherited TBG excess, 7